HEALTH
CARE
MANAGEMENT

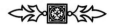

HEALTH
CARE
MANAGEMENT

ORGANIZATION
DESIGN AND BEHAVIOR

THIRD EDITION

Stephen M. Shortell, Ph.D.
A.C. Buehler Distinguished Professor
  of Health Services Management
Professor of Organization Behavior
J.L. Kellogg Graduate School of
  Management
Professor of Sociology
Member, Center for Health Services
  and Policy Research
Northwestern University
Evanston, Illinois

Arnold D. Kaluzny, Ph.D.
Professor
Department of Health Policy and
  Administration
School of Public Health
Senior Associate, Cecil G. Sheps
  Center for Health Services Research
University of North Carolina
Chapel Hill, North Carolina

and Associates

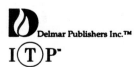
Delmar Publishers Inc.™
I(T)P⁻

NOTICE TO THE READER

Cover design by Timothy J. Conners

Delmar Staff
Senior Acquisitions Editor: William Burgower
Assistant Editor: Debra Flis
Project Editor: Carol Micheli
Production Coordinator: Mary Ellen Black
Art + Design Coordinator: Megan DeSantis and Timothy J. Conners

For information, address Delmar Publishers Inc.
3 Columbia Circle, Box 15-015
Albany, New York 12212

Delmar Publishers' Online Services
To access Delmar on the World Wide Web, point your browser to:
http://www.delmar.com/delmar.html
To access through Gopher: gopher://gopher.delmar.com
(Delmar Online is part of "thomson.com", an Internet site with information on more than 30 publishers of the International Thomson Publishing organization.)
For information on our products and services:
email: info@delmar.com
or call 800-347-7707

COPYRIGHT © 1994 BY DELMAR PUBLISHERS INC.
The trademark ITP is used under license.

Library of Congress Cataloging-in-Publication Data
Health care management : organization design, and behavior / [edited
    by] Stephen M. Shortell, Arnold D. Kaluzny and associates. — 3rd
    ed.
        p.   cm. — (Delmar series in health services administration)
    Includes bibliographical references and indexes.
    ISBN 0-8273-5675-7
    1. Health services administration.   I. Shortell, Stephen M.
    (Stephen Michael), 1944–   . II. Kaluzny, Arnold D.   III. Series.
    [DNLM: 1. Health Services—organization & administration.   W 84.1
    H4364   1993]
    RA393.H38   1993
    362.1'068—dc20
    DNLM/DLC
    for Library of Congress   93-35863
                                                                 CIP

Printed in the United States of America
published simultaneously in Canada
by Nelson Canada,
a division of the Thomson Corporation

5 6 7 8 9 10 XXX 00 99 98 97

INTRODUCTION TO THE SERIES

T his Series in Health Services is now in its second decade of providing top quality teaching materials to the health administration/public health field. Each year has witnessed further strengthening of the market position of each of the principal books in the Series, also reflecting the continued excellence of the products. Each author, book editor, and contributor to the Series has helped build what is widely recognized as the top textbook and issues collection of books available in this field today.

But we have achieved only a beginning. Everyone involved in the Series is committed to further expansion of the scope, technical excellence, and usability of the Series. Our goal is to do more for you, the reader. We will add new books in important areas, seek out more excellent authors, and increase the physical attributes of the book to make them easier for you to use.

We thank everyone, the authors and users in particular, who have made this Series so successful and so widely used. And we promise that this second decade will be dedicated to further expansion of the Series and to enhancement of the books it contains to provide still greater value to you, our constituency.

Stephen J. Williams
Series Editor

Delmar Series in Health Services Administration

Stephen J. Williams, Sc.D., Series Editor

Introduction to Health Services, fourth edition
Stephen J. Williams and Paul R. Torrens, editors

Health Care Economics, fourth edition
Paul J. Feldstein

Health Care Management: Organization Design and Behavior, third edition
Stephen M. Shortell and Arnold D. Kaluzny, editors

Ambulatory Care Management, second edition
Austin Ross, Stephen J. Williams, and Eldon L. Schafer, editors

Health Politics and Policy, second edition
Theodor J. Litman and Leonard S. Robins, editors

Strategic Management of Human Resources in Health Services Organizations
Myron D. Fottler, S. Robert Hernandez, and Charles L. Joiner, editors

SUPPLEMENTAL READER:

Contemporary Issues in Health Services
Stephen J. Williams

To Walter J. McNerney, M.H.A.,
our teacher, friend, and colleague

CONTRIBUTORS

Jeff Alexander, Ph.D.
Professor
Health Services Management and Policy
School of Public Health
University of Michigan
Ann Arbor, Michigan

James W. Begun, Ph.D.
Professor
Graduate Program in Health Administration
School of Allied Health Professions
Medical College of Virginia
Richmond, Virginia

Martin P. Charns, D.B.A.
Director, Management Decision and
    Research Center
Veterans Affairs Medical Center
Boston, Massachusetts

Thomas A. D'Aunno, Ph.D.
Associate Professor
Department of Health Services
    Management and Policy
School of Public Health
University of Michigan
Ann Arbor, Michigan

William L. Dowling, Ph.D.
Vice President
Planning and Policy Development
Sisters of Providence
Seattle, Washington

Ann Barry Flood, Ph.D.
Associate Professor
Center for Evaluative Clinical Sciences
Dartmouth Medical School
Hanover, New Hampshire

Myron D. Fottler, Ph.D.
Professor and Director
Ph.D. Program in Administration-Health
    Services
Department of Health Services
    Administration
School of Health Related Professions
University of Alabama at Birmingham
Birmingham, Alabama

Bruce Fried, Ph.D.
Associate Professor
Department of Health Policy and
    Administration
School of Public Health
University of North Carolina
Chapel Hill, North Carolina

Robert S. Hernandez, Ph.D.
Professor
Graduate Program in Hospital and Health
    Administration
School of Community and Allied Health
    Professions
University of Alabama
Birmingham, Alabama

Arnold D. Kaluzny, Ph.D.
Professor
Department of Health Policy and
    Administration
School of Public Health
University of North Carolina
Chapel Hill, North Carolina

John R. Kimberly, Ph.D.
Henry Bower Professor of Entrepreneurial
    Studies
Department of Management
The Wharton School
University of Pennsylvania
Philadelphia, Pennsylvania

James M. Klingensmith, Sc.D.
Assistant Professor and Director
Health Administration Program
Graduate School of Public Health
University of Pittsburgh
Pittsburgh, Pennsylvania

Peggy Leatt, Ph.D.
Professor and Chair
Department of Health Administration
Faculty of Medicine
University of Toronto
Toronto, Canada

Carol Ann Lockhart, Ph.D.
President, Lockhart Associates
Tempe, Arizona

Beaufort B. Longest, Jr., Ph.D.
Professor and Director
Health Policy Institute
Graduate School of Public Health
University of Pittsburgh
Pittsburgh, Pennsylvania

Roice D. Luke, Ph.D.
Professor
Graduate Program in Health Administration
School of Allied Health Professions
Medical College of Virginia
Richmond, Virginia

Laura L. Morlock, Ph.D.
Professor and Division Head
Division of Health Finance and
    Management
Department of Health Policy and
    Management
Johns Hopkins University
Baltimore, Maryland

Margaret A. Neale, Ph.D.
J.L. and Helen Kellogg Distinguished
    Professor of Dispute Resolutions and
    Organizations
J.L. Kellogg Graduate School of
    Management
Northwestern University
Evanston, Illinois

Dennis D. Pointer, Ph.D.
John J. Hanlon Professor of Health Services
    Research and Policy
Graduate School of Public Health
San Diego State University
San Diego, California

Jeffrey T. Polzer, M.B.A.
Doctoral Candidate, Organization Behavior
J.L. Kellogg Graduate School of
    Management
Northwestern University
Evanston, Illinois

Thomas G. Rundall, Ph.D.
Professor
Department of Social and Administration
    Health Sciences
School of Public Health
University of California
Berkeley, California

Julianne P. Sanchez
Doctoral Student
Department of Sociology
University of Washington
Seattle, Washington

W. Richard Scott, Ph.D.
Professor
Department of Sociology
Stanford University
Stanford, California

Stephen M. Shortell, Ph.D.
A.C. Buehler Distinguished Professor of
    Health Services Management
Professor of Organization Behavior
J.L. Kellogg Graduate School of
    Management
Northwestern University
Evanston, Illinois

Edward J. Zajac, Ph.D.
Associate Professor
James F. Beré Professor of Organization
    Behavior
J.L. Kellogg Graduate School of
    Management
Northwestern University
Evanston, Illinois

Howard S. Zuckerman, Ph.D.
Professor
School of Health Administration and Policy
College of Business
Arizona State University
Tempe, Arizona

FOREWORD

✥

Today's health care executives may have the most challenging management assignment in America. They must "do good" for their communities while "doing well" for their organizations in a time of dramatic change on all fronts—from human resources, to technology, to reimbursement. In a high-pressure environment where demand for services, insistence on cost control, conflict between professions, clamor for the latest technologies, and emphasis on quality all converge, they must pursue goals to ensure both survival and progress. Advancing the welfare of the organization and community requires a sound balance of performance-oriented management and proactive imaginative leadership. To these ends, this new edition of *Health Care Management* is addressed.

Since the second edition was published in 1988, the field of health care management has acquired additional layers of complexity, largely as a result of the explosive growth of the health care industry (of the eight and one-half million individuals employed in this sector, managers and administrators number approximately 350,000). Fueled by virtually insatiable demands for enhanced services and state-of-the-art technology, the national health bill is projected to reach $1 trillion in 1994—14 percent of the nation's gross domestic product—in contrast to its $42 billion in 1965, the year that Medicare was passed by the Congress. The burden of bloat and inefficiency is regarded by many critics as costing the nation over $100 billion annually.

Fortunately, reform may soon be on the way. When it does arrive—as seems certain it will under the Clinton administration—it will exert a profound impact on the way health care organizations are designed and managed and the manner in which health care is financed and delivered. Substantial transformations, analogous to those which dramatically changed health care in the 1960s, will again occur and necessitate major adaptations. Undoubtedly, revised standards of accountability will replace some of the neglectful policies of the past. These measures will, in turn, create a mandate for reinvigorated approaches to management and leadership.

This book, in part, aims to acquaint the reader with the particulars of various new approaches. Professors Shortell and Kaluzny have given us a set of chapters by a distinguished panel of authors that promises to enlighten and stimulate thinking among students and educators, as well as health managers and professionals. The chapters deal with the art and science of health care management and leadership, both conceptual and technical matters. The selections provide the reader with practical assessments, approaches, and insights for understanding health care organizations, fully recognizing that greater technical and informational prowess will be necessary but not sole elements in the education of the successful health manager. A further concern is leadership—a cognitive and creative breadth of compass that includes a strong moral dimension.

How does one cultivate that compass to the degree that permits a resolution of the tensions between "doing good" and "doing well"? One begins by recognizing that this scope of understanding comes not from an unschooled and sedentary mind but from an active one that observes, reads, gathers, and synthesizes an armamentarium of facts and information. It is encouraged by the propensity for a liberal education, with a heightened emphasis on fostering the interdisciplinary frame of mind, and a set of values consistent with the highest ideals of the health professions.

Perhaps the main concern of this book is the key changes that are in the making and are certain to result in further technological and organizational advances in the years ahead. For example, the manager or leader of the twenty-first century in all likelihood will be required to participate in the design of planned health care campuses offering a wide array of sophisticated preventive and diagnostic services as well as rehabilitative, long-term care, and wellness programs. Unprecedented organizational forms and methods of implementing participation and teamwork will require managers who are highly skilled in negotiation and conflict resolution.

With a principal focus on effective management and leadership, the content of the book admirably reflects a balanced concern for organization theory and behavior as well as the improvement of management practices. The text provides numerous suggestions and examples of creative ideas and ways of managing and problem solving. While the editors and authors portray the roles of the health manager as both complex and strenuous, they also offer many examples of specific tasks and decision-making strategies that will help prepare the reader for future environments.

Obviously, no work can be a comprehensive handbook or encyclopedia of how to perform well in the management arena. But this volume does provide a thorough open-systems examination and analysis of the most important structures, processes, checkpoints, and preferred futures that figure prominently in organizational excellence. It recognizes that in the real world suboptimal solutions are often necessary and that there are no royal roads to quality, only deliberately improved ones.

The text offers the double virtues of breadth and detail. It clearly articulates the key fundamentals for each of the book's 15 chapters and then achieves a suitable degree of depth, which leads the reader to improved understandings of the intricacies and workings of health care institutions. The authors are to be commended for providing the field with this thoughtfully conceived and carefully revised and updated treatment of health care management for the 1990s.

Samuel Levey, Ph.D.
Gerhard Hartman Professor
Graduate Program in Hospital
   and Health Administration
College of Medicine and
   Graduate College
The University of Iowa
Iowa City, Iowa

PREFACE

❖

This book is intended for those interested in a systematic understanding of organizational principles, practices, and insights pertinent to the management of health services organizations. While based in state of the art organizational theory and research, the emphasis is on application. While the primary audience is graduate students in health services administration or management programs, the book will also be of interest to undergraduate programs, extended degree programs, executive education programs, and practicing health services executives interested in ready access to the latest developments in organizational and managerial thinking. It is also intended for students of medicine, nursing, pharmacy, social work, and other health professions who will assume managerial responsibilities or who want to learn more about the organizations in which they will spend the major portion of their professional lives.

This third edition of the text contains a number of *new* features, which we believe greatly enhances its value to readers:

- An explicit list of topics is covered at the beginning of each chapter.
- Specific behaviorally-oriented learning objectives are highlighted at the beginning of each chapter.
- Each chapter opens with an "In The Real World" column describing a practical situation facing a health services organization. Many chapters contain several "In The Real World" columns to illustrate the major principles and lessons of the chapter.
- Most chapters incorporate a section called "Debate Time" which poses a controversial issue or presents divergent perspectives to stimulate the reader's thinking.
- A set of comprehensive mangerial guidelines concludes each chapter.
- Each chapter also includes a list of key concepts the reader should be able to define and apply as a result of reading each chapter.

All chapters have been significantly updated and revised. In addition, new chapters have been written on the topics of motivation (Chapter 3), leadership (Chapter 4), conflict management and negotiation (Chapter 5), and strategic alliances (Chapter 11).

The book is organized in five sections or parts. Part One provides an overall perspective on the study of health services organizations and the associated managerial role. Part Two deals with fundamental building blocks of managerial activity involving motivation, leadership, conflict management, and negotiation. Part Three deals with largely internal organizational issues including work design, coordination and communication, and managing power and political processes. Part Four focuses on performance issues related to organization design, strategic alliances, innovation and change, and managing for efficiency and effectiveness. The final section focuses on strategic issues and attempts to anticipate future issues that will challenge health services leaders. With the exception of Part One, which should be read first by all readers because it provides the groundwork for chapters that follow, the remaining sections can be read in any order depending on instructor and course objectives.

We believe that the major strength of the text is the diversity of the talented authors involved. They have brought multiple perspectives, experiences, skills, and expertise to bear on each chapter. As a result, each chapter is at the frontiers of knowledge with clear applications that illuminate the practice of health services management. We hope that readers enjoy this richness as much as we and our colleagues have in creating it.

Stephen M. Shortell   Arnold D. Kaluzny
Evanston, Illinois   Chapel Hill, North Carolina

ACKNOWLEDGMENTS

❖

This third edition has benefitted greatly from feedback from students and faculty over the past five years. Particular thanks are given to Bruce Fried and Tom D'Aunno for extensive critique and suggestions of the second edition. Their suggestions are incorporated into this third edition. However, our colleagues and students remain the ultimate critics. In the preparation of this edition, colleagues including Jim Suver, Jan Riordan, and Peter Weil provided technical consultation for which we are most grateful.

In addition, appreciation is expressed to Alice Schaller at Northwestern University, and Susan Lauffer and Rebecca Riggsbee at the University of North Carolina at Chapel Hill for their overall assistance in manuscript preparation and organization. We also acknowledge the assistance of Bill Burgower and Debra Flis at Delmar and Kelly Ricci at Spectrum for their overall guidance and suggestions in the production of this third edition.

Stephen M. Shortell
Evanston, Illinois

Arnold D. Kaluzny
Chapel Hill, North Carolina

ABOUT THE AUTHORS

Stephen M. Shortell, Ph.D., is the A.C. Buehler Distinguished Professor of Health Services Management and Professor of Organization Behavior in the Department of Organization Behavior at the J. L. Kellogg Graduate School of Management, Northwestern University. Dr. Shortell also holds appointments in the Department of Sociology and the Department of Community Medicine, School of Medicine at Northwestern and is a member of the Center for Health Services and Policy Research.

Dr. Shortell received his undergraduate degree from the University of Notre Dame, his masters degree in public health and hospital administration from UCLA, and his Ph.D. in the behavioral sciences from the University of Chicago.

He has also been the recipient of both the Dean Conley and Edgar G. Hayhow Article of the Year Awards from the American College of Healthcare Executives.

He is an elected member of the Institute of Medicine of the National Academy of Sciences; has served as President of the Association for Health Services Research; and has served as Chairman of the Accrediting Commission for Graduate Education in Health Services Administration.

He is currently conducting research on the strategy, structure, and performance of integrated health systems and is assessing the implementation and impact of continuous quality improvement/total quality management on U.S. health care organizations.

Arnold Kaluzny is a professor in the Department of Health Policy Administration, School of Public Health and an associate of the Cecil G. Sheps Center for Health Services Research and a member of the Lineberger Comprehensive Cancer Center of the University of North Carolina–Chapel Hill. He is a consultant to a number of private research organizations and various international, federal, and state agencies including the World Health Organization, the National Cancer Institute, and the Agency for Health Care Policy and Research. Most recently he serves as the chairman of the Board of Scientific Counselors for the Division of Prevention and Control at the National Cancer Institute. Dr. Kaluzny's research has focused on the organizational factors affecting implementation and change of a variety of health care organizations with specific emphasis given to cancer treatment and prevention and control protocols, continuous quality improvement initiatives in both organizational and primary care settings, and most recently the study of alliances within health care and its implications vis-a-vis health care reform. Dr. Kaluzny received his master's degree in hospital administration from the University of Michigan Graduate School of Business and his doctorate in medical care organization-social psychology from the University of Michigan.

CONTENTS

THE NATURE OF ORGANIZATIONS: FRAMEWORK FOR THE TEXT

ORGANIZATIONS AND MANAGERS
- Organization Theory and Health Services Management (Chapter 1)
- The Managerial Role (Chapter 2)

Need to

MOTIVATE AND LEAD PEOPLE AND GROUPS

by

Satisfying individual needs and values
- Motivating People (Chapter 3) Providing direction
- Leadership: A Framework for Thinking and Acting (Chapter 4)

Encouraging cooperation
- Conflict Management and Negotiation (Chapter 5)

In response to problems of personnel

Commitment
Turnover
Apathy
Conflict among professionals

Need to

OPERATE THE TECHNICAL SYSTEM

by

Determining appropriate work groups and design
- Managing groups and Teams (Chapter 6)
- Work Design (Chapter 7)

Establishing communication and coordination mechanisms
- Coordination and Communication (Chapter 8)

Exerting Influence
- Power and Politics in Health Services Organizations (Chapter 9)

In response to problems of technical performance

Productivity
Efficiency
Quality
Consumer satisfaction

Need to

RENEW THE ORGANIZATION

by

Determining appropriate organization design
- Organization Design (Chapter 10)

Acquiring resources and managing the environment
- Managing Strategic Alliances (Chapter 11)

Managing change and innovation
- Organizational Innovation and Change (Chapter 12)

Attaining goals
- Organizational Performance Managing for Efficiency and Effectiveness (Chapter 13)

In response to problems of the environment

Environmental complexity and uncertainty
Technological and social change
Competitive forces
Multiple performance demands

Need to

CHART THE FUTURE

by

Managing strategically
- Strategy Making in Health Care Organizations (Chapter 14)

Anticipating the future
- Creating and Managing the Future (Chapter 15)

In response to problems of survival and growth

Long-run survival
Long-run performance and growth

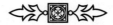

PART ONE

ORGANIZATIONS AND MANAGERS

The unrelenting changes in the health care environment are increasing the demand for organizational and managerial expertise. There is an increased need to manage across organizational boundaries in responding to new treatment technologies, payment mechanisms, consumer preferences, and accountability. The two chapters in this first section take up this challenge by laying the groundwork for the remainder of the book.

Chapter 1, Organization Theory and Health Services Management, addresses the following kinds of questions:

- What are the main forces influencing the organization and delivery of health services?
- What are the major conceptual frameworks and perspectives for thinking about health services organizations?
- What are the major units of analysis that require managerial attention?

The first chapter suggests the importance of viewing health services organizations from different perspectives drawing on a number of different metaphors to stimulate thinking.

Chapter 2, The Managerial Role, focuses on the following kinds of questions:

- What are the major ways of viewing the manager's role?
- What new roles are called for to meet the challenges of the changing health care environment?
- What new skills and knowledge are needed by health services managers to be successful?

This chapter emphasizes the need for leaders who can build consensus and negotiate compromises in an increasingly turbulent environment.

Upon completing the first two chapters, readers should have a clearer understanding of the complexity of the health services manager's role and the need for comprehensive frameworks and approaches that recognize the complexity of the role.

CHAPTER

ORGANIZATION THEORY AND HEALTH SERVICES MANAGEMENT

Stephen M. Shortell, Ph.D.
Professor

Arnold D. Kaluzny, Ph.D.
Professor

CHAPTER TOPICS

The Changing Health Care System
Ecology of Health Services Organizations
A Typology of Health Services
    Organizations
Health Services Organizations as Systems
Units of Analysis
Major Perspectives on Health Services
    Organizations
Metaphors of Health Services
    Organizations
Organization Theory and Behavior: A
    Framework for the Text

LEARNING OBJECTIVES

After completing this chapter, the reader should be able to

1. identify the major forces affecting the delivery of health services
2. understand how these major forces affect the role of the health services manager
3. identify some of the commonalities and differences among major types of health services organizations
4. identify and understand the basic processes that must be accomplished by any organization
5. identify and understand the different units of analysis associated with studying organizations
6. identify, understand, and apply the major perspectives on organizations to real problems facing health services organizations
7. identify, understand, and apply major metaphors of organizations to the challenges facing health services organizations

CHAPTER PURPOSE

In many respects Kaiser Permanente represents a prototype health services organization for our nation's changing health care system. It combines the insurance function with the delivery function while providing nearly all levels of care to a defined population. It provides this care within the constraints of a preestablished budget based on an agreed-upon level of benefits and premiums. It must integrate physicians and a variety of other health professionals across a wide range of treatment settings. It must demonstrate value to its customers—both individual patients and corporate and governmental purchasers. *Value* is created when for a given cost or price to the purchaser additional quality features desired by the purchaser are provided or, conversely, when a given level of quality services can be provided at a lower cost or price relative to others from whom purchasers can obtain the services. Providing greater

IN THE REAL WORLD
LARGE TASKS FOR A LARGE ORGANIZATION: KAISER PERMANENTE'S QUALITY AGENDA

Kaiser Permanente evolved from industrial health care programs for construction, shipyard, and steel mill workers for the Kaiser industrial companies during the late 1930s and early 1940s and was open to public enrollment in 1945. It is the nation's largest and oldest independent prepaid group practice, serving the health care needs of more than 6.5 million members in 16 states and the District of Columbia. In 1990, this not-for-profit practice had total revenues of $8.4 billion and a net income of $381 million. More than 74,700 technical, administrative, and clerical employees and 8,600 physicians make up the business. The practice has 29 medical centers with more than 7,000 licensed hospital beds and more than 200 medical office locations.

Kaiser Permanente encompasses three organizations: Kaiser Foundation Health Plan, Kaiser Foundation Hospitals, and the Permanente Medical Groups. Kaiser Foundation Health Plan contracts with individuals and groups to arrange health care benefits and with Kaiser Foundation Hospitals and the Permanente Medical Groups to provide, respectively, hospital and medical services required to meet its members' covered health benefits. Kaiser Foundation Hospitals owns and operates community hospitals; owns outpatient facilities; provides or arranges hospital services; and sponsors charitable, educational, and research activities. Permanente Medical Groups are partnerships or professional corporations of physicians. The responsibility for providing and arranging the medical care necessary to satisfy Kaiser Foundation Health Plan contracts with individuals and groups is assumed in each region by a Permanente Medical Group. This organizational structure represents a cooperative approach by the professions of medicine and management and assures physicians and managers an opportunity to present their views on all major policy decisions.

In the late 1980s, Kaiser Permanente was one of the early participants in the National Demonstration Project on Quality Improvement in Health Care.[1] Key individuals were drawn from the 11 Permanente Medical Groups and from the Kaiser Foundation Health Plan and Hospitals to attend the educational sessions. Visits were also made to leading quality companies outside the health care industry, and some senior managers attended additional short educational sessions.

Real progress began, however, once the Kaiser Permanente committee (the principal coordinating group of this large, decentralized organization) prepared its Quality Agenda. This document translates the basic understanding of quality into terms that are meaningful for the program and identifies the key actions to be taken.

The Quality Agenda captures part of the strategic vision of Kaiser Permanente.

> To be the value leader in health care, the central focus of Kaiser Permanente must be to provide care of the highest quality, measured by:
> 1. Effectiveness in providing clinical care to individual patients.
> 2. Satisfaction of customers—payers, members, patients, and staff—with services received.
> 3. Efficiency of organization functioning at all levels.
> 4. Appropriate use of resources to improve the health status of its membership.

At this point the top executives also needed to identify the general path to be followed in seeking this vision. The choice had to be consistent with and supportive of what Kaiser Permanente is and wanted to become. The general path had to be intellectually coherent, compatible with the practice of good medicine, proven effective, flexible enough for a geographically and culturally diverse organization, incremental and consistent with Kaiser Permanente's philosophy of being a learning organization, and capable of capturing the hearts and minds of people. There also had to be appropriate outside resources such as models, mentors, and teachers available.

With a vision, agenda, and general path identified, top management began allocating the resources and building an infrastructure to support the new effort and make the goals possible. These tasks cannot usually be performed within an existing organizational structure. Thus, Kaiser Permanente established a quality council for the central office. It is composed of the top executives from the Permanente Medical Group Interregional Services and Kaiser Foundation Hospitals and Health Plan. The quality council is the formal structure through which upper-level managers allocate the needed resources, set priorities, secure the time needed by teams to make major quality improvements, and review their existing personnel, operations, and reward systems. Individual regions, specific service areas, and other major organizational units are also establishing similar quality councils.

It will come as no surprise that, in an organization as large and diverse as Kaiser Permanente, some locations have moved ahead quite rapidly, while others are still rather tentative in their approach. This variation is not surprising nor disappointing. In fact, it has been encouraged—not every location is in the same situation. And, although the central guiding strategy is the same, the details of implementation should not be invariant. The ability of humans to implement and absorb broad, rapid changes uniformly is rather limited.

As Kaiser Permanente begins to expand its efforts and institutionalize what it is learning, upper-level managers must continue to actively participate. They will need to support and nourish quality through providing ongoing resources, developing appropriate data bases on quality, identifying critical projects, reviewing progress, providing rewards and recognition, and funda- mentally changing the approach being used to manage crossfunctional processes. ☒

1. The National Demonstration Project on Quality Improvement in Health Care is an experiment started in 1987 to determine the applicability of quality management methods in health care organizations. In this ongoing experiment, 21 quality management experts are providing their expertise and tools to 21 U.S. health care organizations willing to try them.

SOURCE: Adapted from Lawrence D, Early JF. Large tasks for a large organization. *Quality Progress*. April 1992:47.

value is a challenge for all health services organizations and to the professionals—both clinical and managerial—associated with them. As noted in a Pew Commission Report on Education for the Health Professions:

> Health services management will become even more challenging, because it is the point where increasing service demands, cost containment strategies, interprofessional tensions, technological change pressures, guidelines implementation, and quality improvement mandates all converge. The managerial function in health services is unique because of the relative autonomy of providers and the complexity of assessing the quality of the services rendered . . .[1]

The purpose of this chapter is to describe the primary organizational components of the health care system, use some of the chapter titles as a framework for understanding the commonalities and differences among health services organizations, highlight some of the major approaches and perspectives on the study of organizations, and provide a framework for learning from the chapters which follow.

THE CHANGING HEALTH CARE SYSTEM

Ultimately the goal of health services managers is to help maintain and enhance the health of the public. While individual citizens hold primary responsibility for their health status, there is much that health services managers working in concert with physicians, nurses, and other health professionals can do to assist in the process. This goal may seem strange to some and unrealistic to others. After all, isn't it sufficient simply to care for those that come to you for help and make sure that one's organization retains its financial health in order to provide the requested care? The answer is no. Economic, political, and social forces have moved the health services system beyond the largely reactive acute care paradigm to a more holistic paradigm emphasizing population-based wellness. Some of the major economic, political, and social forces that will influence health care delivery in the next five to ten years are highlighted in Table 1.1. These forces are causing a fundamental shift in the way in which health care is being viewed. The major elements of this *paradigm shift* are outlined in Table 1.2.

At the core of this shift is the movement away from episodic treatment of acute illness events to the provision of a coordinated continuum of services that will enhance the health status of defined populations. In the evolving health care system of capitation, global budgets, and expenditure targets, organizations win by helping health care professionals provide services at that point in the continuum of care where the greatest value (i.e., cost-benefit) is provided. They do not win by filling hospital beds or continuing to have physicians, hospitals, and others go their separate ways. These kinds of changes require new and different ways of organizing and managing health care services. Among the most important are the following:

- Managing a market or network of services. This might be termed *population-based* or denominator-based *management*.
- *Managing* services *across* organizational *boundaries*.
- Actively managing quality and *continuous improvement*.

TABLE 1.1.   Nine Forces Influencing Health Care Delivery and Their Implications for Management

External Force	Management Implication
1. Capitated payment, expenditure targets, or global budgets for providing care to defined populations	• Need for increased efficiency and productivity • Redesign of patient care delivery • Development of strategic alliances that add value • Increased growth of networks and systems
2. Payment based on performance	• Information systems that link financial and clinical data across episodes of illness and "pathways of wellness" • Effective implementation of clinical practice guidelines • Ability to demonstrate continuous improvement of all functions and processes
3. Growth of new technology emphasizing outpatient, workplace, and at home treatment	• Expansion of the continuum of care, need for new treatment sites to accommodate new treatment modalities • Increased capacity to manage care across organizational boundaries • New relationships with physicians and other caregivers
4. Aging of the population	• Increased demand for primary care, wellness, and health promotion services among the 65 to 75 age group • Increased demand for chronic care management among the 75 plus group • Challenge of managing ethical issues associated with prolongation of life
5. Increased ethnic or cultural diversity of the population	• Greater difficulty in understanding and meeting patient expectations • Challenge of managing an increasingly diverse health services work force
6. Changes in the supply and education of health professionals	• Need for creative approaches in meeting the population's need for greater primary care • Need to compensate for shortages in some categories of health professionals (i.e., physical therapy, pharmacy, and some areas of nursing) • Need to develop effective teams of caregivers across multiple treatment sites
7. Social morbidity (AIDS, drugs, homicides, "new surprises")	• Ability to deal with unpredictable increases in demand • Need for increased social support systems and chronic care management
8. Information production and management	• Training the health care work force in new information, production, and management methodologies • Increased ability to coordinate care across sites • Challenge of managing an increased pace of change due to more rapid information transfer • Challenge of dealing with confidentiality issues associated with new information production and management technologies
9. Globalization and creation of the world economy	• need to manage cross-national and cross-cultural tertiary and quaternary patient care referrals • Role of the health services organization in increasing the productivity of the American labor force • Managing global strategic alliances, particularly in the areas of biotechnology and new technology development

TABLE 1.2. Transformation of Health Care

Old Paradigm	New Paradigm
Emphasis on acute inpatient care	Emphasis on the continuum of care
Emphasis on treating illness	Emphasis on maintaining and promoting wellness
Responsible for individual patients	Accountable for the health of defined populations
All providers are essentially similar	Differentiation based on ability to add value
Success achieved by increasing market share of inpatient admissions	Success achieved by increasing the number of covered lives and keeping people well
Goal is to fill beds	Goal is to provide care at the most appropriate level
Hospitals, physicians, and health plans are separate	Integrated health delivery system
Managers run on organization	Managers oversee a market
Managers serve as department heads	Managers operate services across organizational boundaries
Managers coordinate services	Managers actively pursue quality and continuous improvement

Population-based or denominator-based management is not only illustrated by the Kaiser Permanente health system but by a growing number of regional and vertically-integrated delivery systems across the country. These systems are positioning themselves to integrate the insurance component with the delivery component in defined geographic areas. The essential ingredient is the ability to provide cost effective care under capitated or preestablished budgets. This requires integrating all components of service delivery, establishing effective physician relationships, and developing information systems that can tie patients and providers together across the continuum of care. In addition, information on patient care processes and outcomes is required for both external accountability and for internal continuous quality improvement.

The ability to manage across departments and across organizational boundaries is well illustrated by the efforts of the New England Medical Center in Boston to restructure patient care based on an episode of illness. The essential elements of its approach have been to:

1. assess patient needs and expectations
2. reorganize patient care roles based on this assessment
3. train nurses and physicians to provide care across the continuum from acute inpatient care to the physician's office to the patient's home
4. provide care using clinical care protocols
5. use patient outcome and patient satisfaction data to make improvements in care
6. develop an information system which supports the above efforts.

These changes have resulted in improved patient satisfaction in both pediatric and adult hematology-oncology units and the cardiovascular unit at the New England Medical Center.

An example of actively managing quality of care and continuous improvement in processes is provided by Intermountain Health Care in Salt Lake City, Utah. Using an information system called HELP, data were generated indicating that the postsurgical wound infection rate at selected Intermountain hospitals was approximately 2%. While this rate was comparable to the national rate, Intermountain providers asked themselves whether it could be improved further. Using continuous quality improvement tools and methodologies, they diagnosed and remedied the underlying problems and were able to achieve a postoperative wound infection rate of 0.004%.

Drawing on examples such as these, this book focuses on *the new attitudes, the new ideas, the new skills, the new behaviors, and the new mindsets required to manage a continually changing health care system.*

The book is divided into three parts. Part One lays the foundation with chapters that discuss the manager's role, motivational forces, and leadership issues. Part Two emphasizes the knowledge, skills, and understanding required to manage interdependent professional work teams in the provision of services across the continuum of care. Areas covered include negotiation and conflict management, work groups, work design, coordination and communication and power and influence. Part Three deals with the challenges posed by issues of organization design the development of interorganizational networks and strategic alliances, the demands for change and innovation, the emphasis on performance accountability, and the importance of positioning the organization strategically. The book concludes with a discussion of the future issues that will challenge health services executives.

ECOLOGY OF HEALTH SERVICES ORGANIZATIONS

Figure 1.1 depicts the great number and variety of organizations engaged in the process by which services are ultimately delivered to patients. On the financing and payment side, insurance examples include Blue Cross Blue Shield, Aetna, Prudential, and self-insured employers; governmental payers include the federal Medicare program and the federal-state Medicaid program. Providers range from primary care providers such as single specialty and multispecialty physician group practices and health departments to acute care providers such as hospitals and ambulatory surgery centers, and to rehabilitation care providers such as home health care agencies, and rehabilitation centers and to maintenance providers such as nursing homes and hospices. There are also major supplier organizations to the providers including pharmaceutical companies

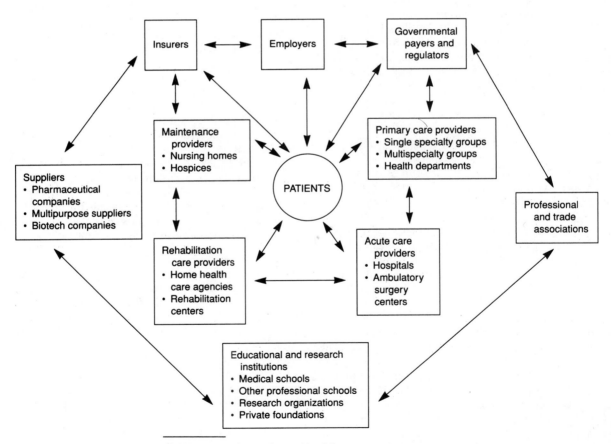

FIGURE 1.1. The ecology of health services organizations.

such as Abbott Labs, Eli Lilly, and Merck; multipurpose suppliers such as Baxter; major equipment suppliers such as the medical divisions of 3M and General Electric; and a growing variety of biotechnology companies such as Amgen and Genentech. In addition, there is a large education and research infrastructure composed of medical schools, other health professional schools, and research organizations including the National Institutes of Health and the Agency for Health Care and Policy Research. There are also many private foundations that provide support for innovations in health care delivery including The Commonwealth Fund, The Hartford Foundation, The Pew Charitable Trusts, The Henry J. Kaiser Family Foundation, The Robert Wood Johnson Foundation, and The W.K. Kellogg Foundation among others. Finally, there are numerous professional and trade associations including the Association for Health Services Research, the American Hospital Association, the American Medical Association, the American Nurses Association, the Association of Academic Medical Colleges, the Association of Academic Health Centers, the American Public Health Association, the Association of University Programs in Health Administration, the American College of Healthcare Executives, the Healthcare Forum, and the Medical Group Management Association.

While the majority of the resources of the health services system are used by provider organizations, it is important to recognize the wide network of organizations that in one way or another compose the health services system. On the provider side alone, there are approximately 500,000 physicians, 1.5 million nurses, 160,000 dentists, 6,780 hospitals, 16,000 nursing homes, 3,350 rehabilitation units, 12,900 home health care agencies, 575 health maintenance organizations (HMOs), and 51 state public health departments. On the educational side, there are approximately 140 medical schools, 50 dental schools, 1,400 nursing education programs, and 60 accredited graduate programs in health services administration. While direct health care expenditures continue to grow—predicted to reach 17% of the gross national product and encompass more than $1 trillion by the year 2000—the actual impact of health care on the American economy through its linkages with other organizations as shown in Figure 1.1 is even more pervasive.

Are Health Services Organizations Unique?

Health services organizations are often described as unique or at least different from other types of organizations, particularly different from industrial organizations. Further, these differences are believed to be significant in the area of management. Among the most frequently mentioned differences are the following:

- Defining and measuring output are more difficult.
- The work involved is more highly variable and complex.
- More of the work is of an emergency and nondeferrable nature.
- The work permits little tolerance for ambiguity or error.
- The work activities are highly interdependent, requiring a high degree of coordination among diverse professional groups.
- The work involves an extremely high degree of specialization.
- Organizational participants are highly professionalized, and their primary loyalty belongs to the profession rather than to the organization.
- Little effective organizational or managerial control exists over the group most responsible for generating work and expenditures: physicians.
- Dual lines of authority exist in many health care organizations, particularly hospitals, that create problems of coordination and accountability and confusion of roles.

Upon careful examination, it is possible to refute or at least question each of these allegedly distinctive attributes. For example, universities also have difficulty in defining and measuring their product. Is it the number of students graduated or the number of credit hours produced? Is quality measured by grade point average? If so, how much of that is the contribution of the student or of the faculty? A number of other organizations such as police and fire departments are concerned with highly variable, complex, emergency work. Other organizations also have limited ability to tolerate errors or ambiguities: for example, air traffic controllers. Are work activities any more interdependent in health care than in a symphony orchestra? What about the high degree of specialization of activities in a large legal firm? As for control over professional members, do universities or research institutes have any more control over their faculty or investigators than health services organizations have over physicians? Finally, many business and industrial organizations have dual lines of authority. In fact, as discussed in Chapter 10, many firms have institutionalized dual authority structures through matrix organization designs. Further, the concept of uniqueness can be harmful if it leads health services managers to believe that their job is so much more difficult or different from others that relatively little can be done to improve performance.

On the other hand, health services organizations may be unusual, if not unique, in that many of them possess all of the characteristics stated above *in combination*. It is one thing to have little control over professionals when they do not need to interact frequently with others in the organization, such as with a number of research and development units in industry. But it is different when physicians, nurses, and other health professionals are highly dependent on each other in providing and coordinating patient care. The independence of professionals from managerial control is also less of a problem in situations where output is readily defined and measured than where clear performance criteria are still under development and yet external bodies hold the organization responsible for the activities of the relatively independent group of professionals. Thus it is the confluence of professional, technological, and task attributes that make the management of health services organizations particularly challenging. Further, health services organizations are highly involved with values on a daily basis. For example, cost containment, which is valued by society at large, may frequently conflict with individual client values such as the desire to recover one's health at almost any cost. In other cases such as abortion, outcomes valued by different parties may be in conflict.

A TYPOLOGY OF HEALTH SERVICES ORGANIZATIONS

A useful way of understanding some of the characteristics of health services organizations is to consider a typology based on a number of issues. Table 1.3 presents such a typology for HMOs, home health care agencies, hospitals, and pharmaceutical companies. These organizations are compared along seven attributes or characteristics: external environment, mission/goals, work groups/work design, organization design, interorganizational relationships, change and innovation, and strategic issues.

This typology is intended to stimulate thinking about differences and similarities between health services organizations and their associated managerial implications. It is important to recognize that there is, of course, substantial variation within different types of HMOs, home health care agencies, hospitals, and pharmaceutical firms. For example, some HMOs own their own hospitals while others do not. While the majority of home health care agencies are for-profit, there is also a sizeable not-for-profit sector. Hospitals, of course, vary greatly in such dimensions as size, degree of teaching activity, and whether or not they belong to organized health systems or alliances. Pharmaceutical companies also vary widely in regard to size, scope of product domain, and emphasis on global markets. Thus what is presented in Table 1.3 represents "modal" characteristics of these organizations with respect to the attribute in question.

It is also important to note that the four organizations are compared *relative to each other*. These comparisons are based largely on judgment and experience since there remains relatively little systematic managerial research on health services organizations except for hospitals and, to a lesser extent, HMOs and nursing homes. The descriptions, therefore, are not intended to be correct in any absolute sense but rather in having some degree of face validity.

External Environment

One key to an organization's success is having a good understanding of its *external environment*. Environments differ in their complexity, susceptibility to change, and competitiveness. Depending on these attributes, organizations might choose different strategies, structures, and processes to compete successfully (see Chapters 7, 10, 13, and 14, in particular). In Table 1.3, HMOs, home health care agencies, hospitals, and pharmaceutical companies are shown to vary somewhat across these attributes. While the environment has become highly competitive for all of them, there

TABLE 1.3. A Typology of Four Health Services Organizations

Attribute	Health Maintenance Organizations (HMOs)	Home Health Care Agencies	Hospitals	Pharmaceutical Companies
External environment	Moderate complexity Moderate change Highly competitive	Relatively simple Moderate change Increasingly competitive	Complex High change Highly competitive	Moderate complexity Moderate change Highly competitive
Mission/goals	Primary care emphasis: keep people well	Quality of life Maintaining functional status	Acute care emphasis: curing illness	Research and development (R&D) emphasis; new product development
Work group/work design	Primary care team; coordinate referrals	Simple design; primarily one-on-one patient contact	Departmental and cross departmental teams; high need for coordination	Separation of functions possible; R&D versus sales; relatively low need for coordination
Organization design	Functional and divisional integrating; primary care physicians and specialists	Functional	Divisional and matrix	Divisional and strategic business units
Interorganizational relationships	Link to expand primary care patient base	Expand patient base and gain economies of scale	Key to becoming part of vertically integrated health systems	Important for global expansion
Change/innovation	Respond to and create new patient care management approaches	Respond to demographic and social changes	Respond to the new paradigm; implement new role within vertically integrated systems	Respond to new product development demands
Strategic issues	Expand the concept of managed care	Demonstrate continuing value, and, therefore, reimbursement for services	Fit into an expanded and changing delivery system	Decrease time to develop new drugs

are some qualitative differences in complexity and the pace of change. For the reasons noted earlier, hospitals are probably undergoing the most upheaval as they reposition themselves as part of vertically-integrated delivery systems. HMOs are affected by continuing purchaser demands for value and pharmaceutical companies by the continued pressure for new drugs that add value in regard to cost benefit. The environment of home health care agencies is simple only in a relative sense. Their environment is largely derived in that home health care agencies depend upon what is done by pharmaceutical companies and the role played by provider organizations such as HMOs and hospitals. To deal with environmental demands, health services organizations are increasingly forming strategic alliances with each other resulting in a dense web of interorganizational networks (see Chapter 11).

Mission/Goals

The organization's *mission* and associated *goals* largely dictate the major tasks to be carried out and the kinds of technologies and human resources to be employed. Organizations, of course, differ widely in their mission and goals as shown by the four selected organizations highlighted in Table 1.3. An organization's mission and goals have both an external and internal purpose. Externally they communicate what the organization is about to those who may want to use its services (e.g., patients) or in some other way have contact with the organization (e.g., regulators and third party payers). They help to provide legitimacy which, in turn, assists in helping the organization acquire needed resources (see Chapter 13). Internally goals serve as a source of motivation and direction (see Chapters 3 and 4).

Work Group/Work Design

How people are grouped together to accomplish the organization's mission is usually a function of the organization's technology and environment. As shown in Table 1.3, this may range from a relatively simple one-to-one relationship between the home health care agency nurse and an individual patient to several teams of care givers that coordinate patient services across multiple treatment settings ranging from the hospital to the home. A major issue is the degree to which tasks are interdependent. For example, in most pharmaceutical companies the research and development (R&D) function can be relatively isolated from the sales division. The factors influencing work group formation and design are further discussed in Chapters 6 and 7.

Organization Design

In contrast with work design, *organization design* focuses on the overall allocation of power and authority, information processing, and decision-making roles within the organization and how individual work groups, departments, or divisions are themselves linked together. As shown in Table 1.3, these can range from functional designs in the case of home health care agencies (i.e., organized around functions such as marketing, reimbursement, and patient care) to more complex divisional and matrix designs typically found in hospitals. As elaborated in Chapter 10, the organization's design should fit its mission, strategy, technology, and environment.

Interorganizational Relationships

As the health services environment grows in complexity and accelerates its rate of change, a key component of many organizations' strategies is to form relationships with each other. Such linkages can help to increase access to resources and new markets, compliment each other's strengths, and accelerate learning. As shown in Table 1.3, such linkages are particularly important for pharmaceutical company expansion efforts into global markets, hospital efforts to survive, HMO efforts to expand membership base, and home health care agencies wishing to expand geographic coverage or achieve greater economies of scale. Chapter 11 highlights the great variety of such relationships and their relative advantages and disadvantages.

Change/Innovation

As never before, health services organizations are being called on to develop their capacity for *change* and innovation. As shown in Table 1.3, these may differ as a function of a given organization's role within the health services system. The commonalities that cut across the capacity for change and innovation are the subject of Chapter 12. For most health services organizations, the abilities to create and manage change and to innovate as needed represent the key differences between short-run existence and long-run viability.

Strategic Issues

There are many levels of strategy ranging from the overall role of the organization in society, to the particular area of business or service that the organization chooses to be in, to how the organization wishes to conduct itself in that area, and finally to the functional means by which the organization accomplishes its objectives. Some key strategic issues facing the selected organizations shown in Table 1.3 range from the HMO's need to expand the concept of managed care, to the home health care agency's need to demonstrate value, to the hospital's need to fit into a more vertically-integrated delivery system, to the challenge of pharmaceutical companies to decrease the time required to move new drugs into the market place. A given organization's approach to these kinds of strategic issues will, of course, vary as a function of its particular environment on the one hand and its internal capabilities and resources on the other. The likely success of a given strategy will depend not only on its content but also on its execution. These issues are addressed in Chapter 14.

As suggested by the typology in Table 1.3, organization theory and behavior can help to explain and, in some cases, predict the commonalities and differences in how organizations function. To make full use of this potential, it is important to consider health services organizations as systems, to describe some basic units of analysis, to highlight the major perspectives on organizations, and to illustrate the usefulness of selected metaphors.

HEALTH SERVICES ORGANIZATIONS AS SYSTEMS

Health services organizations are complex social systems. In managing these organizations, there is a constant tension between the need for predictability, order, and efficiency on the one hand and openness, adaptability, and innovation on the other. The need for predictability, order, and efficiency is consistent with a *closed system* view of an organization. The closed system view assumes that at least parts of an organization can be sealed off from the external environment. As such, the management challenge is how to use internal design, productivity improvement tools, and incentives to maximize internal efficiency.

The need for openness, adaptability, and innovation is consistent with an *open system* view.[2] This view emphasizes that organizations are parts of the external environment and, as such, must continually change and adapt to meet the challenges posed by the environment. The emphasis is on meeting the needs of external customers and stakeholders with relatively less emphasis given to issues of internal efficiency.

Both approaches are needed to understand and manage health services organizations. While each activity, function, or department of a health services organization can be considered by itself with its unique requirements and expectations, the real payoff lies in recognizing the interdependence of most activities and functions. One set of functions and activities are usually the building blocks for another set which, in turn, serve as inputs for still others. These sets of functions, activities, and departments serve as internal environments for each other in addition to being influenced by forces in the external environment. The processes which occur in health services organizations can be described in terms of six primary functions: production, boundary spanning, maintenance, adaptation, management, and governance.[3]

Production

The *production function* provides the product or service and is at the center of most organizational activity. It is represented by the manufacturing of a new drug in a pharmaceutical company, the diagnosis and treatment of patients in a multispecialty group practice, and the alleviation of pain and suffering in a hospice organization. These core production processes can vary on a number of dimensions including complexity, time, use of labor versus capital, and ease with which results can be measured among others.

Boundary Spanning

The *boundary spanning function* focuses on the interface between the organization and its external environment. It is concerned with new developments in technology, reimbursement, regulation, licensure, changing demographics, customer expectations, competitive threats, and related issues. Depending on the size of the organization and its local market environment, these activities will often vary in their complexity and susceptibility to change. Some organizations will establish certain departments that designate specific individuals or functional areas to carry out boundary spanning activities. In other cases, all employees with managerial responsibilities are required to undertake at least some boundary spanning activities.

Maintenance

The *maintenance function* is concerned with both the physical and human infrastructure of the organization. It includes capital acquisition and maintenance as well as employee growth and development. As the rate of change accelerates and as the external environment becomes more threatening, greater demands are placed on the maintenance functions of health services organizations.

Adaptation

The *adaptation function* focuses on change. Using information obtained from the boundary spanning activities of the organization and with knowledge of the organization's production capability and maintenance support systems, the adaptation function helps the organization to anticipate and adjust to needed changes. This may include the need for new programs and services, deletion or modification of existing programs and services, changes in the organization's structure and design, or major changes in the organization's basic strategy. The adaptation function also emphasizes the health services organization's ability to innovate by actively creating changes in its environment. Given the turbulence of the health services environment, the ability of health services organizations to adapt is of growing importance.

Management

Management is a distinct function that cuts across all the other functions and subsystems. In a sense, it is the "head" that organizes, directs, and oversees all of the other functions. It is represented in most health services organizations by the senior management team and key middle managers.

Governance

Although not usually mentioned in traditional texts, *governance* is added as a sixth distinct function because of the important public trust and social accountability responsibilities of health services organizations. It is the function which holds management and the organization accountable for its actions and which helps provide management with overall strategic direction in guiding the organization's activities. The pressure for greater accountability in regard to patient outcomes, treatment effectiveness, patient satisfaction, cost containment, and ethical use of resources is posing significant challenges to the governance function of health services organizations.

UNITS OF ANALYSIS

Figure 1.2 shows the units or levels by which organizations may be analyzed. They include the individual unit, the group/department unit, the organization as a whole, the network of interorganizational relationships, and the larger environment which interacts with all of these units. The figure also suggests the complexity of the manager's job in attempting to integrate the various units in positioning the organization to meet its goals and objectives in the face of environmental challenges.

Traditionally, the individual and group or department units have been the primary focus of *organizational behavior* or what is sometimes referred to as the *micro approach* to understanding organizations. The emphasis is on examining individuals within organizations. Chapters 3–5 deal with clear examples of organizational behavior issues: motivation, leadership, and conflict management. The organizational, interorganizational, and environmental units have typically

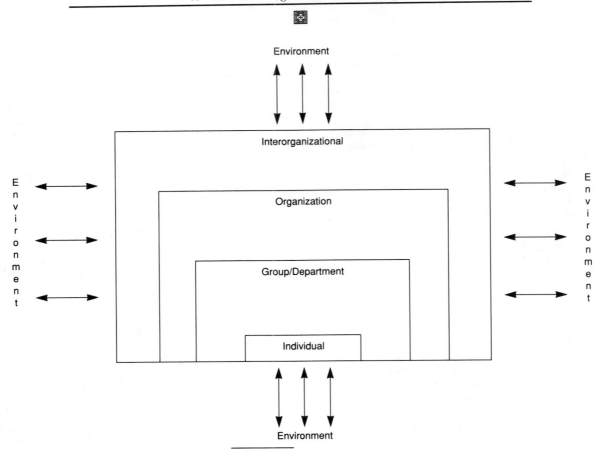

FIGURE 1.2. Units of analysis.

been the focus of *organization theory* or what is called the *macro approach*. This approach primarily treats the organization as a social system while organization behavior focuses on the individual person within the social system. Chapters 10–14 deal with examples of organization theory topics: overall organization design, interorganizational relationships, change and innovation, performance, and strategy. However, the distinction between these areas can be overdrawn, and, indeed, several chapters in this text present combinations of organization behavior and organization theory approaches. These include Chapter 2 dealing with the managerial role and Chapters 6–9 dealing with work groups, work design, coordination and communication, and power and influence.

Kaiser Permanente's efforts to improve quality, as illustrated in the opening scenario, reflects the necessity of examining an organization from the perspective of multiple levels or units. Clearly, quality improvement efforts will require the motivation of individuals to improve performance. Given the interdependence of providing patient care, this will require effective departmental and cross-departmental teams drawing on group dynamics and knowledge of successful work groups. These activities, in turn, will be influenced by the overall design of the Kaiser organization and its ability to adapt to change and to deal with the challenges of an environment calling for increased performance accountability. Its likely success will depend both on the skills and talents of individuals and on the ability of Kaiser Permanente to organize the talent and energy into effective work groups that can exert organizational-wide impact on quality which, in turn, can meet the challenges of the environment. The progression from individual issues to group issues to inter-organizational and environmental issues also corresponds with the need for increased breadth of understanding and vision on the part of the health services executive. The challenge which this progression makes upon the manager is highlighted in Chapter 2.

MAJOR PERSPECTIVES ON HEALTH SERVICES ORGANIZATIONS

Everyone has a theory or a perspective on how organizations function. Based on personal experience, we create "mental maps" of what is connected to what and how things happen. In many respects organization theory consists of the systematic examination of these mental maps of how things work. Over the years, a number of major perspectives of how organizations work have evolved: classical bureaucratic theory, the scientific management school, the human relations school, contingency theory, resource dependence theory, the strategic management perspective, population ecology theory, and institutional theory. These perspectives can be used to gain insight into the structure and functioning of health services organizations.

Bureaucratic Theory

Classical *bureaucratic theory* is consistent with the closed system approach to organizations and is based on five characteristics.

1. The organization is guided by explicit specific procedures for governing activities.
2. Activities are distributed among office holders.
3. Offices are arranged in a hierarchical fashion.
4. Candidates are selected on the basis of their technical competence.
5. Officials carry out their functions in an impersonal fashion.[4]

The bureaucratic organizational form can achieve technical superiority over other forms under certain stable conditions. However, a number of investigators have pointed out dysfunctional consequences of bureaucracy including its lack of individual freedom, rigidity of behavior, and difficulty in dealing with clients.[5–7] While most health services organizations are organized along bureaucratic lines to some degree, other forms of organization are better at dealing with rapidly changing environments. The manager's challenge is to decide which organizational components might best be organized along bureaucratic lines and which might best be organized in other ways. Chapter 6, 7, and 10 deal explicitly with this issue.

The Scientific Management School

Closely related to the bureaucratic approach is the scientific management school.[8–10] This perspective emphasizes span of control, unity of command, appropriate delegation of authority, departmentalization, and the use of work methods to improve efficiency. The scientific management approach consists of

1. programming the job
2. choosing the right person to match the job
3. training the person to do the job

Much of the early work on job design (see Chapter 7) is based on the scientific management school as are some current work methods improvement and operations research approaches.

Returning to the case of Kaiser Permanente, the bureaucratic and scientific management approaches would suggest that the quality improvement goals be explicitly defined and that the requirements for achieving these goals be spelled out in detail and expressed in terms of specific job positions and necessary skills. People should then be screened and selected on the basis of defined criteria. The quality improvement function would be hierarchically organized with one department reporting to an overall head who in turn would report to a Kaiser-wide coordinating body. Various rules, policies, and practices would exist for what problems to study, how to study them, and what kinds of information should be generated. The bureaucratic and scientific management schools would help to contribute needed structure to the organization of Kaiser's quality improvement efforts.

The Human Relations School

The focus of the human relations school is on the individual. Satisfying individual needs is seen as a worthy goal in itself, not merely a means of achieving other organizational goals.[11-15] The approach emphasizes the usefulness of participatory decision making that involves the individual in the organization and the role of intrinsic self-actualizing aspects of work. The approach represents the foundation for many applied organization development efforts and for the reemphasis on empowering individuals associated with total quality management and continuous quality improvement efforts. A number of issues associated with the human relations school are discussed in Chapter 3 on motivation and Chapter 4 on leadership.

Returning to the Kaiser opening scenario, the human relations school would emphasize the importance of empowering individuals in the organization to take greater responsibility for improving all aspects of their work. Employees would be given greater autonomy to identify and solve problems. They would be provided with the training and tools to function in this role. A major challenge which Kaiser would face in implementing this philosophy of management is to get senior and middle managers to let go of the tendency to want to do things themselves to make sure that they get done right. Applying the human relations approach to the issue would require that the Kaiser Permanente culture be consistently supportive of employee empowerment.

Contingency Theory

Contingency theorists[16-21] suggest that a more bureaucratic or "mechanistic" form of organization is more effective when the environment is relatively simple and stable, tasks and technology are relatively routine, and a relatively high percentage of nonprofessional workers are employed. In contrast, a less bureaucratic or more "organic" form of organization is likely to be more effective when the environment is complex and dynamic, tasks and technologies are nonroutine, and a relatively high percentage of professionals are involved. The more organic organizational form involves decentralized decision making, more participative decision making, and a greater reliance on lateral communication and coordination mechanisms to link people and work units. These mechanisms are appropriate when the environment is complex and nonroutine technologies are involved because the organization has a greater need for information, expertise, and flexibility. Organic forms of design are better able to respond to these needs. In contrast, where no such demands are made, there is less need for flexibility and the more traditional bureaucratic approach is likely to be more efficient and effective.

Contingency theorists do not advocate an either/or approach but rather view the process as a continuum from more or less bureaucratic (i.e., mechanistic) to more or less organic. Furthermore, they recognize that different subunits of the organization may be organized differently depending on the specific environments and technologies with which they are involved. Empirical support for contingency theory ideas is mixed depending on whether one is studying the organization as a whole, particular subgroups, or specific individuals.[22] Nonetheless, given the wide variety of health services organizations and different environments in which they operate, the contingency perspective has wide application to health services organizations.[23] The contingency perspective is drawn on throughout this book including Chapters 7, 8, 10, and 13.

In the case of Kaiser Permanente, the contingency perspective would suggest that the quality improvement function might be organized differently depending on the environment faced by each Kaiser facility, the nature of the clinical problems and other issues being addressed, and the types of employee skills available. In smaller Kaiser hospitals operating in more stable markets, it may be possible to develop structured approaches to quality improvement and to do so in an orderly fashion by training most employees in quality improvement tools in advance, conducting pilot projects, learning from them, and gradually diffusing them throughout the organization. In more complex hospitals and clinics operating in more dynamic environments, a more flexible approach may be needed. Some of the training may need to occur in a "just in time" fashion, problems may need to be addressed as they arise, and a more flexible structure may need to be used to make rapid changes as required.

Resource Dependence Theory

The *resource dependence theory* emphasizes the importance of the organization's abilities to secure needed resources from its environment in order to survive.[24-28] Those subunits within the organization that have access to key external resources will hold greater power and influence. While organizations desire to maintain their autonomy and remain relatively independent of their environment, they also recognize the need to form certain coalitions or networks to pool resources and reduce transaction costs. The resource dependence perspective, like the strategic management perspective but unlike the population ecology perspective discussed below, assumes that managers can actively influence their environment to reduce unwanted dependencies and enhance survivability. The resource dependence perspective is drawn on in Chapters 2, 9, 11, 13, and 14.

In regard to Kaiser Permanente, the resource dependence perspective would emphasize the importance of continuous improvement and total quality management for demonstrating value to purchasers of care. To accomplish this Kaiser needs resources from the environment in the form of measurement tools, information systems, and technical expertise to produce valid data on the processes and outcomes of patient care. Kaiser will be able to exert influence over its environment to the extent that it is successful in demonstrating continuous improvement relative to that of other organizations that patients and purchasers can choose.

Strategic Management Perspective

The *strategic management perspective* emphasizes the importance of positioning the organization relative to its environment and competitors in order to achieve its objectives and assure its survival.[29-35] The perspective attempts to link environmental forces, internal organizational design and processes, and the strategy of the firm. It suggests that the firm's strategy needs to be consistent with both the external environmental demands and the organization's internal core capabilities and competencies. It is explicitly concerned with issues of organizational performance, arguing that managers and organizational members have discretion in choosing strategies and structures to match the environment in a way that will enhance the organization's performance. Major subissues of interest include the different processes by which organizations develop strategies, the extent to which organizations are able to successfully change their strategies, and the extent to which organizations vary in their ability to implement strategies. Chapters 11, 13, and 14 of the text highlight many of these issues.

The strategic management perspective would suggest that Kaiser's efforts to improve quality need to be examined from the perspective of its relationship to the central core strategies of the organization. For example, to what extent is Kaiser Permanente attempting to differentiate itself in its marketplace based either on its technical or service quality or both? What other external factors might be influencing this strategy? In turn, to what extent does Kaiser have the internal capabilities to differentiate its services on various quality dimensions? For example, it may be in a better position to do so for primary care and routine secondary care than for certain kinds of more complex tertiary care where its capabilities are less fully developed. Further, the strategic management perspective would argue that, for Kaiser Permanente to be successful as an organization, it is necessary to go beyond quality improvement alone and consider its ability to innovate in developing new programs and services to meet member needs and increased demand.

Population Ecology Theory

Population ecology theorists[36-40] argue that the environment "selects out" certain organizations for survival. Based on theories of natural selection in biology, the focus is on a given population of organizations rather than on an individual organization. Whether a given organization will succeed depends on where it stands in relation to the population of its competitors and the overall environmental forces influencing that population. As environmental pressures increase, only the stronger, more dominant organizational forms will survive; the weaker forms will cease to exist or will survive only as markedly different forms of organization. In the population ecology approach, unlike the resource dependence and strategic management approaches, there are severe limits on the ability of organizations to adapt. This is expressed in terms of "structural inertia." Thus, in this approach, the ability of managers to successfully influence their environments is subsumed to be relatively minor.

The population ecology approach is based on the principles of variation, selection, and retention. Variation involves the continuous development of new organizational forms that add to the variety and complexity in the environment. In health care, examples include freestanding surgery centers, urgent care centers, birthing care centers, hospices, diagnostic imaging centers, and fitness centers.

The selection principle states that some of the new organizational forms will fit the external environment better than others. They will be better able to exploit the environment for resources and will move in the same direction that the environmental trends are moving. In health care, ambulatory surgery centers serve as an example as more surgical procedures are being reimbursed on an outpatient basis and there appears to be a growing trend for consumers to prefer quicker, more accessible, and convenient services.

Retention involves the preservation and ongoing institutionalization of the new organizational form. Those that are valued by the environment in the long run will be retained while others will fall by the wayside. For example, ambulatory surgery centers may experience relatively long survival (at least until it becomes possible to do most surgery in the patient's home), whereas urgent care centers, faced with stiff competition from physician providers, hospital emergency rooms, and growing regulatory requirements, face a less certain future. The winners may be those organizations that manage to carve out specialized market niches viewed as complementary to other organizations and in which they can act as noncompeting sources of patient referrals to other providers.

As health service organizations are faced with increasing cost containment and competitive pressures, the issues raised by the population ecology perspective become particularly important. In recent years a growing number of hospitals and HMOs have gone out of business and, as previously noted, a variety of new organizational forms have arisen. In addition, the hospital industry has been transformed from a largely cottage industry composed of individual hospitals to more than 300 health systems. These systems, both investor-owned and not-for-profit, are working to find specific niches in the market place, focusing in particular on the development of regionally- and locally-integrated networks of care. While the population ecology perspective tends to minimize the manager's role, it adds an important dimension and challenge to the effective management of health services organizations by emphasizing the importance of networking and coalition building and of developing products and services for specific population segments in which the competitive market forces and related pressures are less threatening.[41,42] These issues are further discussed in Chapters 2, 9, 12, 13, and 14.

In the Kaiser Permanente case, the population ecology approach would suggest that efforts at continuous quality improvement are only germane to the extent that they make the Kaiser Permanente organizational form more viable in a changing health care environment. It would emphasize the extent to which the quality improvement principles are congruent with Kaiser's current organizational structure and capabilities. It would suggest that Kaiser has very little flexibility or ability to modify these approaches if they prove to be inconsistent with the Kaiser culture and capabilities. If the Kaiser organizational form experiences difficulty in incorporating the newer continuous quality improvement approaches, the population ecology school would argue that Kaiser becomes more susceptible to being "selected against" by other organizations with which the new approach is more compatible.

Institutional Theory

Institutional theorists emphasize that organizations face environments characterized by external norms, rules, and requirements which the organizations must conform to in order to receive legitimacy and support.[43-45] While technical environments reward organizations for effective and efficient performance, institutional environments emphasize rewarding organizations for having structures and processes that are in conformance with the environment. The rules, beliefs, and norms of the external environment are often expressed in the form of "rational myths."[46] Such myths are rational in the sense of being reflected in professional standards, laws, and licensure and accreditation requirements but are myths in the sense that they cannot necessarily be verified empirically. They are, nonetheless, widely held to be true. Conformity with these myths helps the organization to gain legitimacy and support. This conformance is often referred to as "isomorphism" and causes organizations faced with a similar set of environmental circumstances to resemble each other.[47]

Health services organizations are experiencing a rapid transformation of both their technical and institutional environments.[45] The increased technical pressure for greater efficiency and quality expressed in terms of value is causing health services organizations to change long-established structures. This is reflected in the reorganization of acute care hospitals as they attempt to become components of more vertically-integrated health systems and the development of new norms and beliefs about what constitutes the effective delivery of health care. This transition results in a great deal of internal conflict that must be managed. Chapter 5 addresses the conflict issues. The implications of the institutional theory perspective on health services organization are also addressed in Chapters 9, 11, 13, and 14.

From an institutional theory perspective, Kaiser Permanente's efforts in continuous quality improvement might be viewed as a response to newly emerging norms and practices within the health services sector. These are being fostered by the Joint Commission on Accreditation of Healthcare Organizations (JCAHO) which has adopted continuous quality improvement as the basis for new accreditation requirements. In addition, continuous improvement has been increasingly accepted as a distinguishing feature of an innovative organization with several national awards created to recognize institutions that exert such leadership. Thus, it could be argued that Kaiser Permanente's approach is not motivated so much by substantive concerns over its quality or efficiency of care in a competitive market place but rather by negative perceptions of external groups if it did not pursue continuous quality improvement.

Table 1.4 provides a brief summary of how each major theory or perspective would view Kaiser Permanente's efforts. It is important to note that none of the

TABLE 1.4. How Major Perspectives Would View Kaiser Permanente's Quality Improvement Efforts

Perspective	Point of Emphasis	Contribution
Bureaucratic and scientific management	Explicit goals; hierarchical organization; detailed specifications	Provide needed structure
Human relations	Employee empowerment	Need for a culture supportive of empowerment
Contingency theory	Structure depends on environment, task, technology, and the contingencies facing each unit	Flexible approach needed; adapt efforts to meet the requirements of the situation
Resource dependence	Ability to secure needed resources	Need to demonstrate value through providing reliable and valid data on patient care processes and outcomes
Strategic management	Achieve fit or alignment between the organization's strategy, external environment, and internal structure and capabilities	Need to link quality improvement to core strategies and capabilities of the organization
Population ecology	External environmental pressures are primary determinant of success; little managers can do	Highlights powerful role played by external environment; quality improvement efforts alone may not be sufficient if organization is not well positioned within the environment
Institutional theory	External norms, rules, and requirements cause organizations to conform in order to receive legitimacy; organizations in a similar institutional environment come to resemble each other (i.e., become isomorphic with the environment)	Quality improvement efforts must take into account regulatory and accreditation pressures and public expectations

perspectives are inherently right or wrong. They are different from each other and incomplete. As such, each represents a *partial* view of organizational dynamics and can provide input for constructive disagreement and debate, an example of which is highlighted in Debate Time 1.1. It is important to understand the basic assumptions and premises of each perspective, as they can be drawn on in various combinations to provide a greater understanding of how health services organizations operate.

METAPHORS OF HEALTH SERVICES ORGANIZATIONS

The above perspectives are enriched by recasting them as metaphors of health services organizations as shown in Table 1.5. The eight metaphors are: machines,

tyrants, brains, playing fields, psychic prisons, biological organisms, political systems, and holograms.[51]

Machines

Classical bureaucratic theory is reflected in the image of the organization as a *machine*. In fact, workers may speak of the organization as a "well-oiled machine." This metaphor reflects the image of an organization as interlocking parts with clearly defined roles that are appropriately meshed together to accomplish the organization's work. Being a "well-oiled machine" is important for many of the tasks undertaken by health services organizations including the admission of patients into hospitals, the paperwork associated with billing for patient services, the production of a laboratory test, and the processing of a Federal Drug Adminis-

---

DEBATE TIME 1.1: WHAT DO YOU THINK?

In recent years a number of health services organizations including hospitals, medical group practices, and home health care agencies have either merged, consolidated, or gone out of business. How might this be explained? Population ecology theory, of course, would assert that the environmental variables involving reimbursement rates, competitive factors, technological growth, and societal forces are the primary causes of this organizational restructuring. They would further argue that these organizations and their managers could do relatively little to prevent the eventual outcomes. Basically, the organization was no longer "fit" given the changing environmental forces.

In contrast, the resource dependence and strategic management perspectives argue that organizations have considerable control over their destiny. Through actions taken by organization leaders and members, new strategies, policies and procedures, alliances, changes in structure, and hiring of new or different kinds of people, can be initiated in order to improve the organization's "fit" with changing environmental forces and to assure its viability. They point to examples of organizational "turn arounds" which suggest that the reasons why some organizations are restructured

or closed while others survive has more to do with the vision and talent of the organization and its members than with externally-generated environmental forces. Which view is more correct?

Does The Literature Help?

". . . the corporatization of health care in the United States has been precipitated by a transformation of institutional systems rather than by rational or strategic adaptation by individual organizations to changes in their operating environments."[48]

"Our view is simply that most relevant environmental forces are, in fact, organizationally created and sustained, and thus are subject to organizational influence."[49]

"The basic feature of the natural selection perspective is that the environment selects the most fit or optimal organizations. The organization is thus seen as relatively powerless to affect the selection process. But our review of some of the research on health care organizations suggests otherwise. Furthermore, from a managerial perspective it is difficult to accept so much organizational fatalism and inevitability."[50]

TABLE 1.5. Organizational Perspectives and Metaphors

Organizational Perspectives		Relevant Metaphors
Classical bureaucratic theory	⟶	Machines
		Tyrants
Human relations school	⟶	Brains
		Playing fields
		Psychic prisons
Contingency theory	⟶	Biological organisms
		Brains
Resource dependency theory	⟶	Political systems
Strategic management perspective	⟶	Biological organisms
		Holograms
Population ecology theory	⟶	Biological organisms
Institutional theory	⟶	Biological organisms

tration (FDA) application for approval. The downside is that the "machines" can rapidly become outmoded and inflexible in the face of changing demands and circumstances. An organization whose dominant paradigm is that of a machine sees order and stability where none exists and rapidly becomes technologically and organizationally obsolete.

Tyrants

Organizations can also behave as *tyrants* or as instruments of domination. In pursuit of their missions, they can lose sight of basic human values and exploit their employees and others either unconsciously or by intent. This may be the basis for many physicians' fears of large complex health services organizations such as the growing health services systems and networks. The mental map which many physicians have is that of the organization as tyrant or potential tyrant restricting their freedom and autonomy and making unilateral decisions without soliciting their input. The tyrant metaphor represents the shadow or dark side of organizational functioning that must be carefully guarded against by the organization's leaders.

Brains

The metaphor of organizations as *brains* places emphasis on the importance of learning, intelligence, and information processing. It is based in part on cybernetic theory which stresses four key principles.

1. Systems have the capacity to sense, monitor, and scan significant aspects of their environment.
2. Systems can relate this information to the norms that guide system behavior.
3. Systems can detect significant deviations from these norms.
4. Systems are able to initiate corrective actions when discrepancies are detected.[52]

When these conditions hold, a continuous process of information exchange is created between an organization and its environment allowing the system to operate in a spontaneous self-correcting manner. This operation is characterized by *double-loop learning* which involves an ability to take a second look at a situation by questioning the relevance of underlying assumptions.[53] The brain metaphor is particularly useful for health services organizations in terms of maximizing the ability of individuals and groups to learn from their environment and make use of the information to create innovative programs and services. It is consistent with the human relations school's emphasis on personal growth and development.

Playing Fields

Organizations can also be viewed as *playing fields* or stages upon which individuals perform their "art." For health services organizations this frequently involves a complex performance by many different talented individuals. These professionals—physicians, nurses, therapists, technologists, researchers, executives, and many others—have a highly developed sense of professionalism and professional identity. As such, they frequently clash as one culture emphasizes its beliefs and values relative to others. The result is often "tribal warfare" which must be managed.[54] The challenge is to create a larger overall sense of organizational identity and culture which can embrace the individual cultures of the different health professionals. When this is done, the goals articulated by the human relations school are met, and people are able to work effectively in performing interdependent tasks.

Psychic Prisons

Organizations can also be viewed as places where people are trapped by their own perceptions, ideas, and beliefs whether consciously or unconsciously. Often this is reflected in the tendency to avoid conflict, to avoid anxiety-provoking situations, or to strive to maintain one's sense of identity and self-esteem. These issues can be particularly important in health services organizations because, as noted above, individuals identify strongly with their professional disciplines. When these needs are concretized in a way that allows no room for other perspectives or viewpoints, the result is indeed a *psychic prison* stifling organizational learning, innovation, and the ability to adapt. It is the negative side of the human relations school's emphasis on personal growth and development.

Biological Organisms

In recent years it has become popular to think of organizations as *biological organisms;* that is, as different species which must adapt to their environments in the process of birth, growth, decline, and eventual death. It is concerned with the issue of how the organization becomes fit to survive in its environment. As shown in Table 1.5, contingency theory, strategic management perspective, population ecology theory, and institutional theory each contain major aspects of the biological organism metaphor. Contingency theory primarily emphasizes internal organization design and fit while the strategic management perspective emphasizes the fit of the organization's strategy with its environment. The population ecology approach emphasizes the strength of the external forces that essentially select out various organizational species for survival. Institutional theory suggests that one way in which organizations can succeed is to mimic or match the values and norms contained in the environment in order to maintain necessary legitimacy and credibility with environmental sources of sanctions and power. The biological organism metaphor highlighting the interplay of the organization with the environment over time can provide many useful insights for health services managers. Organizations of different sizes and at different stages in their existence require different resources and different strategies to ensure success.

Political Systems

Organizations, of course, can also be viewed as *political systems* in which various groups and actors vie for control of important resources. Organizations are ruled by whomever controls these resources and decides how they are used to accomplish the interests of various groups. Given the many different kinds of professionals working in or affiliated with health services organizations, the political system metaphor is particularly salient. Physicians, executives, nurses, researchers, and others often vie for control over important resources to push their own view of what is good for the organization. The political system metaphor is closely aligned with the playing field metaphor in which the organization essentially serves as the playing field or battleground for control. When things get out of control, health services organizations can turn into psychic prisons or tyrants. The resource dependence theory is consistent with the political system metaphor as it focuses on the ways in which organizations acquire and control needed resources.

Holograms

A *hologram* is an object in which each of the parts contains the entire essence of the overall object or image. As a result, the overall object or system can continue to function even when specific parts malfunction or are removed. While this metaphor is often used in conjunction with the brain metaphor and can be considered an important aspect of the brain metaphor, we believe that treating it separately provides some special insights. In a holographic structure the intent is to design the whole into the parts and to create a redundancy of parts so that a range of functions can be performed rather than just a single specialized activity. Designing health services organizations as holograms emphasizes the need for flexibility, creativity, change, and innovation. An organization's culture, its design, and its information processing capabilities are facilitators of holographic properties. The metaphor is also consistent with the strategic management perspective's emphasis on viewing the organization as a whole in positioning its various elements to deal with outside forces while at the same time recognizing the interplay between those forces and internal organizational components. The idea is to see the organization's strategy as being expressed in the task and function of an individual worker as well as in the accumulation of worker activities across multiple tasks; that is, the "part-whole relationship." Viewing health services organizations as holograms can provide powerful insights contributing to the need for integrating multiple components of health services delivery into a more coherent whole. A micro example is provided by the cross-training of workers such that more functions and activities are contained in a single individual. A macro example is provided by the efforts of some health services organizations to develop regionally-based vertically-integrated delivery systems to provide more coordinated care across the range of patient needs.

These metaphors are intended to challenge the reader's thinking about health services organizations and to provide a lens for interpreting the chapters which follow. While they are presented in a sequential and categorical fashion, it is important to note that they represent a continuum of perspectives that may overlap each other. Having learned about them, revisit the issues posed in Debate Time 1.1. Have your views of these issues changed?

ORGANIZATION THEORY AND BEHAVIOR: A FRAMEWORK FOR THE TEXT

As discussed in the various perspectives and metaphors above, the essence of management is to motivate people and groups to carry out technical tasks for the attainment of organizational goals and at the same time to renew the organization for long-run survival and growth as it charts the future. These dimensions of the managerial challenge are outlined in Figure 1.3 which provides a basic framework for the book.

The book is divided into five sections. The first is an introductory section that provides an overview of perspectives on the management of health services organizations (Chapter 1) and an analysis of the evolving role of management in these organizations (Chapter 2). This is followed by four sections corresponding to the managerial activities of motivating and leading people and groups, operating the technical system, renewing the organization, and charting the future.

Managers must motivate and lead people to ensure high levels of commitment, stability, and cooperative behavior. This is accomplished by satisfying individual needs and values (Chapter 3), by providing direction (Chapter 4), and by managing conflict and negotiation processes (Chapter 5).

Managers must also operate the technical system in response to problems of technical performance involving productivity, efficiency, quality, and customer satisfaction. This is accomplished by determining the appropriate work groups and work design (Chapters 6 and 7), establishing communication and coordination mechanisms (Chapter 8), and using appropriate influence processes (Chapter 9).

Organizations operate within a constantly changing environment, and managers must renew the organization by determining effective organizational design (Chapter 10), acquiring resources and managing inter-organizational relationships (Chapter 11), by managing change and innovation (Chapter 12), and attaining organizational goals (Chapter 13).

Finally, organizations function through time, and managers must be responsive to problems of long-term survival and growth of the organization. This is accomplished by managing strategically (Chapter 14) and anticipating the future (Chapter 15). The framework presented in Figure 1.3 is intended as a departure point, not a point of closure, for the reader's own synthesis of the material that follows.

THE NATURE OF ORGANIZATIONS: FRAMEWORK FOR THE TEXT

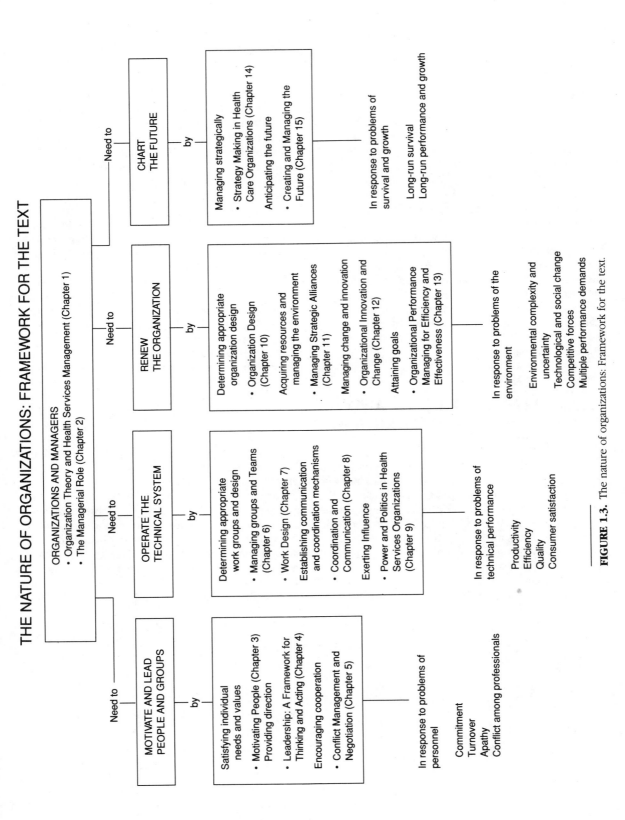

FIGURE 1.3. The nature of organizations: Framework for the text.

KEY CONCEPTS

Adaptation Function
Biological Organisms
Boundary Spanning Function
Brains
Bureaucratic Theory
Change
Closed System
Contingency Theory
Continuous Improvement
External Environment
Governance Function
Holograms
Human Relations School
Innovation
Interorganizational Relationships
Institutional Theory
Machines
Macro Approach
Maintenance Function
Management Function
Managing Across Boundaries
Micro Approach
Mission/Goals
Open System
Organization Behavior
Organization Design
Organization Theory
Playing Fields
Political Systems
Population-Based Management
Population Ecology Theory
Production Function
Psychic Prisons
Resource Dependence Theory
Scientific Management School
Strategic Management Perspective
Tyrants
Work Group/Work Design

Discussion Questions

1. If you were in charge of Kaiser Permanente's continuous quality improvement efforts, which of the major perspectives on organizations (bureaucratic, scientific management, human relations, contingency, resource dependence, strategic management, population ecology, and institutional) would offer you the most assistance? Defend your choice.

2. During the past decade, more than 100 hospitals have closed and several hundred have reorganized. How would you attempt to explain why some closed while others reorganized? In addressing this question, refer to Debate Time 1.1 and consider the resource dependence, strategic management, population ecology, and institutional perspectives on organizations.

3. Several neighborhood health centers have hired you as a consultant to help them form an umbrella organization that in turn would be merged with the local county health department. Which of the metaphors of organizations (machine, tyrant, brain, playing field, psychic prison, biological organism, political system, hologram) would provide you with the greatest insight as you take on this assignment? Defend your choice.

4. State whether you agree or disagree with the following statement: For the most part, health services organizations are no different from most other organizations. Indicate the specific reasons for your agreement or disagreement and develop at least two reasons in addition to those presented in the chapter.

REFERENCES

1. PEW Commission on Education for the Health Professions, Health Care Administration, PEW Charitable Trusts, Philadelphia, 1993.
2. Scott WR. Developments in organization theory, 1960–1980. *American Behavioral Scientist.* 1981;24:407–422.
3. Katz E, Kahn R. *The Social Psychology of Organizations,* 2nd. New York, NY: John Wiley & Sons; 1978.
4. Weber M. *The Theory of Social and Economic Organization.* Glencoe, Ill: Free Press; 1964.
5. Merton RK. Bureaucratic structure and personality. In *Social Theory and Social Structure.* New York, NY: Free Press; 1957.
6. Gouldner A. *Patterns of Industrial Bureaucracy.* New York, NY: Free Press; 1954.
7. Selznick P. *TVA and the Grass Roots.* New York, NY: Harper & Row; 1966.
8. Taylor F. *Scientific Management.* New York, NY: Harper & Row; 1947.
9. Gulick L, Urwick L. *Papers on Science of Administration.* New York, NY: Columbia University Press; 1937.
10. Mooney JE. *Principles of Organization.* New York, NY: Harper and Row; 1947.
11. Barnard CI. *The Functions of the Executive.* Cambridge, Mass: Harvard University Press; 1938.
12. Roethlisberger FJ, Dickson WJ. *Management and the Worker.* Cambridge, Mass: Harvard University Press; 1939.
13. McGregor D. *The Human Side of Enterprise.* New York, NY: McGraw-Hill; 1960.
14. Argyris C. *Integrating the Individual and the Organization.* New York, NY: John Wiley & Sons; 1964.
15. Likert E. *The Human Organization.* New York, NY: McGraw-Hill; 1967.
16. Burns T, Stalker GM. *The Management of Innovation.* London, England: Tavistock; 1961.
17. Woodward, J. *Technology and Organizational Behavior.* Oxford, England: Oxford University Press; 1970.
18. Lawrence P, Lorsch J. *Organization and Environment.* Cambridge, Mass: Harvard University Press; 1967.
19. Thompson JD. *Organizations in Action.* New York, NY: McGraw-Hill; 1967.
20. Perrow C. A framework for the comparative analysis of organizations. *American Sociological Review.* 1967;32:194–208.
21. Schoonhoven CB. Problems with contingency theory: Testing assumptions hidden within the language of contingency "theory". *Administrative Science Quarterly.* September 1981;26:349–377.
22. Mohr LB. *Explaining Organizational Behavior.* San Francisco, Ca: Jossey-Bass; 1982.
23. Strasser S. The effective application of contingency theory in health settings: Problems and recommended solutions. *Health Care Management Review.* Winter 1983:15–23.
24. Hickson DJ et al. A strategic contingencies theory of intraorganizational power. *Administrative Science Quarterly.* 1971;16:216–229.
25. March JG, Olsen JP. *Ambiguity and Choice in Organizations.* Bergen, Norway: Universitetsforlaget; 1976.
26. Pfeffer J, Salancik GR. *The External Control of Organizations.* New York, NY: Harper & Row; 1978.
27. Williamson OE. The economies of organization: The transaction cost approach. *The American Journal of Sociology.* 1981;87:548–577.
28. Ouchi WG. Markets, bureaucracies, and clans. *Administrative Science Quarterly.* 1980;24:129–141.
29. Ansoff HI. *Corporate Strategy: An Analytic Approach to Business Policy for Growth and Expansion.* New York, NY: McGraw-Hill; 1965.
30. Andrews KR. *The Concept of Corporate Strategy.* Homewood, Ill: Dow Jones-Irwin; 1971.
31. Schendel DE, Hofer CW. *Strategic Management: A New View of Business Policy and Planning.* Boston, Mass: Little, Brown; 1979.
32. Porter ME. *Competitive Strategy: Techniques for Analyzing Industries and Competitors.* New York, NY: Free Press; 1980.
33. Porter ME. *Competitive Advantage: Creating and Sustaining Superior Performance.* New York, NY: Free Press; 1985.
34. Shortell SM, Zajac EJ. Health care organizations and the development of the strategic management perspective. In: Mick SS and Associates. *Innovations in Health Care Delivery: Insights for Organization Theory.* Ann Arbor, Mich: Health Administration Press; 1990:144–180.
35. Kimberly JR, Zajac EJ. Strategic adaptation in health care organizations: implications for theory and research. *Medical Care Review.* 1985;42:267–302.
36. Hannan MT, Freeman JH. Structural inertia and organizational change. *American Sociological Review.* April 1984:149–164.
37. Hannan MT, Freeman JH. *Organizational Ecology.* Cambridge, Mass: Harvard University Press; 1989.
38. Delacroix J, Carroll GR. Organizational foundings: An ecological study of newspaper industries of Argentina and Ireland. *Administrative Sciences Quarterly.* 1983;28:274–291.
39. Aldrich H. *Organizations and Environments.* Englewood Cliffs, NJ: Princeton Hills; 1979.

40. Carroll GR. Organizational ecology. *Annual Review of Sociology.* 1984;10:71–93.

41. Alexander JA, Kaluzny AD, Middleton SC. Organizational growth, survival and death in the U.S. hospital industry: A population ecology perspective. *Social Science and Medicine.* 1986;22:303–308.

42. Alexander JA, Amburgey TL. The dynamics of change in the American hospital industry: Transformation or selection? *Medical Care Review.* 1987;44:279–321.

43. Meyer JW, Scott WR. *Organizational Environments: Ritual and Rationality.* Beverly Hills, Ca: Sage; 1983.

44. Scott WR. The adolescence of institutional theory: Problems and potential for organizational analysis. *Administrative Science Quarterly.* 1987;32:493–512.

45. Alexander JA, D'Aunno TA. Transformation of institutional environments: perspectives on the corporatization of U.S. health care. In: Mick SS and Associates. *Innovations in Health Care Delivery: Insights for Organizational Theory.* Ann Arbor, Mich: Health Administration Press;1990:53–85.

46. Fennell M, Alexander JA. Organizational boundary spanning and institutionalized environments. *Academy of Management Journal.* 1987;30:456–476.

47. DiMaggio PJ, Powell WW. The iron cage revisited: Institutional isomorphism and collective rationality in organizational fields. *American Sociological Review.* 1983;48:147–160.

48. Alexander, D'Aunno, op. cit., p. 79.

49. Shortell, Zajac, op. cit., p. 169.

50. Starkweather D, Cook KS. Organization-environment relations. In: Shortell SM, Kaluzny AD, eds. *Health Care Management: A Text in Organization Theory and Behavior.* 2nd ed. New York, NY: John Wiley; 1988:352.

51. Morgan G. *Images of Organization.* Beverly Hills, Ca: Sage Library of Social Research; 1986.

52. Ibid., 87.

53. Argyris C. *Reasoning, Learning, and Action.* San Francisco, Ca: Jossey-Bass; 1982.

54. Neuhauser PC. *Tribal Warfare in Organizations.* Cambridge, Mass: Ballinger Publishing Co.; 1988.

CHAPTER

THE MANAGERIAL ROLE

Howard S. Zuckerman, Ph.D.
Professor

William L. Dowling, Ph.D.
Vice President

LEARNING OBJECTIVES

After completing this chapter, the reader should be able to

1. understand historical perspectives on the managerial role and their underlying concepts
2. recognize the managerial challenges posed by changes in the external environment and within health care organizations
3. understand the changing roles of managers in providing vision and leadership, adapting the organization to its environment, and designing the organization to enact its mission and to achieve its objectives
4. recognize changing skills and knowledge required by managers in light of environmental and organizational dynamics

CHAPTER PURPOSE

The interview with Edward J. Connors sets the stage for a discussion of the managerial role. It nicely captures the breadth, depth, and complexity of the role, reflecting the manager's responsibilities within the organization and in relating the organization to its environment. The interview also recognizes that the managerial role continues to evolve as organizations and their environments change. It is acknowledged that the requisite managerial skills and knowledge must also evolve, but Connors suggests there remains a set of core competencies which must endure. The purpose of this chapter is to understand the managerial role within health services, contributing factors which influence that role, and skills and

IN THE REAL WORLD

REFLECTIONS ON LEADERSHIP

In the fall of 1989, Edward J. Connors, then president of Mercy Health Services and that year's chair of the American Hospital Association (AHA) Board of Trustees, was a featured speaker at the Annual Symposium of the University of Iowa Graduate Program in Hospital and Health Administration where he addressed the theme of leadership in health care. Following the symposium, the editor of *Hospital and Health Services Administration* interviewed Connors about some of the major themes of his remarks. Excerpts from the interview follow:

Q: What is your philosophy of management?

A: The essence of management is to create an environment in which people can function to the optimum of their potential, consistent with the aims of the organization. It may sound trite and simple, and it is quite different from the idea that the essence of management is to plan, direct, evaluate, control, and so on. Woven into that is the concept of service and attention to the disadvantaged. Mercy's expression of its philosophy is called a "preferential option for the poor."

Q: Speaking of trends, what is your perspective on how the institutional sector has responded to the competitive environment?

A: I think there have been only a very few desirable outcomes of the competitive environment. On the positive side, the one or two successes I can think of have focused the attention of the providers on the wants and needs of the consumer. The best of what marketing is all about—not image-building, but determining in a systematic way what people really want—wouldn't have happened if we didn't have some elements of competition.

I think that the sad part of the competitive model is a narrowing of the interests of some institutions rather than a broadening of those interests to meet the comprehensive needs of all persons in the community. In my opinion, the competitive mind-set of hospital leaders has not been a positive force when viewed from the vantage point of the relationship between competition and the challenges of access, cost (and price), and quality of services.

Q: One of the points in your symposium address that intrigued me was the idea of cooperation among health care providers. I think that cooperation has not been much of a factor in strategic planning. How do you as chairman of AHA view the needs inherent in the field of health care which would seem to require greater cooperative efforts?

A: I haven't figured out how collaboration and pure competition can exist side by side, simultaneously. But I think the value that needs to drive health care providers is that of cooperation and collaboration. When you stand back and ask yourself, "Why do hospitals exist in the first place?" the answer, of course, is "to serve people." We have a collective responsibility through some forms of cooperation.

Q: How are we doing in health care in terms of leadership?

A: The major concern I have about leadership in health care is the lack of a vision, an agreement on what we want to end up with as far as a more rational, a more humane, a more affordable system. In the absence of that vision, the leaders are engaged in short-view debates and discussions of adequacy and equity of payment, the amount that will be allocated to Medicare/Medicaid, the issue of whether catastrophic improvements for the aged are going to stick. We have been unable to bring together the elements for the creation of a vision for the future.

Q: How would you describe your role as a leader? Naturally, one's character and values have enormous impact on where an organization goes, where a system goes, where a policy unit goes. Occasionally, the person at the helm makes decisions without being firmly convinced that certain values ought to be engendered in the activity that they are launching. Your organization has a highly articulated mission in which values are very dominant, even the supreme mission aspect. It seems to me that character has to be an underlying force. In your own career and life, how do you view that aspect of your own leadership responsibilities?

A: I think that a leader has to have a fundamental belief in the values of the organization. Values are not really found in mission statements, though it is important for them to be articulated there for purposes of clarity. But they are really found in the hearts, minds, and behavior of people. That is where you find them. I have certain beliefs about health service, and also values as a basis of those beliefs. I don't have much respect for organizations or individuals who are unable or unwilling to articulate where they stand and what values they're bound to. It seems to me that is absolutely essential for a leader—and absolutely essential for me—to internalize and own and understand the value structure not only of health care generally, but of Mercy. You can spot people who just say the words, and who can espouse values that they've never really internalized. That's why our own leadership development program here is absolutely essential.

Q: What do you look for when you pick new leaders for your organization, for the AHA, and so on?

A: Sometimes, as president I advise about who to appoint to this or that. I don't think it is too hard to get a handle on technical and professional competence. I think the track record, the references, and the interviewing techniques are all reasonably good, and I think we tend to do pretty well on that part of it. The other thing we do in our selection/promotion process at Mercy is to have the person give a self-description of how they stand on values—on justice, for example: What does justice mean to you in your work and/or to you as a person?

Q: What does "all men are created equal" mean?

A: Equal opportunity. Equity is different from equal. Early in my career I read an article on leadership skills in the *Harvard Business Review*—something by Katz. The author defines skill as the ability to translate knowledge into action, whether it's hammering a nail or whatever. Then, it goes to say that there are three basic skills for leadership and management: (1) human, (2) technical, and (3) conceptual. These skills are not innate but are capable of being developed. Without human skills a leader doesn't get very far; technical skills are important, of course, but the higher you go in management, the less you need them. The real leader has to have the conceptual skills.

SOURCE: *Excerpted from Reflections on leadership in health care: A conversation with Edward J. Connors.* Hospital and Health Services Administration. *Fall 1990;35:309–323.*

knowledge required to meet the challenges of changing environments and organizations.

ALTERNATIVE ROLE CONCEPTIONS OF THE MANAGER

Traditional Conception

The role of the manager has been conceived in a number of ways, reflecting changes in organizations and in the environments within which organizations operate. Many early writings saw management in terms of skills or activities to be performed within organizations. Within this traditional conception are two distinct schools—the functional and the human relations. Neither of these models is popular in current writings. However, there remains much wisdom and importance within them, and some argue that today's literature in fact reflects their core truths with new words, phrases, and labels.

The functional model of the managerial role is best described as representing the basic activities of management, which include planning, organizing and staffing, directing, and controlling. This classic model assumes that these basic management functions will be performed in any organization, and that they represent the key contribution of management.[1,2] Indeed, in its purest form, the model asserts that these activities *are* the definition of management. Focusing on the formal aspects of management, the functional model emphasizes the application of scientific methods to managerial functions. The more recent contributions of management science and operations research continue to demonstrate the relevance of this model. Critics suggest that the functional view is more a representation of the objectives of managerial work than it is a

description of the work itself. The tone of this approach tends toward prescription, stating norms for what managers should do with limited focus on what they actually do. Emphasizing formal aspects of organizations, this view tends to ignore the informal aspects of the managerial role and excludes external relations.

The human relations perspective has as its central theme the motivation of individuals to the achievement of organizational ends.

The essential task of management is to arrange organizational conditions and methods of operation so that people can achieve their own goals best by directing their own efforts toward organizational objectives.[3]

The social needs of individuals and how they are met at work become key parts of the understanding and knowledge required for effective management. In this context, the informal organization is not an unofficial, irrelevant, and sometimes troublesome component of an organization; rather, it is a centrally important element of organizational success. The model is thus focused on the obligations of management to create and sustain effective work groups; an atmosphere of openness, trust, and supportiveness; and a system of participation in decision making.

Every aspect of a firm's activities is determined by the competence, motivation, and general effectiveness of its human organization. Of all the tasks of management, managing the human component is the central and most important task, because all else depends on how well it is done.[4]

The human relations school is driven by an ideology that focuses on the importance of individuals and the moral and economic benefits that accrue from enabling them to share in shaping their own destiny. Presumably, this in turn may lead individuals to adopt the organization's goals as their own. To build this motivational force, management tactics have included leadership processes, development of intrinsic rewards, team building, participative decision making, and communication processes. Like the functional model, the human relations approach tends to be prescriptive in nature, specifying what managers ought to do. Further, it also ignores the external environment, focusing solely on the internal workings and processes of organizations.

Political-Personal Conception

The political-personal conception emphasizes the centrality of power and personal tactics in understanding the managerial role. This conception is often framed in terms of the "heroic manager" or the "great man or woman" and centers around the charisma of individuals or the politics of *power*. The individualist theme is an old, and still popular, conception of the manager. This enduring view stresses the importance of the *leadership* and the resources of the individual manager. This heroic conception can come close to

rejecting, or at least being quite suspicious of, the contribution of management education and hints that leaders are more likely to be born than made. Livingston, for example, argues that management education has limited value and that the capacity to find the right problems to work on and a natural management style, neither of which can be taught in management education programs, are the critical abilities. While avoiding the position that great managers are born, his descriptions revolve around personal characteristics and qualities needed to manage effectively.[5] Zaleznik suggests that "there are no known ways to train 'great' leaders," his view of a leader being someone with a mission who is willing to use an organization to achieve it.[6] Writings that promote the heroic construct see a certain hardness and unswerving purposefulness in the behavior of the manager. The challenges facing Lee Iacocca are often cited to illustrate the actions of an heroic manager.

In its fundamental assumptions, the heroic model is free of reference to organizations per se, formulated as it is on the attributes of the individual manager. This

IN THE REAL WORLD
A TIME FOR HEROICS: LEE IACOCCA MOVES TO CHRYSLER

Before . . . [my first day at Chrysler] was over, I noticed a couple of seemingly insignificant details that gave me pause. The first was that the office of the president, where Cafiero worked, was being used as a thoroughfare to get from one office to another. I watched in amazement as executives with coffee cups in their hands kept opening the door and walking right through the president's office. Right away I knew the place was in a state of anarchy. Chrysler needed a dose of order and discipline—and quick.

Then there was the fact that Riccardo's secretary seemed to be spending a lot of time taking personal calls on her own private phone! When the secretaries are goofing off, you know the place has dry rot. During the first couple of weeks in a new job, you look for telltale signs. You want to know what kind of fraternity you've joined. These are the signs I remember, and what they told me

about Chrysler made me apprehensive about what I was getting myself into.

It turned out that my worries were justified. I soon stumbled upon my first major revelation: Chrysler didn't really function like a company at all. Chrysler in 1978 was like Italy in the 1860's—the company consisted of a cluster of little duchies, each one run by a prima donna. It was a bunch of mini-empires, with nobody giving a damn about what anyone else was doing.

What I found at Chrysler were thirty-five vice-presidents, each with his own turf. There was no real committee setup, no cement in the organizational chart, no system of meetings to get people talking to each other. I couldn't believe, for example, that the guy running the engineering department wasn't in constant touch with his counterpart in manufacturing. But that's how it was. Everybody worked independently. I took one look at that system and I almost threw up. That's when I knew I was in really deep trouble . . .

There was so much to do and so little time! I had to eliminate the thirty-five little duchies. I had to bring some cohesion and unity into the company. I had to get rid of the many people who didn't know what they were doing. I had to replace them by finding guys with experience who could move fast. And I had to install a system of financial controls as quickly as possible.

These problems were urgent and their solutions all pointed in the same direction. I needed a good team of experienced people who could work with me in turning this company around before it completely fell apart. My highest priority was to put that team together before it was too late . . .

Fortunately, the cancer at Chrysler did not reach all the way down. Although I had to replace almost all the officers, there was plenty of dynamic young talent beneath them. As we started getting rid of the less competent people, it was a lot easier to find the good ones. To this day, I can't believe that the former management didn't notice them.

I'm talking about people with fire in their eyes; you can practically tell they're good just by looking at them . . .

One of the luxuries we had to eliminate was a large staff. Ever since Alfred P. Sloan took over the presidency of General Motors, all management functions in our industry have been divided into staff and line positions—just like the Army. Line guys are in operations. They have hands on involvement and specific responsibilities, whether it's in engineering, manufacturing, or purchasing . . .

With all the firings, we ended up stripping out several levels of management. We cut down the number of people who needed to be involved in important decisions. Initially we did it out of the sheer necessity to survive. But over time we found that running a large company with fewer people actually made things easier. With hindsight it's clear that Chrysler had been top-heavy, far beyond what was good for us. That's a lesson our competitors have yet to learn—and I hope they never do!

SOURCE: From IACOCCA: AN AUTOBIOGRAPHY by Lee Iacocca with William Novak. Copyright © 1984 by Lee Iacocca. Used by permission of Bantam Books, a division of Bantam Doubleday Dell Publishing Groups, Inc.

is not the case, however, with the managerial strategist conception, built on the notions of organizational power and politics. While individual skills and personality can affect the amount of influence a manager has, "power is first and foremost a structural phenomenon, and should be understood as such."[7] Large, complex organizations often contain multiple influential decision makers, who have their own interests, values, and goals that often, perhaps inevitably, conflict. In such organizations, goals and objectives are defined by a process of continuous bargaining among changing coalitions of these decision makers.[8] Further, these coalitions have different degrees of influence and power in different situations and on different issues. This formulation seems especially applicable in professional organizations in which various professional groups work in their own directions, seeking to implement

their own professional values.[9] To the extent that organizational and professional goals are integrated, such *integration* occurs among conditions of diverse values and competing interests only as a result of a political process.[10] Power to influence policy tends to be diffused, and the locus and balance of power often shift in response to different issues and as different persons and groups move through the organization. In such settings managers must deal with separate interest groups, each with its own basis of power. However, not all groups are created equal, and some will be more powerful than others. Thus, managers must understand the sources of power (including that of managers) and the circumstances under which power might be used, withheld, or transferred. Managers in complex organizations are seen as "superb politicians" and "power brokers," understanding their own internal and external bases of power as well as those of others, anticipating the demands of and likely coalitions among competing groups, and developing negotiating and bargaining *strategies* to balance conflicting interests.

Organizational Conception

The organizational conception produces a different and more complex view of the manager by taking into account factors both within the organization and its environment and considering their respective effects. This view, which takes an open system perspective, involves three levels of the organization—technical, managerial, and institutional.[11] The technical level is concerned with activities that produce the organization's outputs; that is, where the work gets done. The managerial level administers the technical level, secures the needed resources for the organization, and finds customers for the products or services. The institutional level represents that portion of the environment from which the organization must secure its resources, its markets, and its legitimacy. In this context, the manager stands at the intersection of the internal (technical) and external (institutional) levels and is faced with the sometimes conflicting requirements and demands that arise from within and without the organization.

Organizations may be viewed as having several subsystems of activities necessary to their organizational survival.[12] The production system involves those activities that produce the products or services of the organization, emphasizing technical proficiency and efficient production methods. The supportive system aids the production system by securing necessary resources, allocating resources, and disposing of the organization's outputs. The maintenance system centers on the human organization and is focused on maintaining stability and predictability of behavior among individuals and groups. Activities include selection of personnel, socialization practices, and reward and sanction mechanisms. The adaptive system faces outward, focusing on the organization's ability to adapt to its environment. Through such functions as market research, research and development, and planning, this system seeks to understand the environment and translate the meaning of environmental changes to the organization. Katz and Kahn's fifth subsystem, the managerial, may

be seen as overarching, attempting to coordinate and direct the other subsystems, resolve conflicts between levels, and mediate external demands with organizational resources.

This organizational conception is the most comprehensive of the historical alternatives, transcending both organizational and environmental domains. Given the growing complexity of organizations and the continuing turbulence of the *external environment,* this broad formulation would appear to portend new challenges for the role of the manager. Interestingly, the reflections in the Connors interview are consistent with this broader view of the managerial role.

NEW MANAGERIAL CHALLENGES

As we have seen, conceptions of the managerial role have evolved over time. This evolution will continue as organizations and the environments within which they operate change, thereby affecting the role of the health care manager.

Looking first to the environment, it is clear that the American public has lost confidence in the U.S. health care system. Health care is no longer seen as a public service, but rather health care institutions are viewed as pursuing their own private interests. A national survey reports that almost 90% of the respondents think that the health care system needs fundamental change or complete rebuilding and is considered to be too expensive, uncoordinated, and fragmented.[13] Access to care remains a major issue, with approximately 37 million Americans uninsured or underinsured. This figure has grown by 25% since the early 1980s. Further, of the uninsured or underinsured, 75% are employed or are the dependents of those who are employed, a bitter irony in a country in which the health insurance system has evolved largely around the workplace.

The cost of health care remains the predominant issue. Health care costs have continued to rise, largely unabated, despite a variety of regulatory and competitive alternatives put forth in attempts to stem the tide. Yet health care now accounts for over 13% of the gross domestic product and costs continue to increase at double-digit rates. These facts are obviously of great concern to government, insurers, consumers, and employers. For example, to the extent that health insurance premiums raise the prices of American products

DEBATE TIME 2.1: WHAT DO YOU THINK?

Contrary to what we would like to believe, the manager's personal values and views about what would be best for the organization don't count for much in day-to-day organizational life. This is because management is essentially a political process. The manager's role is to balance (some would say juggle) the many, often contradictory, pressures on the organization from external and internal stakeholders, some of which may be groups or organizations. Each stakeholder has something the organization needs—whether dollars, patients, regulatory approvals, a willingness to work for the organization, or whatever. This enables stakeholders to make demands on organizations that further their own self-interest. Often, these demands are conflicting. For example, physicians may want a hospital to purchase the latest equipment for them to use in treating their patients while purchasers want the hospital to cut its costs. Some stakeholders have a lot of power to press for their agendas; others have less. Those that the organization needs the most and those with the most power tend to get more of what they want. The manager has little choice but to respond to these pressures. Skillful managers try to orchestrate the diverse demands so as to accommodate as many as possible while maintaining a reasonable degree of harmony within the organization. This is fundamentally a matter of accommodation and compromise, although a consensus can sometimes be found. The manager's role is essentially political—a broker of power. The manager's job is to balance the competing pressures to maintain harmony in the organization. A manager's own goals and values may have little to do with it.

and impede the ability of U.S. firms to compete in international markets, American industry will continue to focus attention on the cost of health care. It is especially within the context of cost that we witness the shift in power from the provider to the purchaser sector. Changes in payment systems have sought to alter the incentives to and the behavior of health care organizations and professionals.

Attendant to the cost issue is concern about the quality of care. There remains great variation in treatment patterns and limited understanding of the relationships among practice patterns, processes of care, and clinical outcomes. Significant effort is being expended to develop clinical guidelines and protocols and to establish mechanisms for assessing effectiveness and efficacy. It has also become clear that the definition and measurement of quality is no longer the exclusive domain of professionals and professional organizations. Rather, those who use and pay for care and services will insist that their voices be heard and that they participate in the definition and measurement processes.

The profound issues of access, cost, and quality, and the accompanying demands for greater *accountability,* are largely instrumental in the evolving reforms of the U.S. health care system. There are, however, other issues which add to the turbulence and uncertainty of the external environment. For example, changing demographics, notably the aging of the population, bring new and different demands for service and exemplify the need for a shift from acute to chronic care. Epidemiological changes, changes in the composition of the work force, and continuing technological imperatives likewise contribute to shifting external dynamics. Structural changes within the health care industry—the shift from inpatient to outpatient care, expansion of managed care, changing demographics of the medical profession, growth of group practice—also contribute to a new and different environment for health care organizations and their managers.

At the same time, important changes within health care organizations are occurring. For example, structural reconfigurations have resulted in larger, more complex, and often multiunit organizations such as hospital systems. Hospital systems now account for almost 50% of all nonfederal community hospitals.[14] These organizations present an array of issues including resource allocation, decision-making processes, domains of authority and responsibility, coordination and communication, balance between integration and differentiation, to name but some. Other forms of increasingly prevalent *interorganizational relationships* and arrangements, such as strategic alliances and joint ventures, add to organizational complexity.[15] As organizations seek to adapt to a changing environment characterized by constraints and limits, new strategies are emerging, many of which call for different relationships between the organization and key professionals such as physicians. The ability to effectively develop, implement, and sustain such new relationships will be crucial to organizational and professional success. At the same time, an array of occupational groups seek to define their domains of activity relative to one another, leading to tension and often conflict. These combinations of relationships will also result in redistribution of power within health care organizations.

The combination of environmental and organizational changes, briefly noted here and more fully considered in Chapter 1, present new opportunities, conflicts, and challenges for managers of health care organizations. As will be discussed in the following sections, the managers of the future will be faced with an often bewildering array of demands and pressures to adapt to a turbulent, often hostile, external world while seeking to maintain internally those structures and processes designed to ensure achievement of the organization's purposes consistent with its underlying values.

NEW ROLES FOR MANAGERS

The preceding sections demonstrated how our understanding of organizations, the environments within which they operate, and the roles of managers have changed over time. Our early conceptions of organizations and managers were developed in the context of a relatively stable and placid environment. Thus, the environment as an influence on organizations was given rather little attention in what was essentially a closed system view of organizational dynamics with emphasis on the internal workings. The role of the manager was, in turn, bounded by the "walls" of the organization. This is clearly exemplified in the traditional conceptions of the managerial role, which focused on planning, organizing, staffing, directing, and controlling, or in the case of the human relations approach, on ensuring that workers were satisfied and happy and that internal processes were free of strain and conflict. Increasingly, it was recognized that managers and their organizations interact with their environment, thereby challenging the traditional view of the managerial role.[16-18] It is clear that a broader view

DEBATE TIME 2.2: WHAT DO YOU THINK?

Although we like to think of the top managers of a health care organization as master strategists who envision and lead their organizations to a new and better future, in reality that view of the management role greatly overstates the case. This is because most of what health care organizations do or become is determined not by management but by fundamental external forces and trends. The aging of the population, advances in technology, or changing societal expectations are such fundamental and pervasive forces that health care organizations cannot realistically envision or strategize direction or roles that are inconsistent with them—at least not if they want to survive. The same can be said of other external forces, such as tightening reimbursement, the growth of managed care, and the shift to outpatient settings. At most, organizations have a little "wiggle room" in how they adapt to these forces, but adapt they must. Hence, it is more accurate and realistic to take a more limited view of what managers really contribute than what the "experts" and the literature suggest. This more limited view is consistent with some theories that recognize that organizations are open to (i.e., not able to buffer themselves from) external forces and are subject to significant influence from outside, whether they like it or not. This is certainly the case with health care organizations, and so their future is largely determined by the changing environment, not by how they are managed.

must take into account the responsibilities of managers within the organizations, that is, having to do with the workings, operations, processes, and structures of organizations, as well as consider the dynamics of the two-way interplay between organizations and environments.

These ideas suggest that managers of the 90s and beyond, and certainly managers of health care organizations, will need to manage organizations in new ways and focus attention on the external environment and its relation to the organization while attending simultaneously to the internal needs as well. To try to capture the implications of these new organizational directions for managers, we will consider the managerial role as a "trinity," requiring managers to serve as designers, as strategists, and as leaders, as shown in Figure 2.1.* It is intended that this formulation be pervasive, cutting across different types of organizations as well as being applicable to different levels of organizations. However, the degree of emphasis on the three dimensions of the trinity may vary as a function of such factors as the stage of an organization's development, its location within its life cycle, or the nature of the environment in which it operates. For purposes of illustration, many of the examples will draw from senior level managers but are presumed to be generally applicable at other levels as well. We also concur with Mintzberg that the managerial role need not be conceived as being housed within the person of a single individual; rather, the role represents a gestalt involving a number of people who must be integrated in order to result in the full explication of the role.[19]

As designer, the manager must attend to the structure and internal operations of the organization. As strategist, the manager is concerned with the *adaptation* of the organization to its environment. As leader, the manager seeks to provide vision and strategic direction to the organization. In the sections to follow, we will examine these three dimensions of the managerial role, provide illustrations of the responsibilities and realities facing managers and the organizations they serve, and consider the implications of the emerging new roles.

* This material is adapted from Zuckerman HS. Redefining the role of the CEO: challenges and conflicts. *Hospital & Health Services Administration.* Spring 1989;34:25–38.

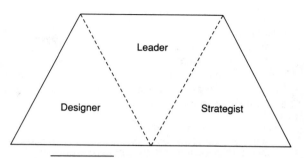

FIGURE 2.1. Trinity of managerial roles.

The Manager as Designer

Organizations of the 90s and beyond will provide the manager as designer with many challenges. Managers must address such matters as *organizational structure, innovation and change,* managing the production functions, information systems, continuous quality improvement, managing human resources, and changing roles of and relationships with professionals and governance.

In designing organizations for the future, structures must be flexible and adaptive. Organizations face operating environments characterized by increasing turbulence and instability. Consequently, these organizations must develop flexible internal designs that permit them to react to uncertain environmental conditions.[20] Demands from the external environment, coupled with internal needs of the organization, will require that there be a balance of integration and differentiation in the design. Health care organizations must strike a balance among facilitating achievement of overall goals, enhancing coordination, and taking advantage of organizational synergies and economies (integration) while encouraging innovation and creativity and enabling rapid response to environmental changes (differentiation). These issues are discussed further in Chapters 7, 8, 10, and 12.

Managing the production functions will continue to be a major focus for managers of health care organizations. For example, the issue of cost will continue to command managerial attention. As indicated earlier, external forces will undoubtedly press health care organizations on the matter of controlling the rate of increase in costs. Regardless of the eventual direction of health care reform and changes in the system of financing, managing costs will be fundamental in a competitive environment, in a regulated price structure, or under capitated systems. Managers will further explore means to increase productivity, reduce excess capacity, and improve utilization of physical, financial, and human resources.

> In an international competitive marketplace, the requirements for a change and for improvement are almost astronomical and it's easy in healthcare to be a little bit—to feel a little bit—removed from that by saying, "Well, we don't really compete with healthcare in the European market or Japan." But that's not true because we contribute. Regardless of whether we're directly competing in those markets or with those markets, we clearly contribute to the cost of American products in a world economy.[21]

Central to the design of organizations will be the development and management of information systems. Such systems will be crucial for effective management of costs and quality, for analysis of organizational performance, and for assessment and monitoring of environmental conditions. It will become increasingly important to integrate clinical and financial information and to shift emphasis to *health* records, consistent with the changing dimensions of organizational responsibility. The role of information technology in the organization and the requirements of the information systems fall appropriately within the domain of managers.[22] Thus defining information needs is a critical responsibility of those who will use the information, namely those in management positions.

Commitment to quality is a hallmark of successful organizations. An organization reflects such commitment by taking good care of its customers with superior products and exceptional service, by constantly innovating, and by developing its people through trust and respect for the creative potential of each person in the organization.[23] Recognizing the centrality of quality not only internally but also in terms of the perceptions and expectations of key external constituencies and stakeholders is leading health care organizations toward the principles of continuous quality improvement (CQI) and total quality management (TQM). These principles represent a paradigm shift from quality inspection and assurance to the continuous and relentless improvement of the processes of care provision

and not merely the improved actions of individuals.[24] Quality is defined as meeting the needs of customers, which requires broadly-based participation throughout the organization. Problems are characterized as typically systemic rather than individual, and changes to operating systems are based on data, use of multidisciplinary teams, and group processes. Health care organizations will come to reconceive the human resource function, seeing it as an investment not a cost. In so doing, there will be a fuller recognition of the importance of enabling individuals to realize their potential.

Within the organization, new roles, responsibilities, and relationships will emerge among managers, governance, and physicians. Those in governance are finding their roles to be more demanding and challenging. In the face of environmental turbulence and organizational complexity, trustees and directors find themselves dealing with conflicting pressures regarding social imperatives, public expectations, community need, cost control, quality improvement, financing, and technological development. As governance evolves, the requisite changes in roles, responsibilities, authorities, and relationships are not always clear. Effective boards will have to manage diverse stakeholders, involve physicians in the governance process, learn to govern emerging organizational forms such as integrated systems of care, and develop greater understanding of strategy formulation and implementation.[25] Boards must actively build assets, be willing to take risks, provide strategic direction for the organization, serve as mentors for management, and be prepared to be held accountable for the activities of the organization. These responsibilities will lead to revisiting such fundamental questions as board membership, structure, operating processes, and expectations.[26,27] In many ways, these expanding responsibilities and accountabilities parallel those of managers. Thus it is anticipated that these two groups will jointly examine such questions as, do we seek expertise or representation among governance members? how effective are our decision-making processes? are we sufficiently focused on achieving desired outcomes?

A critical challenge for managers lies in the effective integration of physician and organizational interests. This will require new models for physician-organization interrelationships, new thinking about such relationships, and greater involvement of physicians in governance and management of the enterprise. The imperatives of managing costs, improving quality, enhancing productivity and resource utilization, and designing strategies to enable health care organizations to adapt to their environments cannot be achieved without physician involvement. Physicians must play a key role in formulating policy, making decisions, allocating resources, and developing and implementing strategy. Certainly, the advent of managed care leads organizations and physicians to recognize that they must operate in common, sharing the risks and developing mechanisms to go into the marketplace together.[28] The destinies of physicians and organizations are inextricably intertwined and while relationships will assume various forms as they evolve, they must be nurtured and cultivated in order to deal with environmental and organizational imperatives.

There is already evidence of physicians playing larger roles in organizational governance and management.[29] In the face of increased competition for patients and market share, physicians see the growing importance of the managerial role and seek to be positioned to influence decision making about the delivery of care. This is accompanied by growing disillusion regarding the practice of management in the current economic and political environment and changing lifestyle concerns, particularly among younger physicians. The transition into management is not always easy for physicians. Management requires a tolerance for ambiguity, a long-term perspective, and deferred gratification, in some contrast to the perspective usually associated with medicine. Further, physician managers often face opposition both from physicians and from nonphysician managers. New knowledge and skills must also be developed to facilitate the transition and to enhance the likelihood that physician managers will be successful in their new roles.

The Manager as Strategist

Given the dramatic changes in the external environment described earlier, it is incumbent on managers to maintain a continuing outward look to identify and evaluate developments which may affect the organization. Signals from the environment must be monitored and analyzed, giving careful attention to the potential implications to the organization and its stakeholders.

In their role as strategists, managers must view the relationship between their organization and its environment as two-way; that is, managers seek not only to react to but also influence the environment. This point is of particular relevance in light of the move toward important reforms of the health care system. Managers serve as advocates of the organization, of the constituencies it represents, and of the population it serves.[30] As key members of what are fundamentally community service agencies designed to serve the public interest, managers of health services organizations should be involved in the formulation and implementation of public policy.[31] They have a responsibility, therefore, to actively participate in such policy decisions as they affect the public interest.

In observing and assessing the environment, managers will expand their field of vision to put health care in a larger context. That is, while health care has many unique attributes, it is also true that there are similarities and commonalities with other industries.[32] In fact, other industries that share structural, strategic, and service characteristics have undergone transformations not unlike that being experienced by health care. Managers will draw from the lessons, both positive and negative, to be learned from the experience of such other industries. For example, it is instructive to observe the structural and strategic changes in industries such as airlines and banking as they sought to adapt to changing environmental conditions. Structural changes included new entrants, mergers, and consolidations, while strategic shifts involved greater emphasis on cost accounting and cost management, investment in information system development, and use of networking and strategic alliances. In addition, health care managers will employ a variety of techniques, such as scenario analysis, to assess the environment under differing conditions and will seek to understand the organizational implications of alternative strategies.

". . . scenarios are a tool to do a variety of things. One is to get you to think: Do you agree or don't you agree with these? Are there others that you think are more likely? The scenarios summarize the best thinking of a core of leading health futurists in the U.S., and in effect we may be wrong. On the other hand, this may be an accurate portrayal of a good range of scenarios to think about. Either way it's important for healthcare managers, healthcare executives to have a sense of what are the threats and opportunities, so we can ask ourselves: What do I want to create?[33]

Health care managers will employ a variety of strategies in light of changing environmental forces. Horizontal integration, or linking organizations at the same stage of the production process (e.g., hospital-hospital), to achieve economies of scale, improve utilization of resources, enhance access to capital, increase political power, and extend the scope of the market will continue. Vertical integration, or linking organizations at related stages of the production process, to ensure sources of supply and markets for services and products will expand. Vertical integration enables organizations to move toward providing multiple levels of care and a more comprehensive range of services. Yet a third alternative involves diversified activities which may or may not be related to health care. Diversification, which may focus on new products or services, new production technologies, or entry into new markets, seeks to generate new sources of revenue and provide opportunities for growth and expansion.[34] Regardless of which strategy or combination of strategies is selected, adaptation to a changing environment requires a shift away from a product orientation to a market orientation. Strategic managers must seek to understand the characteristics, needs, and demands of the various populations which the organization serves. Market research will play a prominent role in answering such questions and providing the bases on which programs, services, and products can then be developed and marketed.

A key strategic opportunity and challenge for managers will be the emergence of integrated systems for delivering and financing health care services. As suggested by a growing number of industry observers, such systems are likely to be local or regional, based on market areas, and serving a defined population. Emphasis will be placed on health care and not only medical care. These systems will be integrated vertically as well as horizontally and clinically as well as administratively. They will be "seamless," designed to enable entry at multiple and convenient points. These systems will offer multiple levels of care across a connected continuum of services, enabling the movement of patients up and down the production process to the most appropriate placement both clinically and financially. Financing and delivery will be linked, an important factor in positioning organizations for the advent of managed care. Governance and management structures, as well as resource allocation decision processes, will reflect the focus on the regional system. Physicians will be key, integral participants in such systems, sharing the risk and the power inherent in such organizations. Information systems will receive substantial attention and be designed to reflect the emphasis on health, be organized around episodes, and to move across the component units of the organization. Operationally, integrated systems will emphasize continuous quality improvement, development of human resources across the system, and effective management of cost and utilization. There will thus be a unity, symmetry, and synergy in the strategy, structure, and operations of such systems. These integrated organizations will not merely be *structured* as systems, but rather will *function* as systems, thereby building the potential to achieve the benefits of "systemness" as described by Shortell.[35] Importantly, such systems should be well situated for the new and broader accountabilities to be faced by organizations, which will include public accountability for the health status of the population served.

The Manager as Leader

As leader, the manager may well seek to transform the organization to meet the new realities of this decade and beyond. Despite the exigencies of external pressures and internal complexity, it will be incumbent on managers to retain a broad view, keep the long-term perspective in mind, and seek to add value to the organization over time. Managers play key roles in ensuring that members of the organization know, understand, and accept the core *values* of the organization. As keepers of the organization's values, managers must live the values of the organization, showing their relevance in decision making and integrating them into the organization's reward system.[36] The extent to which managerial decision making reflects the basic values of the organization is of fundamental importance to its long-term viability.[37,38] To have meaning, organizational behavior must be consistent with these values; saying so doesn't make it so.

Phrases such as "the customer comes first" has meaning only if customers are treated with respect and dignity. "We are a people-oriented company" has no meaning if people are treated as expendable. "We are a risk-taking, innovative company" has no meaning if the organization does not reward risk-taking and innovation.[39]

As underscored in the Connors interview, managers must lead in living the values of the organization, in being responsive to the needs of key stakeholders, and in enacting the *mission* of the organization. In a recent report entitled "Bridging the Leadership Gap in Healthcare," the *Healthcare Forum* concludes that, in order to transform health care, we must transform our leaders.[40] Believing that health care will be and should be significantly different in the twenty-first century, opinion leaders participating in the study called for a system characterized by greater emphasis on preven-

tion and healing; universal, cost-efficient, community-based managed care; and national health reform with a public-private partnership. Leaders of such a *transformation* will be called upon to redefine health care, focusing on healing, changing lifestyles, and the holistic interplay of mind, body, and spirit. Such leaders must develop a *shared,* collective *vision* of the future, fusing a social mission to the public and the community to organizational goals, objectives, and actions.

Wouldn't that be marvelous? I mean to keep people healthy, that's what we are supposed to be doing. And wouldn't it be marvelous if we were paid to do that rather than to do procedures, to fix a fender, to replace an engine. I think these are exciting times and I think the next ten years are going to be dramatic in terms of the direction that healthcare is going. We're talking about healing rather than curing. That's something remarkable isn't it?[41]

IN THE REAL WORLD:

A TIME FOR STRATEGY: MICHAEL BICE REORIENTS LUTHERAN HEALTH SYSTEMS

The genesis of the ongoing organizational transformation activity in Lutheran Health Systems can be traced to the summer of 1982. At the time, I was the System's chief operating officer and had arrived at several conclusions about the organization. I believed it had very significant potential, but it did not have either the will or the resources to be an effective long-term player. It had an organizational structure which was relatively unchanged for 30 years; an organizational overhaul was clearly called for. It had a strong historical culture which served primarily as a barrier to change. It was a "society of administrators" with a major norm of conformance. Finally, it was slow to react to environmental changes, and thus, was not perceived to be in the mainstream of healthcare . . .

I carefully sought out support from the young future leaders of the organization, many of whom were disgruntled with the old order. I recruited members of senior management from outside of the organization who were at least open to organizational change. Consultants—external auditors,

attorneys, and strategic planners—were used judiciously in an effort to lay the groundwork and present a case for large-scale cultural change. The "old guard" wasn't ignored. Rather, I sought out long-time employees who, while loyal to the organization, also were frankly concerned about where it was heading.

I then spent most of the next eighteen months building my knowledge base of corporate culture change and also selling the concept to our Board of Directors, Corporate Officers, field managers, and department heads. During this period of time, I made approximately 25 presentations on my assessment of the Society's culture. Support for organizational change grew and put me in an increasingly combative posture relative to the incumbent President. The matter came to a head in June of 1984, when I was promoted to the position of President and Chief Executive Officer. Upon reflection, the field generally supported this change, but still had no clear understanding of the implications of my program of organizational transformation . . .

In a rapidly changing healthcare environment, leverage to move the organization forward was not hard to find. In 1984, the introduction of a new Medicare payment system accelerated the decline in usage of many of our rural facilities, and we ended the year in poor financial shape. Eight facilities were earmarked for divestiture. The impact of changes in farming and energy have placed many of our communities in severe economic distress. Thus, changes in Federal healthcare payment, together with economic decline, have been used to convince field managers that they must change their behavior if they are to survive. Market, and not operational orientation, has been stressed as a pathway to the future . . .

It's clear that from this point forward, the field can make or break this effort. No amount of cajoling or negative incentives will lead to the widespread acceptance of this transformation. Rather, the field managers need to perceive this program as in their best interests as well as the corporation's. In fact, they should see it as representing an appropriate response to a rapidly changing environment. Fortunately, many do. The remainder will come on board, given time, and given a continuing commitment to the program by the senior management of the company.

Large-scale cultural change is an imposing undertaking and substantive change will not come about overnight. The chief executive officer must make a multiple year commitment to the effort. Enormous amount of time and travel are involved, and to the extent possible, the individual should embody the desirable attributes of the new culture. Continuing, personal, hands-on involvement is essential . . .

SOURCE: *Excerpted from Bice M. The organizational transformation of Lutheran Health Systems. in Kilman RH. Corporate Transformation. San Francisco, Ca: Jossey-Bass; 1988:435–450.*

We thus see the managerial role in three dimensions—designer, strategist, and leader. While treated separately, the implications of these developments in fact cut across the trinity, as we will see in the next section.

IMPLICATIONS OF NEW MANAGERIAL ROLES

Rosabeth Moss Kanter argues that new conceptions are required to understand the changing managerial role.[42] As organizations change to adapt to new internal and external pressures, many of the traditional tools of management—hierarchy, motivation, bases of power, and channels of communication—likewise must change. Indeed, she contends that such tools may no longer be effective. Rather, managers will have to reinvent their profession as they move into "postentrepreneurial organizations" to adapt to these new demands. Her formulation of organizations and the changing role of managers calls for the application of flexibility and creativity in order to achieve results. Kanter envisions organizations marked by a greater number and variety of channels for taking action or exerting influence and in which influence will shift from vertical to horizontal relationships. Such organizations are visualized as flexible clusters of activity rather than as rigid hierarchical and authoritative structures. This view is consistent with that offered by Drucker, who foresees a shift from control and chain of command models to peer networks and commitment models.[43] Likewise, the gap between the managers and the managed will shrink as control over information, assignments, and access to external relationships become more diffused. External relationships will become a greater source of internal power and influence, recognizing the growing link of organizations and environments. Environmental scanning and assessment will be important at multiple levels of the organization. Interestingly, career development will become less circumscribed as alternative

DEBATE TIME 2.3: WHAT DO YOU THINK?

It sounds good to talk about empowering others, sharing power, and "teaching people to lead themselves," in part because these ideas appeal to basic values that emphasize the inherent importance of each and every individual. But in the final analysis, the buck has to stop somewhere in organizations, and that's with top management. This is not to say that developing others in the organization and delegating or sharing decisions with them doesn't work. These can be extremely effective management tools in the right circumstances. But in reality, some subordinates just are not comfortable with more responsibility or don't have the skills to solve problems as well as the manager could. In addition, empowering multi-disciplinary, cross-organizational teams to grapple with problems, rather than referring them up the management hierarchy for solution, can be time consuming, creates confusion across departments, and obfuscates who is accountable for results. Perhaps most important, it must be remembered that in the real world not all the actors in an organization share the organization's goals, or, even if they do, the natural inclination to seek to further one's own interests through the organization may be more motivating. As a result, managers could delegate decision-making opportunities only to find the participants "running away with the store." Selective empowerment and carefully proscribed delegation can be effective tools. But organizations work best when top management retains final decision-making authority and everyone knows it and when the most critical or difficult decisions are not left in the hands of others all over the organization.

paths emerge, allowing for more innovation and opportunity.[44] Further, these new organizations will be characterized by motivation which relies less on traditional rewards such as promotion, raises, or bonuses based on individual performance and more on commitment to common vision, mechanisms for developing shared vision, value-adding activities, and importance of teams. Such organizations also will be characterized by commitment to learning and mentoring, to enhancing the role and value of individuals, and to increasing the contribution to the life of the organization.[45,46]

In these postentrepreneurial organizations, there will be shifts of power among and between managers and alteration of the types of power available. There will be greater reliance on influence without authority and less on authoritative power based on position in a hierarchy. Managers will recognize the necessity to juggle multiple constituencies and to negotiate, broker, bargain, and sell rather than make unilateral decisions. Success will depend heavily on networking, multiple sources and channels of information, and the ability to span traditional organizational boundaries.[47] Managers will be concerned with their ability to integrate, to facilitate, and to add value to the organization. As we consider these propositions, it becomes clear that the implications cut across the trinity of managerial roles. That is, as designer the manager must recognize the shift in the role of organizational structure and the need for greater flexibility. As strategist, the importance of external linkages and interorganizational dependencies become increasingly apparent but are, in turn, related to decision-making processes within the organization. As leader, the manager must ensure that the culture of the organization evolves so as to be consistent with the changing internal and external realities.

In the *Healthcare Forum* report cited earlier, managers of the future are called upon to transform their organizations.[48] In so doing, they will need to display, as individuals, a deep personal commitment coupled with the ability to align others with the vision of the organization. Such managers will challenge long-held assumptions, seek new pathways for learning, and craft the organization to promote creativity and participation.[49,50] In this context managerial strength lies "in the ability to maximize the contributions of others by helping them to effectively guide their own destinies, rather than the ability to bend the will of others to the leader's."[51] Leading others to lead themselves within organizations will be a particular challenge in health care organizations, where the commitment to one's profession often exceeds commitment to the organization.

> One of the old assumptions used to be that when you teach people to lead, that you teach them to lead other people. The challenge today in healthcare, and for many of our leaders, is just to manage themselves, to manage and lead themselves. And then from there, to truly let go and empower others so that their talents can come to the forefront.[52]

The concept of shared vision is a critical attribute of those who would seek to transform organizations. Shared vision answers the question, What do we want to create? Such a vision creates a sense of commonality, gives a coherence and connection to diverse activities, and establishes commitment and responsibility because it reflects the individual's personal vision, not merely a view handed down from the top. "Visions are powerless unless they are derived from and embraced by those individuals who will collectively achieve them."[53] Thus the transformational manager will foster the nurturing and creation of a shared vision for the organization and will seek to generate a certain amount of "creative tension" between the current reality and the idealized vision in order for people to be motivated to improve.[54] Such creative tension recognizes that "an accurate picture of current reality is just as important as a compelling picture of a desired future."[55] However, managers in their role as leaders must continuously strive to maintain the vision of a desired future. It is easy to become discouraged by the seeming difficulty of bringing the vision to reality. The demands of the day can lead people to lose sight of the vision and the connection of those within the organization seeking to achieve the vision. Thus managers must themselves believe in the vision and their ability to change current realities, for "vision becomes a living force only when people truly believe they can shape their future."[56]

> Visions are values projected into the future, so if you don't know what you stand for, what you believe in, it's very difficult to develop a compelling vision. A vision should be a very loud pronouncement of what's important to you. Leaders who are involved in helping to set and develop a vision need to have a very clear

sense of what their core values are and need to find a way to align those with the values of others.[57]

In addition to the individual and personal commitment of managers to the notion of shared vision, there is an organizational dimension which serves to promote the ability of the organization to learn faster than competitors. Indeed, this may be the only competitive advantage that counts in the future as "over the long run, superior performance depends on superior learning."[58] Such superior learning, however, cannot simply be "adaptive," that is, only focusing on coping with and responding to an organization's environment. Rather, learning must be "generative," seeing the world in terms of interrelated systems and seeking to create and influence the environment. Generative learning emphasizes continual experimentation and feedback as organizations examine themselves and the ways in which they make decisions and solve problems.

In building the social architecture of an organization, managers must design around the purpose, vision, and core values by which organizational members will live and ensure that policies, strategies, and structures are consistent to effectively guide the organization. A key element of the architecture is the creation of learning processes, such as scenario analysis and continuous quality improvement, that enable and encourage systems thinking, seeking to examine interrelationships, ongoing processes and patterns, and underlying causes of behavior. In so doing, organizations can become "learning laboratories," characterized by experiential learning, in which management teams learn to learn together.[59] "The ability of an organization or manager to learn is not measured by *what* the organization or manager knows (that is, the *product* of learning) but rather by *how* the organization or manager learns—the *process* of learning."[60] Thus, building *learning organizations* will require that managers discover how to tap into their organization's commitment and potential at all levels. Managers must develop individuals who see the organization as a system, who have a personal commitment to a shared vision, and who learn how to experiment and collaboratively reframe problems.

Health care managers also will be called upon to focus on the community and national agenda, playing a key role in developing innovative, long-term solutions for providing affordable health care to the public they serve. In so doing, the process requires rethinking the ways in which health care is viewed and accomplished. Such a rethinking argues that managers will be "responsible not only for the productive performance of the organization but must also consider the additional dimension of being a citizen of the community."[61] It suggests (as did Connors) that organizations will need to refocus attention on the health of the community served, not merely on delivery of medical care. Further, it presumes that health care organizations increasingly will be held accountable for the health status of the populations they serve.[62]

> Maybe what we need is more thought about how as a community we come together to create a better place to live. And I think that is an area where hospitals and healthcare also have a responsibility. I think with the competitive model that has been in place for the last eight years or longer, a lot of the good will toward hospitals and public institutions has evaporated. We are seen as competitive organizations, rather than as organizations whose roots are in nonprofit service.[63]

This broadening shift in thinking has profound implications for organizations and may briefly be illustrated in such areas as managing quality and cost, physician-organization relations, and development of integrated delivery systems. As applied to managing quality and cost, the acknowledgment that most problems are systemic suggests that there be a collective rather than an individual responsibility to fix such problems. Thus, multidisciplinary teams will become involved in addressing issues formerly seen as the exclusive domain of professionals. Clinical problem solving will require participation beyond clinicians. In so doing, historical understandings about professional and administrative roles, authority, autonomy, and accountability will be challenged and reconceptualized.[64] Such shifts will lead to modifications in organizational objectives and reward systems, with emphasis on process as well as outcomes, on longer time frames for change, on an orientation toward internal and external customers, and greater focus on participation, *empowerment,* and teams.[65]

> . . . What I particularly appreciate about the total quality improvement or continuous quality

improvement approach is it allows us to integrate those core values with our commitment to people and dignity, and gives us a framework within which to live. It pulls the values down off the wall, off the piece of paper, and gives us a framework to make them live. How we implement them in a daily way in the organization will be by focusing on continuous improvement, by focusing on empowering people, bringing them into the process, making the process owners part of it, and focusing on teams as a way of managing. All of these things come from those kinds of processes and it unleashed tremendous energy in the organization.[66]

As organizations, their managers, and physicians address the future, the acknowledgement of interdependencies, mutual interests, and shared values will be fundamental.[67] Effective physician-organization relationships have been shown in situations where there is a history of cooperation and collaboration, a desire to work together, and a recognition of their interdependent destinies.[68] Management stability was found to be important in establishing trust and confidence, as was a genuine respect for and liking of physicians by health care executives. Also identified as successful were those situations in which there was shared decision making with early physician involvement; an effort to manage change; a commitment to open, honest, and candid communication; and a willingness to admit mistakes and try alternative approaches to problems. Attempts were made to work together as business partners, using an array of structural mechanisms and support of physicians in practice management, information systems, and enhancement of their patient base. Perhaps the most distinguishing characteristic of effective relationships was the strength of physician leadership and commitment to leadership development programs—helping others to lead themselves. The many issues involving physicians and other health care professionals are further discussed in Chapter 9.

The development of integrated delivery systems represents another important challenge for the manager. In this development, key for the manager will be such concepts and approaches as integration, networking, alliances, *commitment versus control* models, interorganizational relationships, interdependence, and collaboration. For example, such systems presume that an organization's

MANAGERIAL GUIDELINES

1. Conceptualizations (models) of the management role help managers make sense of the complex reality in which they function. No one model provides all the answers; rather, different models offer different but useful insights about the context, ends, and functions of management.

2. Managers must consciously size up the amount and sources of power possessed by key individuals and groups in the organization and be aware of the agendas each is inclined to press for.

3. Based on an understanding of the power and agendas of the individuals likely to be affected by a decision under consideration, the manager needs to decide how these individuals should be involved and how to structure the decision-making process so that their views are balanced with other important perspectives.

4. Translating potential conflicts over desired outcomes into cooperation or collaboration requires that the manager search for common ground among the different interest groups.

5. Organizations need to adapt to the changes in their environment. They must also secure inputs from and sell outputs to external sources. Hence, effective management involves managing external interactions as well as "running a tight ship" internally.

6. The environment of health care organizations is increasingly complex, fast-changing, and demanding. Managers must design effective processes and structures for keeping up with external changes affecting the organization, determining their implications, and deciding how the organization should respond.

7. Building consensus, forming coalitions, and negotiating compromises are activities that are becoming more and more important for managers as the number of external and internal parties health care organizations must deal with increases.

8. The difficult issues health care organizations face today require involvement in decision making by representatives of governance, management, medical staff, and functional or program specialists. Hence, managers should design or find educational opportunities in which all of these parties can learn together as a team.

9. Managers should view the relationship between an organization and its environments as a two-way street. Each is able to influence the other to some extent. By actively managing external

ability to continuously improve the effectiveness of managing interdependence is the critical element in responding to new and pressing competitive forces. Unlike in previous eras, managerial strategies based on optimizing operations *within* functional departments, product lines, or geographical organizations simply will not be adequate in the future.[69]

Cutting across the managerial roles, these emerging interdependent organizations will lead to greater role complexity as managers must adjust rapidly and more frequently to new situations and cope with ambiguity and fluid structures and decision-making processes. It will often be the case that these systems are not owned or controlled by any one organization; rather multiple players will be involved and bound together because of commitment to a unifying vision and common values, as well as exigencies of the marketplace.[70] In such interdependent systems and networks of organizations, there must be managerial commitment to sharing power and sharing risk. Lateral communications, relationships built on trust and respect, extensive sharing of information, joint decision making, and clarity in purpose and expectations will characterize these collaborative efforts.[71] As noted earlier, managers in these organizations will thus balance constituencies rather than control subordinates.

Many of us view the 1980's as the decade of the deal. I think the 90's will be a decade of collaboration, and the reason I say that is I think the pressure caused by

---

MANAGERIAL GUIDELINES

relations, managers should try to make the environment more favorable or moderate external pressures on the organization.

10. Managers must see to it that the organization's data collection capabilities and information systems encompass external as well as internal information and enable integration of data on demographics, the market, costs, utilization, and quality.

11. Articulation and communication of the mission and values of the organization and a clear sense of direction are critical management responsibilities. Equally important is assessing which parties are "on board" and which do not fully accept the organization's direction.

12. Managers should consciously model and act in concert with the values they seek to develop in the organization. Behavior by others consistent with these values should be encouraged and recognized.

13. Managerial training and leadership development should encompass both opportunities to learn about trends and issues in health care and opportunities to strengthen management skills, especially skills that enhance the facilitation of effective interactive processes.

14. Managers should establish forums in their organizations where the management team can discuss new concepts of management and the beliefs and values that underlie these conceptualizations.

15. Managers must understand and then act on the knowledge that power or the ability to get things done in the organization of the future will come more from empowering, inspiring, and supporting others and from teamwork and not so much from the manager's own authority or decision making. Through the sharing of power, the manager's effectiveness will be enhanced.

16. To inspire and motivate, the organization's mission or vision must be compelling in two respects: it must clearly demonstrate a fit between the organization's directions and external demands such that the organization is positioned to be successful, and the mission must be seen as worthwhile in the sense of being based on worthy values.

17. Managers must establish a culture, processes, and structures that help the organization become a learning organization, constantly striving to reexamine old assumptions and old ways of doing things.

---

the availability of capital, the pressure to reduce capacity and the pressure to return to a community-focused healthcare system is going to require that organizations that may have competed with each other in the 80's and the 90's are going to have to find ways to work together.[72]

NEW SKILLS AND KNOWLEDGE FOR MANAGERS

As this chapter has suggested, health care managers of the 90s and beyond will be obliged to manage organizations in new ways, focusing attention on the external environment and its relation to the organization while attending to the organization's internal needs and providing vision and strategic direction. To meet these evolving obligations, the managerial role has been cast as a trinity of designer, strategist, and leader. A review of the content of these emerging roles and consideration of their implications make clear that managers will need to develop new skills and knowledge to effectively meet their responsibilities. The *Healthcare Forum* referenced earlier spoke of "transformational competencies" which would be needed to bridge the leadership gap in order to guide health care organizations toward the future.[73] A recent report by the Pew Health Professions Commission emphasized many of the emerging trends in health care which have been discussed in this chapter and in Chapter 1 and suggested that several new competencies would be required of health care managers. The report suggested that integrated networks for the organization and delivery of care, an orientation toward health and wellness, increasingly constrained resources, a stronger customer focus, information-driven decisions and actions, and attention to both patient and system outcomes will characterize the health care system.[74]

Managers must learn to facilitate the process of change, remaining flexible in responding and adapting to an ambiguous and unstable environment. Change must be seen as a mechanism for new opportunities and calculated risk taking. Managers in this new environment must be skilled in team building, group processes, participative decision making, conflict management, negotiation, communications, and coalition building. A networking perspective will be necessary as managers seek integration of organizations and clinical professionals. This will require systems thinking, the ability to understand interrelationships and patterns in solving complex problems. Managers of the 90s and beyond will need to understand and be involved in interorganizational relationships and dynamics, power bases and structures, and the policy and political process. Demands for accountability and *performance* will require managers to be familiar with concepts and techniques of epidemiology, statistics, health status, and outcomes. Mastery of information systems and technology will be pivotal. Managers will be obliged to understand and practice the principles of continuous quality improvement, maintaining a "never-satisfied atti-tude," and learn to provide mechanisms to support ongoing processes to improve clinical and service outcomes. Sensitivity to the relationship between cost and quality will call for managers to be adept at budgeting, resource management, managing within limits and constraints, and formulating downsizing strategies. Problem-solving skills likewise will be critical. Managers will need to become more conversant with health services management research and its utilization in assessment, evaluation, and decision making. Emphasis will be placed on the manager as innovator, able to provide the transformational leadership and create the collective and shared vision of the future necessary to move the organization in new directions. In so doing, transformational managers must be able and willing to redefine health care in broad terms and be cognizant of their organization's responsibility to the public and community served.

The role of the health care manager in the 90s and beyond will be complex, multidimensional, and demanding. But it also will be exciting and rewarding, offering opportunities to serve both public and organizational interests while seeking to balance the value orientations of "mission and margin." As suggested by McNerney,

There is more to management than crisp efficiency. In the health field, perhaps more than in any other, management involves moral issues and ethical choices. It involves deep commitment and personal courage. It involves a resolve to be just and right, not only a resolve to win.[75]

KEY CONCEPTS

Accountability
Adaptation
Commitment versus Control
Empowerment
External Environment
Innovation and Change
Integration
Interorganizational Relationships
Leadership
Learning Organization
Organizational Structure
Performance
Power
Shared Vision
Strategy
Transformation
Values and Mission

Discussion Questions

1. Managers generally respond to the question, What do you do? in one of several ways. They may describe their work in terms of generic management functions, the activities or tasks they perform, the ends they seek to achieve, the issues or problems they deal with, or the knowledge and skills they use. Think of several examples pertinent to health services organizations of each way of describing what managers do.

2. Adapting an organization to its environment, articulating and gaining support for a strategic vision and values, and designing the internal structures of the organization are key management roles in health services organizations. Is each role equally important? What determines this? What knowledge and skills do you think are most helpful in carrying out each of these three roles?

3. How important is it for a manager to be proficient in every aspect of management? Can you think of managers who are particularly competent in some areas but not in others? What do you see as your greatest strengths? Weaknesses? How can managers compensate for areas they are not particularly proficient in?

4. Assume that you are the chief executive officer of a large urban health system that is struggling for its survival in the face of increasing local competition involving managed care pressures. What role should physicians play in deciding what strategies to pursue? How do you as the leader of the organization facilitate their involvement? What role would other actors play? What are some of the alternative strategies that you might pursue? How are the strategic alternatives facing large urban health systems likely to differ from those encountered by smaller suburban health systems?

REFERENCES

1. Fayol H. *General and Industrial Administration.* New York, NY: Pitman; 1949.
2. Taylor FW. *The Principles of Scientific Management.* New York, NY: Harper & Brothers; 1911.
3. McGregor DA. *The Human Side of Enterprise.* New York, NY: McGraw-Hill; 1960.
4. Likert R. *The Human Organization: Its Management and Value.* New York, NY: McGraw-Hill, 1967.
5. Zaleznick A. Managers and leaders: are they different? *Harvard Business Review.* 1977;55(3):67–78.
6. Ibid.
7. Pfeffer J. *Power in Organizations.* Marshfield, Mass: Pitman; 1981.
8. Cyert RM, March JG. A behavioral theory of organizational objectives. In: Haire M, ed. *Modern Organizational Theory.* New York, NY: John Wiley & Sons; 1959.
9. Bucher R, Stelling JG. *Becoming Professional, XLVI.* Beverly Hills, Ca.: Sage Library of Social Research; 1977.
10. Mintzberg H. *Mintzberg on Management.* New York, NY: Free Press; 1989.
11. Parsons T. *Structure and Process in Modern Society.* New York, NY: Free Press; 1960.
12. Katz D, Kahn R. *The Social Psychology of Organizations.* 2nd ed. New York, NY: John Wiley & Sons; 1978.
13. Blendon RJ, Edwards JN, Hyams AL. Making the critical choices. *Journal of the American Medical Association.* 1992; 267:2509–2520.
14. American Hospital Association. *Annual Guide Issue.* Chicago: The Association, 1991.
15. Zuckerman HS, D'Aunno TA. Hospital alliances: Cooperative strategy in a competitive environment. *Health Care Management Review.* Spring 1990; 15:21–30.
16. Parsons, op. cit.
17. Katz, Kahn, op. cit.
18. Mintzberg, op. cit.
19. Mintzberg H. *The Nature of Managerial Work.* Englewood Cliffs, N.J.: Prentice-Hall; 1973.
20. Lewis P, Fandt PM. Organizational design: Implications for managerial decision-making. *SAM Advanced Management Journal.* Autumn 1989:13–16.
21. *Bridging the Leadership Gap in Healthcare.* Healthcare Forum Leadership Center; 1991.
22. Marting WE, Dehays DW, Hoffer JA, Perkins WC. *Managing Information Technology: What Managers Need to Know.* New York, NY: Macmillan Publishing Co; 1991.
23. Darling JR. Total quality management: The key role of leadership strategies. *Leadership and Organizational Development Journal,* 1992;134:3–7.
24. McLaughlin CT, Kaluzny AD. Total quality management in health: Making it work. *Health Care Management Review.* Summer 1990;15:7–14
25. Shortell SM. New directions in hospital governance. *Hospital and Health Services Administration.* Spring 1989;34:7–23.
26. Kovner A. Improving hospital board effectiveness: An update. *Frontiers of Health Services Management.* Spring 1990:3–27.
27. Umbdenstock R, Hageman W, Amundson B. The five critical areas for effective governance of not-for-profit hospitals. *Hospital and Health Services Administration.* Winter 1990; 35:481–492.
28. Haggland MM. Compensation, social trends alter hospital-MD relations. *Hospitals.* November 1991;65:20–25.
29. Nash DB. Hospitals and their medical staffs: High anxiety. *Frontiers of Health Services Management.* Spring 1988;4:24–26.
30. Zuckerman HS. Redefining the role of the CEO: Challenges and conflicts. *Hospital and Health Services.* Spring 1989; 34:1 25–38.
31. Vladeck BC. Health, health care executives, and their communities. *Hospital and Health Services Administration.* September/October 1986;31:7–15.
32. Zuckerman, op. cit.
33. *Bridging the Leadership Gap,* op. cit.
34. Clement JP. Vertical integration and diversification of acute care hospitals: Conceptual definitions. *Hospital and Health Services Administration,* Spring 1988;33:99–110.
35. Shortell SM. The evolution of hospitals systems: Unfulfilled promises and self-fulfilling prophesies. *Medical Care Review.* Fall 1988;45:177–213.
36. Rossy GL. The executive's role in ethics: The view from business and industry. *Healthcare Executive.* September-October 1987;2:17–21.
37. Bice MO. Corporate cultures and business strategy: A health management company perspective. *Hospital and Health Services Administration.* September-October 1984;31:7–15.
38. Kaluzny AD, Shortell SM. Creating and managing our ethical future. *Healthcare Executive.* September-October 1987;2:29–32.
39. Zuckerman, op. cit.
40. *Bridging the Leadership Gap,* op. cit.
41. Ibid.
42. Kanter RM. The new managerial work. *Harvard Business Review.* November-December 1989;89: 85–92.
43. Drucker PD. The coming of the new organization. *Harvard Business Review,* January-February 1988;88:45–53.

44. Kanter, op. cit.
45. Drucker, op. cit.
46. Senge PM. *The Fifth Discipline.* New York, NY: Doubleday; 1990.
47. Kanter, op. cit.
48. *Bridging the Leadership Gap,* op. cit.
49. Bass BM. From transactional to transformational leadership: Learning to share the vision. *Organizational Dynamics.* Winter 1990;18:19–31.
50. Matey DB. Significance of transactional and transformational leadership theory on the hospital manager. *Hospital and Health Services Administration.* Winter 1991;36:600–605.
51. Manz CC, Sims HP, Jr. *SuperLeadership.* New York, NY: Berkley Books; 1990.
52. *Bridging the Leadership Gap,* op. cit.
53. Stata R. The role of the chief executive officer in articulating the vision. *Interfaces.* May-June 1988;18:3–9.
54. Bryson JM. *Strategic Planning for Public and Nonprofit Organizations.* San Francisco, CA: Jossey-Bass; 1990.
55. Senge, op. cit.
56. Ibid.
57. *Bridging the Leadership Gap,* op. cit.
58. Senge, op. cit.
59. Ibid.
60. McGill ME, Slocum JW, Lei D. Management practices in learning organizations. *Organizational Dynamics.* Summer 1992;21:4–17.
61. Miller I. Executive leadership, community action, and the habits of health care politics. *Health Care Management Review.* Winter 1992;17:81–84.
62. Shortell SM, McNerney WJ. Criteria and guidelines for reforming the U.S. healthcare system. *New England Journal of Medicine.* 1990;322:463–467.
63. *Bridging the Leadership Gap,* op. cit.
64. McLaughlin, Kaluzny, op. cit.
65. Kaluzny AD. Revitalizing decision making at the middle management level. *Hospital and Health Services Administration.* Spring 1989;34:39–51.
66. *Bridging the Leadership Gap,* op. cit.
67. Derzon RA. The odd couple in distress: Hospitals and physicians face the 1990's. *Frontiers of Health Services Management.* Spring 1988;4:4–19.
68. Shortell SM. *Effective Hospital-Physician Relationships.* Ann Arbor, Mi: Health Adminstration Press; 1991.
69. Rockart JF, Short JE. IT in the 1990s: Managing organizational interdependence. *Sloan Management Review.* Winter 1989:7–17.
70. Drucker, op. cit.
71. Zuckerman HS, Kaluzny AD. Strategic alliances in health care: The challenges of cooperation. *Frontiers of Health Services Management.* Spring 1991:3–24.
72. *Bridging the Leadership Gap,* op. cit.
73. Ibid.
74. Health professions education: Schools in service to the nation. *Report of the Pew Health Professions Commissions.* September 1992:53–67.
75. McNerney WJ. Managing ethical dilemmas. *Journal of Health Administration Education.* Summer 1985;3:331–340.

THE NATURE OF ORGANIZATIONS: FRAMEWORK FOR THE TEXT

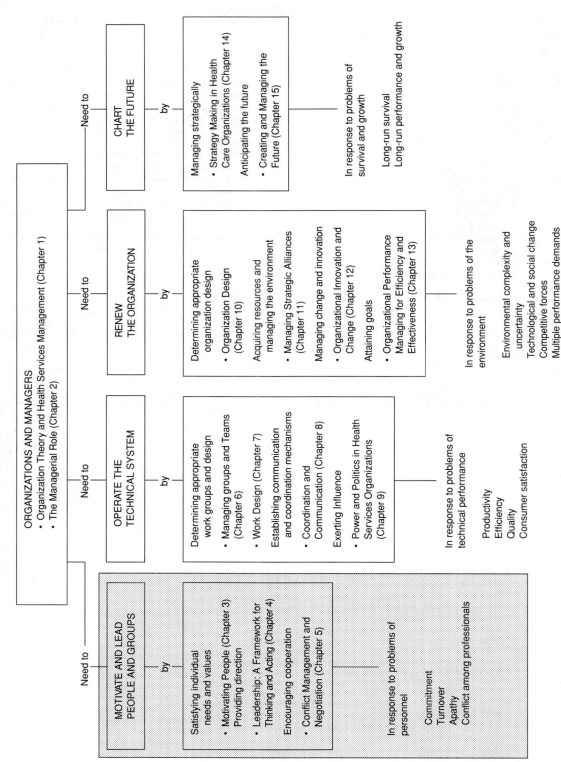

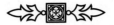

PART TWO

MOTIVATING, LEADING, AND NEGOTIATING

Chapters 3–5 deal with fundamental issues related to motivation, leadership, and negotiation. These processes are fundamental building blocks for working effectively with individuals and groups. Understanding multiple sources of motivation, different approaches to leadership, and various ways of managing conflict and negotiations are key determinants of successful managerial performance.

Chapter 3, Motivating People, focuses on a variety of issues related to motivation. The chapter addresses the following questions:

- What are some of the common myths associated with motivating people?
- What are the major content and process approaches to understanding motivation?
- What are some of the more effective ways of dealing with motivational problems?

The chapter emphasizes multiple approaches for dealing with motivational issues.

Chapter 4, Leadership: A Framework for Thinking and Acting, addresses the multiple ways in which leadership has been defined and various approaches to understanding leadership effectiveness. Specific questions examined include:

- What is known about the different perspectives regarding effective leadership?
- What are the special leadership challenges facing health services organizations?

- What skills are needed to be successful health care leaders?

The chapter sets forth an integrative model of leadership for the reader's consideration.

Chapter 5, Conflict Management and Negotiation, highlights the major forms of conflict that occur in health services organizations and various approaches for dealing with them. Special attention is devoted to structuring and managing negotiation processes. Among the key questions addressed are:

- What are the major causes of conflict in health services organizations?
- What are the pros and cons of different approaches for managing conflict?
- What are the primary concepts and approaches associated with effective negotiation?

The chapter emphasizes multiple approaches to managing conflict and the importance of preparation for effective negotiation.

Upon completing these three chapters, readers should have a fuller understanding of the relationships among motivation, leadership, and conflict management and negotiation. Readers should have a firm grasp of the various approaches to dealing with these issues and understand which approaches are most likely to be effective under different circumstances.

CHAPTER

3

MOTIVATING PEOPLE

Thomas A. D'Aunno, Ph.D.
Associate Professor

Myron D. Fottler, Ph.D.
Professor and Director

CHAPTER TOPICS

LEARNING OBJECTIVES

After completing this chapter, the reader should be able to

1. define motivation and distinguish it from other factors that influence individuals' performance
2. recognize popular but misleading myths about motivation
3. understand that motivation depends heavily on the situations in which individuals work
4. understand managers' roles in motivating people
5. identify key characteristics of the content of peoples' work that motivates them
6. identify important processes involved in motivating people
7. assess and deal with motivational problems

CHAPTER PURPOSE

The decision to fire or salvage is a dilemma many health care managers face, and it is not limited to decisions involving lower-level employees. The objective of this chapter is to understand how to motivate individuals to perform effectively in health services organizations. The chapter consists of four major sections. The first section defines motivation and distinguishes it from other factors that can affect performance. This section also describes common but misleading myths about motivation. As antidotes to these myths, we emphasize that motivation is situational. That is, there are several characteristics of individuals and the settings in which they work that managers should take into account in trying to moti-

---

IN THE REAL WORLD
THE DEMOTIVATED ATTENDANTS

St. Mary's Hospital is a Roman Catholic hospital in the Southeast run by the Daughters of Charity system. Until recently, the hospital ran a School of Nursing which had produced about 40 new diploma nurses each year. As a result of the high costs of operating the school, a decision was made to close the school two years ago.

Prior to the closing of the School of Nursing, two attendants (a nurse's aide and a porter) had been in charge of maintenance for 12 years. They received virtually no supervision and the facility was always spotless. During that time period, they were commended verbally and in writing for the high quality of their work. The vice president of Human Resources attributed their high motivation and good work to the pride and ownership they felt in what they viewed as "their" area.

When the School of Nursing was closed, the two attendants were transferred to the hospital. In the hospital they were viewed as new employees, moved around on a regular basis, and no longer had autonomy and ownership of a specific area.

The quality of their work suffered. They were written up by supervisors on several occasions for attitudinal problems, lack of motivation, and inadequate work performance. Instead of the praise, recognition, and positive reinforcement they had previously received from the director of the now defunct School of Nursing, the two attendants were now receiving criticism from several supervisors.

The vice president for Human Resources faces a dilemma. The easy solution is simply to fire them, as several supervisors have suggested. On the other hand, these have been good and loyal employees of the hospital for many years. Through no fault of their own, their job structure and environment was changed. She would therefore like to salvage them and make them motivated and productive employees once again. Although she's not quite sure how to do it, she realizes the problem is not that the two employees are simply unmotivated by nature since they had demonstrated extremely high motivation for a long period of time prior to their transfer to the hospital.

SOURCE: Adapted from Lutz S. Employee suggestions net $20 million in savings. *Modern Healthcare.* 1990; 20(9):21–22.

vate people. The section concludes by examining the role that managers can play to maintain or increase motivation. The next two sections identify the most important factors that managers can influence to improve or maintain the motivation of employees and co-workers. The focus is on those approaches that seem most promising, and we refer readers to more extensive reviews.[1,2] Finally, the last section examines common motivational problems and discusses how to assess them. Several alternatives for dealing with motivational problems are explored.

MOTIVATION AND MANAGEMENT

Defining and Distinguishing Motivation

The beginning of wisdom in motivating people is to recognize what *motivation* is and is not.[3] We define motivation as a state of feeling or thinking in which one is energized or aroused to perform a task or engage in a particular behavior.[4] This definition focuses on motivation as an emotional or cognitive state that is independent of action. This focus clearly distinguishes motivation from the performance of a task and its consequences. Notice, too, that motivation can be a state of either feeling or thinking or a combination of the two. For some individuals motivation is more a matter of feeling than thinking, while, for others, the reverse is true.

Myths about Motivation— and Some Antidotes

There are several popular but misleading myths about motivating people. Our view is that these myths are more harmful than helpful and, as a result, need to be confronted early in this chapter. Four particular myths are addressed below.

Myth #1: Motivated workers are more productive. To illustrate this myth, consider this conversation:[5]

> Supervisor: George just isn't motivated any more!
> Foreman: How can you tell?
> Supervisor: His productivity has fallen off by more than 50%.

Motivation should not be confused with performance. People can be highly motivated but still perform poorly. Performance depends not just on motivation but also on ability and a host of situational factors such as the availability of resources needed to perform a job well. In other words, motivation is just one of several factors that managers need to consider in trying to improve or sustain individuals' performance. Nonetheless, it is often a critical factor.

Myth #2: Some people are just motivated and others aren't. This myth is based on the view that motivation is a personality trait or characteristic that remains relatively stable from time to time and place to place. If this view were taken to its extreme, it would suggest that managers should carefully select only those employees who have the trait of motivation, for managers could otherwise do little to influence motivation and behavior.

In contrast, we take the view that motivation is more specific to situations (i.e., influenced by factors in an individual's environment) than it is a stable personality trait or characteristic.[6] There is strong empirical support for the view that situations significantly shape individual behavior.[7] For example, as illustrated in the case at St. Mary's Hospital, individuals who are motivated at certain times and in particular situations can lose their motivation if their work conditions change.

We argue that, even if motivation were a somewhat stable personality trait, it would still be important for managers to ensure that employees have work conditions that will reinforce their tendency to be motivated or change their tendency to be unmotivated. In short, motivation and behavior are produced by a complex interaction of situational and individual factors.

Myth #3: Motivation can be mass produced. A major myth about motivation is that it can be mass produced, for example, in speeches by charismatic leaders to large groups of people. Though this approach sometimes works, it is most often the case that, to motivate people effectively, managers need to treat them as individuals. Contrary to the myth of mass production, we assert that individuals vary widely from each other in many ways. As a result, it is a central and recurring theme of this chapter that managers must motivate employees and co-workers on an individual basis, taking each person's situation into account. At least three important types of individual and situational differences should be considered:

1. job position or occupation
2. career stage
3. personal factors

Job position or occupation. One of the most distinctive features of health care organizations is the number of different occupational groups and job categories involved. These groups range from nurse's aides and porters to nurses, physical therapists, and physicians. Health care occupations vary along dimensions such as the amount and type of training they require, their power and status, and what types of individuals are attracted to them. Managers should understand how their ability to motivate individuals may vary according to their occupation or job category. For example, union contracts often prohibit certain types of changes in job design and responsibilities; managers need to know what occupational groups are covered by such contracts and how they affect certain approaches to motivation.

Career stage. A second important way in which individuals vary is their career stage. To illustrate, consider a recent graduate of a health services management program. He may be highly motivated by assignments that provide opportunities for learning about the different divisions of a health care organization. In contrast, his colleague who has more experience may wish to work on a single project from start to completion. Managers need to be sensitive to such career stage needs, motives, and values.

Personal factors. Perhaps more than we recognize, people at work are influenced by a variety of factors from their personal lives. For example, personal factors sometimes parallel career stages. A recent graduate may have few family ties that would limit her interest in work that involved travel, whereas a manager with young children may be less motivated by opportunity for travel on the job. Other important personal influences that can affect motivation include family illness, divorce, substance abuse, health problems, child care, and financial stress. These are clearly delicate areas for managers to tread. Yet, managers need to be aware that such personal factors can affect work motivation. On the one hand, it may be harmful to pry into the personal lives of employees and co-workers. On the other hand, it may be very helpful to be sensitive to needs at work that stem from their personal lives.

Myth #4: Money makes the world go 'round. We do not deny that many, if not most, individuals care about and are motivated by money. But too often managers think only of money when trying to motivate people. Unfortunately, money is likely to be in short supply for health care managers, at least in the next several years. Fortunately, money is not always the most important motivator; indeed, it seldom is. In the next sections, the importance of several other factors in motivating people that do not require cash will be discussed.

Manager's Role

The situational perspective described above implies that managers should take an active role in systematically assessing the motivation of their employees and co-workers. Individuals' motivation can vary over time and with the kind of work they are performing. Thus managers need to periodically assess motivation and performance, taking into account the occupational, career stage, and personal factors discussed above. Such assessments should include informal interviews with employees and co-workers in which open-ended questions are asked about individuals' needs, motives, perceptions, and values.[8] These assessments need not be lengthy. What matters more is that they are timely; employees feel comfortable in openly expressing their concerns, and managers use the opportunity to do problem solving and goal setting. In short, managers can play a critical role by not only assessing their employees' motivation but by taking the lead to alter conditions that can increase motivation.

What factors make people energized or aroused to work? Further, what factors influence how individuals' energy is directed and to what tasks, how intense their arousal is, and how long they persist in these states? These are the key questions that managers need to address to motivate people. Research attempts to explain work motivation through two basic types of theories: content and process. *Content theories* are concerned with *what* energizes behavior, while *process theories* focus on *how* behavior is energized.

CONTENT PERSPECTIVES

Content perspectives on motivation focus in large part on needs and need deficiencies. Researchers agree that people have a multitude of needs with varying degrees of intensity. Such needs create a state of disequilibrium within the person which, in turn, creates a desire to meet the need or needs he is experiencing. Consequently, individuals search the environment for potentially satisfying goals. Once attained, these goals will lead to a reduction in the disequilibrium or the fulfillment of their needs. Motivation can be increased to the degree that peoples' needs can be satisfied on the job.

Thus, content perspectives try to answer the question, What factor or factors motivate people? Some assert that motivation is a function of pay, working hours, and working conditions. Others suggest that autonomy and responsibility are the causes of motivation.[9] Still others believe either or both sets of factors could be important in a given situation.

The motivation framework in Figure 3.1 is a good starting point for understanding how needs can motivate people. The motivation process often begins with needs that reflect some deficiency within the individual. For example, the employee might feel underpaid or lacking recognition *vis-a-vis* other employees. In response to these unsatisfied needs, the employee searches for ways to satisfy them. She may ask for a raise or promotion, work harder to try to earn either, or seek another position outside the organization. Next, she chooses one or more options. After imple-

menting the chosen option or options, she then evaluates her success. If her hard work resulted in a pay raise or a promotion, she will probably continue to work hard. If neither has occurred, she will probably try another option.

The Need Hierarchy

Theory Overview

Many theorists advanced the concept of a *need hierarchy,* but Abraham Maslow developed the most popular version in the management field in the 1940s.[10] He proposed that people want to satisfy various needs and that these needs can be arranged in a hierarchy of importance as shown in Figure 3.2.

Maslow's hierarchy of needs assumes there are five need levels that must be satisfied sequentially. The *physiological* needs include such things as air, food, and sex. They represent basic issues of survival and biological function. In organization settings, such needs are generally satisfied by adequate wages and a satisfactory work environment that provides adequate lighting, temperature, and ventilation.

The *security* needs include a secure physical and emotional environment. Examples include the need to be free from worry about money and job security. In the workplace, security needs are satisfied by job continuity (no layoffs), a grievance system (to protect against arbitrary action), and an adequate health insurance and retirement package (for security against illness and eventual retirement).

Belongingness needs involve social processes. They include the need for love and affection and the need to be accepted by one's peers. For most people, they are satisfied by a combination of family and community relationships outside the job and friendships on the job. A manager can promote the satisfaction of these needs by encouraging social interaction and by making employees feel part of a team or work group. Sensitivity to an employee's family problems can also help employees meet this need.

Esteem needs are actually comprised of two different sets of needs: the need for a positive self-image or self-respect and the need for recognition and respect from others. Managers can help address esteem needs by providing signs of accomplishment such as job titles, public recognition, and praise (i.e., extrinsic rewards).

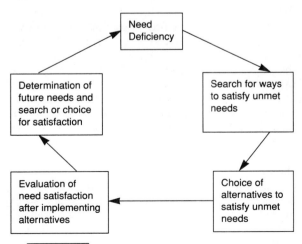

FIGURE 3.1. A framework for employee motivation.

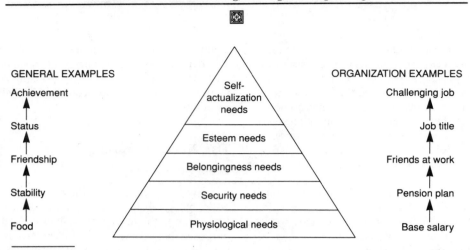

GENERAL EXAMPLES

Achievement

Status

Friendship

Stability

Food

ORGANIZATION EXAMPLES

Challenging job

Job title

Friends at work

Pension plan

Base salary

Self-actualization needs

Esteem needs

Belongingness needs

Security needs

Physiological needs

FIGURE 3.2. Maslow's hierarchy of needs. Adapted from Maslow AH. A Theory of Human Motivation. *Psychological Review.* 1943;50:370–396.

They may also provide more challenging job assignments and other opportunities for employees to feel a sense of accomplishment.

Self-actualization needs, at the top of the hierarchy, involve realizing one's potential for continued growth and individual development. These are most difficult for a manager to identify and meet due to individual differences in goals. However, allowing employees to participate in decision making and the opportunity to learn new things about their work may promote self-actualization.

Maslow suggests that the five need categories constitute a hierarchy. People are motivated first to satisfy the lower level needs beginning with physiological needs. As long as these remain unsatisfied, the individual is motivated only to fulfill them. When these needs are satisfied, they cease to motivate people and they move up the hierarchy and become sequentially concerned with each higher level in turn. The process continues until the self-actualization level is reached.

Research Support and Evaluation

The need hierarchy has a certain intuitive logic, but research indicates various shortcomings in the theory. While the progression principle suggests a systematic approach to satisfying needs from lowest to highest levels, research provides little evidence that a step-wise hierarchy actually exists. For example, some research shows that the five levels of need are not always present and the order of the levels is not always the same as Maslow proposed.[11,12]

Nor has research confirmed the deficit principle, in which unmet needs systematically motivate behavior.[13] Needs do not fall into a neat five-step hierarchy.[14,15] There are some rather obvious exceptions to the theory to necessitate caution. For example, outstanding artists have continued their creative work while sacrificing health and security. Soldiers risk death for an ideal. Some employees strive for excellence despite their low-wage, dead-end jobs. Others employed in higher-wage jobs offering numerous opportunities for growth and development fail to take advantage of such opportunities. While their lower-level needs are being met, they do not strive to meet higher-level needs identified by Maslow's need hierarchy.

A major reason why the literature shows little support for Maslow's theory is because the needs are ambiguous and overlap, rather than being distinct and independent.[16] In some studies, the lower-level needs formed a cluster and the higher-level needs formed a cluster.

The major problem with Maslow's need hierarchy is that it cannot be turned into a practical guide for managers who are trying to enhance work motivation. The research evidence is just not there to support such rules of thumb as "If you satisfy employees' physiological and safety needs through job security and a competitive compensation system, then employees will be motivated mainly by needs for affiliation or self-actualization." It would be helpful if the advice were accurate, but it is not.

Application

Though managers cannot apply Maslow's needs hierarchy mechanistically, it is not unreasonable to conclude that unmet needs do motivate *most* employees *most* of the time. Maslow did identify some of the major categories of human needs that *may* motivate different employees at different times. In practical terms, organizations should provide employees with wages sufficient for food and shelter; reasonable protection of jobs, health, and safety; a satisfactory physical and social environment at work; and rewards or recognition that reinforce individual esteem. Managers should also recognize and support growth needs by providing opportunities for career advancement, encouraging personal self-development, and creating environments in which individuals can explore their individual talents and dreams.

The major implication of Maslow's theory for management is that organization policies and practices must pay attention to all of these needs if the organization hopes to have employees working up to their full potential. For example, allowing understaffing so that registered nurses work such long hours they do not get enough sleep probably reduces their desires for providing high quality patient care (achievement) and creativity. During periods of retrenchment, being arbitrary and capricious about employees' job security interferes with cooperation, initiative, and other desirable behaviors. On the other hand, paying exclusive attention to the more basic physiological and security needs while ignoring the needs for achievement and self-esteem would defeat organizational purposes. Maslow's theory keeps managers aware of employees' higher level needs when considering motivation strategies.

It should also be noted that people's needs change over time. The needs, wants, and desires of individuals in their sixties differ from those of individuals in their twenties. Moreover, all employees have a variety of needs motivating them, and these differ by individual. One study found that the individual's position in the organizational hierarchy affects need satisfaction significantly with lower-level personnel less satisfied with their level of need achievement than higher level personnel.[17] The manager's task is to develop situations that permit as many employees as possible to satisfy as many wants as possible. The astute manager will recognize what specific needs are important to motivate each individual. When possible, the manager will alter his or her supervisory style, economic and non-economic rewards, job assignments, and related factors, to maximize need fulfillment of as many people as possible.

ERG Theory

Theory Overview

As a result of the above criticisms of Maslow's approach to employee motivation, Clayton Alderfer proposed an alternative hierarchy called the ERG theory of motivation.[18] The letters E, R, and G stand for existence, relatedness, and growth. The ERG theory collapses Maslow's need hierarchy into three levels. *Existence* needs correspond to the physiological and security needs of Maslow's hierarchy. *Relatedness* needs focus on how people relate to others and encompass Maslow's need to belong and need to earn the esteem of others. *Growth* needs include both the need for self-esteem and self-actualization.

While the ERG theory assumes a hierarchy of needs as suggested by Maslow, there are three important differences. First, the ERG theory suggests that more than one level of need can motivate behavior at the same time. Unlike Maslow, the emergence of relatedness and growth needs does not require satisfaction of the existence needs. For example, people can be motivated by a desire for money (existence), friendship (relatedness), and the opportunity to learn new skills all at once.

Second, the ERG theory has a frustration regression element that is missing in Maslow. Maslow maintained that each lower-level need must be satisfied before an individual can progress to a higher need level. In contrast, the ERG theory suggests that if needs remain unsatisfied at higher levels (i.e., growth), the individual will become frustrated, regress to a lower level, and begin to pursue those things again. For example, an employee receiving "adequate" pay (as defined by the employee) may attempt to seek opportunities for personal growth on the job. If these needs are frustrated, the employee may regress to being motivated to earn more money.

Third, the ERG theory suggests that needs are not fixed. The opportunities available in the organization may affect employee needs. Relatedness and growth needs may become more intense in an organization where there is ample opportunity to meet them.

Research Support and Evaluation

Research suggests that the ERG theory may be a more valid account of employee motivation in organizations than Maslow's needs hierarchy.[19,20] However, managers should not rely too heavily on any single perspective on motivation. The key insights from both Maslow and Alderfer are that some needs are more important than others and that people may change their behavior after any particular set of needs have been satisfied.

Application

The major managerial implication of the ERG theory is that health care managers should assume that *all* employees have the potential for continued growth and development. This suggests the desirability of offering ongoing opportunities for training and development, transfer, promotion, and career planning to all employees.

Two-Factor Theory

Theory Overview

Another well-known content perspective on employee motivation is the two-factor theory developed by Frederich Herzberg on the basis of 200 interviews with accountants and engineers in Pittsburgh.[21,22] He asked them to describe occasions when they felt especially satisfied and highly motivated and other occasions when they had been dissatisfied and unmotivated. Surprisingly, he found that entirely different sets of factors were associated with satisfaction and high motivation and with dissatisfaction and low motivation. He found that the key factors in satisfaction and motivation were achievement, recognition, the work itself, responsibility, and advancement. He labeled these factors *mo-*

tivators since their presence increases job satisfaction and motivation but their absence does not lead to dissatisfaction. Herzberg also found that if a second group of factors, *hygiene factors* were negative or absent, dissatisfaction results. These hygiene factors included company policy and administration, supervision, salary, interpersonal relations, and working conditions. The presence of positive hygiene factors, by themselves, prevents dissatisfaction but does not lead to satisfaction and motivation.

Note that the factors influencing the satisfaction dimension—motivation factors—are specifically related to the work content (i.e., intrinsic factors). The factors presumed to cause dissatisfaction—hygiene factors—are related to the work environment. According to Herzberg, changing the environment alone will not enhance employee motivation.

Research Support and Evaluation

Herzberg's two-factor theory has several limitations and weaknesses. His sample was not representative of the general population. The findings in his initial interviews are subject to different interpretations, some of which differ from the one he offered. Subsequent research often failed to uphold the theory in that some factors, such as salary, appear to be associated with both satisfaction and dissatisfaction.[23-25] Research also shows that both categories of factors serve to motivate. In one study of managerial and professional workers, the hygiene factors were as frequently associated with self-reports of high performance as were the motivators.[26]

Other researchers question whether the individual factors are mutually exclusive. For example, salary is defined as a hygiene factor, but for many highly paid executives and professionals, salary may be viewed as a form of recognition. Logic suggests that, in reality, these factors do not operate separately from one another in a given person. The desires for advancement and for recognition—both motivators—are connected to feelings and attitudes about salary—a hygiene factor.

Still other researchers criticize the theory for being too simple. Lee flatly states that "the evidence to date clearly eliminates Herzberg's theory as a general or universal theory of work motivation."[27] Steers and Porter, on the other hand, take a more positive view: "It appears that a fruitful approach to this controversial theory would be to learn from it that which can help us to develop more improved models rather than to accept or reject the model totally."[28]

Application

Despite the above criticisms, the two-factor theory has had a major impact by increasing managers' awareness of motivation and its importance. Herzberg argued there are two stages in motivating employees. First, the manager must make sure the hygiene factors are not deficient. Pay and security must be appropriate, working conditions must be safe, and supervision must be acceptable. By providing hygiene factors at an appropriate level, the manager does not stimulate motivation but does avoid dissatisfaction.

The manager should then proceed to stage two—giving employees the opportunity to experience motivation factors such as achievement and recognition. The result is predicted to be a high level of satisfaction and motivation. Herzberg goes a step further than most theorists and describes exactly how to use the two-factor theory in the workplace. Specifically, he recommends that jobs be redesigned and enriched to provide higher levels of the motivation factors.

Herzberg's theory has great value for health care managers because it identifies a wide range of factors involved in employee motivation. Consideration of all of these factors is useful in any attempt to enhance motivation and to diminish demotivating factors in an organization. The theory has also had a major influence on job design in many health services organizations because it has made managers more aware of the importance of job challenge and responsibility in motivation. (Also see Chapter 7.) The recent trend toward the employment of multiskilled health practitioners is one manifestation of this awareness.[29,30]

Learned Need Theory

Theory Overview

The theories of Maslow, Alderfer, and Herzberg identify a number of individual needs and then attempt to arrange them in some kind of order of importance. Other content views of employee motivation focus more on the important needs themselves without concern for ordering them. The three needs most often discussed are the needs for *achievement, power,* and *affiliation.* Far more importantly, it has been argued that these needs and the behaviors associated with the efforts to satisfy them can be learned.[31,32]

John W. Atkinson proposed that everyone enjoys an "energy reserve" that can be released depending upon individual incentives to achieve desired goals.[33] He also proposed the above three basic human drives. David C. McClelland gave form to these three drives and related them to performance in organizations.[34]

The first basic drive is the need for achievement and refers to the individual's need to accomplish complex tasks, compete, and resolve problems. It reflects the desire to achieve a goal more effectively than in the past. People with a high need for achievement are assumed to have a desire for personal responsibility, a tendency to set moderately difficult goals, a need for specific goals and immediate feedback, and a preoccupation with their task.

The second basic drive, a need for power, refers to the individual's desire to influence or control others' behavior. It also represents the desire to control one's environment. Individuals high in power needs are thought to be more suited to management than achievers. In this view, "power" implies being responsible for control of others and for influencing behavior in complex situations.

The third drive, the need for affiliation, reflects an individual's desire to associate with others in friendly circumstances. It is similar to Maslow's belongingness need. Those high in affiliation prefer friendly, participative work environments where the quality of group interaction with co-workers is more highly valued than achievements or influence. People with a strong need for affiliation are likely to prefer (and perform better in) a job that entails a lot of social interaction. Few of these individuals manage effectively in most organizations because they tend to emphasize friendship at the expense of organizational productivity and effectiveness.

Research Support and Evaluation

McClelland concluded that, although the need for achievement is the main motivation for those who wish to start and develop their own small businesses, the need for power is a crucial motivator of top executives in larger, more complex organizations. Most successful managers exercise their power in a controlled and disciplined way on behalf of others and create a strong sense of team spirit among their subordinates. One study found that managers as a group tend to have a stronger power motive than the general population and that successful managers tend to have stronger power motives than less successful managers.[35] Other research has shown that people with a strong need for power are likely to be superior performers, have good attendance records, and occupy supervisory positions.[36]

Persons with high achievement needs tend to flourish in very competitive situations, enjoy challenges, and thrive in complex and stimulating environments such as those found in most health care organizations. McClelland argued that these achievers would be best suited to situations where independent responsibility and autonomy prevail. The implication is that, while many achievers are found in professional positions such as physicians, they are not always among the best managers in highly bureaucratic organizations. Since such organizations are based on diffused authority and group activities, achievers are often uncomfortable in situations of group responsibility and control.

An important aspect of McClelland's theory is that all three needs are acquired. Individuals develop these needs to varying degrees through life experiences. They are learned drives evolving from one's background and environment. Indeed, since a high need for achievement is important for professional and managerial success in nonbureaucratic organizations, McClelland devised a training program for increasing one's need for achievement. Studies found that employees who complete this achievement training tend to make more money and receive promotions faster than other employees.[37,38] Moreover, achievement training may also affect organizational outcomes. In one case, three different groups of small business employees were given 70 hours of achievement training and assistance. Median profits for these businesses increased from $280 per month to $670 per month.[39]

Application

Other managerial implications of McClelland's work are far reaching. For individuals already set in their ways, matching work environments with their needs is crucial to their motivation and career success. Employees established in health care organizations undergoing rapid change may need counseling or education to help them adapt to the new environment. For example, an affiliation-oriented manager may not fare well in an entreprenuerial environment that emphasizes achievement.

Further, organizations might focus on identifying and selecting individuals with high levels of achievement motivation or other desired values and behavior. Irvine (CA) Medical Center, for example, uses both psychological testing and structured interviewing in employment selection and promotion decisions.[40] These approaches determine the prospective candidate's service orientation, performance, motivations, and ability to work as a team member. The result has been a collaborative, achievement-oriented culture with shared values among the employees.

An Assessment of Content Theories

It is well accepted that motivation has important origins in human needs. Need theories of motivation assume that people attempt to satisfy such needs and wants. A simplistic view is that all a manager or supervisor has to do to release their employee's motivation potential is to identify their needs and then take steps to satisfy them. Unfortunately, there is no simple set of needs and need satisfiers that would be universally applicable. First, as noted above, people differ on the basis of age, sex, race, and other demographic and background characteristics. No one set of motivators is likely to be appropriate for all employees since their needs will be different. Second, the organizational context and culture differ both across organizations and within organizations. The learned needs of a given individual may vary depending on the incentives present in his or her organization. Third, for a given individual, needs change over time. This has already been implied by the needs hierarchy theorists. The relative importance of various needs are continuously changing, thus forcing managers to aim at a moving target. Fourth, employees in different positions in an organizational hierarchy will undoubtedly differ in terms of their configuration of needs and potential motivators. Fifth, resource constraints or lack of such constraints may also impact the relative importance of various needs.

Despite these caveats, content theories of motivation help health care managers focus on individual needs in the motivation process. All provide useful insights into factors that may promote motivation in a given situation. Moreover, they are not separate and discrete views of motivation but share much in common with one another. Figure 3.3 compares the needs identified by the four content theories described in this section. It should be noted that, while they do not necessarily agree on whether there is a hierarchy of needs or whether individuals attempt to satisfy multiple needs simultaneously, some of their basic concepts are similar and overlap with one another.

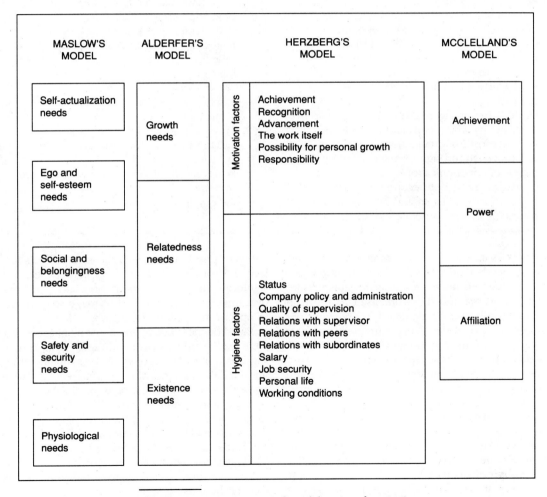

FIGURE 3.3. A comparison of need theories of motivation.

MANAGERIAL GUIDELINES

1. Employees often have unmet needs that they attempt to satisfy through work. These include physiological, security, social esteem, self-control, power, and achievement needs. Such unmet needs will vary from individual to individual based on a wide variety of factors. No two persons will have the same proportion of each of these needs.

2. At any given point in time, people attempt to satisfy a wide variety of needs. They exchange their labor for rewards that they value because these rewards respond to their needs. Such rewards may be intrinsic or extrinsic to the job. Intrinsic motivation is particularly important for health care professionals.

3. Health care managers can motivate people by determining what needs and rewards they view as most important. This can be accomplished through formal and informal means of communication.

4. Rewards may be both economic and noneconomic. They should be relevant to the priority needs of particular employees or employee groups. What is a hygiene factor for one person may be a motivator for another. However, satisfied needs are not motivators for anyone.

5. Employees should be selected on the basis of how well their needs, motivations, and qualifications match the requirements of each position. Written examinations and oral interviews may be used to assess the degree of job-applicant match.

6. Redesigning jobs is another alternative for increasing this match. Redesigning offers much potential for increased motivation to the extent that it involves building in responsibility, decision making, control, autonomy, challenge, and opportunities for achievement.

7. Training programs that emphasize enhancement of the achievement motive can enhance motivation.

8. Managers should be concerned with both hygiene factors and motivators as defined by the employees themselves.

Employees in health services organizations have a variety of needs motivating them. For example, one study of registered nurses found achievement, interpersonal relations, and the work itself to be major motivators while another identified autonomy or personal control, promotional opportunities, and work scheduling to be most important.[41,42] While the specifics differed, in both studies two of the three key factors were motivators identified by Herzberg. The task of health care managers is to identify the specific needs of their employees and then develop opportunities that permit these employees to satisfy their needs.

Employees' needs can be identified by attitude surveys and continuous two-way oral communication with various subgroups of employees.[43,44] When possible, the manager should also attempt to recognize what needs are important in the motivation of each individual employee and to match those needs to the requirements of positions to which those individuals are assigned.[45] Studies of job redesign typically find significant increases in motivation and performance over time.[46,47] Needs themselves may also be modified by special motivation training courses.[48]

Based on identified needs, astute managers will alter their leadership and communication style, economic rewards, noneconomic rewards, job assignments, training and development emphases, and feedback to maximize the need fulfillment of as many subordinates as possible. For example, some will need to be left alone to work independently. Others will need more structure, goals, and feedback. Since employees have different needs, they need to be managed in different ways. The managerial guidelines given below provide a convenient summary of the managerial implications of content theories.

Though content theories provide useful insights into motivational factors, they do not constitute a complete theoretical or managerial approach to employee motivation. They do not shed much light on the process of motivation. For example, they do not explain why employees might be motivated by one factor rather than by another at a given level or how their different needs might be satisfied. These questions involve behaviors or actions, goals, and feelings of satisfaction which are addressed by various process theories of motivation. It is to these theories that we now turn.

PROCESS PERSPECTIVES

In this section, we examine five approaches to motivation that, although they differ from each other, share a focus on the processes involved in motivation. In contrast to the approaches examined in the previous section that concern the content of work and its influence on motivation, these approaches attend to the context in which work is done as well as individuals' reactions—especially thoughts and feelings—to work.

Equity Theory

Theory Overview

Adams proposed a theory of work motivation that assumes that individuals value and seek fairness, or *equity,* in their relationships with employers.[49] Relationships are fair when people perceive that their outcomes (e.g., pay) are proportionate to their perceived contributions or inputs (e.g., task performance). Further, people evaluate fairness by comparing themselves to others. In other words, people contrast their perceived inputs and outcomes with their perceptions of others' inputs and outcomes. To the extent that this ratio is seen as unequal, individuals experience tension.

Adams proposed two kinds of inequity. Underpayment refers to the case when someone perceives that she is receiving fewer rewards from a job than another person making a comparable contribution. In contrast, overpayment occurs when someone perceives that she is receiving more rewards than another person making a comparable contribution.

Adams also proposed that people are motivated to reduce tensions that result from perceived inequity. The greater the perceived inequity and resulting tension, the greater the motivation to reduce it. In other words, from the perspective of equity theory, work motivation stems from the need to reduce tensions caused by inequity.

Depending on the magnitude of the perceived injustice and individual as well as situational circumstances, people may use one of several approaches to reduce inequity and restore balance in their relationships with employers. These approaches include altering their perceptions of their own or others' inputs or outcomes, changing their inputs or outcomes, getting others to change their inputs or outcomes, and leaving the inequitable situation altogether.[50]

Research Support and Evaluation

There are a relatively large number of studies testing various aspects of Adams' equity theory. Most of these have concentrated on the effects of perceived inequity in pay on quality and quantity of work performance when people are paid either hourly or on a piece-rate. Results from most studies support equity theory's hypotheses about the effects of underpayment.[51] The results from studies examining hourly payment are also stronger than results from studies examining piece-rate payment.[52] On the other hand, studies of overpayment inequity provide mixed support for Adams' theory.

Despite the empirical support for equity theory, it has several limitations that managers should consider. The theory does not help to identify which of several approaches to restoring equity an individual will take. In actual work situations, there are typically several ways that perceived inequities can be addressed. One can simply convince oneself that an inequity is not worth worrying about or will be reduced at the next annual review.

Further, the theory does not specify who people are likely to compare themselves with to assess their equity with employers. Do people compare themselves more often with immediate co-workers, or are comparisons with colleagues in other organizations equally or more important? For example, do primary care physicians compare their income to that of specialists such as orthopedic surgeons, or do they only consider the pay levels of other primary care physicians?

Another problem is that studies have not examined how perceptions of equity vary over time and how such variation affects motivation.[53] Most studies take a short-term view of equity issues, and the theory provides little guidance about how to deal with variation over time in work situations. Finally, it is not clear how this theory can be used to motivate people who perceive no important inequities in their work. That is, the theory proposes that people are motivated to reduce tensions created by perceived inequities in inputs and outcomes. It provides no guidance for managers once they have addressed perceived inequities other than to try to be as fair as possible.

Application

Despite the limitations just noted, we believe that equity theory provides some useful guidelines for health care managers. First, it is important to note that people compare themselves to others in many situations and in many ways. Such comparisons affect not only their motivation but other aspects of their behavior as well. When people experience uncertainty, they are especially likely to turn to others, consciously or unconsciously, to provide them with cues about what to do. Equity theory would be useful even if its only contribution were to remind us of the importance of social comparison.

Second, managers need to directly address perceptions of inequities so that individuals are not motivated to reduce their contributions or inputs or to leave their jobs. It may be that perceptions of inequity can be changed simply by explaining differences between jobs or other conditions that make it necessary to reward or treat people differently. In other cases, managers may need to consider pay raises or increases in other ways to reward people. In still other cases, there may be nothing that a manager can do to restore perceptions of equity. But, if such concerns are not addressed, it is clear that they can be a source of motivational problems.

Finally, we have argued that it is important to motivate people on an individual basis. Equity theory reminds us that even this approach has limits. To the extent that people are treated as individuals, perceptions of inequity are likely to increase because people will be comparing themselves to others who are being treated differently; such differences can trigger perceptions of inequity.

Expectancy Theory

Theory Overview

Expectancy theory has several variations that all trace their roots to cognitive psychology in the early 1950s. Georgopoulos, Mahoney, and Jones and Vroom were the first to apply expectancy theory to work motivation.[54,55] Vroom's expectancy model was particularly influential. Since this early research, expectancy theory has become perhaps the most prominent theory of work motivation. The theory assumes that people are rational decision makers who will expend effort on work that will lead to desired rewards. Further, the theory assumes that people know what rewards they want from work and understand that their performance will determine the extent to which they attain the rewards they value.

Though there are several variations of expectancy theory, they all share four central components.[56] First, there are *job outcomes*. These include both rewards (e.g., pay raises, promotions, recognition) and negative experiences (e.g., job loss, demotion).

Second, there are *valences*. These are individuals' feelings about job outcomes. Like job outcomes, they can range from positive to neutral to negative, and they vary in strength as well as direction.

The third component is *instrumentality,* which refers to the perceived link between performance and outcomes. In other words, instrumentality is the extent to which individuals believe that attaining a job outcome depends on, or is conditional on, their performance. For example, if a nurse thought that an outcome (pay raise) depended highly on his performance rather than some other factor (hospital patient volume), the instrumentality for the outcome would be high.

Finally, *expectancy* is the perceived link between effort and performance. That is, to what extent do individuals believe that there is a relationship between how hard they try and how well they do.

Motivation is the end product of valence, instrumentality, and expectancy. People are motivated when a combination of factors occurs: they value an outcome (i.e., valence is high and positive), they believe that good performance will be rewarded with desired outcomes (i.e., instrumentality is high), and they believe that their efforts will produce good performance (i.e., expectancy is high). In contrast, motivation is likely to be low if the components of expectancy theory have low values. If people do not care about their job outcomes, they have less reason to work for them. Or, if organizations do not link outcomes to performance (e.g., pay raises are linked to seniority rather than performance), people have less reason to care about their performance. Similarly, if effort and performance seem unrelated, there is less reason to try hard. Each of these factors can decrease motivation, and if all are present, it is improbable that motivation will be high.

Research Support and Evaluation

Empirical support from many studies of expectancy theory is quite good.[57] Nonetheless, the theory seems to receive more support in studies that examine the levels of effort an individual will expend on different tasks than in studies that examine the strength of motivation across different people.[58]

Expectancy theory rests clearly on the assumption that people are highly rational and consciously engage in decisions to work harder on tasks that they believe will maximize their gains while minimizing their losses. Though this assumption works quite well for many people in many situations, it is not universally valid. People have unconscious motives. Moreover, their calculations about the links between effort and performance and performance and reward are not always accurate.

Further, there are some studies that indicate that the strength of the theory may vary depending on personality factors.[59] For example, the theory may hold more strongly for people who have a high internal, rather than external, locus of control. Such people tend to believe that their lives are under their own control more than the control or influence of external events. As a result, people with a high internal locus of control believe that there are strong links between their efforts and performance and their performance and outcomes. These beliefs, as noted above, are central to the theory's predictions about motivation.

Application

Despite these limitations, expectancy theory provides very useful guidelines for managerial action.[60] These include

1. Incentives or job outcomes should be chosen so that they are attractive to employees. Perhaps the best way to do this is to ask employees directly about their preferences using surveys or interviews.
2. The rules for attaining incentives must be clear to all involved. For example, expected levels of performance should be spelled out in as much detail as possible. Such rules should be stated in job descriptions and employee orientations. These rules should also be reviewed periodically, both informally and formally. We add here a note from equity theory: the rules should be perceived as fair.
3. People must perceive that their efforts will lead to the desired level of performance.

There are many practical limitations involved here simply because several factors can intervene to weaken the link between effort and performance. For example, people may be trying hard but lack the resources (e.g., equipment) to do well, or as is often the case in health care, there is a great deal of interdependence between people so that performance depends on all their efforts. Work done in groups or teams often has this feature. When this is the case and co-workers' efforts are lacking, an individual's perceptions of the link between their efforts and group or unit performance can be easily diminished. In any case, managers need to make it clear that, insofar as they are able, they will not hold people accountable for performance problems that stem from factors not in their control.

Reinforcement Theory

Theory Overview

Reinforcement theory, also known as operant conditioning or behavior modification, is based on the work of B.F. Skinner. The theory has three components: stimulus, response, and consequence. A stimulus is any condition or variable that elicits a response, such as a request from a supervisor for some information. A response is a behavior performed contingent on a stimulus. A consequence is anything that follows a response that changes the likelihood that the response will occur again following a stimulus.

In turn, there are three types of consequences: rewards (termed positive reinforcement), which increase the likelihood of a response; punishments, which decrease the likelihood of a response; and negative reinforcement, which is the removal of a reward or punishment to increase the likelihood of a response.

Further, research shows that four types of connections between responses and consequences can increase the frequency of a response. These include

1. Fixed interval. People are rewarded at a fixed time interval. For example, people paid on an hourly basis are on a fixed-interval reward schedule.
2. Fixed ratio. People are rewarded on the basis of a fixed number of responses. For example, physicians who are paid on a fee-for-service basis are rewarded on this schedule.
3. Variable interval. Responses are rewarded at some time interval which varies.
4. Variable ratio. Reward is based on behavior, but the ratio of reward to responses varies.

In short, from the perspective of reinforcement theory, motivation results when people are rewarded contingent on performance, based on the above schedules. In general, research indicates that responses are maintained best on ratio schedules.

Research Support and Evaluation

Research from a variety of settings indicates that reinforcement schedules work. As noted, the results may vary depending on the type of reinforcement schedule that is used, but performance is better when rewards are given contingently. This result is, of course, consistent with the views of expectancy theory.

Reinforcement theory has drawn sharp criticism since Skinner published his first work in this area.[61] One critique is that it encourages managers and others to manipulate employees through the design of reinforcement schedules over which employees have no control. Similarly, if employees have no input into selecting rewards, reinforcement may be ineffective. The antidote for these criticisms seems clear: employees need to have input into the design of reinforcement systems. Again, this guideline is consistent with an expectancy theory perspective.

A second common critique is that reinforcement theory presents a flat, one-dimensional view of human nature and motivation. That is, the theory says little about human emotion or cognition. People are often portrayed as somewhat mindless robots in pursuit of rewards. This critique is similar to a critique of expectancy theory: that is, it views people as very rational in pursuit of valued outcomes. The difference here is that critics of reinforcement theory argue that it does not even give people credit for thinking.

Application

The primary lesson from reinforcement theory is that performance, if not motivation, is better when rewards are given contingently. The effectiveness of reinforcement schedules will vary; thus it is best to take a pragmatic approach and see what works best in a given situation.

Goal Setting

Theory Overview

Locke proposed a motivation theory that focuses on the role of goals and *goal setting.*[62] He and his colleagues define a goal as something that an individual is consciously attempting to attain.[63,64] Goals are powerful because they direct people's attention, focus effort on tasks related to goal attainment, and encourage people to persist in such tasks. Further, Locke proposed that the more difficult and specific the goal, the greater will be the motivation to attain it. In short, a goal provides guidelines for how much effort to put into work.

Several conditions must be met for goals to have a positive influence on performance. First, people must be aware of goals and know what must be done to attain them. Second, goals must be accepted as something that people are willing to work for. People must be committed to goals. In other words, goals can fail to motivate people if they are seen as too difficult or too easy or if an individual does not know what tasks are required for goal attainment.[65]

Research Support and Evaluation

The empirical support for key parts of goal setting theory is impressive. Nearly 400 studies—mostly experimental—show that specific, difficult goals lead to better performance than specific, easy, vague goals such as "do your best" or no goals at all.[66]

There is also support for the view that commitment to goals is critical to effective performance.[67] In turn, commitment to goals is generally higher when people think they can attain the goals and when they value them.[68] Further, monetary rewards increase goal commitment if people value money and the amount is sufficiently large.

One surprising finding is that assigning goals to individuals generally leads to the same level of commitment and performance as when individuals participate in setting goals or when they set goals for themselves. Perhaps assigned goals work well because they come from authority figures or because assigned goals, if difficult, are more challenging.[69] We are concerned about applying these results to health care professionals, however, given that many of them are trained and socialized to set their own goals. In this case, managers just need to be sure that goals are specific and difficult regardless of who sets them.

Research also shows that goal setting is more effective, and usually only effective, when feedback is given to individuals so that they can monitor their performance in relation to goals. Indeed, goal setting without feedback seems to have little long-term effect on performance.[70] On the other hand, feedback without goal setting is also ineffective. People need both goals and feedback on progress toward goals to be motivated. Finally, for goal setting to be effective, people must have the ability to reach or approach the goals.[71] Once again, this result is consistent with expectancy theory.

The strength of this perspective is its simplicity and ease of application. It seems to be generalizable; its principles can be applied in any circumstance. Moreover, as noted above, it has a very strong base of empirical support.

There are, of course, some important unanswered questions. How do people become committed to goals, and why do they select certain goals and not others?[72]

Application

The implications for managers are relatively straightforward:

1. Set or encourage people to set goals that are difficult and specific; revise and update goals as necessary. Prompts such as daily, weekly or monthly "to do" lists are examples of useful techniques.
2. Provide timely and specific feedback to people on their progress toward goals.
3. Build commitment to goals by helping people believe they can attain goals and by selecting goals that are congruent with their values.
4. Consistent with reinforcement theory, rewards should be given contingent on goal attainment.
5. Make sure that individuals have the ability to achieve goals they or you set.

An Assessment of Process Theories

Each process theory has limitations that make it incomplete for understanding and motivating behavior. On the other hand, taken together the theories offer a powerful set of guidelines for health care managers (see Managerial Guidelines below). Process theories share the view that the content of work is often not enough to motivate people; they need reinforcement, expectations, fairness, and goals to be energized to perform their best.

Indeed, taken together, process theories suggest a cycle of managerial action as follows:

1. Goals should be set at the time of hiring or at periodic performance evaluations.
2. Expectations about goal attainment and consequences should also be set at this time.
3. Perceptions of fairness should be checked periodically.
4. Reinforcement should be given contingent on performance.

This cycle used in concert with the guidelines suggested from content perspectives can go a long way toward increasing motivation in health care organizations.

MANAGERIAL GUIDELINES

1. Check employees' perceptions of the fairness of their work and rewards. Address perceived inequities as best as possible, given resource constraints. Unfortunately, perceptions of inequity are especially likely when managers try to take individuals' different needs into account.
2. Select rewards that are attractive to employees.
3. Make sure that the rules for attaining rewards are clear to everyone.
4. Make sure that people understand that their efforts will lead to the desired level of performance.
5. Reward people contingent on performance; try various reinforcement schedules to see what works best in your setting.
6. Set or encourage people to set goals that are difficult and specific; revise and update goals as necessary.
7. Provide timely and specific feedback to people on their progress toward goals.
8. Build commitment to goals by helping people believe that they can attain them and by selecting goals that are consistent with their values.

MOTIVATIONAL PROBLEMS

Nature and Causes

A major challenge for all health care organizations is to avoid employee motivation problems and to remedy such problems if they do occur. Despite their best efforts, most organizations do experience some problems of employee motivation. The symptoms may involve apathy, low quality work, and complaints from supervisors and patients.

The causes of motivational problems often fall into three categories. First, there may be inadequate performance definition. This means the employees do not fully understand what is expected of them. There is no clear definition of what is expected of employees nor any continuous orientation of employees toward effective job performance. Symptoms of this problem include a lack of goals, inadequate job descriptions, inadequate performance standards, and inadequate performance assessment.

Second, there may be impediments to employee performance. Among the most important of these may be bureaucratic or environmental obstacles, inadequate support or resources, and a mismatch between the employee's skills and job requirements. An example is a hospital experiencing significant understaffing in nursing. Since the nursing staff is probably overworked, stressed-out, and burned-out, efforts to provide a motivating environment will fail unless and until adequate staffing is provided.

Third, there may be inadequate performance-reward linkages. Rewards may be economic or noneconomic. Symptoms of this problem are inappropriate rewards that are not valued by employees, inadequate rewards for performance, delay in receipt of rewards, a low probability of receiving rewards, and inequity in the distribution of rewards.

Determining the specific causes of a particular employee motivation problem is difficult. The most effective approach is for health care executives to develop communication skills, interpersonal skills, and interview skills so that two-way communication with employees is continued. The emphasis is on listening and encouraging employees to speak frankly. As a result, the problems and frustrations of particular employees—both individuals and groups—are well-understood by both their immediate supervisors and higher-level managers. Many organizations have found that an upward communication system utilizing interviews has paid off in terms of reduced absenteeism and turnover, increased productivity, and higher profits.[73]

Employee attitude surveys can also be useful in collecting information about employee beliefs and attitudes as long as they are anonymous and there is assurance the results will be acted upon.[74,75] First, such surveys are valuable for identifying the problems and impediments to performance that need to be reviewed and modified. Second, they are useful for learning the value that employees attach to a number of different outcomes such as money, recognition, autonomy, and affiliation. Discrepancies between employee and management views provide a basis for exploring ways to modify employee beliefs or job conditions to create a better match of employee values and job attributes. Third, attitude surveys are useful for learning the nature of employee beliefs about contingencies. In particular, surveys should reveal the extent to which employee beliefs about expectancies and instrumentalities (i.e., probability of receiving reward and adequacy in meeting needs) match those managers believe exist for these employees. Unfortunately, this diagnosis of employee attitudes and needs is deficient in most health services organizations. One survey found only 43% of health care employees felt their organization seeks their opinions and suggestions. Worse yet, only 26% felt their organizations act on their input.[76]

Potential Solutions

Table 3.1 outlines the three motivational problems discussed in the beginning of this section together with potential solutions. It is important to recognize that most motivational problems have more than one cause and more than one solution. In fact, the latest theory and research suggest that successful employee motivation programs should include several integrated and mutually reinforcing motivational approaches.[77] At a minimum, these approaches should include positive reinforcement with behavior modification if necessary, high challenge or difficult goals, valued rewards contingent upon performance expectancy of success, employee feedback, employee involvement or participation, job redesign, and low situational constraints. The long-run goal should be to develop and retain a "culture of performance." Epic Healthcare is an example of one company's attempt to create such a culture.

In situations where motivational problems exist, the cause is often an inadequate linkage between performance and rewards valued by the employee (see Problem III of Table 3.1). One solution is *behavior modification,* a technique for applying the concepts of reinforcement theory in organizational settings.[78] First, the manager specifies behaviors that are to be increased or decreased. Then these target behaviors are measured to establish a baseline against which the

TABLE 3.1. Common Employee Motivation Problems and Potential Solutions

Motivational Problems	Potential Solutions
1. Inadequate performance definition (i.e., lack of goals, inadequate job descriptions, inadequate performance standards, inadequate performance assessment)	• Well-defined job descriptions • Well-defined performance standards • Goal-setting • Feedback on performance
2. Impediments to performance (i.e., bureaucratic or environmental obstacles, inadequate support or resources, poor employee-job matching)	• Improved employee selection • Job redesign or enrichment • Enhanced hygiene factors (i.e., safe and clean environment, salary and fringe benefits, job security, staffing, time-off-job, equipment)
3. Inadequate performance-reward linkages (i.e., inappropriate rewards, inadequate rewards, poor timing of rewards, low probability of receiving rewards, inequity in distribution of rewards)	• Behavior modification or positive reinforcement (individual or group) • Pay for performance • Enhanced achievement or growth factors (i.e., employee involvement-participation, job redesign or enrichment, career planning, professional development opportunities) • Enhanced esteem or power factors (i.e., autonomy or personal control, autonomous work teams, self-management, modified work schedule, recognition, praise or awards, opportunity to display skills or talents, opportunity to mentor or train others, promotions in rank or position, information concerning organization or department, preferred work activities or projects, letters of recommendation, preferred work space) • Enhanced affiliation or relatedness factors (i.e., work teams, task groups, business meetings, social activities, professional and community group participation, personal communication or leadership style)

IN THE REAL WORLD
EMPLOYEE MOTIVATION AT EPIC HEALTHCARE

Could you justify spending $6 million to achieve more than $20 million in savings or new revenue gains? That's the tradeoff executives of Epic Healthcare Group achieved when they offered $5 million in prizes to employees who made revenue-generating or money-saving suggestions.

Epic Excellence Ideas is one of several bonus and incentive programs intended to motivate workers within the employee-owned hospital chain. It is a grand-scale version of the traditional employee suggestion box. Of the 9,000 Epic employee-owners, 84% participated in the program. They joined 7-member teams at each of Epic's 38 hospitals. More than 5,000 ideas were generated, and 2,153 have been approved by the teams. They range from starting a substance-abuse outpatient program to converting an unused labor and delivery room to an outpatient surgery suite.

Each team provided financial analysis of its idea before presenting it to the hospital's Idea Action Committee composed of three to seven people. Ideas valued at more than $50,000 had to go through Epic's 4-member steering committee.

For accepted ideas, team members received credits redeemable for catalog merchandise. The eight teams receiving the most credits gained even greater rewards. Each team member and spouse were flown to St. Louis for a 60-second shopping spree at an electronic and consumer merchandise warehouse. The program was not only a morale booster, but it also honed the employees' teamwork, financial, and operational skills.

In addition to the Epic Excellence program, employees received incentive bonuses of $4.4 million for meeting or exceeding quality and financial performance objectives in 1989. These awards are now given annually.

SOURCE: Adapted from Lutz S. Employee suggestions net $20 million in savings. *Modern Healthcare.* 1990;20(9):21–22.

---

effectiveness of behavioral modification will be assessed. The manager then analyzes the situation to ascertain what rewards employees value most and how best to tie these rewards to the target behaviors. Next, rewards are given so that desired behaviors have pleasant consequences and undesirable behaviors have unpleasant consequences. Finally, the target behaviors are measured again to determine the value of the program.

The most publicized example of behavior modification has been at Emery Air Freight when management desired more efficient packing of large shipping containers. Through a system of self-recorded feedback and rewards, Emery increased container usage from 45% to 95% of capacity and saved over $3 million during the first three years of the program.[79]

One extension of behavior modification is *pay for performance*. This links the desired behavior or outcomes to one specific positive employee outcome—higher pay. During the past decade, pay for performance has boomed in popularity. Between 70% and 80% of U.S. companies offer some type of pay for performance incentive.[80] A 1991 survey indicated that almost half of more than 1,200 hospitals have implemented incentive-based pay systems, a fivefold increase since 1983.[81] However, in most cases it applies primarily or exclusively to management personnel.

One way to classify such plans is according to the level of performance targeted—individual, group, or total organization. Within these broad categories, literally hundreds of different approaches for relating pay to performance exist. Failure often occurs because the rewards are too small, the links between performance and rewards are weak, and supervisors resent performance appraisal.[82–84] Successful programs establish high standards of performance, develop accurate performance appraisal systems, train supervisors in the mechanics of performance appraisal and the art of giving feedback, and use a wide range of pay increases.

Well-conceived and well-designed pay-for-performance plans tend to work because they clearly articulate standards of performance and provide a strong motivation for employees to focus on meeting these standards. Health care administrators who have launched pay-for-performance plans have found them to have high employee acceptance and to be effective management tools for increasing cost efficiency, productivity, and quality of care.[85,86] The goals and performance standards that are rewarded have more intrinsic meaningfulness to employees if they are tied to the strategic goals of the organization.[87]

Unlike many Wall Street brokers who are motivated primarily by money, many health care workers choose their profession for reasons other than salary. Consequently, health care organizations need to identify and respond to a wide variety of noneconomic needs which may motivate their employees (see Table 3.1). There are a wide variety of employee involvement-participation programs that are based on the belief that employees at all levels in the organization can and will contribute useful insights to the effective functioning of the organization given an opportunity. The most common programs are gain-sharing suggestion systems, quality circles, union-management committees, total quality management programs, and autonomous work groups.[88,89] Employee participation in making critical job and organizational decisions is the one common element in all of these programs.

Employee involvement-participation appears to be highly-desired in health care organizations. Methodist Hospital in Houston surveys its employees annually. The most recent survey showed employees wanted higher salaries and more participation.[90]

Employees also desire participation linked to incentives. *Gainsharing* encourages employees to find ways to increase productivity and to cut costs in exchange for receiving a share of the savings realized. This has been very successful in motivating employees at Charity Health Care Systems in Cincinnati.[91] To be successful, gainsharing programs require top management to start disseminating relevant information and giving employees the time and tools to get involved.

Quality circles offer another employee involvement-participation option. A quality circle consists of a small number of volunteers, typically eight to ten nonmanagement employees from the same department, who meet a few hours each week to examine productivity and quality problems. Members identify a problem, study it, and present their recommendations for change to management. These problems often involve subtle difficulties that may be noticed only by those who actually perform the work.

The research results concerning the effectiveness of quality circles are mixed. In one recent review of the research, about half of the studies of quality circles reported uniformly positive results in all criteria (i.e., productivity, quality, absenteeism, and job attitudes).[92] One quarter of the studies found some beneficial effects, and the other quarter reported no beneficial changes. Similar mixed results have been found for quality circles in health care organizations.[93] Specific recommendations for increasing the probability of quality circle success include management support for genuine participation, a pilot program, a long-term view, modest expectations, willingness to adapt some proposals, training of participants, voluntary participation, defined scope and limit, and evaluation.[94]

Employee recognition programs offer another method of linking employee participation and rewards. Surveys of nonhealth employees show most believe simple positive feedback from management and recognition for a job well done serve as valued rewards capable of motivating employees.[95,96] Such feedback and recognition may also take more tangible forms as noneconomic award programs. Examples include trophies, wall plaques, certificates, letters or handwritten personal notes of thanks, visits or telephone calls by top executives, and luncheon invitations.[97] For such awards to be effective motivators, they must recognize only high-performing employees.

Job redesign is yet another strategy that can lead to increased intrinsic motivation (also see Chapter 7). It is based on the premise that altering certain aspects of the job to satisfy employees' psychological needs will motivate them to exert more effort. According to Hackman and Lawler, satisfaction of higher order needs (which is the essence of intrinsic motivation) occurs when the employee experiences these psychological states.[98] First, the job allows the employee to feel personally responsible for a significant segment of his work outcomes. Autonomy or personal control is the key job dimension contributing to feelings of personal responsibility for job outcomes. Second, the job involves doing something that is perceived as meaningful by the individual. The three core dimensions that can make jobs more meaningful are task identity (i.e., completion of a whole task), skill variety (i.e., utilization of different skills), and task significance (i.e., substantial impact). Third, the job provides the employee with knowledge of results. Feedback from the job itself or from another individual is the core job dimension which provides knowledge of results.

Job redesign aims to enrich a job so that the employee is more motivated to do the work. It is most appropriate when there is a demonstrated need to redesign jobs—for example, due to employee downtime, and it is feasible to redesign jobs given the present structure of jobs, legal constraints, technological constraints, and the characteristics and values of employees. Job redesign in health care is feasible but may be subject to more legal and professional constraints than most other industries.[99]

Job redesign may apply to either individual positions or to groups of employees. For employees with high growth needs, job redesign can pay off. Research in both nonhealth care organizations and health care organizations has generally supported the validity of the job characteristics model in enhancing employee motivation for employees who strongly value personal feelings of accomplishment and growth.[100,101] However, the actual success of any job redesign effort is likely to depend on other reinforcing or nonreinforcing factors such as the reward system and top management support.[102]

In terms of efficiency and practicality, some jobs can be done only by a group. An example is a surgical team in a hospital operating room. Anesthesiologist, surgeon, nurse, and technicians must work interdependently. This is true of most health care occupations. In fact, more organizations in general have implemented work redesign projects for *autonomous work groups* (AWGs) than for individuals.[103] These groups decide how members will work together. Generally when an AWG is created, the group members themselves control the planning and decision-making process within the group, select its own leader, and set its own quality and quantity output levels. AWGs provide opportuni-

ties for employees to exercise more control over their daily work life.

While research is sparse, there is some evidence of positive benefits such as job satisfaction and productivity in such groups.[104] The best known American success story is the Saturn General Motors Plant in Spring Hill, Tennessee where AWGs emphasize teamwork, efficient use of resources, and a tireless effort to improve quality.[105]

In contrast to employee involvement-participation approaches, AWGs involve participation together with changes in job design and organization design. This tends to affect more employees and create a longer-lasting impact on the organizational culture. The specific benefits of AWGs found in certain U.S. corporations include more integration of individual skills, better performance in terms of quantity and quality, reduced absenteeism and turnover, and a growing sense of confidence and accomplishment among team members.[106]

While a large number of experiments are now occurring in health care organizations, most are so recent that empirical evidence of the effectiveness of AWGs is not yet available. There is, however, some evidence to suggest that AWGs will increase employee involvement, commitment, and intrinsic motivation.[107]

Overall Assessment

As we have seen, there are many approaches to dealing with motivational problems among employees. None are foolproof. Whether a particular approach succeeds in a particular setting depends first on whether it was properly matched with the primary causes of low motivation. Second, it depends on how and whether the program was introduced and implemented so that resistance was minimized and commitment maximized. For example, favorable reaction is likely to be greatest if the affected employees have some voice in choosing and implementing a particular motivation program. Third, it depends on whether the program is compatible with other aspects of the organization's culture.[108,109] The simultaneous introduction of several mutually-supportive and mutually-reinforcing motivation programs are probably most effective in overcoming motivation problems, assuming they are

IN THE REAL WORLD

A VISION OF EXCELLENCE AT AMI PALMETTO GENERAL HOSPITAL

AMI Palmetto General Hospital in Hialeah, Florida, recently implemented the Visions of Excellence program to integrate employee relations, customer service, and commitment to patient care quality. Monthly themes and activities are designated by a Visions of Excellence committee to deliver messages to all employees regarding organization goals, communication, customers (i.e., physicians, patients, patient families), challenges, and excellence. Some successful themes and activities have been Physician Appreciation Month, Commitment Pledge Month, Employee Exchange Day, Patient Satisfaction Means Success, and the Employee Honor Roll.

The Visions committee originated as a voluntary task force with the mission of "redefining the organization's culture." This required management to commit to certain beliefs such as recognizing and rewarding employee contributions in a participative environment where individuals are treated with respect and allowed to participate in problem solving. The committee believes that employee commitment to the organization is more likely when all employees are rewarded for attaining specific goals in a participative environment.

Each level of management participates in a series of skills workshops on such topics as identifying supports and barriers to effective teamwork, sharing information, developing action plans based on strategic plans, productivity measures, and the service culture. The purpose of each workshop is to help managers develop mutual goals and plans to achieve success. Each level of management, in turn, is encouraged to train its own team in similar workshops so that everyone is part of the process.

Employees are asked what they want the organization to be and what they are willing to do to get it there. Employee responses are then integrated into the program document. Volume and quality indicators of performance that are clear and understandable to employees at all levels are preferable to complicated indicators. Each month several employees are selected from employee nominations for recognition as employee achievement award winners. The winner is given a plaque, cash, and a selected parking place for a month.

An employee relations program, a customer service program, and a commitment to excellence have a greater chance of long-term survival if they are interrelated. One of the three without the others will be lame. To expect employees to provide excellent customer service, top management must believe that how employees are treated will affect how they treat customers. Everyone on the organization serves an external customer or an internal customer. A commitment to excellence must be accompanied by an answer to the question, What's in it for me? The employee relations program and the reward system must answer that question. Likewise, good customer service is just window dressing without an excellent technical product to go along with it.

The Visions of Excellence program has demonstrated several benefits. Efficiency, productivity, service quality, employee morale, teamwork, and favorable letters from patients have increased. Costs, physician complaints, and turnover have decreased. The workforce has become focused on what needs to be done for success.

SOURCE: Adapted from Pujol JL, Tudanger E. A vision of excellence. *HRM Magazine.* 1992;35(6):112–116.

all relevant to the causes of the problem. An example is the program at AMI Palmetto Hospital.

Two reviews of the literature have compared the relative effectiveness of several motivation programs. One concluded that financial incentives were most effective, while goal setting was also quite effective.[110] Participative decision making and job redesign were relatively less certain to produce significant improvements. The other study suggested that employee training and goal setting were most likely to improve motivation or productivity, followed closely by changes such as AWGs and carefully designed financial incentives.[111] Job redesign is less powerful but still has a significant impact on productivity. This review also suggests that combined interventions are more effective than single-method approaches. Yet almost any of these approaches can be effective if they are matched to the motivational problem, are carefully implemented, involve all parties, and are implemented in a culture that emphasizes employee motivation and performance.

MANAGERIAL GUIDELINES

1. The major reasons for low employee motivation are lack of understanding concerning expectations, organizational impediments to performance, and lack of valued rewards for performance.
2. A variety of upward communication methods are available to assist health care managers in determining the nature and causes of employee motivation problems including direct supervisor communication, interviews, and employee attitude surveys.
3. Expectations can be clarified through well-defined job descriptions, performance standards, goal setting, and feedback on performances.
4. Motivational impediments can be removed by addressing relevant hygiene factors in the environment as well as better matching of employee and job through improved selection and job redesign.
5. Inadequate performance-reward linkages can be addressed through behavior modification, pay for performance, and provision of desired motivators related to achievement or growth or esteem or power needs of employees.

KEY CONCEPTS

Achievement
Affiliation
Autonomous Work
   Group
Behavior Modification
Belongingness Needs
Content vs. Process
   Motivation Theories
Equity
Esteem Needs
Existence
Expectancy
Gain Sharing
Goal Setting
Growth
Hygiene Factors
Instrumentality

Job Outcomes
Job Redesign
Motivation
Motivators
Need Hierarchy
Pay for Performance
Physiological Needs
Power
Quality Circles
Reinforcement
Relatedness
Security Needs
Self-actualization Needs
Self-actualization
Valence

Discussion Questions

1. How can content and process motivation theories best be combined in practice?
2. How can managers distinguish a motivational problem from other factors that affect an individual's performance?
3. How can motivational theories be used to select the best potential solution for a given individual's needs?

REFERENCES

1. Kanfer R. Motivation theory and industrial and organizational psychology. In: Dunnette MD, Houghin LM, eds. *Handbook of Industrial and Organizational Psychology*. Palo Alto, Ca: Consulting Psychologists Press, Inc.; 1990:75–170.
2. Steers RM, Porter LW. *Motivation and Work Behavior*. New York, NY: McGraw-Hill; 1987.
3. Mohr LB. *Explaining Organizational Behavior*. San Francisco, Ca: Jossey-Bass; 1982.
4. Steers and Porter, op. cit.
5. Muchinsky PM. *Psychology Applied to Work: An Introduction to Industrial and Organizational Psychology*. Belmont, Ca: Wadsworth, Inc.; 1987:341–378.
6. Kanfer, op. cit.
7. Davis-Blake A, Pfeffer J. Just a mirage: The search for disposition effects in organizational research. *Academy of Management Review*. 1989; 14(3):385–400.
8. Zima JP. *Interviewing: Key to Effective Management*. Chicago, Ill: Science Research Associates, Inc.; 1983.
9. Kovach KA. What motivates employees: Workers and supervisors give different answers. *Business Horizons*. 1987;30:58–65.
10. Maslow AH. A theory of human motivation. *Psychological Review*. 1943;50:370–396.
11. Pinder C. *Work Motivation*. Glenview, Ill: Scott, Foresman; 1984.
12. Steers and Porter, op. cit.
13. Schwartz HS. Maslow and the hierarchial enactment of organizational reality. *Human Relations*. 1983;36(10):933–956.
14. Wahba MA, Budwell LG. Maslow reconsidered: A review of research on the need hierarchy theory. *Organization Behavior and Human Performance*. 1976;15(2):317–333.
15. Mitchell V, Mowdgill P. Measurement of Maslow's need hierarchy. *Organization Behavior and Human Performance*. 1976;16(2):334–349.
16. Lee JA. *The Gold and Garbage of Management Theory and Prescriptions*. Athens, Oh: Ohio University Press; 1980.
17. Hurka SJ. Need satisfaction among health care managers. *Hospital and Health Services Administration*. 1980;25(3):43–54.
18. Alderfer CP. *Existence, Relatedness, and Growth*. New York, NY: Free Press; 1972.
19. Alderfer CP. An empirical test of a new theory of human needs. *Organization Behavior and Human Performance*. 1968;16(2):142–175.
20. Pinder, op. cit.
21. Herzberg F, Mausner B, Snyderman B. *The Motivation to Work*. New York, NY: John Wiley; 1959.
22. Herzberg F. One more time: How do you motivate employees? *Harvard Business Review*. 1987;65:109–120.
23. House RJ, Wigdor LA. Herzberg's two-factor theory of job satisfaction and motivation: A review of the evidence and a criticism. *Personnel Psychology*. 1967;20(3):369–389.
24. Vroom VH. *Work and Motivation*. New York, NY: John Wiley; 1964.
25. Pinder, op. cit.
26. Schwarb DP, Devitt WH, Cummings LL. A test of the adequacy of the two-factor theory as a predictor of self-report performance effects. *Personnel Psychology*. 1971;24:293–304.
27. Lee, op. cit., 101.
28. Steers and Porter, op. cit., 395.
29. Blayney KD, ed. *Healing Hands: Customizing Your Health Team for Institutional Survival*. Battle Creek, Mi: W.K. Kellogg Foundation; 1992.
30. Vaughan DG, Fottler MD, Bamberg R, Blayney K. Utilization and Management of multiskilled health practitioners in U.S. hospitals. *Hospital and Health Services Administration*. 1991;36(3):347–419.
31. McClelland DC. *The Achieving Society*. Princeton, NJ: Van Nostrand; 1961.
32. McClelland DC. *Power: The Inner Experience*. New York, NY: Irvington; 1975.
33. Atkinson JW. *An Introduction to Motivation*. New York, NY: Van Nostrand; 1961.
34. McClelland, *The Achieving Society*, op. cit.
35. McClelland DC, Burnham DH. Power is the great motivator. *Harvard Business Review*. 1976;54(2):100–110.
36. Cornelius E, Lane F. The power motive and managerial success in a professionally oriented service company. *Journal of Applied Psychology*. 1984;69:32–40.
37. Nicholls JG. Achievement motivation: Conceptions of authority, subjective experience, task chores, and performance. *Psychological Review*. 1984;91:328–346.
38. Kiechel W. The workaholic generation. *Fortune,* April 10, 1989:50–62.
39. Miron D, McClelland DC. The impact of achievement motivation in small business. *California Management Review*. 1979;22:34–46.
40. Eubanks P. Hospitals probe job candidates' values for organization fit. *Hospitals*. October 20, 1991;65(20):36–38.
41. Longest BB. Job satisfaction of registered nurses in a hospital setting. *Journal of Nursing Administration*. 1974;4(3):46–52.
42. Ford RC, Fottler MD. Studies of nurses attitudes during the 1980's: What have we learned? In: Ray DF,

ed. *Proceedings of the annual meeting of the Southern Management Association.* Mississippi State, Ms: Southern Management Association; 1992:130–132.

43. Farnham A. The trust gap. *Fortune.* December 4, 1989:56–78.

44. Reibstein L. A finger on the pulse: Companies expand use of employee surveys. *The Wall Street Journal.* October 27, 1986:27.

45. Chusmir LH. How fulfilling are health care jobs? *Health Care Management Review.* 1986;11(1):27–32.

46. Griffin RW. Effects of work redesign on employee perceptions, attitudes, and behavior: A long-term investigation. *Academy of Management Journal.* 1991;34(2):425–435.

47. Hackman JR, Oldham G. *Work redesign.* Reading, Mass: Addison-Wesley; 1980.

48. Durand DE. Modified achievement motivation training: A longitudinal study of the effects of a condensed training design for entrepreneurs. *Psychological Reports.* 1983;52:901–911.

49. Adams JS. Inequity in social exchange. In: Berkowitz L, ed. *Advances in Experimental Social Psychology, II.* New York, NY: Academic Press; 1965.

50. Campbell JP, Pritchard RD. Motivation theory in industrial and organizational psychology. In: Dunnette MD, ed. *Handbook of Industrial and Organizational Psychology.* Skokie, Ill: Rand McNally; 1976:63–130.

51. Greenberg J. Approaching equity and avoiding inequity in groups and organizations. In: Greenberg J, Cohen RL, eds. *Equity and Justice in Social Behavior.* New York, NY: Academic Press; 1982.

52. Muchinsky, op. cit.

53. Kanfer, op. cit.

54. Georgopoulos BS, Mahoney BS, Jones NW. A path-goal approach to productivity. *Journal of Applied Psychology.* 1957;41:345–353.

55. Vroom V. *Work and Motivation.* New York, NY: Wiley; 1964.

56. Mitchell TR. Motivation: New directions for theory, research, and practice. *Academy of Management Review.* 1982;7:80–88.

57. Muchinsky, op. cit.

58. Kennedy CW, Fossum JA, White BJ. An empirical comparison of within-subjects and between-subjects expectancy theory models. *Organizational Behavior and Human Performance.* 1983;32:124–143.

59. Weiner B. *An Attributional Theory of Motivation and Emotion.* New York, NY: Springer-Verlag; 1986.

60. Pritchard RD, De Leo PJ, Von Bergen CW. A field experimental test of expectancy-valence incentive motivation techniques. *Organizational Behavior and Human Performance.* 1976;15:355–406.

61. Skinner BF. *Contingencies of Reinforcement: A Theoretical Analysis.* New York, NY: Appleton-Century-Crofts; 1969.

62. Locke EA. Effects of knowledge of results, feedback in relation to standards, and goals on reaction-time performance. *American Journal of Applied Psychology.* 1968;81:566–574.

63. Locke EA, Latham GP. *Goal Setting: A Motivational Technique that Works.* Englewood Cliffs, NJ: Prentice Hall; 1984.

64. Locke EA, Latham GP. *A Theory of Goal Setting and Task Performance.* Englewood Cliffs, NJ: Prentice Hall; 1990.

65. Muchinsky, op. cit.

66. Locke, Latham, op. cit., 1990.

67. Erez M, Zidon I. Effect of goal acceptance on the relationship of goal difficulty to performance. *Journal of Applied Psychology.* 1984;69:69–78.

68. Locke EA, Latham GP, Erez M. The determinants of goal commitment. *Academy of Management Review.* 1988;13:23–39.

69. Locke, Latham, op. cit., 1990.

70. Becker LJ. Joint effect of feedback and goal setting on performance: A field study of residential energy conservation. *Journal of Applied Psychology.* 1978;63:428–433.

71. Locke EA. Relation of goal level to performance with a short work period and multiple goal levels. *Journal of Applied Psychology.* 1982;67:512–514.

72. Hollenbeck JR, Klein HJ. Goal commitment and the goal-setting process: Problems, prospects, and proposals for future research. *Journal of Applied Psychology.* 1987;82:212–220.

73. Imberman W. Letting the employee speak his mind. *Personnel.* 1976;53(6):12–22.

74. York DR. Attitude surveying. *Personnel Journal.* 1985;64(5):70–73.

75. Taglinferri LE. Taking note of employee attitudes. *Personnel Administrator.* 1988;33(4):96–102

76. Lutz S. Hospitals stretch their creativity to motivate workers. *Modern Healthcare.* 1990;20(9):20–33.

77. Locke EA, Latham GP. Work motivation and satisfaction: Light at the end of the tunnel. *Psychological Science.* 1990;1(4):240–246.

78. Luthans F, Kreitney R. *Organization Behavior Modification and Beyond: An Operant Conditioning Approach.* Glenview, Ill: Scott, Foresman; 1985.

79. At Emery Air Freight: Positive reinforcement boosts performance. *Organizational Dynamics.* 1973:41–50.

80. Waldman S, Roberts B. Grading "merit pay." *Newsweek.* Nov. 14, 1988, Vol. 112, 45–46.

81. Rondeau KV. Pay for performance: Compensating senior executives. *Trustee.* 1992;45(1):12–13.

82. Labor letter. *The Wall Street Journal.* February 20, 1980:A1.

83. Lawler EE. Pay for performance: A strategic analysis. In: Gomez-Mejia LR, ed. *Compensation and Benefits.* Washington, D.C.: Bureau of National Affairs; 1989;3:136–181.

84. Rollins T. Pay for performance: The pros and cons. *Personnel Journal.* 1987;66(5):104–107.

85. Berger S, Moyer J. Launching a performance-based pay plan. *Modern Healthcare.* 1991;21(33):64.

86. Wagner RG. Merit pay as a motivational tool in healthcare. *Hospital Topics.* 1988;66(6):10–15.

87. Fottler MD, Blair JD, Phillips RL, Duran CA. Achieving competitive advantage through strategic human resources management. *Hospital and Health Services Administration.* 1990;35(3):341–363.

88. Lawler EE. Choosing an involvement strategy. *Academy Of Management Executive.* 1988;2(3):197–204.

89. Cotton JL, Volrath DA, Frogett KL, Lengnick-Hall MD, Jennings KR. Employee participation: Diverse forms and different outcomes. *Academy of Management Review.* 1988;13(1):8–22.

90. Lutz, op. cit., 32.

91. Eubanks P. Gainsharing gives employees rewards for innovations. *Hospitals.* 1991;65(1):46–47.

92. Barrick MR, Alexander RA. A review of quality circle efficacy and the existence of a positive finding bias. *Personnel Psychology.* 1987;40(4):579–592.

93. Phillips RL, Duran CA, Blair JD, Peterson MF, Savage GT, Whitehead CJ. Quality circles in health-care organizations: Pitfalls and promises. In: Metzger H, ed. *Handbook of Healthcare Human Resources Management.* Rockville, Md: Aspen Systems; 1990:137–146.

94. Ibid.

95. Rawlinson H. Make awards count. *Personnel Journal.* 1988;67(10):139–146.

96. Koch J. Perpetual thanks: Its assets. *Personnel Journal.* 1990;69(1):72–73.

97. Huseman RC, Hatfield JD. *Managing the Equity Factor.* Boston, Mass: Houghton-Mifflin; 1989.

98. Hackman JR, Oldham GR. *Work Redesign.* Reading, Mass: Addison-Wesley; 1980.

99. Blayney, op. cit.

100. Guzzo RA, Jette RD, Katzell RA. The effects of psychologically based intervention programs on worker productivity: A meta analysis. *Personnel Psychology.* 1985;38(3):275–291.

101. Alpander GG. Relationship between commitment to hospital goals and job satisfaction: A case study of a nursing department. *Health Care Management Review.* 1990;15(4):51–62.

102. Fried Y, Ferris GR. The validity of the job characteristics model: A review and meta analysis. *Personnel Psychology.* 1987;40(3):287–322.

103. Wall TD, Kemp NJ, Jackson PR, Clegg WW. Outcomes of autonomous work groups: A long-term field experiment. *Academy of Management Journal.* 1986;29(2):280–304.

104. Ibid.

105. Gwynne SC. The right stuff. *Time.* October 29, 1990:74–84.

106. Bassin M. Teamwork at General Foods: New and improved. *Personnel Administrator.* 1988;33(5):62–70.

107. Alpander, op. cit.

108. Hames DS. Productivity-enhancing work innovations: Remedies for what ails hospitals? *Hospital and Health Services Administration.* 1991;38(4):545–557.

109. Mohrmann SA, Lawler EE. Quality of worklife. *Research in Personnel and Human Resources Management.* 1984;2:219–260.

110. Locke, op. cit., 1982.

111. Guzzo, et. al., op. cit.

CHAPTER

4

LEADERSHIP:
A FRAMEWORK
FOR THINKING
AND ACTING

Dennis D. Pointer, Ph.D.
Professor
Julianne P. Sanchez
Ph.D. Student

CHAPTER TOPICS

Core Concepts
Leadership Effectiveness and Success:
  What We Know
Leadership: An Integrative Framework
Several Distinctive Aspects of Leading in
  Health Services Organizations

LEARNING OBJECTIVES

After completing this chapter, the reader should be able to

1. better appreciate why leadership skills are so important
2. understand what leadership is and what it is not
3. understand the distinction between management and leadership
4. understand the leadership role and how it is executed in health services organizations
5. understand the major leadership perspectives as well as some emerging theories and concepts
6. consider how different leadership perspectives can be combined into a more integrative framework
7. appreciate several distinctive challenges of leading in health services organizations
8. continue developing leadership knowledge and skills

CHAPTER PURPOSE

We want to help you gain an understanding of one of the most fundamental concepts in organization and management theory: LEADERSHIP. Leadership is one of the most important things managers do. It is the means by which things are accomplished in organizations. A manager can establish goals, strategize, relate to others, communicate, collect information, make decisions, plan, organize, monitor, and control; but nothing happens without leadership.

In this chapter we will first explore the concept of leadership. As the exercise presented by the consultant may have demonstrated, leadership is very difficult to get a firm grip on. Second, we will describe what scholars working in the field have come to know about the factors related to leadership effectiveness and success. Third, we will develop an integrative model of leadership. Our objective is to blend together key features of the different perspec-

IN THE REAL WORLD

WE'RE SEARCHING FOR A LEADER, BUT WE MAY NOT FULLY UNDERSTAND WHAT LEADERSHIP IS!

You are a board member of a 250-bed short-term general hospital that has just begun the process of working with an executive search consultant to recruit a new Chief Executive Officer (CEO). The present occupant of the position will be voluntarily retiring in five months after 23 years of service. The headhunter has a unique background. She holds a Ph.D. in organization behavior and taught this subject in a health administration program for ten years prior to starting her own executive search firm. In addition to all of the other types of experience, knowledge and skills necessary for being a successful hospital CEO, the board wants to recruit someone who is an "exceptional leader." They have communicated this desire to the search consultant and selected her because they felt she could help them find such a person.

The consultant is meeting with board members, over dinner, for the first time since being

retained. While coffee and dessert are being served, she begins talking with the board about why they feel leadership ability is so important in this search. She concludes by saying, "If we are going to locate someone with the type of leadership style and skills you want, we've got to have a shared notion of just what it is we are looking for. If you all define leadership in different ways and have varying ideas about what an exceptional leader is, we're in for some difficulties as this process unfolds. I have a few questions that I want you to think about. Take the next ten minutes to jot down some notes on a piece of paper. Don't feel like you have to compose elegant prose; just go for substance. This exercise may seem a bit academic. Indeed, I asked these questions of students before we began the leadership module in my organization behavior and management course at the university. During the years I have taught this material, I've found that they're very helpful in getting people to begin thinking a bit more rigorously about leadership. Let me warn you up front that these are not easy questions to answer. After you're finished, we will spend the next half hour or so discussing your ideas."

Here are the questions.

- What is leadership? Rough out a 1- or 2-sentence definition that captures the essence of the term.
- Is leadership synonymous with management, or is leading just one of many things that a manager does? In what ways are they different, or how are they the same?
- Think of some individuals whom you feel are really exceptional leaders. What, if anything, do they have in common?
- Think of some individuals who are truly lousy leaders. What, if anything, do they have in common?
- How does leadership affect the performance of what's being led (whether it's an individual, a group, or an entire organization)? That is, in what ways does leadership make a difference?
- Have you ever known people who were successful leaders in one situation and failures in others? Why is this so?

To our readers: Pause a few moments, take out a piece of paper and answer these questions. We realize that it's far easier not to expend the effort and just press ahead. However, prior to being exposed to our thinking about leadership, we feel it's important that you clarify your own. You might want to share your answers, and frustrations in composing them, with fellow students. One of the real benefits of this exercise is gaining an appreciation of how varied peoples' notions of leadership are. Save your responses to these questions. You will want to look at them again after you've completed this chapter.

tives that have been presented in the literature. Fourth, we will discuss several distinctive aspects of leadership in health service organizations. Finally, we will offer some suggestions regarding how you can continue improving your leadership knowledge and skills.

CORE CONCEPTS

Can you imagine the following ad being run in the "Help Wanted" section of *Modern Healthcare*?

Of course not!

Leadership is one of the most highly valued management abilities. Health services organizations and their assortment of divisions, departments, units, and groups are presumed to thrive under great leadership and face considerable difficulty or even fail when it's poor. Everyone is on the lookout for those who have the ability to lead. People who can convince others they are leaders generally get hired and promoted. Managers without the leadership "right stuff," no matter how good they are at performing other aspects of their jobs, often face career stagnation or, worse yet, find themselves looking for a different position and maybe even a new line of work. Think for a moment about yourself. How would you like to be tagged as a non-leader or someone who has no leadership potential? How would this label affect your ability to either get or keep a management position, irrespective of level, in a health services organization?

As important as leadership seems to be, when asked to define and describe it, people seem to have trouble. Perhaps you experienced difficulty when attempting to answer the first questions in the opening case. Leadership is one of the most elusive management concepts. Here's how one major textbook in the field approaches a definition.

> It is neither feasible nor desirable at this point in the development of the discipline to resolve the controversy over the appropriate definition of leadership. For the time being, it is better to use the various conceptions of leadership as a source of different perspectives on a complex, multifaceted phenomenon.[1]

Hardly adequate! The inability to define something makes it nearly impossible to study it, learn about it, or improve one's ability to do it.

We want to begin by presenting a very stripped-down definition of leadership including only the essentials with which most scholars working in the field would have little disagreement. Leadership is the process through which an individual attempts to intentionally influence another individual or a group in order to accomplish a goal.

Simple enough, but the core concepts embedded in this seemingly simple sentence warrant some emphasis and elaboration. First, leadership is a process. It is a verb, an action word, not a noun. Leadership manifests itself in the doing; it is a performing art. Second, only individuals lead. The *locus of leadership* is in a person. Inanimate objects don't lead, groups don't lead, organizations don't lead; only people lead. When looking for and at leadership, our subject is the individual. Third, the *focus of leadership* is other individuals and groups. Leadership can't exist absent this connection between someone who is leading and those who, for whatever reason, choose to follow. The follower might be just one other person, a group, members of an organization, or the population of a nation. Fourth, leadership entails influencing. *Influence* is leadership's center of gravity and most critical element. Who is influenced? Followers (individuals and groups), as we've just noted, are influenced. What is influenced? The cognitive target of influence is their thoughts; the affective target is their feelings; and the behavioral target is their actions or deeds. For what purpose are followers influenced? This brings us to our fifth point; the objective of leadership is *goal accomplishment*. Leadership is instrumental; it is done for a purpose. Sixth, and last, leadership is intentional; it's not accidental. All of us unknowingly influence others hundreds of times each day. These, however, are not acts of leadership; they are just "happenings."

We think our definition is precise and useful, but it can be pointed in many directions. Leadership is exercised in a lot of different places and in a wide variety of situations. For example, you are engaged in leadership when attempting to persuade that person sitting next to you in accounting to join you at the student center for lunch after class. Keep in mind, all of the key elements are here—you, the locus of leadership; that person, the follower; and an act of intentional influence in order to accomplish a goal. We are interested, however, in a particular type of leadership—that engaged in by managers in organizations. To further develop our definition, we need to briefly explore this context.

Organizations exist to accomplish tasks that are so large or complex that they can't be undertaken by individuals and small groups. They do this by sequentially subdividing work over and over again. For example, the delivery of acute inpatient care in a community is a task that is so large and complex an organization must undertake it. A hospital assumes this task and proceeds to divide it up. Nursing services does some parts of it, ancillary services does other parts, professional services does others, and so on. For example, the delivery of nursing care is also such a large and complex task that it too must be subdivided. It is parceled out among different divisions (e.g., medicine, surgery, pediatrics, obstetrics/gynecology). Thus, organizations sequentially subdivide tasks until they are small and simple enough to be performed by an individual. In the process the hospital is divided into a series of components, all of which must be managed.

Figure 4.1 presents a schematic organizational chart typical of a short-term general hospital. We've focused on one segment of a vertical slice that is composed of four components. In each component there is a *managerial office,* associated with which are sets of expectations called *roles.* Roles are constellations of things managers are expected to do because they hold the office.[2] Roles are attached to the office, not the particular person occupying it. Occupants of the office may come and go, but the roles remain; and they remain the same. There are a wide variety of ways to describe the roles of a manager, several models of which were presented in Chapter 2. The critical point is that leadership is only one of the many roles managers are expected to perform because of the office they hold in the organization. Leadership and management

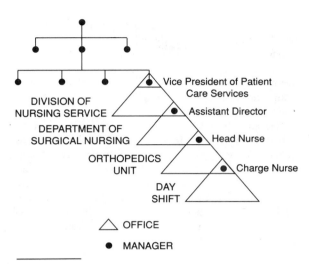

Vice President of Patient Care Services

DIVISION OF NURSING SERVICE

Assistant Director

DEPARTMENT OF SURGICAL NURSING

Head Nurse

ORTHOPEDICS UNIT

Charge Nurse

DAY SHIFT

△ OFFICE

● MANAGER

FIGURE 4.1. Organizational components and managerial offices.

are not the same thing; they aren't synonyms. This is an irrefutable and terribly important notion. Keep the concepts of manager (an individual who holds an office attached to which are multiple roles), and leadership (one of these roles) straight. A lot of folks don't, and it leads to considerable confusion.

Execution of the *leadership role* is the way managers get things done; if this is absent or performed poorly, the organization is impaired. While leadership is not the only role of the manager, it is certainly the central one. Other roles such as information processing, decision making, and visioning are converted into tangible results by leading.

Put Figure 4.1 under a magnifying glass and you have Figure 4.2. It focuses on one managerial office in the hospital's chain of command, an assistant director of nursing service. This manager is a subordinate in one component of the organization (the division of nursing service), reports to a vice president, and is a peer of others having the same reporting relationship. Simultaneously, the manager holds a superordinate office in that component of the organization for which he is responsible, the department of surgical nursing. Reporting to the assistant director are other managers (head nurses), each of whom is responsible for a different unit.

We will use this one office as an illustration to introduce several key points about leadership. First, leadership is multidirectional. The assistant director leads not only subordinates in the component of the organization of which he is the manager but also peers, his superior, and individuals or groups outside of the organization. Only when we conceptualize leadership as intentional influence and when the proper distinction between managing and leadership is drawn does this notion become clear. For example, the assistant director of nursing intentionally influences or leads (but does not manage) his peers in chairing a departmental work group to implement a new scheduling system and his superior in providing direction prior to an upcoming budget review and negotiation session with the hospital's chief operating officer. Additionally, he might engage in the leadership role when working with individuals and groups outside of the organization such as suppliers, physician office staffs, and colleagues in other organizations. Not only does the assistant director lead in all directions, he is simultaneously led from these same directions—from above by his superior, from the side by peers, from below by subordinates, and from outside the organization. Leadership's arrows of influence point in two directions simultaneously.

Second, although leadership is multidirectional, it's the downward focus that has received the greatest amount of attention and study. When one thinks of leadership, the first thing that generally comes to mind is the relationship between managers and their subor-

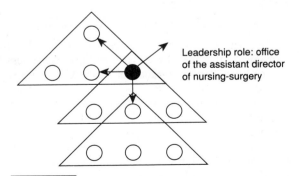

Leadership role: office of the assistant director of nursing-surgery

FIGURE 4.2. Directionality of the manager's leadership role.

dinates. The vast majority of leadership research (which we will review in the next section) has this focus. Most leadership is pointed downward, primarily towards one's direct reports (in the case of the assistant director, head nurses) and secondarily towards subordinates in lower and lower layers of the organization.

Third, when one engages in leadership, irrespective of its direction, the focus is generally other managers. In our illustration, it's only at the level of the charge nurse that nonmanagers are led. For the most part, managers lead other managers.

Fourth, the extent to which leadership attempts are successful depends on the amount of *power* associated with a particular managerial office and the person holding it. Leadership, influence, power, and *authority* are interrelated concepts. The latter three are the focus of Chapter 9, but we need to address them briefly here. Power is influence potential. The more power a person possesses, the greater is the potential she will be able to influence another individual or a group. The key concept here is potential; one can have appreciable amounts of power and not use it. Leadership, on the other hand, is actual influence, or power in use. Power can come from many sources. An important one in organizations is the office held, where power is the result of formal authority. Some other sources of power are information, knowledge, skills, abilities, and experience (expert power); connections with other individuals and groups who possess power (referent power); control of incentives (reward or coercive power); and one's own persona (charismatic power).

LEADERSHIP EFFECTIVENESS AND SUCCESS: WHAT WE KNOW

We turn now to reviewing what is known about those factors that are related to leadership effectiveness and success. The importance of this issue is underscored by the following two questions which scholars in the field have been trying to help practicing managers answer for almost half a century: If you want to select an effective and potentially successful leader, what should you look for and at? If you want to improve your own leadership effectiveness and success, what factors should you focus upon?

As noted in Debate Time 4.1, there are several ways to go about answering these questions. The vast major-

ity of the theorizing and research on leadership can be classified into three different perspectives—trait, behavioral, and contingency.[3] These perspectives are described below along with the review of some of the major studies that have been undertaken in each. Additionally, several emerging leadership theories and concepts are introduced.

Readers should note that what follows is not an exhaustive review of the literature. The objective is to provide you with an introductory tour of the leadership terrain with key references provided for those who wish to explore the area further. Also, none of the basic work within these perspectives has been conducted in health services organizations. So, for the rest of this section, bear with us as the foundation is laid for later application to health services.

The Trait Perspective

Since individuals lead, it's natural and reasonable to look for those characteristics of individuals that might separate successful from unsuccessful leaders or effective from ineffective leadership. And, indeed, this is where the search began. Early work on the *trait perspective* was biographical and focused almost exclusively on military commanders and those holding political office. In the late 1930s psychologists became interested in the area and began investigating relationships between individual characteristics and leadership effectiveness in organizations. Even though critiques of this work in the 1940s suggested that such relationships were weak and not generalizable across different situations, the hunt continued.[4] Every attribute imaginable has been studied.[5]

The most comprehensive review of this literature was conducted by Roger Stodgill in his classic work *Handbook of Leadership*.[6] Stodgill examined 287 studies undertaken from 1904 through 1970. He classified the hundreds of different traits that had been studied into six categories: physical (e.g., age, height, appearance); personality (e.g., self-confidence, independence, dominance); intelligence (e.g., fluency, decisiveness); social background (e.g., educational attainment, social status); social (e.g., cooperativeness, integrity); and task-related (e.g., initiative, persistence, need for achievement).[7]

Stodgill and others were able to identify a small number of traits that seemed to be present in leaders,

DEBATE TIME 4.1: WHAT DO YOU THINK?

At this point you should have a fairly clear idea of what leadership is and what it is not in addition to possessing a better feel for the organizational context in which the role is performed by managers. It's clear that all managers are not equally effective or successful leaders. The question is, What sets of factors explain the variability? There has been a raging debate regarding this issue in the literature during the last 50 years or so. There are three very different points of view. What's yours?

The nature argument:

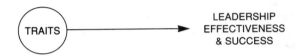

The greatest proportion of the variability in leadership effectiveness and success is due to traits and dispositions that individuals are endowed with at birth or that they develop very early in life. By the time a person assumes a management position, these characteristics are set and nearly impossible to change in any significant way. Some people have traits that predispose them to be successful leaders; others don't.

The nurture argument:

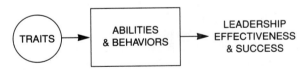

The greatest proportion of the variability in leadership effectiveness and success is due to abilities and behaviors that can be learned. Personal traits and dispositions provide the foundation upon which abilities are acquired and behaviors are developed, but they are only

the foundation. Individuals who are exceptional leaders make themselves; they are not made.

The situational argument:

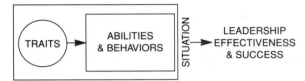

The greatest proportion of the variation in leadership effectiveness and success is due to the characteristics of the situation in which managers find themselves. Sets of traits, abilities, and behaviors are important, but they are very situation-specific. In one situation certain traits, abilities, and behaviors may predispose a manager to be an effective leader; in a different situation the result could be ineffectiveness and failure.

- If you agree with the nature argument, which personal traits and dispositions are most associated with leadership effectiveness and success?
- If you agree with the nurture argument, which abilities and behaviors are most associated with leadership effectiveness and success? What are the best ways to acquire these abilities and develop these behaviors?
- If you agree with the situational argument, which factors are most important?
- Think back for a moment to the opening case. Let's say that each of the three members of the board search committee agrees with a different argument. What would be the consequences?
- People often espouse a situational argument. However, their actual "theory in use" is generally a blend of the nature and nurture arguments. Do you find this to be the case, and if so why?

as compared to followers, and good leaders, as compared to poor ones.[8] Intelligence, dominance, self-confidence, high energy level, and task relevant knowledge were on most lists. However, the findings were inconsistent and relationships were weak; correlation coefficients generally ranged from 0.20 to 0.35. We could spend pages reviewing the different studies, describing their findings, and noting their limitations, but the "bottom line" is that there are no individual traits that predict leadership effectiveness or success, or which differentiate those who lead from those who follow.[9]

It is hard to argue that individual traits have no effect whatsoever on leadership effectiveness and success, as it is counter to experience, logic, and common sense. Researchers began to appreciate that traits had an impact, but not in the way originally imagined. First, traits are best thought of as predispositions. A particular trait, or set of them, tend to predispose (although do not cause) an individual to engage in certain behaviors which may or may not result in leadership effectiveness. Traits and behaviors are only loosely coupled. Second, multiple traits are associated with a given behavior, and more than one behavior is linked to an individual trait. Third, it is one's behavior and not one's traits *per se* that is most related to leadership effectiveness and success. "What seems to be most important is not traits but rather how they are expressed in the behavior of the leader."[10] These three observations go a long way in explaining why a set of universal leadership traits has not been uncovered; yet research employing this perspective continues.[11]

The Behavioral Perspective

Interest in leadership behaviors emerged due to the inability of traits to explain variations in effectiveness. Researchers reasoned that, if traits couldn't explain such variations, maybe the behaviors that flowed from them could. Most of the work has focused on identifying dimensions that could be employed to describe and categorize different leadership behaviors, developing models of leadership style (a style being defined by a combination of behaviors), and examining how specific leadership styles are related to effectiveness. Additionally, behaviorists began to develop more rigorous ways to conceptualize and measure leadership effectiveness.

The first study recognized as employing a *behavioral perspective* was conducted by Kurt Lewin, Ronald Lippitt, and their associates at the University of Iowa in the 1930s.[12] They compared three styles of leadership—autocratic, democratic, and laissez-faire—in groups of preteen boys. Leaders of the groups were confederates of the researchers and instructed on how to perform the various styles. Democratic leaders coordinated activities of the group and facilitated majority rule decision making on important decisions; autocratic leaders directed the activities of the group and made important decisions absent input from members; laissez-faire leaders (who accidentally emerged during the course of the study) provided neither facilitation nor direction. This work was significant because it focused on behavior rather than traits, identified and described different leadership styles, and found that variations in style had an impact on followers.

There were several major studies of leadership undertaken immediately after the conclusion of World War II; one of the most widely cited was conducted by a group of investigators at Ohio State University.[13] The question addressed was, How does the behavior of a leader impact upon work group performance and satisfaction? Instruments were designed to measure leadership behavior as perceived by managers themselves, in addition to their peers, superiors, and subordinates. Two dimensions of leader behavior were identified: *initiating structure,* or the degree a manager defined and organized the work that was to be done and the extent attention was focused on accomplishing objectives established by the manager; and *consideration,* or the extent the manager exhibited concern for the welfare of the group and its members, stressed the importance of job satisfaction, expressed appreciation, and sought input from subordinates on major decisions. Initiating structure and consideration were not conceptualized as opposite ends of the same continuum, but rather separate and independent dimensions. A manager's behavior could range from high to low on both. As depicted in Figure 4.3, the two dimensions combine to form four distinct leadership styles. Researchers hypothesized that group performance would be maximized when a manager had a leadership style that was high on both consideration and initiating structure. However, numerous follow-up studies found little consistency between the type of leadership style and group satisfaction or performance.[14,15] As with the trait research, it appeared that some other factor was confounding results. One criticism of this work was that managers' perceptions of their own leadership style and those of peers, superiors, and subordinates were often dissimilar.[16]

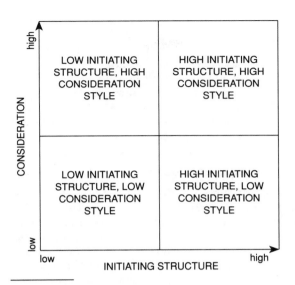

FIGURE 4.3. Ohio leadership study: Behaviors and styles.

In related work, Rensis Likert and colleagues at the University of Michigan specified two leadership behaviors: job-centered and employee-centered.[17] They were defined similar to consideration and initiating structure in the Ohio studies. Investigations conducted in a wide variety of industries found that effective supervisors were employee-centered and focused on the needs of the group in addition to establishing high performance goals jointly determined by leaders and followers.[18,19]

While the Ohio and Michigan studies provided the theoretical underpinning for the behavioral perspective, several other works are frequently referred to in most reviews of this literature.

Blake and Mouton drew upon previous research and formulated the *managerial grid* popularized in their book of the same name.[20] Their model, originally developed as a consulting tool, was extensively employed in leadership development programs during the 1960s and 1970s. The grid has two dimensions: production orientation and people orientation. In expressing a production orientation, leadership behaviors are directive and focused on accomplishing assigned objectives and tasks. In expressing a people orientation, leadership behaviors focus on enhancing the quality of manager-follower and follower-follower interactions. The model suggests that a manager's be-

havior can range from low to high on both dimensions, resulting in five different leadership styles.

- *High production and low people oriented style:* Leadership behavior focuses exclusively on goal and task accomplishment, and maximizing productivity through explicit direction and tight control.
- *High production and high people oriented style:* Leadership behavior is goal and task centered but seeks a high degree of follower involvement.
- *Low production and high people orientation:* Leadership behavior focuses on creating fulfilling relationships even if goal and task accomplishment suffer.
- *Low production and low people orientation:* Leadership behavior is focused on neither goal and task accomplishment nor on fulfilling the needs of followers; minimal energy is expended on execution of the leadership role.
- *Moderate production and moderate people orientation:* Leadership behavior focuses on balancing goal and task accomplishment, and follower need fulfillment.

Blake and Mouton contended that the high production and high people oriented style was most effective and resulted in the best outcomes (group productivity and satisfaction) irrespective of the situation faced. Little research supports this assertion, but there is some evidence that this style is preferred by managers and perceived by them to be most effective.[21]

Robert Tannenbaum and Warren Schmidt portrayed leadership behavior as a *continuum* that ranged from manager-centered to follower-centered.[22] In the manager-centered style, considerable authority is exercised and followers have little opportunity to participate in making decisions that affect them; leadership behavior is autocratic and directive. In the follower-centered style, the manager exercises a minimum amount of authority, and followers have considerable freedom to set their own goals and determine how tasks should be executed; leadership behavior is democratic and participative. Tannenbaum and Schmidt, contrary to previous models, conceptualized leadership behavior as bipolar. One was either manager-centered, follower-centered, or somewhere in between. The authors explicitly stated that there was no one style that would be equally effective in all situations. Additionally, they noted that the effectiveness of a particular style depended upon three factors: characteristics of the manager (e.g., their traits or dispositions, skills, and values), characteristics of followers (e.g., their skills, knowledge, experience; readiness to assume responsibility, understanding of goals and tasks), and characteristics of the situation (e.g., time availability, nature of the problem). This model underscored that leadership effectiveness depended on contingencies and suggested some important ones. However, it did not specifically indicate how a manager should go about selecting the most effective style in a specific circumstance. Below, we summarize the important components of the behavioral perspective.

Leadership behavior focused on the objectives to be accomplished and the tasks to be performed	Autocratic Initiating structure Job centered Production orientation Manager centered	Iowa study Ohio study Michigan study Managerial grid Leadership continuum
Leadership behavior focused on fulfilling follower needs and facilitating participation	Democratic Consideration Employee centered People orientation Follower centered	Iowa study Ohio study Michigan study Managerial grid Leadership continuum

The Contingency Perspective

In the early 1960s it became increasingly apparent that variations in leadership effectiveness and success could not be adequately explained by either traits or behaviors. Attention turned to incorporating situational characteristics, or *contingencies,* into leadership models. Recall that this notion was first forwarded in the 1940s. A number of leadership contingency models have been developed. We will introduce you to only

three of them here: leadership match, path-goal, and leadership effectiveness and adaptability (LEAD). This selection is made because the leadership match and path-goal models have been the subject of considerable empirical research, and the LEAD model has been extensively employed as a teaching and leadership development tool. We will conclude this section with a discussion of attribution theory which deals with the manager as a contingency.

Leadership Match Model

The first comprehensive contingency model of leadership was developed by Fred Fiedler. His model is complex, and only a highly simplified description of it is provided here. Readers interested in a more thorough treatment should refer to the original sources.[23-25] The underlying notion of this model is that managers are unable to alter their style to any appreciable degree. Leadership effectiveness depends not on fitting one's style to the situation but rather on selecting a situation that is conducive to one's style.[26]

Based on behavioral studies, two leadership styles were specified: task-oriented and employee-oriented. Fiedler developed a unique and controversial way in which to measure them. After completing a 20-item questionnaire, a person was assigned a least preferred co-worker (LPC) score. The score reflected the degree of regard a respondent held for that co-worker she preferred least. Managers with low LPC scores (disregard for the least preferred worker) were classified as having a task-oriented leadership style. Managers with a high LPC score (favorable evaluations of the co-worker they least preferred) were classified as possessing an employee-oriented style.

Fiedler identified three situational factors: manager-follower relationship, which could be good or poor; task structure, which could be either high or low; and manager position power, ranging from strong to weak. The combined effect of these three factors produce situations that are favorable, moderately favorable, or unfavorable to the manager.

Based upon studies conducted with hundreds of groups in a variety of organizations, it was determined that managers with a task-oriented leadership style were most effective in situations that were either favorable or unfavorable. Managers with an employee-oriented leadership style did better in situations that were moderately favorable. However, there have been a number of criticisms of this work, including questions regarding the validity of the LPC questionnaire and concerns that situational factors and leadership style may not be independent of one another.[27,28]

Path-Goal Model

The *path-goal leadership model* is based on the expectancy theory of motivation discussed in Chapter 3.[29,30] Expectancy theory is interested in the factors that affect an individual's choice of behavior, or why someone is motivated to do one thing rather than another. The focus is on effort, performance, rewards, motivation, and the relationships between them (expectancies, instrumentalities, and valences). While the expectancy theory of motivation focuses on describing such relationships, the path-goal model of leadership is interested in the factors that effect them. Initial formulation of this model was forwarded by Martin Evans in the early 1970s and then refined by Robert House and Terrance Mitchell. It has undergone constant revision over the years.[31-34]

From the perspective of the path-goal model, the manager exercises influence to increase the motivation of a follower attempting to accomplish a specific goal, in a particular context, during a finite period of time. As depicted in Figure 4.4, a follower's level of motivation is a result of her perceptions of expectancies, instrumentalities, and valences. Such perceptions are affected by three sets of contingencies: leadership behavior or style, features of the work environment, and characteristics of the follower.

In most leadership situations, follower characteristics and features of the work environment are not under the direct control of the manager; in the short run, they are fixed. Follower characteristics include such things as needs and motives (e.g., the degree to which achievement, power, affiliation are important to the person), ability (knowledge, skills, and experience) to perform the task, and the extent to which individuals feel they have control over critical contingencies that affect their performance in a given situation. Features of the work environment include such things as the extent to which the task is structured or unstructured, amount of time available to complete the task, nature and degree of interdependence among work group members, and a host of organizational characteristics.

The contingency most under a manager's control is his own leadership style. The dimensions that define leadership style are presently conceptualized as instrumental behavior (defining objectives and specifying the task to be performed), supportive behavior (providing support to and fulfilling needs of followers), participative behavior (seeking followers' input on decisions

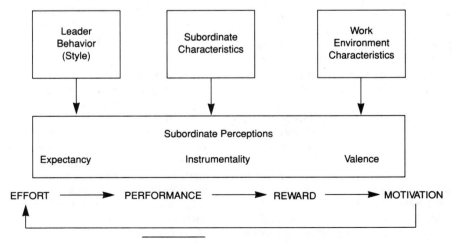

FIGURE 4.4. The path-goal model.

that affect them), and achievement-oriented behavior (establishing goals and setting expectations that challenge followers).

Given the number of contingencies and the numerous ways in which they can interact with one another, empirical tests have focused only on pieces of the model, and like most leadership research, the results have been conflicting.[35] Additionally, because of its complexity, the model is difficult to employ in real-life situations. However, several general observations and suggestions can be forwarded.[36]

- One of the most important aspects of leadership behavior is stimulating the release of and focusing follower effort on motivation.
- Often the path between effort, performance, and rewards is crooked, narrow, unpaved, and filled with barriers. The manager must do everything possible to turn what is often a cowpath into a well-designed freeway.
- In leading, the manager should appreciate that individuals' valences are heterogeneous (i.e., people value various rewards differently). The manager should understand what a follower values and construct rewards accordingly.
- Leadership behavior should help followers define expectancies. Questions that need to be addressed include: How should a follower direct his/her effort so that it results in adequate, if not exemplary, performance? What additional knowledge, skills, and experiences does a follower need to perform assigned tasks?
- Leadership behavior should focus on clarifying instrumentalities. It is important that followers understand the specific type and amount of reward that will flow from a given level of performance.
- The manager should be mindful of how work environment characteristics affect follower expectancies, instrumentalities, and valences and the implications of these effects for the selection of a leadership style. For example, when a task is very unstructured, a follower may not know how to perform the job successfully (e.g., instrumentality is low). In such instances, a higher level of instrumental leadership behavior may be required.

LEAD Model

The *LEAD model* was developed by Paul Hershey and Kenneth Blanchard while they were affiliated with the Center for Leadership Studies at Ohio University.[37] Differing degrees of task and relationship oriented behavior (defined in a way similar to the Ohio, Michigan, and Blake and Mouton studies) produce four different leadership styles: style 1, high task and low relationship; style 2, high task and high relationship; style 3, low task and high relationship; and style 4, low task and low relationship.

Hershey and Blanchard argued that the single most important contingency in selecting a *leadership style* that is effective is follower task-relevant maturity. Maturity is a function of motivation, having energy and being willing to expend it in order to accomplish the assigned task; responsibility, being willing and able to assume responsibility for planning, organizing and completing the task; and competence, possessing the necessary knowledge, skills, or experience to perform the task proficiently. A mature follower is highly motivated, willing and able to assume responsibility, and possesses the necessary competencies. An immature follower lacks motivation, is not willing or able to assume responsibility for the task, and doesn't have the necessary competencies. Maturity is situational and task-specific; a follower may be very mature performing one task and quite immature in executing another.

Hershey and Blanchard provide suggestions regarding which styles are most effective or successful with followers having varying degrees of task-relevant maturity. Here are two extreme examples.

- If the maturity of the follower is very low, the model suggests using a style that is high task-oriented and low relationship-oriented (style 1). The follower is unmotivated, not willing or able to assume responsibility, and doesn't possess the competencies necessary to perform the task. Therefore, if the task is to get done, leadership must be very directive. A low degree of relationship-oriented behavior is recommended so as not to reinforce the follower's state of immaturity.
- If the maturity of the follower is exceedingly high, the model suggests using leadership style

4—low task- and relationship-oriented behavior. Here the follower is extremely motivated, is very responsible, and possesses all the competencies necessary to perform the task. The follower does not need and, in fact, would likely not appreciate task directiveness; she knows what to do and how to do it. High relationship-oriented behavior is not needed because followers get their "stokes" or reinforcement from each other and from performance of the task itself. In this case, task and relationship responsibilities are totally delegated to the follower.

This is a highly abbreviated and simplified description of a model that has many more features than we can possibly discuss here. For example, the authors provide a dynamic interpretation that focuses on sequences of leadership behaviors to enhance follower maturity. They have designed a package of questionnaires that provide feedback regarding the extent to which individuals perceive themselves employing the four different leadership styles, how others (subordinates, peers, superior) perceive a manager's leadership style, and how one's selection of different leadership behaviors aligns with the most appropriate style suggested by the model given the maturity of followers in a series of cases.

There has been virtually no research to confirm the linkage between follower maturity, execution of the "appropriate" style as suggested by the model, and leader effectiveness.[38] However, managers and students alike find the model simple to use, practical, and intuitively appealing.

Attribution Theory

One important leadership contingency factor is a manager's own frame of reference. *Attribution* (sometimes referred to as perceptual or cognitive) *theory* holds that a manager's selection of a leadership style depends on the way follower behavior is perceived and interpreted.[39,40] Managers notice some things and are totally unaware of others. Furthermore, what's noticed is always filtered through the manager's unique cognitive frame and reshaped by it. Based on these perceptions, a manager attributes causes to the follower's behavior. There are two general types of attributions: internal (e.g., lack of follower effort or ability) and external (e.g., bad luck, inadequate task design by others, poor supervision).

A manager's choice of leadership behavior is significantly influenced by such attributions. For example, a manager might employ one leadership style if he attributes a follower's poor performance to task overload and use a different one if he feels the cause is laziness. Attribution theorists argue that, in many cases, a manager's choice of leadership style might be due more to the manager's perceptual and cognitive frame than the "reality" of the situation itself; indeed, reality is only what one perceives it to be. The basic notion of attribution theory is a simple one. An important determinant of leadership style is the manager's perceptions and attributions.[41] The resulting admonition is that managers need to be aware of these inherent biases and develop ways to minimize them.[42]

The Contingency Perspective: Selected Implications

Noted below are several implications that transcend the specific models of leadership described in this section.

- The contingency perspective helps us appreciate that leadership effectiveness and success is situational. Leadership behaviors and styles focus on influencing specific followers, be they individuals or a group, in a specific context, performing a specific task in order to accomplish a specific objective at a particular point in time. All of these things—contingencies—vary from one situation to another. The most effective leadership style in one situation is not likely to be the most effective in another.
- Three sets of contingencies seem to be most closely related to leadership effectiveness or success: characteristics of the manager, characteristics of followers, and characteristics of the immediate context in which the manager and followers interact.
- Given the large number of contingency factors and the complex ways in which they are

interrelated, it's highly unlikely that a "general theory" of leadership effectiveness or success will be formulated anytime soon.

- Much of leadership behavior has to do with stimulating and then focusing follower motivation.
- Leadership effectiveness depends, more than anything else, on a manager having a full and diverse repertoire of styles and being able to flexibly move among them; possessing the ability to diagnose the most critical contingencies of a given situation; based on the diagnosis, being able to select an effective leadership style for that situation; and having the ability to execute the chosen style well.
- The way in which a specific leadership situation is diagnosed depends, in no small measure, on the manager's perceptions and attribution of causes to follower behavior.
- Taken to the extreme, contingency driven leadership—behaving differently toward the same followers in different situations or differently toward different followers in the same situation—may appear erratic and arbitrary. This can be confusing and frustrating for followers unless managers are very explicit about how they are behaving and the reasons why they are behaving in a particular way.

Emerging Theories and Concepts

The trait, behavioral, and contingency perspectives have traditionally been the basis of most leadership theory and research. In the past decade, some new perspectives have been developed.

Transformational Leadership

James McGregor Burns, in his classic work *Leadership,* identified two types of politicians: transactional and transformational.[43] There is a growing body of literature that draws a distinction between these leadership orientations in organizations.[44] Whereas *transactional leadership* attempts to preserve and work within the constraints of the status quo, *transformational leadership* seeks to upset and replace it.

For the most part, the models of leader behavior that we have examined so far view managers as involved in exchange relationships with followers, the defining characteristic of which is, I'll provide what you want, if you'll give me what I want. Transactional leadership entails recognizing what followers want and giving it to them if their performance warrants. "In these exchanges transactional leaders clarify the roles followers must play and the task requirements followers must complete in order to reach their personal goals while fulfilling the mission of the organization."[45] You'll note that this sounds very much like the path-goal model of leadership in which the manager attempts to influence follower expectancies, instrumentalities, and valences. The objective of leadership is to get followers to comply with the rules of the game as it is currently being played. The result of such transactions, contend proponents of the theory, is ordinary levels of performance.[46] Performance improvements, if they occur at all, are marginal and achieved incrementally over a long period of time.

Transformational leaders, on the other hand, are more concerned with changes than exchanges. Seeking to alter both the objective and nature of manager-follower interactions, followers are motivated to take on difficult goals they normally would not have pursued and accept the value that work is far more than the performance of specific duties for specific rewards. The relationship between the manager and followers is not contractual, but empowering. Advocates of the transformational orientation suggest that it produces extraordinary levels of performance that flow from enrollment in a cause rather than compliance with a set of rules.[47]

Transactional and transformational leadership is differentiated by the type of goals pursued, the nature of manager-follower relations, and the values to which managers and followers adhere. Provided below is a comparison of these two orientations.

Dimension	Trans- actional	Trans- formational
goal	maintain status quo	upset status quo
activity	play within the rules	change the rules

Dimension	Trans-actional	Trans-formational
locus of reward	self (maximize personal benefits)	system (optimize systemic benefits)
nature of incentives	tit for tat	the greater good
manager-follower interaction	mutual dependence	interdependence
needs fulfilled	lower level (physical, economic, and safety)	higher level (self actualization)
performance	ordinary	extraordinary

Presently, the transformational approach to leadership is little more than a rough framework. Foundational concepts have not been rigorously defined, a comprehensive model has not been developed, and there is virtually no empirical research supporting its primary assertions.

Charismatic Leadership

Charisma is derived from a Greek word meaning divinely inspired gift or state of grace. It is a characteristic that has been attributed to those with truly exceptional leadership abilities for centuries. The concept was first introduced into the organizational literature by Max Weber who defined charismatic authority as being based on "devotion to the specific and exceptional sanctity, heroism, or exemplary character of an individual person."[48] The concept has received renewed interest by leadership scholars who have focused on a small subset of individuals able to exercise extraordinary levels of influence.[49,50] *Charismatic leadership* is

> . . . a distinct social relationship between the leader and follower, in which the leader presents a revolutionary idea, a transcendent image . . . the follower accepts this course of action not because of its

rational likelihood of success, but because of an effective belief in the extraordinary qualities of the leader.[51]

It has been increasingly recognized that charisma is not a characteristic of the manager *per se*, but rather a result of the interaction of many factors—manager and follower traits, manager and follower behaviors, the relationship between the manager and followers, situational dynamics, and the nature of the goal being sought. The following characteristics have been identified in the literature:[52–58]

- nature of the goal: revolutionary or transformational
- manager traits: self confidence, dominance, need for influence or power, strong conviction in beliefs, creativity, high energy level, enthusiasm
- leadership behaviors: ability to conceptualize and convey transcendent vision or ideology, ability to inspire and build confidence, use of unconventional means, rhetorical fluency
- follower traits: dependence, need to transcend self and situation
- follower behaviors: dedication, commitment
- manager-follower interaction: projection of idealized traits and behaviors on the leader by followers, identification (psychological fusion) of followers with leader, empowerment of followers by leader
- nature of the context: crisis, uncertainty, transformation, deprivation

As you can see, the present notion of charisma incorporates, and weaves together, concepts included in the trait, behavioral, and situational perspectives. Because charisma is (by definition) rare, and due to the complex dynamics involved, it is exceedingly difficult to study. As a result there has been little empirical research in this area, although sets of hypotheses have been suggested.

Toward a Broader Conceptualization of Leadership Effectiveness

There has been a discernible trend over the last decade to reconceptualize what constitutes leadership effectiveness or success and the factors that account for it.[59] The contention (although not always explicitly stated) is that past theorizing and research, in its quest for methodological rigor and empirically testable relationships, has been far too narrow. Writers such as Warren Bennis, James Kouzes and Barry Posner, Gareth Morgan, Tom Peters, Peter Senge, and Peter Vail suggest that high performance leadership depends on such things as systems thinking, visioning, facilitating learning, and follower empowerment.[60–66]

Systems thinking.[67] Managers lead in systems. While their surface features may vary, all systems have a number of common attributes. Effective leaders possess a highly refined understanding of their form, operating dynamics, and the way in which they achieve stability and undergo change. Most of us like to believe that we are systemic thinkers when we're really not. Peter Senge notes that

> Since we are part of the lacework ourselves, it's doubly hard to see the whole pattern. . . . Instead we tend to

focus on snapshots of isolated parts of the system and wonder why our deepest problems never get solved.[68]

Systems thinking requires mastering a conceptual framework and associated set of analytical tools or techniques that allows us to understand these patterns and how they can be changed.

Visioning.[69] The most effective managers lead by pulling, not by pushing. They have the ability to formulate rich images of future states that are both possible to achieve and highly desirable. Such images, ranging from dreams to specific goals, may be the product of the manager, followers, or both. When communicated powerfully (often through symbols and metaphors) and shared by all members of a system, a vision releases and focuses a huge amount of energy; and it fosters genuine commitment and enrollment, rather than just compliance. In order to lead, one must be going somewhere and accomplishing something that is worthy of a follower's effort—a vision is the target that beckons.

IN THE REAL WORLD
THE LEADERSHIP GAP IN HEALTH CARE

In 1991 the Healthcare Forum, with support from Eastman-Kodak, undertook a study of leadership practices and values in health service organizations.[74] Questionnaires were sent to 2,500 health care opinion leaders, approximately 400 of which were returned. The study sample included representatives of provider, insurer, and supplier organizations in addition to physician leaders, consultants, and academics. Respondents were asked to rate 36 leadership competencies and values on a 1 (low) to 7 (high) scale with respect to their current prevalence and future importance. Findings suggested that there was a significant disparity between current competencies or values and those that will be required to effectively lead health care organizations in the next century. Shown below are the areas where disparity was greatest. Note that there is substantial overlap between these competencies or values and the emerging leadership concepts identified in the previous section.

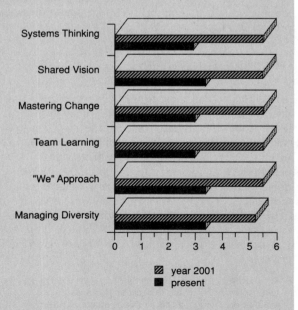

year 2001
present

Facilitating learning.[70] Organizations and the environments in which they operate are not static; they constantly undergo change. Increasingly such change is revolutionary rather than evolutionary. Change of the revolutionary variety has been characteristic of the health services industry during the last decade. In periods of revolutionary change, ways of thinking and doing that have been very successful in the past lose much of their value; they undergo rapid and significant depreciation. In such instances, organizations face two supreme challenges if they are to thrive. First, they must unlearn what is no longer relevant. Second, they must develop new mental maps, acquire new knowledge, and develop new sets of skills. Effective leaders facilitate follower unlearning and relearning.

Empowering followers.[71,72] Rosabeth Kanter observes that, "Powerlessness corrupts. Absolute powerlessness corrupts absolutely."[73] The essence of leadership is getting things done. Yet there is pitifully little that managers can do by themselves. Effective leaders view followers as the primary source of organizational creativity, energy, and value added. They create a climate and the systems that empower followers so they are willing and able to make their maximum potential contribution. Followership is the reciprocal of leadership. Effective and successful leadership is dependent upon effective, successful, and empowered followers. Team-oriented approaches for providing patient care and programs to continuously improve quality (such as total quality management (TQM) and continuous quality improvement (CQI) have attracted increasing attention in health services organizations. Both require high levels of follower empowerment if they are to be successful.

LEADERSHIP: AN INTEGRATIVE FRAMEWORK

More than a half century of research has identified a number of factors that seem to be related to leadership effectiveness and success. Figure 4.5 provides a summary and interpretation of these findings. Given the concepts that have been covered in previous sections of this chapter, the model should be relatively self-explanatory. Accordingly, only selected aspects of it are highlighted here.

A manager's leadership style is the patterns of behavior in which that manager engages to intentionally influence followers in order to accomplish a specific goal in a particular situation. We suggest that leadership style can be defined by three sets of behavioral dimensions.

- Focus is the direction of a manager's influence attempts. External leadership focuses outside the boundary of the organizational component for which the manager is responsible (toward superiors, peers, or individuals and groups outside the organization). Internal leadership is directed downward toward subordinates.
- Objective is what a manager hopes to accomplish in exercising influence. Transformational leadership seeks to alter both the nature of goals sought and manager-follower interactions; the objective is to transcend the status quo. Transactional leadership attempts to optimize the outcome of manager-follower exchange relationships by achieving stated goals in the most efficient manner within the "rules" as presently defined.
- Approach is the way in which a manager influences followers. In exercising directive (initiating structure, job-centered) leadership, a manager defines the task and specifies how it is to be performed. The focus is on goal accomplishment, and little attention is paid to manager-follower or follower-follower relationships. In exercising facilitative (consideration, employee-centered) leadership, a manager involves followers in making decisions that affect them and pays considerable attention to fulfilling their needs.

A manager's behavior can vary between "high" and "low" on each of these three sets of dimensions, the specific combination of which defines one's leadership style in a given situation.

Selection of a leadership style is influenced by two sets of factors—the manager's traits and dispositions and knowledge and skills—and the characteristics of followers and the situation, which are filtered through the manager's distinctive cognitive frame. The manager's leadership style affects the motiva-

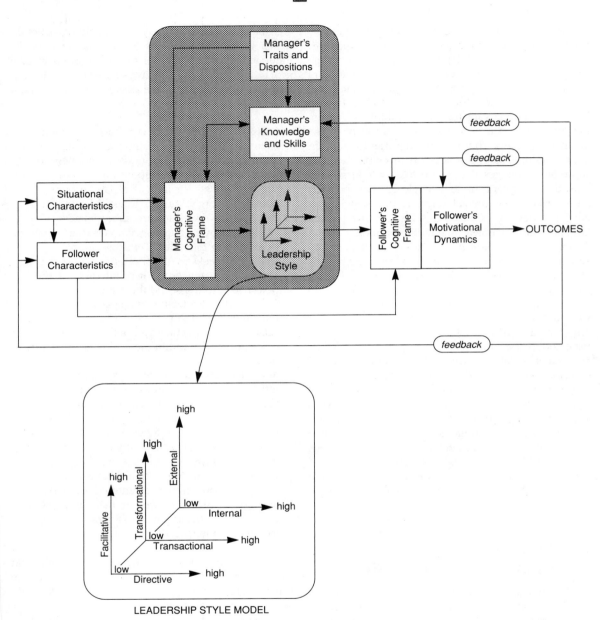

LEADERSHIP STYLE MODEL

FIGURE 4.5. Leadership: An integrative framework.

tional dynamics (expectancies, instrumentalities, and valences) of followers mediated by their own cognitive frame. The outcomes of leadership attempts include follower efficiency, effectiveness, creativity, satisfaction, turnover, and absenteeism. The feedback loops depicted can be either positive (reinforcing a given characteristic) or negative (dampening or extinguishing it).

All models leave out more than they include in addition to overly simplifying complex relationships and dynamics. This one is no exception. Our model is admittedly crude and incomplete, but we hope it will stimulate you to continue thinking about how pieces of the "leadership jigsaw puzzle" might fit together.

SEVERAL DISTINCTIVE ASPECTS OF LEADERSHIP IN HEALTH SERVICES ORGANIZATIONS

There are many distinctive aspects of leadership in health services organizations; we have chosen to address only two of them here, professionalism and gender. First, health services organizations are populated by professionals who either perform or directly supervise most of the "real work" that gets done in them; they do patient care. Professionals control the organization's core input, transformation, and output processes. Second, managerial positions in health services organizations at all levels are being increasingly filled by women.

Leading Clinical Professionals

Professionals, because of the complexity and importance of the work they perform, are granted exceedingly high levels of autonomy regarding what they do and how they do it. Different occupations have varying degrees of autonomy, and hence, possess differing degrees of professionalism. The epitome in health services organizations is, of course, the physician. We will focus on physicians here as a prototypical example, although the notions forwarded can easily be applied to other categories of clinical professionals (e.g., nurses).

For a moment, entertain the notion that physicians possess a distinctly different mentality, cognitive frame, or paradigm than do managers. This mentality, of course, is not "hard wired." Rather, it is like mental operating system software programmed through a long and intensive education and socialization process. The programing begins in medical school, continues through residency training, and is reinforced every day by the nature of the work physicians do. Noted below are several critical aspects of this clinical mentality as contrasted to the mentality of managers.[15]

Aspect	*Managerial Mentality*	*Clinical Mentality*
primary allegiance	to the organization	to their client
responsibility	shared	personal
authority relationships	hierarchical (vertical)	collegial (horizontal)
time frame	long/future	short/ present
feedback	delayed and vague	immediate and concrete
tolerance for ambiguity and uncertainty	high	low

In general, the primary allegiance of physicians is to their individual patients for whom they must bear total personal responsibility. They prefer, and are accustomed to, working in collegial-type relationships where power is symmetrical rather than in those where it flows primarily from the organizational office held. Through dealing with courses of illness that are generally time limited, [physicians are trained] to focus on the short run; the feedback they receive regarding their performance is generally very immediate and concrete (i.e., the patient either improves or gets worse, lives or dies); and their tolerance for ambiguity and uncertainty is quite low. Managers, on the other hand owe their allegiance to the organization rather than to any one physician or set of patients. Because of the high degree of interdependence necessary for accomplishing managerial tasks, accountability is generally diffuse or shared, and the power they exercise is often defined primarily by the office held. Managerial time frames are long (it takes forever to accomplish anything significant), and the feedback is often delayed and vague. As a consequence, managers have a high degree of tolerance for ambiguity and uncertainty. This is a highly stylized and exaggerated characterization, to be sure.

Two of the most frustrating and vexing aspects of leadership is when your behavior is misinterpreted by followers and followers do not respond at all like you

MANAGERIAL GUIDELINES

1. Identify and work with a mentor during the early stages of your career. Leadership is a performing art; becoming proficient at it requires continual and intensive coaching from an experienced practitioner who is invested in your development. There is a growing body of evidence which suggests that establishing an effective mentoring relationship is one of the most important things separating successful from unsuccessful leaders and managers.[86] If you would like to read more about how to work with a mentor, we recommend *Mentoring at Work: Developmental Relationships in Organizational Life.*[87]

2. Become a reflective practitioner of leadership. Reflection is the key to really learning from experience. Just as a winning sports team reviews its game film, so should the manager. Get in the habit of replaying and analyzing the leadership situations in which you have been involved some time before each day ends. It's important that you look at both your successes and failures. What happened? Play the tape in your mind. Did you get the result anticipated? If so, why? If not, why not? What could/should you have done differently? What lesson have you learned from this experience? Such reflection requires considerable discipline; the

effort, however, will pay handsome dividends.

3. Seek to better understand yourself. All accomplished artists have a very refined and rich feel for their tools. The primary (some would say only) tool of leaders is themselves. One particularly efficient way to gain enhanced self-understanding is through the feedback provided by self-administered questionnaires, instruments, and inventories. There are a lot of different ones available, and we suggest that you seek the advice of a faculty member who teaches organization behavior regarding those that may be most useful.

4. Seek feedback from followers. Rest assured that your intentions and leadership behavior will be perceived by followers in idiosyncratic ways. Our perceptions of self are always somewhat at odds with how others perceive us. To be an effective and successful leader you must understand the impact you are having on others. The best way to gain such understanding is to ask and to do so constantly. How am I coming across? What am I doing that helps you to be as effective, creative, or satisfied as you can be? What types of things am I doing that create road blocks and sap your energy or enthusiasm? Additionally, it's virtually impossible to lead if

---

expected, or hoped, they would. When the follower is a physician, the notion of *clinical mentality* helps explain why. Refer back to the integrative model of leadership (Figure 4.5) presented in the previous section. The cognitive frames of managers and physicians are quite different from one another. There are several important, and rather obvious, implications. First, physicians are likely to perceive and interpret a manager's leadership behavior in idiosyncratic ways and quite different than what might have been intended. Remember that the impact registered on physicians comes not from what you intended, or even your behavior, but rather is a result of what they perceive and the attributions they make. Second, physicians have distinctive

motivational dynamics. Their expectancies, instrumentalities, and valences differ considerably from those of managers. Remember, to motivate physicians (exercise influence to release and focus energy) you have to do so on their terms, not your own. Third, managers, because of their mentality and distinctive cognitive frame, are prone to misinterpreting the intentions or behaviors of physicians and attributing negative cause to them (e.g., not in the best interest of the organization). "I just can't understand why Dr. _____ did that." What this generally means is the physician acted in a way differently than the manager would have in that situation. Our retort is, why would you expect otherwise? Remember to interpret and attribute the

MANAGERIAL GUIDELINES

you don't have an indepth understanding of who is following. Invest the time and energy in getting to know each follower upon whom your effectiveness and success depends. What are their aspirations? What are their wants and needs? What do they view as their most important competencies (knowledge, skills, experiences), and how could the organization make better use of them? What motivates them the most?

5. Keep reading and studying. Experience is, perhaps, the single best teacher of leadership. However, there are not enough hours in the day, days in the year, or years in life to acquire all the experience we need. Some of it has to be gained vicariously, and the best vicarious teacher is reading. Additionally, reading provides the essential models, concepts, and ideas that can help us to become much more effective and efficient experiential learners, avoiding the trap where years of experience is just one year's worth repeated many times over. We've included The Manager's Essential Leadership Bookshelf to get you started.

THE MANAGER'S ESSENTIAL LEADERSHIP BOOKSHELF

There are thousands of books on leadership with hundreds of new ones published every year, all forwarding their own recipes for success. None of us have the time, energy, patience or money to consume even a small proportion of what is being written. Here's our picks, a handful of books that we have found to be the most sound, interesting, and useful. Although there are clearly others that might warrant inclusion, we recommend these to you without reservation.

Atchison TH. *Turning Health Care Leadership Around: Cultivating Inspired, Empowered and Loyal Followers*. San Francisco, Ca: Jossey-Bass; 1990.

Bennis W, Nanus B. *Leaders*. New York, NY: Harper and Row; 1985.

Covey SR. *Principle Centered Leadership*. New York, NY: Simon and Schuster; 1990.

DePree M. *Leadership is an Art*. New York, NY: Doubleday; 1989.

Gardner J. *On Leadership*. New York, NY: The Free Press; 1990.

Kelley R. *The Power of Followership: How to Create Leaders People Want to Follow, and Followers Who Lead Themselves*. New York, NY: Doubleday/Currency; 1991.

Kouzes JM, Posner BZ. *The Leadership Challenge: How to Get Extraordinary Things Done in Organizations*. San Francisco, Ca: Jossey-Bass; 1990.

Senge P. *The Fifth Discipline: The Art and Practice of the Learning Organization*. New York, NY: Doubleday/Currency; 1990.

Vail P. *Managing as a Performing Art*. San Francisco, Ca: Jossey-Bass; 1989.

---

causes of physician behavior from the perspective of the physician's mentality before attempting to understand it from your own.

Most of the writing in this area suggests that a style uniformly high in consideration, relationship orientation, and participation should be employed in leading professionals.[76-78] The degree of task orientation would then depend on the task-relevant maturity of the professional or professional group in that particular situation. If they understand the goal to be achieved, accept and are motivated to undertake it, and possess the competencies to do so (i.e., high maturity), task orientation should be low. When this is not the case, a greater degree of directiveness is warranted. It's im-

portant to reiterate that professional task-relevant maturity is situational. A professional might be very mature in one situation (e.g., doing her professional work) and quite immature in another (e.g., working on a hospital committee to design an independent practice association).

Leadership and Gender in Health Services Organizations

While issues related to gender and leadership are not necessarily distinctive to health services organizations, they are certainly very important. In 1991 females comprised 23% of the affiliates of the American College of Healthcare Executives (ACHE), up from 14% in 1985. Approximately 11% of ACHE members who were women held CEO positions.[79] These figures are likely to change in the future given the mix of individuals entering the field. Between 1979 and 1988, the composition of graduate programs in health administration in terms of gender has changed dramatically. In 1979, 60% of the graduating class were male and 40% were female. By 1988, males constituted 40.6% of the graduating class and females composed 59.4%.

Several recent reviews of the literature suggest that, while females may demonstrate different patterns of leadership behaviors than males, gender is not a particularly good predictor of leadership effectiveness and success.[81,82] This finding should not be surprising given problems associated with trait and behavioral theories of leadership, described previously. However, there does appear to be some evidence that individuals who ranked higher in male sex role orientation (describing themselves as having more masculine characteristics) were perceived to be better leaders than those with feminine, androgynous, or undifferentiated gender roles.[83] Keep this finding in as foreground as you read further.

In 1990 the ACHE, in conjunction with the Graduate Program in Hospital and Health Administration at the University of Iowa, conducted a comparative study of women and men health care managers. The sample consisted of 1,108 College affiliates, about half female and half male who entered the field between 1971 and 1985.[84] The study produced a number of interesting findings regarding gender differences in career attainment, compensation, professional satisfaction, and work patterns. Those dealing with leadership are summarized in Table 4.1.

With respect to general leadership qualities, the majority of respondents view males and females to be equal. Where differences in perceptions existed, both males and females overwhelmingly ranked males as being superior. The same general relationship emerged in other key factors associated with leadership effectiveness (e.g., support from those who are led—superiors, peers, and subordinates) and behaviors often associated with successful leaders (e.g., risk taking and competitiveness). Although not directly related to leadership, a striking disparity was perceived regarding chances for career advancement in health

services organizations by both men and women. Fully 72% of the females and 46.4% of the males perceived men possessing significantly better advancement opportunities than women. We encourage you to look over Table 4.1 carefully. The findings are quite significant and have some important implications regarding gender differences and leadership in health services organizations.

Overall, there seems to be a stereotypical view of women possessing fewer of the qualities considered essential for exercising the leadership role of the manager in health services organizations. We underscore that this is a stereotypical perception, because evidence from other industries cited previously suggests that gender is a very poor predictor of leadership effectiveness or success. There is a *gender* leadership *gap* in health services organizations, and it seems to be the result of a gender bias on the part of both women and men. The traditional solution is to close this gap by assimilation; helping women managers to think and act more like men. Many management educational and training programs, reinforced by organizational cul-

TABLE 4.1. The Gender Gap in Health Administration

| | Female Responses | | | Male Responses | | |
| | (respondents opinion regarding which gender exhibits more of a given attribute) | | | | | |
	men	women	equal	men	women	equal
Leadership qualities*	21.0	8.0	71.1	38.3	0.6	61.1
Support from superiors*	43.2	3.7	53.2	17.1	8.4	74.6
Support from peers**	24.5	15.0	61.1	23.0	9.6	67.4
Support from subordinates***	23.3	15.6	61.1	23.0	9.6	67.4
Risk taking inclinations*	37.6	13.8	48.7	53.9	3.7	42.4
Competitiveness at work*	39.0	7.4	53.6	31.1	17.6	51.3
Advancement opportunities*	72.2	1.1	26.7	46.4	5.8	47.8

* chi square significant at $p < .001$
** chi square significant at $p < .01$
*** chi square significant at $p < .05$
SOURCE: Gender and Careers in Healthcare Management: Findings of a National Survey of Healthcare Executives. Research Series Number 3. Chicago, Ill: American College of Healthcare Executives; 1991:41.

ture, implicitly embrace this approach. Elsie Cross notes, in addressing both gender and racial bias, that

> . . . white women and people of color cannot—nor should they attempt to—become like white men. The best I can hope for is that others will feel that I can "think like a man". . . . But I can never be more than an imitation white man. And in becoming an imitation, I give up the richness, the creativity, the strength that comes from who I really am.[85]

Like Cross, we feel that assimilation is counterproductive. Irrespective of the trait focused upon (gender, race, ethnicity, sexual orientation), assimilation results in a reduction of diversity at a time when it is needed most in health services organizations. Managerial and leadership heterogeneity is essential for finding different ways to solve new problems and seize new opportunities in times of revolutionary change.

KEY CONCEPTS

Attribution Theory
Authority
Behavioral Perspective
Charismatic Leadership
Consideration
Clinical Mentality
Contingency Perspective
Gender Gap
Goal Accomplishment
Influence
Initiating Structure
Leadership Continuum
  Model
Leadership Focus
Leadership Locus

Leadership Match Model
Leadership Role
Leadership Styles: S1, S2,
  S3, S4
LEAD Model
Managerial Grid
Managerial Office
Managerial Roles
Office
Path-Goal Model
Power
Situation Favorableness
Trait Perspective
Transactional Leadership
Transformational
  Leadership

Discussion Questions

1. Reread the opening case and answer the questions again. Compare your answers written before and after reading this chapter. What are the differences? How have you altered your thinking about the nature of leadership and the factors that contribute to leadership effectiveness and success?

2. You are interviewing for a position and your prospective superior asks you to describe your leadership style. How would you do so? This is a fairly typical question asked of candidates for management positions, irrespective of level, so it is a good idea to have a reasonably well thought out and articulate answer. Draft a one or two paragraph statement. Share your statement with fellow students.

3. There are those who contend leadership is highly romanticized. That is, there's a tendency to ascribe far more to leadership as a cause than is actually warranted.[88] While leadership certainly makes a difference, it may not make as much differences as either managers, followers, or onlookers generally think it does. Successful performance of a group, organization, or nation is the result of many factors interacting in complex ways. However, it is generally far easier and more reassuring to attribute such success to the leadership abilities of an individual. What do you think?

4. Several distinctive aspects of leading in health services organizations have been presented in this chapter. What are some other characteristics of health services organizations that pose challenges for effectively executing the leadership role of the manager? In thinking about this question, consider distinctions between different types of health services organizations—acute care hospitals, long-term care hospitals, nursing homes, health maintenance organizations (HMOs), and group practices.

5. What do you *think* about the data from the ACHE study presented in the section on gender and leadership? How do you *feel* about these findings? From your perspective, what are the implications of these data? Discuss the differences between males and females in your class regarding cognitive and affective reactions to these findings and the nature of the implications they see as most significant. What are some specific approaches that health services organizations might employ to stimulate and capture the benefits of greater leadership diversity?

REFERENCES

1. Yuki GA. *Leadership in Organizations*. Englewood Cliffs, NJ:Prentice-Hall; 1981:5.
2. Katz D, Kahn RL. The taking of organizational roles. In: *The Social Psychology of Organizations*. New York, NY: John Wiley and Sons; 1966.
3. Jago AG. Leadership: Perspectives in theory and research. *Management Science*. 1982;28:315–336.
4. Jennings WO. A review of leadership studies with a particular reference to military problems. *Psychological Bulletin*. 1947;44:54–79.
5. Stodgill RM. Personal factors associated with leadership: A survey of the literature. *Journal of Applied Psychology*. 1948;32:35–71.
6. Stodgill RM. *Handbook of Leadership*. New York, NY: Free Press; 1974.
7. Bass BM. *Stodgill's Handbook of Leadership*. New York, NY: Free Press; 1981.
8. Sartle CL. *Executive Performance and Leadership*. Englewood Cliffs, NJ: Prentice-Hall; 1956.
9. Lord RG, et al. A meta analysis of the relation between personality traits and leadership: An application of validity generalization procedures. *Journal of Applied Psychology*. 1986;71:402–410.
10. Van Fleet DD, Yukl GA. A century of leadership research. In: Rosenbach WE, Taylor RL, eds. *Contemporary Issues in Leadership*. Boulder, Co: Westview Press; 1989:67.
11. Coska LS. A relationship between leader intelligence and leader rated effectiveness. *Journal of Applied Psychology*. 1984;14:22–34.
12. Lewin K, et al. Patterns of aggressive behavior in experimentally created social climates. *Journal of Social Psychology*. 1939;10:271–276.
13. Stodgill R, Coons A, eds. *Leader Behavior: Its Description and Measurement*. Columbus, Ohio: Bureau of Business Research, Ohio State University; 1957.
14. Fleishman EA. Twenty years of consideration and structure. In: Fleishman EA, Hunt JG, eds. *Current Developments in the Study of Leadership*. Carbondale, Ill: Southern Illinois University; 1973:1–37.
15. Halpin AW. The leadership behavior and combat performance of airplane commanders. *Journal of Abnormal and Social Psychology*. 1954;39:82–84.
16. Korman AK. Consideration, initiating structure and organizational criteria: A review. *Personnel Psychology*. 1966;19:349–361.
17. Likert R. *New Patterns of Management*. New York, NY: McGraw-Hill; 1961.
18. Katz D, et al. *Productivity, Supervision and Morale in an Office Situation*. Ann Arbor, Mich: Institute for Social Research, University of Michigan; 1950.
19. Katz D, et al. *Productivity, Supervision and Morale Among Railroad Workers*. Ann Arbor, Mich: Institute for Social Research, University of Michigan; 1951.
20. Blake J, Mouton R. *The New Managerial Grid*. Houston, Tex: Gulf Publishing; 1978.
21. Blake RR, Mouton JS. Theory and research for developing a science of leadership. *Journal of Applied Behavioral Science*. 1982;18:275–291.
22. Tannenbaum R, Schmidt W. How to choose a leadership pattern. *Harvard Business Review*. 1973;51(3):162–180.
23. Fiedler FE. *A Theory of Leadership Effectiveness*. New York, NY: McGraw-Hill; 1967.
24. Fiedler FE, Chemers MM. *Leadership and Effective Management*. Glenview, Ill: Scott, Foresman; 1974.
25. Fiedler FE, et al. *Improving Leadership Effectiveness*. New York, NY: John Wiley; 1976.
26. Hall DD, Norgaim KE. The leadership match game: Matching the man to the situation. *Organizational Dynamics*. 1976;4:6–16.
27. Stinson JE, Tracy L. Some disturbing characteristics of LPC scores. *Personnel Psychology*. 1974;27:477–485.
28. Nebeker DB. Situation favorability and perceived environmental uncertainty: An integrative approach. *Administrative Science Quarterly*. 1975;20:281–294.
29. Vroom VH. *Work and Motivation*. New York, NY: John Wiley; 1964.
30. Porter LW, Lawler EE. *Managerial Attitudes and Performance*. Homewood, Ill: Richard D. Irwin; 1968.
31. Evans MG. Leadership and motivation: A core concept. *Academy of Management Journal*. 1970;13:91–102.
32. Evans MG. The effects of supervisory behavior on the path-goal relationship. *Organizational Behavior in Human Performance*. 1970;5:277–298.
33. House RJ. A path-goal theory of leader effectiveness. *Administrative Science Quarterly*. 1971;16:321–323.
34. House RJ, Mitchell TR. Path-goal theory of leadership. *Journal of Contemporary Business*. 1974;3(4):81–98.
35. Schreisheim CA, von Glinow MA. The path-goal theory of leadership: A theoretical and empirical analysis. *Academy of Management Journal*. 1977;20:398–405.
36. House RJ, Baetz ML. Leadership: Some empirical generalizations and new directions. *Research in Organization Behavior*. 1979;1:385–386.
37. Hershey P, Blanchard KH. *Management of Organizational Behavior: Utilizing Human Resources*. Englewood Cliffs, NJ: Prentice-Hall; 1977.
38. Graeff CL. The situational leadership theory: A critical review. *Academy of Management Review*. 1983;8:271–294.
39. Shaver KG. *An Introduction to Attribution Processes*. Hillsdale, NY: Erlbaum Books; 1983.
40. Mitchell TR, et al. An attributional model of leadership and the poor performing subordinate: Development

and validation. *Research in Organization Behavior.* 1981;3:197–234.

41. Lord RG, et al. A test of leadership categorization theory: Internal structure, information processing and leadership perception. *Organizational Behavior and Human Performance.* 1984;34:343–378.

42. Mitchell TR. Attributions and actions: A note of caution. *Journal of Management.* 1982;8(1):65–74.

43. Burns JM. *Leadership.* New York, NY: Harper and Row; 1978.

44. Tishy NM, Devanna MA. *The Transformational Leader.* New York, NY: John Wiley; 1986.

45. Kuhnert KW, Lewis P. Transactional and transformational leadership: A constructive/developmental analysis. *Academy of Management Review.* October 1987;12:649.

46. Liden RC, Dienesch RM. Leader-member exchange model of leadership: A critique and further development. *Academy of Management Review.* 1986;11:618–634.

47. Bass BM. *Leadership Beyond Expectations.* New York, NY: Free Press; 1985.

48. Eisenstadt SN. *Max Weber: On Charisma and Institution Building.* Chicago, Ill: University of Chicago Press; 1968:46.

49. Bass, op. cit.

50. House RJ. A 1976 theory of charismatic leadership. In: Hunt JG, Larson LL, eds. *Leadership: The Cutting Edge.* Carbondale, Ill: Southern Illinois University Press; 1977:189–207.

51. Dow TE. The theory of charisma. *Sociological Quarterly.* 1969;10:315.

52. Shils EA. Charisma, Order and Status. *American Sociological Review.* 1965;30:199–213.

53. Dow, op. cit., 306–318.

54. Hummel RP. Psychology of charismatic followers. *Psychological Reports.* 1975;37:759–770.

55. Berlew DE. Leadership and organizational excitement. *California Management Review.* 1974;17:21–30.

56. Conger JA, Kanungo RN. Toward a behavioral theory of charismatic leadership in organizational settings. *Academy of Management Review.* 1987;12:637–647.

57. Oberg W. Charisma, commitment and contemporary organizational theory. *Business Topics.* 1972;20(2):18–32.

58. Wilner AR. *The Spellbinders: Charismatic and Political Leadership.* New Haven, Conn: Yale University Press; 1984.

59. Conger, Kanungo, op. cit.

60. Management's new gurus. *Business Week.* August 31, 1992:44–52.

61. Bennis WG, Nanus BI. *Leaders.* New York, NY: Harper and Row; 1985.

62. Kouzes JM, Posner BZ. *The Leadership Challenge: How to Get Extraordinary Things Done in Organizations.* San Francisco, Ca: Jossey-Bass; 1988.

63. Morgan G. *Riding the Waves of Change: Developing Managerial Competencies for a Turbulent World.* San Francisco, Ca: Jossey-Bass; 1988.

64. Peters T. *Thriving on Chaos: Handbook for a Management Revolution.* New York, NY: Alfred A. Knopf; 1987.

65. Senge PM. *The Fifth Discipline.* New York, NY: Doubleday/Currency; 1991.

66. Vail PB. *Managing as a Performing Art: New Ideas for a World of Chaotic Change.* San Francisco, Ca: Jossey-Bass; 1989.

67. Kauffman Jr DL. *Systems One: An Introduction to Systems Thinking.* Minneapolis, Minn: SA Carlton; 1980.

68. Senge, op. cit., 7.

69. Kouzes, Posner, op. cit., 79–129.

70. Senge, op. cit., 233–272.

71. Peters, op. cit., 387–478.

72. Kelley RE. *The Power of Followership: How to Create Leaders People Want to Follow and Followers Who Lead Themselves.* New York, NY: Doubleday/Currency; 1991.

73. Ibid., 285.

74. *Bridging the Leadership Gap in Healthcare.* San Francisco, Ca: Healthcare Forum; 1992.

75. Freidson E. The clinical mentality. In: *Profession of Medicine: A Study of the Sociology of Applied Knowledge.* New York, NY: Dodd/Mead; 1972: 158–184.

76. Benveniste G. *Professionalizing the Organization.* San Francisco, Ca: Jossey-Bass; 1987.

77. Raelin JA. *The Clash of Cultures: Managers and Professionals.* Boston, Mass: Harvard Business School Press; 1986.

78. Shapiro A. *Managing Professional People.* New York, NY: Free Press; 1985.

79. Some answers to questions about female healthcare executives. Chicago, Ill: American College of Healthcare Executives; unpublished data, no date noted: 1.

80. Health administration employment: A survey of early career opportunities. A Korn/Ferry International-AUPHA Report. Arlington, Va: Association of University Programs in Health Administration; 1990:18.

81. Morrison AR, et al. Executive women: Substance plus style. *Psychology Today.* August 1987:18–21.

82. Rice RW, et al. Leader sex, leader success and leadership process. *Journal of Applied Psychology.* 1984;69:15–27.

83. Goktepe J, Schneier C. Role of sex, gender roles and attraction in predicting emergent leaders. *Journal of Applied Psychology.* 1989;74:165–167.

84. *Gender and Careers in Healthcare Management: Findings of a National Study of Healthcare Executives,* Research Series Number 3. Chicago, Ill: American College of Healthcare Executives; 1991.

85. Cross EY. Making the invisible visible. *Healthcare Forum Journal.* January-February 1992:29.

86. Dreher GF, Ash RA. A comparative study of mentoring among men and women in managerial, professional and technical positions. *Journal of Applied Psychology.* 1990;75:539–546.

87. Kram KE. *Mentoring at Work: Developmental Relationships in Organizational Life.* Glenview, Ill: Scott, Foresman; 1985.

88. J. R. Meindl, et al., "The Romance of Leadership," *Administrative Science Quarterly,"* 30 (1985), pp. 78–102.

CHAPTER

5

CONFLICT MANAGEMENT AND NEGOTIATION

Jeffrey T. Polzer, M.B.A.
Ph.D. Candidate

Margaret A. Neale, Ph.D.
Professor

CHAPTER TOPICS

LEARNING OBJECTIVES

After completing this chapter, the reader should be able to

1. identify reasons that conflict is prevalent in health care organizations
2. understand several different types of conflict and the levels at which conflict occurs
3. identify several different conflict management techniques, based on various concerns of the disputants
4. identify the basic concepts and dimensions of negotiation
5. appreciate the importance of planning for a negotiation and know the key issues to consider when preparing to negotiate
6. identify and understand special types of conflict management situations, such as multi-party negotiations and third-party intervention

CHAPTER PURPOSE

The situation at Chiefland Memorial Hospital illustrates a conflict over medical and administrative jurisdictions that is certainly not unique to Chiefland. Although the meeting described in the case represents a relatively formal approach to dealing with the conflict, imagine all of the disputes about these issues that had arisen during the several months leading up to this crisis. *Conflict* is pervasive in health services organizations, as in all organizations. Conflict occurs every day in a wide variety of situations ranging from emotional disputes between two colleagues, to disputes between departments about lines of authority, to legal disputes involving several organizations. In this chapter, we will focus primarily on the types of conflict that confront managers on a day-to-day basis.

IN THE REAL WORLD

CONFLICT AT CHIEFLAND MEMORIAL HOSPITAL

James A. Grover, retired land developer and financier, is the current president of Chiefland Memorial Hospital Board of Trustees. Chiefland Memorial is a 200-bed voluntary short-term general hospital serving an area of approximately 50,000 persons. Mr. Grover has just completed a meeting with the administrator of the hospital, Edward M. Hoffman. The purpose of the meeting was to seek an acceptable solution to an apparent conflict-of-authority problem within the hospital between Hoffman and the Chief of Surgery, Dr. Lacy Young.

The problem that concerns Dr. Young involves the operating room supervisor, Geraldine Werther, R.N. Ms. Werther schedules the hospital's operating suite in accordance with policies that she believes to have been established by the hospital's administration. One source of irritation to the surgeons is her attitude that maximum utilization must be made of the hospital's operating rooms if hospital costs are to be reduced. She therefore schedules in such a way that operating-room idle time is minimized. Surgeons complain

that the operative schedule often does not permit them sufficient time to complete a surgical procedure in the manner they think desirable. More often than not, insufficient time is allowed between operations for effective preparation of the operating room for the next procedure. Such scheduling, the surgical staff maintains, contributes to low-quality patient care. Furthermore, some of the surgeons have complained that Ms. Werther shows favoritism in her scheduling, allowing some doctors more use of the operating suite than others.

The situation reached a crisis when Dr. Young, following an explosive confrontation with Ms. Werther, told her he was firing her. Ms. Werther then made an appeal to the hospital administrator, who in turn informed Dr. Young that discharge of nurses was an administrative prerogative. In effect, Dr. Young was told he did not have authority to fire Ms. Werther. Dr. Young asserted that he did have authority over any issue affecting medical practice and good patient care in Chiefland Hospital. He considered this a medical problem and threatened to take the matter to the hospital's board of trustees.

As the meeting between Mr. Grover and Mr. Hoffman began, Mr. Hoffman explained his position on the problem. He stressed the point that a hospital administrator is legally responsible for patient care in the hospital. He also contended that quality patient care cannot be achieved unless the board of trustees authorizes the administrator to make decisions, develop programs, formulate policies, and implement procedures. While listening to Mr. Hoffman, Mr. Grover recalled the position belligerently taken by Dr. Young, who had contended that surgical and medical doctors

holding staff privileges at Chiefland would never allow a layman to make decisions impinging on medical practice. Young also had said that Hoffman should be told to restrict his activities to fund raising, financing, maintenance, and housekeeping—administrative problems rather than medical problems. Dr. Young had then requested that Mr. Grover clarify in a definitive manner the lines of authority at Chiefland Memorial.

As Mr. Grover ended his meeting with Mr. Hoffman, the severity of the problem was unmistakably clear to him, but the solution remained quite unclear. Grover knew a decision was required—and soon.

SOURCE: *Adapted from Champion JM, James JH.* Critical Incidents in Management. *Homewood, Ill: Richard D. Irwin, Inc.; 1980.*

THE IMPORTANCE OF CONFLICT MANAGEMENT

The field of conflict management has grown dramatically in the last decade, reflected both by the amount of research conducted on this topic and the increased importance placed on teaching conflict management techniques. This increase in popularity, particularly concerning negotiation, has been fueled by several general environmental trends that are especially noticeable in the health services industry.[1] First, the marketplace is growing increasingly global as firms face competition from foreign companies. For example, pharmaceutical firms such as Burroughs-Wellcome, Inc. increasingly find themselves conducting business in different countries as their current markets become more competitive. This increased diversity in potential business partners heightens the need for managers to be able to negotiate effectively with people who have different backgrounds, interests, and values.

Secondly, at the firm level, there has been a vast increase in corporate restructuring throughout the 1980s and into the 1990s. Managers in corporations that are going through structural transformations need negotiation skills to ensure their position within the new organization. At an individual level, the workforce is growing increasingly mobile. Many employees proactively manage their career paths, often within multi-

ple organizations. Increased mobility demands better negotiation skills of those changing jobs and those employing these people.

Finally, the shift from a manufacturing-based to a service-based economy means that typical negotiations are likely to be more difficult, because desired outcomes are more ambiguous and therefore harder to specify in negotiated agreements.[2] For example, physicians, administrators, and patients may each have different definitions for "low-quality patient care," an issue at the heart of the conflict in the Chiefland Hospital dispute. This ambiguity is clearly present in many areas of the health services field, increasing the importance of good negotiating skills as negotiations become more difficult.

We will explore negotiation in depth later in the chapter. Before we focus on ways to resolve conflict, though, we will discuss various types of conflict and some of the typical reasons conflict occurs in organizations.

THE CAUSES OF CONFLICT
The Role of Resource Scarcity

Conflict arises for many reasons and can be characterized in numerous ways. At a very basic level, most conflict occurs because of a fundamental problem inherent in every organization. Organizational members desire several types of resources, including power, money, information, advice, and praise.[3] However, resource scarcity dictates that the members of an organization will not all be able to receive the level of resources they desire. Therefore, conflict arises between organizational members regarding the distribution of desired resources.

It is useful to distinguish conflict from *competition* because many people confuse the two concepts. While conflict is a typical result of resource scarcity, organizational members also compete for resources. However, conflict and competition are distinct concepts. In both cases, the goals of the parties are incompatible. In situations involving resources, this means that the parties cannot both acquire their desired level of resources. However, competition is characterized by parallel striving toward a goal that both parties cannot reach simultaneously, while conflict is characterized by mutual interference. Conflict occurs when a concern of one party is frustrated, or perceived to be frustrated, by another party.[4] Parties can compete and still remain relatively independent of each other. Conflict, on the other hand, requires some interaction or contact between the parties.

Conflict can also occur for reasons that are less tangible than resource acquisition. People may have conflicting perceptions, ideas, or beliefs as well as conflicting resource allocation goals. For example, one subordinate may perceive that another subordinate receives more praise, even when both subordinates actually receive the same objective amount of praise; two administrators may have different ideas about what an employee dress code policy should entail; and people may have different beliefs about the appropriateness of a certain medical treatment or procedure. A basic but important point to be drawn from these examples is that conflict always occurs because of the differences between people, even though these differences occur on a variety of dimensions.

Beneficial versus Detrimental Effects of Conflict

Because differences between people are unavoidable, conflict will always exist in organizations and groups. The question that must be addressed by suc-

cessful managers is how to handle the conflicts that they will inevitably face. Should managers try to create a work environment in which there is as little conflict as possible or is some important purpose served by having certain levels of ambient conflict? This boils down to the question of whether conflict is good or bad, and therefore, whether it should be encouraged in work groups or discouraged and suppressed. This is the focus of Debate Time 5.1.

In trying to ascertain whether conflict is good or bad, functional or dysfunctional, something to be explored or suppressed, part of the puzzle may lie in differentiating various types of conflict. It may be that some types of conflict are important for successful organizational performance while other forms of conflict are associated with problematic organizational performance. In the next section, we will consider three different types of conflict—content conflict, emotional conflict, and administrative conflict—and their unique impact on organizational functioning.

Jehn's Typology of Conflict

Conflict within an organization can be characterized by type regardless of the level at which it occurs. Karen Jehn devised a typology that includes three types of conflict. *Task content conflict,* the first type, refers to disagreements about the actual task being performed by organizational members. The focus in this type of conflict is on differing opinions pertaining to the task, rather than the goals of the people involved.[6] For example, everyone in a group medical practice may agree that the group should have a marketing campaign, but members may disagree about the content of the advertisements and whether advertising should be run on radio, television, or in newspapers.

Emotional conflict is an awareness of interpersonal incompatibilities among those working together on a task. It involves negative emotions and dislike of the other people involved in the conflict. The third type of conflict is *administrative conflict* and is defined as an awareness by the involved parties that there are controversies about how task accomplishment will proceed.[7] Disagreements about individual responsibilities and duties are examples of administrative conflict. For example, members of a group practice may disagree about who should decide what type of advertising to

DEBATE TIME 5.1: WHAT DO YOU THINK?

POINT: *Conflict is a necessary and useful part of organizational life.* Not all conflict is unhealthy. Low levels of conflict can often stimulate the parties involved and heighten their attention. Novel or creative solutions frequently result from conflict when people search for ways to satisfy a diverse set of interests. In fact, the absence of conflict can be as indicative of problems as too much conflict. For example, Irving Janis originated the concept of groupthink, which occurs when too little conflict is expressed within decision-making groups.[5] Very low levels of conflict may indicate that unavoidable differences are being suppressed or that the people involved do not have perspectives that differ enough to contribute to a well-thought out decision.

COUNTERPOINT: *Conflict is dysfunctional.* Especially in the United States, most people think of conflict as a negative phenomenon. They are usually correct. High conflict levels are typically detrimental and can be destructive. Instead of allocating resources to the production of the goods or services that are the mission of the organization, conflict requires that managers spend time and energy trying to resolve the conflict. In fact, one study discovered that managers spend almost 20% of their time in activities directly related to the resolution of disputes—time that could be much more productively applied directly to achieving the mission of the organization.

In addition, conflict is associated with higher levels of stress. Such an environment can reduce the psychological well-being of employees and make it difficult for them to develop trusting, supportive relationships within the organizational context. It is for this reason that managers spend so much of their time managing and resolving conflict.

---

use or who should be responsible for working with an advertising agency.

In general, the research conducted by Jehn and others suggests that a moderate amount of task content conflict is critical to the effective functioning of groups. Groupthink, for example, is probably more likely to occur when there is an implicit avoidance of all conflict, but especially task content conflict. Administrative conflict and, to a greater extent, emotional conflict are likely to be the culprits when groups become dysfunctional or impaired because a high degree of conflict inhibits their ability to interact. All three of these types of conflict may occur between individuals, groups and individuals, or different groups as people perform the tasks that make up organizational life. These various levels at which conflict can occur are the focus of the next section.

LEVELS OF CONFLICT

It is useful to consider the level at which conflict occurs, along with the type of conflict, when trying to decide how to manage it. That is, conflict can occur within an individual (*intrapersonal conflict*), between individuals (*interpersonal conflict*), within a group (*intragroup conflict*), and between groups (*intergroup conflict*). The alternatives available for resolving the conflict may depend on the level in the organization at which it exists.

Individual Level

Individual conflict occurs when the locus of the dispute is the individual. Intrapersonal conflict may occur for a variety of reasons. People are often faced with a choice between two options that may vary in attractiveness. In characterizing conflict at this level, it is valuable to think about the relative attractiveness of each option. When two options are equally attractive, approach-approach conflict occurs within the person. This conflict results from the person's effort to differentiate between the two alternatives. For example, a health maintenance organization (HMO) executive may have two equally viable and attractive plans for expanding enrollment. It is difficult to choose either of the options because selecting one necessarily means the other must be turned down.

On the other side of the coin, avoidance-avoidance conflict occurs when a person has to choose between equally unattractive options. If a nursing home is trying to reduce costs, one of two good nurses may have to be laid off. The decision is made more difficult because the options are equally unattractive.

The most prevalent type of intrapersonal conflict is approach-avoidance conflict, which occurs when multiple options each have favorable and unfavorable features. Conflict that is initially approach-approach conflict often turns into approach-avoidance conflict when the person making the decision looks at the alternatives more critically in an attempt to differentiate them. Unattractive components of each option may be found that were overlooked initially, such as additional costs associated with each option for expanding HMO membership enrollment. A person may arrive at a different decision depending on which features of each option the person focuses. After the decision is made, post-decision regret frequently occurs, as the alternative that the person passed up looks increasingly better as more information is gathered about the chosen option.

Group Level

When most people think about conflict, the examples that first come to mind are at an interpersonal level, between two or more people. Conflict at this level typically occurs because of incompatible goals, ideas, feelings, beliefs, or behaviors, as illustrated by the examples in the first section of this chapter. This level of conflict is usually characterized by interdependence between the parties, whereby the choice of each party affects the outcome of the other party. The choice that is optimal for one party may result in a poor outcome for the other, leading to conflict. This is the most common level of conflict that comes to the surface in organizations.

Paralleling individual conflict, group conflict can occur between members of the same group (intragroup conflict) or between members of different groups (intergroup conflict). Intragroup conflict is similar in many ways to interpersonal conflict, with the former type being more complex because of the higher number of people involved. However, this is not the only difference. When a group is involved that has an identity above and beyond its individual members, several things can occur as a result of the influence of the group on its members. A formal definition of what we mean by a "group" may help to clarify the ideas that follow. In this context, a group is defined as

> an organized system of two or more individuals who are interrelated so that the system performs some function, has a standard set of role relationships among its members, and has a set of norms that regulate the function of the group and each of its members.[8]

As this definition of a group implies, the interactions of the group members are influenced by their roles within the group and by the norms of the group. Members of the group may not always be amenable to these influences, leading to conflict between the individual member and the group. Conflict between the members of a group may result in decreased coordination, communication, and productivity.[9] Intragroup conflict will come up again later in this chapter in the section on multi-party negotiations.

Intergroup conflict can have a profound impact on the perceptions and behaviors of people. When acting as a member of a group, people tend to divide others into an ingroup and an outgroup. The ingroup consists of all the other members of the salient group. The outgroup consists of those outside the boundaries of the ingroup. Some examples of the characteristics people frequently use to divide people into in- and out-groups include gender, race, religious preference, geographic location, organizational membership, departmental membership, and functional position within an organization. Most people are members of numerous groups based on demographic, organizational, or other demarcations. This creates abundant opportunities for intergroup conflict to arise. Intergroup conflict occurs whenever the disputants identify with or represent different groups that are relevant to the conflict during the conflict episode.

Intergroup conflict may have a variety of causes, many of which are the same as those that cause interpersonal conflict, such as resource scarcity, differing beliefs, or incompatible goals. The distinction is simply that the relevant unit from which the differences stem is the group rather than the individual. Intergroup conflict can have a variety of consequences both within and across the groups involved in the conflict. Within the groups, cohesiveness, task orientation, loyalty to the group, and acceptance of autocratic leadership may

IN THE (EXPERIMENTAL) REAL WORLD

INTERGROUP CONFLICT AT ROBBER'S CAVE

Consider the experience of a group of young boys at the Robber's Cave Camp—a camp specifically set up to examine intergroup conflict. During the first days of camp, the boys—coming from different schools—were allowed to develop friends through a variety of campwide activities. The boys were then assigned to one of two cabins. The make-up of each cabin was such that about 60% of an individual's best friends were in the other cabin. Within a few days, however, the interaction patterns shifted dramatically. The boys tended to interact almost exclusively with others in their own cabins.

The boys were then involved in a series of competitive activities in which the two cabins were on opposite teams. To increase the conflict, the winners of each competition were awarded prizes. Quickly, the amount of hostility and stereotypes escalated. Raids and ambushes were planned, and leaders emerged in each cabin who were effective at combat. There was a huge increase in intragroup solidarity.

The researchers then set up a party in which one cabin, the Red Devils, arrived considerably earlier than the other group, the Bulldogs. The food at the party was of two very different levels of attractiveness: half of the food was fresh and appealing; the other half was old and unappetizing. Because of the competition between the two groups, the Red Devils ate most of the good food and left the unattractive food for their competitors. When the Bulldogs arrived, they were so upset that the conflict quickly escalated from name-calling to a full-fledged food fight. ■

SOURCE: Adapted from Sherif M. *Intergroup Conflict and Cooperation.* Norman, Okla: University Book Exchange; 1977.

increase. Between the groups, distorted perceptions, negative stereotypes of outgroup members, and reduced communication may result. A mentality of "us versus them" often forms and grows stronger as the conflict escalates.[10] As seen at Robbers Cave, the strength of group affiliations as a contributing factor to conflict is often overlooked but should always be considered when trying to determine the causes of conflict.

MANAGING CONFLICT

It is clear that conflict is commonplace, and that for organizational members to function productively, they must manage conflict effectively. There are many strategies for managing conflict, including those that are planned as well as those that emerge as conflict is experienced. Some conflict management techniques apply to conflict on all levels, while others are relevant for a limited number of types and levels of conflict. In this section, we will briefly introduce the dual-concern model as a typology of conflict management techniques, focusing on four ways that people handle conflict—accommodation, pressing, avoidance, and negotiation.

The Dual Concern Model

Kenneth Thomas has developed a two-dimensional model of conflict management techniques that reflects a concern for both an individual's own outcomes as well as an opponent's outcomes. Depending on these two dimensions of concern, a negotiator might prefer one of five different strategies for handling conflict. If concern for both self and other's outcomes are low, this model predicts that one might prefer an *avoidance* strategy. If concern for one's own outcome is high and concern for the other's outcome is low, then one should prefer a competing, or *pressing,* strategy. If concern for one's own outcome is low and concern for the other's outcome is high, then *accommodation* or capitulation is probably the preferred strategy. If concern for both one's own outcome and the other's outcome is high, then collaboration is the appropriate strategy. Finally, if one has intermediate concern for both one's own and the other's outcomes, then one is likely to prefer a compromise strategy. The Dual Concern model is graphically represented in Figure 5.1.

If we think about how differing preferences for these five strategies might be expressed by an organizational actor in various situations, four different conflict management techniques can be identified. Accommodation, pressing, avoiding, and *negotiation* (incorporating compromise and collaboration) are described in greater detail in the following sections.

Accommodation

Capitulating to or accommodating the other party is one popular way to deal with conflict. Accommodation does not necessarily require any interaction among the parties and can simply entail giving the other side what they want. It is one of the least confrontational methods for dealing with conflict. Capitulation has the advantage of being efficient in that, by giving the other

party what he wants, the conflict ends quickly. Other advantages are that the relationship between the parties may be preserved and that the other party may feel a sense of indebtedness, which may come into play in the future. The adage, it is better to give than to receive, seems to recommend accommodation, although it is not clear that this advice was meant for organizational members in an increasingly competitive environment. While capitulation may be recommended in some situations, people are unlikely to get what they want by relying on others accommodating them. They may rarely achieve outcomes that are good for them if they use capitulation too often. In most situations, there are better ways to manage conflict.

Pressing

When individuals have as their primary objective the achievement of their interests and are unconcerned about whether other parties get what they want (or even wish to "beat" the other side), they often rely on a series of strategies that are typically described as contentious. These strategies include a variety of tactics

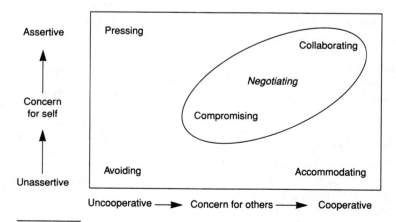

FIGURE 5.1. Dual concern model. Adapted from Thomas, K. "Conflict and Conflict Management," in *Handbook of Industrial and Organizational Psychology,* ed. M.D. Dunnette (Santa Monica, CA: Goodyear Publishing Company, 1976), 900. Used by permission of Marvin D. Dunnette.

such as irrevocable commitments, threats or promises, and persuasive argumentation.[11]

Irrevocable commitments occur when one party credibly guarantees to continue behaving in a certain way that once begun will not be changed. An excellent example of an irrevocable commitment is the game of Chicken. Chicken involves two participants who are driving their cars at breakneck speed on a direct collision course with each other. The loser in this game is the one who first turns aside—the "chicken"—thereby avoiding a head-on collision and almost certain death for both players. In this game each side tries to convince the other that they are committed to their course of action—driving straight toward the other car. More generally, irrevocable commitments occur when two parties engage in a test of wills in which neither side is willing to concede. A typical example of the risk of such games and tactics can be seen in the escalation of losses and acrimony that can occur when couples divorce.

Irrevocable commitments are useful because they do not require agreement of the other party to work nor do they require that the committing party be of equal or greater power. In the case of irrevocable commitments, weakness can become strength. Consider Gandhi's power, stemming from his weakness in the face of the other party's strength, to compel the British to modify their policies in India.

Threats and promises are both meant to convey intention. The typical promise is designed to induce some particular behavior by describing what will happen if such an action occurs. For example, one might promise to trade future support on issue A for current support on issue B. Promises do not give information about what will happen if compliance does not occur. Threats, on the other hand, convey what will happen if the preferred behavior does not happen. As such, one might threaten to vote against my interests unless I vote *for* her interests. Threats and promises are designed to have the same effect, but the mechanism by which the effects come about are different. Promises rely on the benefits of compliance while threats work because of the costs of noncompliance. In fact, compared to promises, threats provide more information because they describe how an individual intends to behave in response to a broader variety of actions. Promises only tell me what you will do if I take one

particular action. They tell me nothing about what you would do if I take no action or another action.

Compared to threats and promises, persuasive argumentation is a less controlling tactic, although one that requires considerable skill. Through persuasive argumentation, I can influence you to give up something that you hold dear, change a situation you currently enjoy, or lower your aspirations. Consider the difficulty of persuading employees to work fewer hours rather than laying off other organizational members. When undertaking this tactic, one typically appeals to the unattractive alternatives that will ensue if the situation is left unchanged.

Avoidance

The most common response to conflict on any level is to avoid it. In many situations, people avoid conflict when both they and their organizations would benefit if they managed it more proactively. For example, issues involving quality of care are sometimes ignored because people fear the conflict associated with addressing them. However, avoidance does have its merits. If the issues involved in the conflict are trivial and the parties do not care much about their own outcome or the other party's outcome, avoidance may be the best strategy. The costs incurred by confronting the problem may be greater, at least in the short run, than the benefits that accrue from having the conflict resolved. Avoidance may also be the best way to deal with conflict when someone else can resolve the problem more effectively or when the problem would be better dealt with in the future after the involved parties have cooled down. If avoiding conflict becomes a habit, however, important issues, when they arise, may never get addressed.

Negotiation

Unlike other conflict resolution tactics, negotiation is a process through which multiple parties work together on the outcome. People negotiate every day, although they do not always think of their activities as negotiations. This becomes clearer, however, when negotiation is defined as the process whereby two or more parties decide what each will give and take in an exchange between them.[12] This broad definition encompasses a preponderance of activities that people do every day, both within and outside organizations. Negotiations typically, but not always, involve some type of direct interaction between the parties, with the interaction being face to face, verbal, or written. The parties in a negotiation are interdependent in that they both desire something the other party has control over.

An interesting aspect of negotiation that distinguishes it from other forms of conflict resolution is the considerable amount of attention it has received in both applied and scholarly settings. One result of this trend is that we now know more about the behavior of negotiators and the structural factors that influence them than we did in the past. In the next section, we will provide a framework for thinking about negotiations that can be applied equally well to almost any negotiation situation, whether it involves a husband and wife or two nations. By analyzing the structure of a negotiation, negotiators should be able to improve their preparedness for, the process of, and the outcome of the negotiation.

NEGOTIATION

Basic Concepts

A negotiator never *has* to negotiate; there are always alternatives to reaching an agreement through a negotiation. Many were discussed above, such as avoiding the situation or giving the other party what they want. However, when a person in an interdependent situation (i.e., the person desires something the other party has control over and vice versa) does not reach a negotiated agreement with the other party, that person has to settle for another alternative regarding the desired resource controlled by the other party. For example, if a hospital is trying to hire a nurse but does not reach an agreement on an employment contract with a particular nurse, the hospital has to either accept the alternative of not having the position filled or choose the alternative of trying to hire another person for the job. From the nurse's point of view, if an agreement is not reached with the hospital, he will have to settle for another alternative, perhaps accepting a job with another hospital or continuing the job search.

Whether they have thought about them or not, the parties in a negotiation have alternatives that they will implement if the negotiation ends in an impasse. The negotiator will obviously choose her best alternative to an agreement if an impasse is reached, so this alternative will be our focus. Specifically, a negotiator's *Best Alternative To a Negotiated Agreement (BATNA)* is an important consideration because it is a source of power in the negotiation.[13] Being able to walk away from the negotiation if a satisfactory agreement does not appear to be forthcoming can be a valuable negotiating tool. Besides the opportunity to use this information strategically, it is also important to know when you actually should walk away. Knowing your best alternative allows a comparison to be made between the value of your best alternative and the value of various agreements that might be reached, which in turn allows you to know which agreements are desirable and which should be turned down.

A BATNA is put into action by determining a *reservation price*. A reservation price can be thought of as a bottom line, or the point at which you are indifferent between an impasse and an agreement.[14] A reservation price should be stated in terms of whatever units are being negotiated. In many negotiations the units of exchange are dollars so that, for example, a negotiator might have a reservation price of $18,000 when buying a car (i.e., the buyer will pay no more than $18,000 for a car). A BATNA and a reservation price, although closely related, are distinct concepts. The connection between the two is that a reservation price should equal the value placed on your best alternative *plus* whatever transaction costs you will incur to enact your best alternative.[15] For example, the expenses that would be involved in hiring another nurse should be taken into consideration in determining a reservation price for a negotiation with a nurse candidate.

An *aspiration level* is what a negotiator would ideally like to achieve in the negotiation. It can also be referred to as a target or goal. An aspiration level should be challenging but attainable. A goal that is too challenging is not motivating because it is not within the realm of possibilities, while one that is too easy also loses its motivating potential once it is surpassed. Typically an aspiration level is stated in the same units as the reservation price (e.g., dollars).

The three concepts just discussed focus on one party rather than the constellation of parties involved in a negotiation. When the parties in a negotiation come together, additional structural features come into play.

The most prominent feature is the *bargaining zone.* The bargaining zone is found by combining the reservation prices of each negotiator and determining whether they overlap, and if so, the extent of the overlap. A positive bargaining zone occurs if a set of agreements exists that both parties prefer over impasse.[16] It is easier to understand this concept with the aid of a diagram. Imagine that a nurse and a hospital are negotiating over the nurse's salary. The nurse's reservation price is $30,000 and the hospital's reservation price is $35,000. This is outlined in Figure 5.2. The bargaining zone is the range of agreements between and including $30,000 and $35,000. If there is no overlap region between the reservation prices of the parties, then a negative bargaining zone exists. Because there are no agreements that are acceptable to both parties, no resolution is possible. It is important for a negotiator to gather information about the size of the bargaining zone during the course of the negotiation.

The Distributive Dimension of Negotiation

Of the two dimensions of negotiation, only the *distributive dimension* is necessarily part of every negotiation. The *integrative dimension,* on the other hand, is never applied in many negotiations. Negotiation always

TABLE 5.1.   Claiming Value: Distributive Bargaining Strategies

1. Know your BATNA.
2. Determine your bottom line or reservation price.
3. Set a goal or aspiration level that is (a) significantly better than your bottom line and (b) optimistically realistic.
4. Think of what objective standards might be acceptable to the other party.
5. Plan your opening. An initial offer should not be too extreme, but it should prevent the other party from "anchoring" the negotiation.
6. Develop reciprocity. Avoid making unilateral concessions.

involves the allocation, or distribution, of some set of resources. The distributive dimension is often referred to as that part of negotiation in which value is claimed. In every negotiation, regardless of the amount of resources to be distributed, an integral task for the negotiators is to determine how much each party will take from the "pie" of resources. Single issue negotiations are the most common example of purely distributive negotiations. The amount of resources is fixed, and whatever one party gains is always at the expense of the other party. Resolving negotiations that are distributive often entails compromise by both parties, as each party concedes a little at a time in a reciprocal manner until they reach an agreement. Negotiators should consider several strategies that may help them claim as large a share of the resources as possible. These strategies are outlined in Table 5.1.

Many negotiators presume that all negotiations are purely distributive and that their task as negotiators is to get as much as they can from the fixed amount of resources to be divided. A common assumption is that the interests of the other party are diametrically opposed to their own interests, and therefore there is a direct conflict over the resources in question. This is called the "fixed-pie bias."[17] Based on this assumption, they view negotiation as an adversarial process. The integrative dimension of negotiation is often overlooked because of this bias.

The Integrative Dimension of Negotiation

The most basic assumption underlying the integrative dimension of negotiation is that one party can

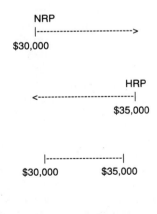

FIGURE 5.2.   Bargaining zones.

gain without the other party necessarily having to lose. Another way to say this is that there are ways for the parties to mutually benefit. To do this, the parties need to take more of a problem-solving, cooperative approach rather than the contentious, competitive approach that typically characterizes purely distributive negotiations. In effect, the parties try to "expand the pie" of resources, or create value. A key element that should be present for a problem-solving orientation to work is trust between the parties. Trust is crucial because information sharing is at the heart of the negotiation process, and if information is not openly and accurately shared, albeit in a reciprocal manner, it is unlikely that integrative solutions can be found. Negotiating along the integrative dimension, or trying to find mutually beneficial solutions, can be difficult because it frequently requires finding creative or novel solutions that may not have been considered prior to the negotiation.

There are several ways to achieve integrative solutions. Most of them are based on differing interests underlying the conflict on the surface. Although this may sound strange because differences are the reason for the conflict, it is differences *in preferences* that allow integrative negotiation to occur. An example from the Chiefland Memorial Hospital case at the beginning of the chapter may help to clarify this point. In general, both hospital administrators and physicians would be in favor of lower costs for the hospital and higher quality service. However, the two parties differ in the importance they place on these two objectives. Administrators place more importance on lowering costs, while physicians place greater importance on increasing the quality of service. Conflict occurs because increasing quality is thought to require incurring more costs. The underlying interests of both parties may be met, though, if the parties view the problem within the context of a longer time horizon. Increasing quality may raise costs in the short run, but this higher level of quality service may lower costs in other areas, such as malpractice suits, in the future.

There are many techniques for finding integrative solutions. Logrolling entails trading issues that are of differing importance to the two parties.[18] Cost cutting occurs when one party finds a way to make the conces-

sions of the other party less costly. This is often accomplished by one party offering the conceding party some sort of compensation that is related to the issues being negotiated. Cost cutting differs from nonspecific compensation, in which the party that concedes is paid by the other party in some currency that is unrelated to the negotiated issues. Obtaining added resources may sometimes be possible so that both parties can meet their goals. Frequently, the time and effort spent negotiating over a given set of resources may instead be spent finding ways to increase the amount of available resources.[19] By undertaking one or more of these strategies, the parties in a negotiation may both be better off than if they simply compromised on the issues.

There are many obvious and some not-so-obvious benefits of finding integrative solutions in negotiations. Increasing the amount of resources to be distributed may be necessary for both parties to be able to reach their reservation prices. In these cases, an impasse is likely unless some integrative solution is found. An obvious benefit to finding integrative agreements is that a party's outcomes may be increased because a larger amount of resources is available to be distributed.

Less obviously, a party may also benefit from the opponent receiving a higher outcome. An opponent's satisfaction with the negotiation should increase as the outcome gets better. This should have a positive effect on the relationship between the two parties and should make the agreement more stable. If the other party is required to implement a decision that was reached as part of the negotiated agreement, successful implementation is more likely if the opponent is happy with the outcome, rather than disgruntled. Of course, the importance a party places on an opponent's outcome may vary with the expectation or probability of future interaction or with the types of issues that are being negotiated (e.g., some issues may require implementation, while others may not). The point here is that most people think only of their own outcome when they determine whether they were successful in a negotiation when several benefits, however indirect, may accrue to them if the other party also achieves a good outcome. Several specific strategies for reaching integrative agreements are outlined in Table 5.2.

TABLE 5.2. Creating Value: Integrative
Bargaining Strategies

1. Know your BATNA. Try to ascertain the other side's BATNA.
2. Analyze your own and the other party's reservation prices to determine the bargaining zone.
3. Set priorities on your interests and those of the other party.
4. Construct multi-issue packages of offers that take into account differences between your own and the other party's priorities.

The Mixed-Motive Nature of Negotiation

When thinking about the distributive and integrative dimensions of negotiation, it is crucial to keep in mind the mixed-motive nature of negotiations. Creating value by finding integrative solutions requires primarily cooperative behavior, while claiming value along the distributive dimension of the negotiation requires primarily competitive behavior. Many people make the mistake of thinking they can segment a negotiation into integrative and distributive components so that, for example, the parties can first integratively expand the pie and then negotiate the distribution of the enlarged pie. In fact, it is very unlikely for these to happen sequentially. Instead, the processes of integration and distribution occur simultaneously.

Negotiators must simultaneously balance cooperative and competitive behavior, so that they enlarge the pie *while* they claim an acceptable share of the enlarged pie. It is this "fundamental tension between cooperation and competition" that is the heart of negotiation, and that makes negotiation both an art and a science. The way that the value is created affects the way it is divided; the process of creating value is entwined with the process of claiming it.[20] This is especially true if the motives and behaviors of the other party are unpredictable before the negotiation or are hard to read during the negotiation.

The Role of Information Sharing

Cooperative or competitive orientations are easy to talk about in general terms, but how do they manifest themselves in actual behavior during a negotiation? One of the core behavioral components of negotiation is information sharing. It is through the sharing of information that parties learn about their opponent's preferences on the issues, BATNA and reservation price, willingness to concede, interest in adding other issues to the negotiation, and in general, their opponent's overall orientation. Although the total amount of information that is shared during the negotiation is likely to affect the quality of the outcome reached by the parties, examining the subtleties of the parties' information sharing patterns may be more revealing. First, if one party shares much more information than the other party, the party that receives the greater amount of information may have an advantage because they may know more about how far the other party can be pushed or what the chances are of finding an integrative solution. For example, if only one party knows the other's reservation price, the party with this information knows the size of the bargaining zone while the other does not. This could have a profound impact on the outcome of the negotiation.

One clarification here is that sharing information is not the same as talking. One side may talk more than the other party but share a lesser amount of important information. If negotiation is viewed solely as a persuasive process, then the party that talks more may be expected to do more persuading, and thus achieve a better outcome. However, persuasion is typically not included in what we refer to as information sharing. Information that is relevant in this analysis concerns the interests of the party, and thus the side that gives away less of this information may have an advantage.

Even if the amount of information shared by the parties is symmetric, the order in which it is shared may influence the outcomes of the parties. If one party gives away all of his information before the other party gives away any of her information, the party that delays sharing information may have an advantage, knowing more about the issues and the structure of the negotiation than the other party at an earlier point in the negotiation. Ideally, information should be shared in a reciprocal fashion so that one party gives away information incrementally while receiving equivalent amounts of information from the other party.

There are several strategies aimed at getting more information from the other party. Some of them, such as asking questions, are simple but often overlooked. These strategies include

- building trust between the parties so that information is more likely to be shared
- asking questions
- giving away some information unilaterally in the hope that the other party will reciprocate
- making multiple offers simultaneously so the other party's interests can be inferred from the acceptability of each offer
- searching for post-settlement settlements (agreements that occur based on an extended search after an initial agreement is reached)[21]

Of course, the accuracy and specificity of information obtained by the other party is crucial. Discerning the accuracy of the information given by the other party is primarily a matter of trust, both on the part of the party giving information (trusting that the other party will not take advantage of true information) and on the part of the party receiving information (believing the information given by the other party).

Compatible Issues

There is one other type of issue we have not yet mentioned that is frequently overlooked when people think of negotiation. *Compatible issues* are those for which the parties have the same preferences. The parties have no conflict over these issues, perhaps making it seem odd that we include them in a chapter about conflict management. However, they are often included in negotiations because the negotiators do not know they have the same preferences on these issues and they make assumptions about the preferences of the other party.

Specifically, as mentioned earlier, many negotiators have a fixed-pie bias, meaning that they systematically assume their task in a negotiation is to split a fixed amount of resources.[22,23] The incompatibility bias inhibits negotiators in a related way, as they assume that the other party's preferences on the issues are necessarily in direct conflict with their own preferences and that they have no common interests.[24] Because of these biases, issues that are included in a negotiation for which the negotiators want the same outcome are often not identified as compatible, and a substantial number of negotiators settle for an outcome on these issues other than the one they both want.

Multi-Party Negotiations

Most of the examples that are used to illustrate negotiations are dyadic, involving two parties. Although there are certainly many negotiations that involve only two parties, a substantial portion of negotiations involve three or more parties (which we refer to as multi-party). In health care, frequent examples involve negotiations among state or federal payment agencies, hospitals, and physicians. While many of the concepts of negotiation generalize from dyadic to multi-party negotiations, there are important differences between these types of negotiation.

The biggest difference is the increased complexity that occurs when parties are added to the negotiation. This complexity falls into two categories. First, interpersonal complexity increases as more people become involved in the interaction. For each person, there are more signals, gestures, and other types of communications from others to interpret. The second type of complexity involves the issues themselves. There are now multiple sets of preferences to be worked through rather than just two sets. For example, regarding the same subset of issues, two parties may have compatible preferences, two other parties may have opposite preferences but place a different amount of importance on these issues, while the preferences of two other parties may be diametrically opposed. Sharing the information to determine these preferences becomes much more difficult with multiple parties, and even if perfect information is shared, it is still a complex task to determine an optimal solution that is acceptable to everyone.

The bargaining zone in a negotiation with multiple parties is defined as the set of agreements that exceed every party's reservation price. It can be very difficult to determine whether a bargaining zone exists, much less the size of the bargaining zone. Furthermore, there may be people involved in the negotiation who would prefer that no agreement be reached, so that their purpose at the negotiation table (whether disguised or not) is to impede the process of the negotiation. Building trust may be more difficult between multiple parties, especially if coalitions form within the group of negotiators.

Coalition formation can have a major effect on the negotiation process and outcome. Coalitions may be based on longstanding relationships outside of the negotiation, or they may form during the negotiation based on similarity of preferences. They may form either to try to reach a specific agreement or to try to block a specific type of agreement. What is best for the coalition may not be what is best for the entire group. Negotiators in a multi-party situation should think about who they would like to form a coalition with, who might like to form a coalition with them, and who is unlikely to want to include them in a coalition.

Proactive behavior may be especially helpful in building a coalition because it should be easier to form a coalition initially than to break up an existing coalition and reform another one. However, coalitions, especially those formed around specific preferences in the negotiation, are likely to be unstable. When considering that the typical reason for joining a coalition is to increase your own outcomes, it is not surprising that people readily switch allegiances when they get better offers from other potential coalition partners. As such, coalitions may shift repeatedly during the course of a negotiation.

Decision rules for reaching agreement may also be necessary in multi-party negotiations. Possible decision rules include unanimity, majority rule, or some other special rule detailing how many people must agree in order to reach a settlement. Some parties may also have veto power, which affects the power balance in the negotiation. These latter considerations may be influenced by the context within which the negotiation takes place. For example, if all the parties are working in the same organization (e.g., physicians employed by the same hospital), there may be hierarchical considerations, existing norms guiding the selection of a decision rule, or pressure from superiors to reach an agreement. Conversely, in a group negotiation in which the parties represent several different organizations (e.g., physicians having their own organizations), many of the parties may have more freedom to withdraw from the negotiation or force an impasse because they may have better alternatives with other sets of organizations. Also, few norms may exist if the negotiation itself is the first time the parties have been together in a group.

The above factors should be considered when preparing for and participating in a multi-party negotiation. If properly managed, the increased complexity inherent in this type of negotiation does not have to be an impediment and can in fact be used strategically if other parties are less prepared for or less able to cope with the complexity.

Fairness and Ethics in Negotiation

Negotiators often make claims about fairness to support their arguments. Fairness is not a unidimensional concept, however, and the application of different norms of fairness can lead to different outcomes. For this reason, it is important to think about which different norms of fairness can be applied in particular situations so that generalized claims for fairness are not used inappropriately. In a negotiation context, fairness will be discussed as it applies to the allocation of resources, which is the typical result of negotiation.

The most prevalent *fairness norm* in our society is *equality,* in which every party gets the same absolute amount of resources.[25] A second fairness norm that is used in most organizations to determine compensation is *equity,* whereby each person gets allocated an amount of resources proportional to his inputs.[26,27] Defining what relevant inputs consist of and measuring these inputs can often lead to additional conflict, but once norms are in place in organizations regarding these issues, allocating resources equitably is often regarded as fair. Equity can be invoked in many negotiations other than organizational compensation situations as well. A third popular norm of fairness upon which allocations can be based is *need,* so that parties receive an amount of resources proportional to their need for them.[28] As with inputs in the equity norm situation, determining the relative needs of each party can be tricky. Besides these three pure allocation norms of fairness, people may combine two or three of these norms to determine a fair allocation. Negotiators should consider which of these norms is applicable when they or one of their opponents claim that the negotiated outcome should be "fair."

Many people think of fairness and ethics in negotiation as somewhat entwined. Fairness may not always refer to the norm used for resource allocation, as discussed above, but instead may refer to the process by which people negotiate. For instance, people often say that if a negotiator is "unethical," she is not negotiating fairly. This triggers the same kind of problem that is triggered when determining fair allocations, in that people are not always in agreement about what constitutes ethical behavior. This is especially relevant for negotiation because there are many typical negotiating strategies, such as bluffing or avoiding an answer to a specific question, that fall in a gray area concerning the ethicality of such behavior. Furthermore, many people believe that what is ethical is partially determined by context. For example, in some cultures bribes are an accepted way of doing business when negotiating. Others adhere to a more absolute form of ethicality, believing that actions are either ethical or unethical regardless of the situation.

We are not going to state any rules about what is ethical or unethical. Instead, our purpose in discussing ethics is to increase the reader's awareness of several issues. First, however it is defined, unethical behavior is typically the result of self-interest.[29] People act unethically because they benefit from it. When negotiating, regardless of your particular beliefs about ethics, it is important not to assume that the other party has the same beliefs you do or that they will behave (or restrict their behavior) in the same way you will. Also, unethical behavior can have consequences, especially regarding reputations, such that unethical behavior may help negotiators in the short run but may come back to haunt them in the long run. Negotiations can be full of ethical dilemmas. Thinking through and determining your own standards before you get into difficult situations is advised, as is being cautious, especially when making assumptions about the other party's ethical standards.

Preparing to Negotiate

Preparing for a negotiation often has as much to do with achieving a successful outcome as does the actual negotiation. But what exactly should a negotiator do to prepare for the negotiation? In this section, we offer several suggestions for how to increase the probability of a successful negotiation by preparing appropriately.

The least obvious, and perhaps most important, activity that should be worked on before the negotiation is to develop a BATNA, which was discussed earlier. If negotiators can develop a better and more certain alternative to a negotiated outcome, they will have more power in the negotiation and be likely to reach a better outcome. Determining a reservation price, based partially on the BATNA, is the next step to knowing in advance when you will be willing to walk away from the negotiation rather than reach agreement.

Concerning the negotiation more directly, a negotiator should think about what issues are likely to be included in the negotiation if they have not been specified in advance by either party. What additional issues could you bring to the negotiation? What issues might your opponent want to include? Whatever the set of issues includes, the negotiator should determine the importance of each issue relative to the other issues. This facilitates the process of comparing different offers made by the other party and trading low-priority issues for high-priority issues. Collecting information about the other party's alternatives and the importance that party places on each issue is a priority during a negotiation. It follows that negotiators can enhance their position if they can discover some or all of this information about their opponent before the negotiation. Sometimes this information can be gathered directly from the other negotiator prior to negotiating, while in other situations it may be learned from other sources.

Another important piece of information to gather is how many negotiators the other party will be bringing to the table. This question, along with the determination of how many negotiators your party should bring to the negotiation, is the focus of Debate Time 5.2. A negotiator should also determine before the negotiation how important the relationship with the other party is. What future effects are likely to be caused by reputations that are developed in this negotiation? How much is the other party likely to be concerned about the relationship? The extent to which the decisions that are reached during the negotiation need to be implemented by either party after the negotiation is an important factor related to the relationship between the parties. If you have to rely on the other party to implement part of the deal, it is obviously not good to have the other party unhappy with the agreement or with you. Determining the time constraints faced by each party can be useful, as the party who has the longer time before needing to reach an agreement has an advantage, if both parties know about the time constraints of the other.

Even the end of a negotiation should be prepared for. If negotiators do not reveal all of their information during the negotiation, they should think about whether they want to share any of this information after the negotiation. It is usually advisable to keep some information confidential even after the negotiation so the other party does not grow concerned about whether she received a good outcome in the negotiation. The better-prepared party in a negotiation is often the most successful during the negotiation. As in school, doing your homework before the negotiation is half the battle when it is time to take the test.

MANAGING CONFLICT THROUGH THIRD PARTY INTERVENTION

In many conflict situations, the disputants are unable to resolve the conflict. A third party that is not directly involved in the conflict can frequently intervene in one of several different ways to help resolve the conflict. There are many formal, institutional third parties that can be turned to outside of any particular organization. The court system in the United States is a very large example of a third party. Arbitrators are third parties that resolve differences between parties on many different issues, such as professional baseball salaries. The focus of this chapter, however, is on the manager's role as a third party in the day-to-day conflicts that occur in organizational life, rather than on formal third party systems. To the extent that conflict is disruptive in organizations and hampers productivity, managers can increase the effectiveness of their organizations by intervening in conflict situations. Of course, the time the manager spends trying to resolve the disputes of other people is a cost to the organization, which needs to be balanced with the benefit derived from decreased conflict.

Dispute Intervention Goals

After making the decision to intervene in a conflict, the manager has a wide range of third party intervention strategies to choose from. The particular role the manager plays in the dispute may depend on what he

---

DEBATE TIME 5.2: WHAT DO YOU THINK?

POINT: The more people I can bring with me to the negotiation table, the better off I will be. There are many benefits to be realized from including several people in a negotiation party. The more people that are at the negotiation, the more ideas they should be able to think of for ways to reach an integrative outcome. If expertise in different areas is helpful during the negotiation, it may be beneficial to have more "experts" on hand. Multiple roles, such as spokesperson, notekeeper, or financial analyst, can be performed more effectively at the table if a different person performs each function. A higher degree of critical thinking may occur when more people apply different perspectives to the problem being negotiated. Finally, if one party has more people at the negotiation than the other party, the bigger party may be perceived as having more power and may achieve better outcomes as a result.

COUNTERPOINT: I am better off negotiating by myself. The most obvious reason to negotiate alone is that time is a valuable resource, and bringing other people to a negotiation that one person can handle is unnecessarily expensive. There are also more subtle reasons, stemming from intergroup conflict, that more people in each party may not result in better outcomes in a negotiation. When there is a team of negotiators on each side of the table, the intergroup boundaries between the parties may be much stronger than if each party consisted of just one person. When an "us against them" mentality occurs in a negotiation, which may be more likely with groups than with individuals, several negative consequences may result, including increased competitiveness, decreased trust, and a decreased level of information sharing. These may in turn result in outcomes that are inferior to those that may have been reached by individual negotiators bargaining in a more cooperative and trusting manner.

MANAGERIAL GUIDELINES

1. Managers need to analyze the amount and type of both beneficial and detrimental conflict that currently exists in their organization so that they can focus on eliminating the detrimental conflict.
2. Health care managers should evaluate the level at which conflict usually occurs in their organization. Are there strong group boundaries (e.g., between departments or functional areas) that contribute to conflict, or is most conflict at the individual level?
3. When managers are involved in conflict, they should think explicitly about how much concern they have for the other party, as well as how concerned they are about their own outcomes for the issues involved in the conflict. This should help to determine what conflict management strategy will be most appropriate.
4. When negotiating, managers need to determine the exact issues that are currently being negotiated and identify any other issues that might be included in the negotiation. Also, the importance of each issue to both the manager and the other party should be compared to determine where mutually beneficial tradeoffs might occur.
5. Managers should think carefully about what ethical standards they feel comfortable with *before* they enter situations that involve ethical considerations.
6. Managers should not underestimate the importance of preparing for a negotiation. Failing to adequately prepare is probably the single biggest mistake made by negotiators.
7. If managers are going to intervene in a conflict as a third party, they need to consider how much control they want to have over both the process and the outcome of the dispute. Distinguishing between these types of control will facilitate effective intervention implementation.

is trying to accomplish and on the constraints imposed by the situation. When intervening in a dispute between subordinates, a manager has a high level of authority, making any type of intervention an option. This is not the case when a manager intervenes in a dispute between two peers. The amount of conflict between the parties may also influence the manager's selection of intervention strategies. The importance of the issues in dispute, the amount of time pressure faced by the manager, the relative power of the disputants, and the relationships between the parties and between the manager and the parties may all affect the manager's choice of intervention strategies.[30] The manager may also be concerned with how satisfied the disputants will be with the resolution and their perceptions of fairness regarding the intervention.

Types of Intervention Strategies

The types of intervention strategies a manager can undertake can be usefully categorized along two dimensions—the control the third party has over the process of the dispute and the control the third party has over the outcome of the dispute. Suppose a medical group practice manager is trying to manage the conflict between primary care physicians and specialists involving sharing revenue generated by the group practice. The control the manager desires over the process and outcome is likely to be affected by the factors discussed in the preceding paragraph. When the manager desires high control over both the process and outcome of the dispute, she may act as an *inquisitor*. In this type of intervention, the manager gathers information on the dispute by asking questions of the physicians, rather than letting them present the information as they would like. The manager then makes a decision about the outcome of the dispute and communicates this to the physicians. As in the court system, a manager acts as a judge or *arbitrator* when he controls the outcome but not the process of the dispute. The parties are free to present their sides of the dispute as they wish, after which the manager makes the decisions necessary to end the dispute. *Mediators* have control over the process of the dispute but have no authority, or do not use their authority, to control the outcome. Acting as mediator, the group practice manager may control the flow of information between the physician groups by separating them and acting as a go-between or may guide the discussion between them when they are together. The outcome, however, will ultimately be decided by the leaders of the respective physician groups.

The manager who chooses not to have high process or outcome control can choose from several options. The most efficient approach from the manager's perspective is to ignore the conflict and hope the disputants will resolve it by themselves. Managers can also delegate responsibility for getting the dispute resolved to someone else. Another option is to threaten the disputants to increase their motivation to resolve the conflict.

Managers have many options to choose from in determining which third party intervention strategies best fit their needs. It is possible that, for the same dispute situation, a manager may change intervention strategies if the previously chosen strategy does not work. When this happens, a manager will usually progress from strategies involving less control to strategies involving more control.

Although conflict is pervasive, it can be successfully managed through an understanding and application of various conflict management techniques and negotiation skills. By managing conflict more effectively, health services executives make important contributions to organizational effectiveness while improving the productivity and satisfaction of the people with whom they work.

KEY CONCEPTS

Accommodation
Administrative Conflict
Arbitrator
Aspiration Level
Avoidance
Bargaining Zone
Best Alternative To a
    Negotiated Agreement
    (BATNA)
Compatible Issues
Competition
Conflict
Cooperation
Distributive Dimension
    of Negotiation
Emotional Conflict

Equality Fairness Norm
Equity Fairness Norm
Inquisitor
Integrative Dimension of
    Negotiation
Intergroup Conflict
Interpersonal Conflict
Intragroup Conflict
Intrapersonal Conflict
Mediator
Need Fairness Norm
Negotiation
Pressing
Reservation Price
Task Content Conflict

Discussion Questions

1. What types of skills do managers need to successfully manage conflict in their organizations? Which of these skills do you possess? What might be your greatest weakness as a conflict resolver? What can you do to strengthen your weak areas?

2. Related to Debate Time 5.1, what are some indications that a health services organization is experiencing dysfunctional levels of conflict? What systems can be put in place to monitor these indicators?

3. What third party intervention strategies are likely to be favored by managers acting as third parties? What third party intervention strategies are likely to be favored by the disputants? If these answers are different, what can a manager do to satisfy all the parties involved? What factors may affect your answers to these questions?

4. Regarding intergroup conflict, which groups do you most frequently represent or identify with in your interactions? How might this change depending on the type of health services organization with which you might be employed?

5. If you were James Grover in the Chiefland Memorial Hospital case presented at the beginning of the chapter, what actions would you take to resolve the dispute between Hoffman and Young? Specify the steps you would take to resolve this conflict and give reasons why your recommended course of action is the best way to handle the dispute.

REFERENCES

1. Neale MA, Bazerman MH. *Cognition and Rationality in Negotiation*. New York, NY: Free Press; 1991:2.
2. Ibid.
3. Homans G. *Social Behavior: Its Elementary Forms*. New York: Harcourt, Brace; 1961.
4. Thomas K. Conflict and conflict management. In: Dunnette M, ed. *Handbook of Industrial and Organizational Psychology*. New York, NY: Rand-McNally; 1976.
5. Janis I. *Groupthink: Psychological Studies of Policy Decisions and Fiascoes*. Boston, Mass: Houghton-Mifflin; 1982.
6. Jehn KA. The impact of intragroup conflict on effectiveness: A multimethod examination of the benefits and detriments of conflict. Unpublished dissertation, Evanston, Ill: Northwestern University; 1992.
7. Ibid.
8. Northcraft GB, Neale MA. *Organizational Behavior: The Managerial Challenge*. Homewood, Ill: Dryden Press; 1990.
9. Deutsch M. An experimental study of the effects of cooperation and competition upon group process. *Human Relations*. 1949;2:199–232.
10. Sherif M. *Intergroup Conflict and Cooperation*. Norman, Ok: University Book Exchange; 1977.
11. Pruitt DG, Rubin JZ. *Social Conflict*. New York, NY: Academic Press; 1986.
12. Rubin J, Brown B. *The Social Psychology of Bargaining and Negotiation*. New York, NY: Academic Press; 1975.
13. Fisher R, Ury W. *Getting to Yes*. Boston, Mass: Houghton-Mifflin; 1981.
14. Raiffa H. *The Art and Science of Negotiation*. Cambridge, Mass: Belknap; 1982.
15. White SB, Neale MA. The role of negotiation aspiration and settlement expectancies on bargaining outcomes. *Organizational Behavior and Human Decision Processes*. In press.
16. Neale, Bazerman, op. cit.
17. Bazerman MH, Magliozzi T, Neale MA. The acquisition of an integrative response in a competitive market. *Organizational Behavior and Human Decision Processes*. 1985;35:294–313.
18. Pruitt, Rubin, op. cit.
19. Pruitt DG. Achieving integrative agreement. In: Bazerman MH, Lewicki RJ, eds. *Negotiating in Organizations*. Beverly Hills, Ca: Sage; 1983.
20. Lax DA, Sebenius JK. *The Manager as Negotiator*. New York, NY: Free Press; 1986.
21. Raiffa H. Post settlement settlements. *Negotiation Journal*. 1985;1:9–12.
22. Bazerman, Magliozzi, Neale, op. cit.
23. Thompson LL. Information exchange in negotiation. *Journal of Experimental Social Psychology*. 1991;27(2):161–179.
24. Ibid.
25. Rawls J. *A Theory of Justice*. Cambridge, Mass: Harvard University Press; 1971.
26. Adams JS. Toward an understanding of inequity. *Journal of Abnormal and Social Psychology*. 1963;67:422–436.
27. Homans, op. cit.
28. Deutsch M. Equity, equality, and need: What determines which value will be used as the basis of distributive justice? *Journal of Social Issues*. 1975;31:137–149.
29. Murnighan JK. *Bargaining Games*. New York, NY: William Morrow and Company, Inc.; 1992.
30. Neale, Bazerman, op. cit.

THE NATURE OF ORGANIZATIONS: FRAMEWORK FOR THE TEXT

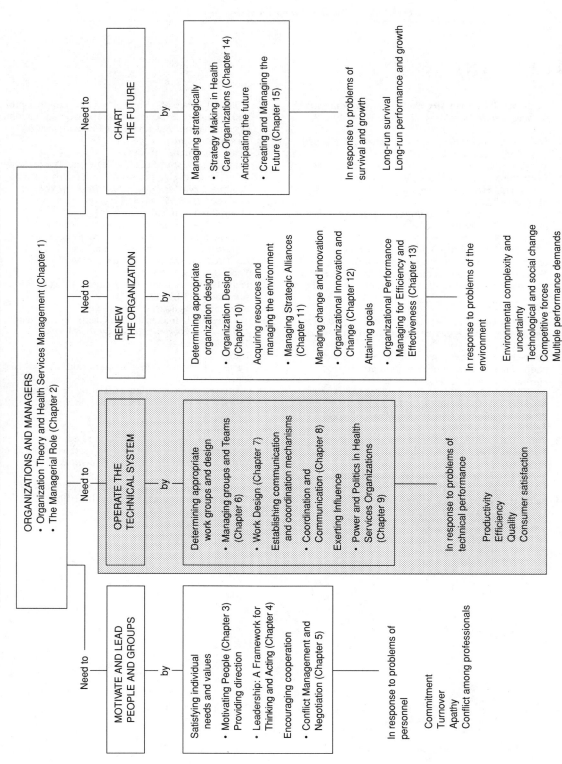

ORGANIZATIONS AND MANAGERS
- Organization Theory and Health Services Management (Chapter 1)
- The Managerial Role (Chapter 2)

Need to

MOTIVATE AND LEAD PEOPLE AND GROUPS

by

Satisfying individual needs and values
- Motivating People (Chapter 3)
Providing direction
- Leadership: A Framework for Thinking and Acting (Chapter 4)
Encouraging cooperation
- Conflict Management and Negotiation (Chapter 5)

In response to problems of personnel

Commitment
Turnover
Apathy
Conflict among professionals

Need to

OPERATE THE TECHNICAL SYSTEM

by

Determining appropriate work groups and design
- Managing groups and Teams (Chapter 6)
- Work Design (Chapter 7)
Establishing communication and coordination mechanisms
- Coordination and Communication (Chapter 8)
Exerting Influence
- Power and Politics in Health Services Organizations (Chapter 9)

In response to problems of technical performance

Productivity
Efficiency
Quality
Consumer satisfaction

Need to

RENEW THE ORGANIZATION

by

Determining appropriate organization design
- Organization Design (Chapter 10)
Acquiring resources and managing the environment
- Managing Strategic Alliances (Chapter 11)
Managing change and innovation
- Organizational Innovation and Change (Chapter 12)
Attaining goals
- Organizational Performance Managing for Efficiency and Effectiveness (Chapter 13)

In response to problems of the environment

Environmental complexity and uncertainty
Technological and social change
Competitive forces
Multiple performance demands

Need to

CHART THE FUTURE

by

Managing strategically
- Strategy Making in Health Care Organizations (Chapter 14)
Anticipating the future
- Creating and Managing the Future (Chapter 15)

In response to problems of survival and growth

Long-run survival
Long-run performance and growth

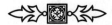

PART THREE

OPERATING THE TECHNICAL SYSTEM

The four chapters of this section focus on operating critical components of the technical system within health care organizations. This involves determining the appropriate work design, establishing communication and coordination mechanisms, and assuring and improving performance. The following chapters characterize these functions in order to enhance technical aspects of productivity, efficiency, quality, and consumer satisfaction.

Chapter 6, Managing Groups and Teams in Health Services Organizations, focuses on the effective management of groups and teams. The chapter addresses the following questions:

- Why are groups and teams important?
- How does group structure and process affect performance?
- What are the causes of intergroup conflict, and what strategies are available for its management?

Chapter 7, Work Design, considers the design of work in organizations. The emphasis is on defining different types and components of work and assessing the interconnected nature of work within a variety of health services organizations. The chapter addresses the following questions:

- What is work? Is it different from working?
- How does work design affect individual motivation and productivity?
- How does the interconnectedness of work affect individuals and work groups?

Chapter 8, Coordination and Communication, deals with the essential means through which managers link together the various people and groups within the organization and link the organization to other organizations. The following questions provide the major focus of this chapter:

- What is the role of intraorganizational coordination? How is it similar or different from interorganizational coordination?
- What are the mechanisms available to achieve intra- and interorganizational coordination?
- What are the major components and barriers of effective communications?

The last chapter in this section, Power and Politics in Health Services Organizations, discusses the means by which power distributions can be identified, the conditions under which conflict among groups may result, the uses of power to resolve conflict, and the strategies and tactics that are commonly employed to do so. The chapter addresses the following questions:

- What are the sources of power?
- What are the conditions that promote the use of power, politics, and informal influence?
- What approaches are available for consolidating and developing power by managers, physicians, and other groups of health care providers?

Upon completing these four chapters, the reader should be able to understand the nature of work and the processes affecting work within health services organizations.

CHAPTER

MANAGING GROUPS AND TEAMS

Bruce J. Fried, Ph.D.
Associate Professor

Thomas G. Rundall, Ph.D.
Professor

CHAPTER TOPICS

Types of Groups and Teams in
Organizations
A Model of Work Group Performance
Group Structure
Group Processes
Intergroup Relationships

LEARNING OBJECTIVES

After completing this chapter, the reader should be able to

1. describe the importance and types of groups and teams in health services organizations
2. distinguish between different approaches to assessing work group performance
3. analyze the effects of a work group's structure on group performance
4. explain the relationship between work group norms and group productivity
5. identify the key roles assumed by individuals in work groups
6. describe key aspects of group process including communications structures, decision making, and stages of group development
7. define the major causes and consequences of intergroup conflict and identify alternative strategies for managing conflict

CHAPTER PURPOSE

As illustrated by the unfolding events involving the Interagency Program on Sexual Abuse, groups are a mainstay of organizational life and will become more important in coming years. The work of health services organizations is increasingly being carried out by groups and teams, and we simply cannot escape the necessity of working in groups. Almost all clinical and managerial innovations are dependent to some degree on effective group performance. For example, as patient care technology becomes more specialized, there will be increasing need for team structures to coordinate the work of individual specialists. Quality improvement methods, such as continuous quality improvement, are highly dependent upon well-functioning cross-functional teams.[1]

Work groups are permanent structures, not temporary aberrations, within health services organiza-

IN THE REAL WORLD

FORMING AND MANAGING AN INTERORGANIZATIONAL TASK FORCE: A CASE IN GROUP MANAGEMENT

Glendale Children's Center is a large multipurpose mental health center in a large urban community. The Center provides a comprehensive range of services to children and families, including inpatient treatment, family therapy, outpatient services, community educational services, and a variety of specialized programs aimed at specific ethnic and cultural groups. Good relationships are maintained with the government child protection services, hospitals, law enforcement agencies, and other human service organizations. The Center is staffed by several full- and part-time psychiatrists, psychologists, nurses, social workers, teachers, child care workers, and child care aides. The Center also maintains contracts with several pediatricians and family physicians.

The Center recently received a generous grant to begin an interorganizational effort aimed at coordinating services for sexually abused chil-

dren. This topic has received increased attention over the years from private foundations and from various levels of government. National and local changes in government are likely to increase the visibility of this issue.

The situation in this community was not unlike that found in many other areas. Various public and private agencies, as well as clinicians in private practice, were involved in assessing and treating children who had been sexually abused. Referral networks were unclear, and there was a chronic problem of getting children into treatment programs. The shortage of programs was in part related to the lack of clinicians interested in dealing with this problem as well as the shortage of individuals with specific training in this area. Funding was provided to begin a program that would coordinate a fragmented set of services currently provided in the community and to identify services that might be needed.

After consulting with representatives of other agencies, the program was intended to produce initiatives in six areas

1. developing referral networks and designing and implementing common intake and referral procedures
2. providing educational and training services to professionals throughout the city
3. providing educational services to community members and nonprofessionals
4. providing consultation services to hospitals and other community agencies
5. developing and implementing new needed services, preferably on an interorganizational basis
6. engaging a group of key agencies in ongoing monitoring of the system of care

In accepting the grant, the Center committed itself to involving a wide group of agencies in this effort.

Katherine Kalmbach, a social worker, was hired to manage this program, now called the Interagency Program on Sexual Abuse. This individual had clinical experience in this area and had worked in various community programs. Her first task was to establish an advisory committee to engage the support of community agencies and to develop the program's mission and priorities. The following individuals agreed to serve on this committee:

• Joe Samuels is a child protection supervisor with the state government child protection agency. His main role is to supervise child protection workers who investigate sexual abuse and other child neglect and abuse cases. He himself was a child protection worker for ten years before moving into a supervisory role. The role of his agency is clear: child protection. He has had reservations about the efficacy of treatment for offenders, although he is quite supportive of treatment for children. He is strongly in favor of interagency collaboration and will often speak for prolonged periods about the problems in the mental health and social

services system. Along with Frances Jenkins, the support of Joe Samuels is viewed as critical to the success of the program.

• Charles Long is an officer with the city police department. His main interest in being involved in this group is in seeing offenders prosecuted; he possesses great expertise in the legalities surrounding child abuse and neglect. In particular, he would like to see more children come forward as reliable witnesses in court. He has a tremendous amount of important information to contribute to this group, although he tends to be reserved in these situations and somewhat intimidated by the presence of professionals.

• Fred Ewell is a psychologist at Thames Treatment Center, a private psychiatric hospital. He has a decidedly psychoanalytic bias and strongly opposes attempts to "force" people into treatment. He feels that therapy is worthless unless the motivation comes from within the individual. He is quite outspoken on this point. Fred is well respected as a clinician in the community and speaks frequently on treatment issues. In terms of sexual abuse, he is active in a national organization known as Free Choice. This group questions the ability of children to recall accurately events that may have happened several years ago.

• Frances Jenkins is the director of the city's division of the state child protection agency. Like Mr. Samuels, her role is child protection. She supports the concept of an interagency coalition and has for 30 years been an outspoken advocate for children's rights. However, she is cautious about committing other people in her agency to the coalition, and she is very protective of her own time. In general, she feels this is a worthwhile initiative but doubts its eventual success because community agencies are already stretched to the limit. Her support is deemed essential to the eventual success of this initiative.

• Dr. Jane O'Flaherty is a psychiatrist who sees a number of sexually abused children and is a community activist for children's rights. She is somewhat of a renegade in the psychiatric community. She supports an eclectic approach to treatment and is skeptical of those who take a narrowly psychoanalytic approach to treatment. She is also a supporter of treating offenders and recognizes the abuser as an individual in need of treatment.

- Walt Williams is an attorney in private practice. He has been asked to join the group because of his expertise in family and criminal law.
- Rev. Benjamin Sellig is the pastor of a Methodist church who has a special interest in the topic of sexual abuse.
- Don Bunker is a popular city councilman who is now serving his fifteenth year in office.

The initial meeting of this group was polite and surprisingly productive. In a two-hour period, they produced a draft mission statement for the program and a set of priorities. Disagreements were minimal. Group members identified themselves and committed themselves to working with this team. Earlier misgivings about time commitments and possible philosophical differences seemed nonexistent. Other individuals were identified in the community who should work with the Advisory Committee, and a work plan was established. Each member agreed to chair or co-chair a committee formed around one of the six functions of the Advisory Committee. Each member would also be responsible for identifying community members to participate on each committee. It was agreed that each committee would produce a work plan for its area and present it at the next meeting in three weeks. Ms. Kalmbach agreed to produce a draft of the mission statement and priorities which would also be reviewed.

The program director deliberately used a group approach to developing this program. She recognized that the problem of sexual abuse is extremely complex; to accomplish the objectives of the program requires the participation of individuals with different levels of expertise as well as individuals with key political ties to the community. She was pleased with the willingness of these individuals to participate and was delighted at the productivity and camaraderie evidenced at the first meeting of the group. The second meeting, therefore, came as a surprise, when the following events transpired:

- Frances Jenkins did not attend the meeting. She sent a newly hired 24-year-old child protection worker to permanently replace her on the committee. She sent a note regretting her inability to devote adequate time to the committee.
- The group spent half of the meeting arguing about the mission statement. At the end of the first half hour, the original mission statement was in shreds, and the committee asked Ms. Kalmbach to forget about the mission statement and move on to other matters.
- Fred Ewell got into a heated debate with Dr. Jane O'Flaherty and Walt Williams on the issue of helping children to testify in court. Don Bunker expressed genuine disbelief of Fred Ewell's views, and Dr. O'Flaherty said it would be very difficult for her to sit in the same room with him.
- Joe Samuels reported that his committee on developing treatment services reached an impasse because he and Dr. O'Flaherty could not agree on the issue of treating sexual abuse offenders.

The meeting was saved by Rev. Sellig who convinced committee members to "cool off" for two weeks and reconvene. Meanwhile, Katherine Kalmbach was dismayed and wondered how she would fulfill the mandate of the committee.

tions. When managed well, work groups can be highly creative and productive and contribute in a positive way to organizational effectiveness. When poorly managed, the organization and its patients or clients can face disastrous consequences.

Given the strategic importance and ubiquity of work groups in health services organizations, it is appropriate that managers concern themselves with the management of work groups. While there are many types of work groups, concepts of group organization, process, and effectiveness are applicable across a wide spectrum of groups including

- boards of directors and their committees and subcommittees
- nursing teams
- operating room teams
- strategic planning teams
- treatment teams
- interorganizational planning teams

Most organizational members participate in a variety of formal work groups and, as such, may assume numerous roles depending on the group and their role in the group. What is important is that an awareness of group concepts is key to organizational performance.

Notwithstanding the importance of work groups in organizations, there is likely no other aspect of organizational life that causes as much ambivalence as working in groups. While many of us enjoy the interactions and synergies that result from group participation, groups often create misunderstandings and bring out latent conflicts between individuals. Interprofessional rivalries and status differences are often played out in groups causing anger, dissatisfaction, lower productivity, and frequently, a sense that individuals' knowledge and skills are underutilized. Anyone who has spent time in work groups is often aware of the destructive potential of personality clashes; these are often severe in the relatively intimate environment of work groups.

The importance of the work group structure and group processes has been recognized for at least 50 years. The Hawthorne experiments firmly established the proposition that an individual's performance is determined in large part by relationship patterns that emerge within the group.[2] The work group has a pervasive impact on individual behaviors and attitudes because it controls so many of the stimuli to which the individual is exposed in performing organizational tasks.[3,4]

This chapter focuses on the effective management of groups and teams in organizations. It does this by building on Chapters 3–5, dealing with issues of motivation, leadership, and conflict management respectively, and also touches on issues of work design, communication and coordination, and organization design, which are subsequently discussed in Chapters 7, 8, and 10 respectively. Following a discussion of the types of groups found in health services organizations, attention is given to issues of group cohesiveness, including concerns with professionalism, status differences, communication, and group size and composition. The following section deals with the question of group productivity and why certain groups are more productive than others.

TYPES OF GROUPS AND TEAMS IN ORGANIZATIONS

Various types of groups are found in organizations, including reference groups, membership groups, informal groups, and formal groups as shown in Table 6.1.[5] *Reference groups* are groups of individuals whose purpose is to share particular experiences or to assess members' own personal attitudes or behavior. These groups need not formally convene to be considered a group. For example, a student wanting advice on accepting a job offer may seek out the opinions of other students. Typically, we construct reference groups from individuals having certain desirable characteristics.

There are two types of *membership groups* in organizations: informal groups and formal groups. *Informal groups* are established to satisfy members' personal needs. While the focus in this chapter is on formal work groups, it is also important to understand that individuals in organizations are often members of informal groups. Membership in informal groups are those in which membership is voluntary; they usually evolve gradually among employees with common in-

TABLE 6.1. Types of Groups in Health Services Organizations

Type	Definition	Examples
Reference groups	Groups of people with whom individuals compare themselves in order to assess their own personal attitudes or behavior	Co-workers, friends, relatives
Friendship groups	Groups of people who form together to satisfy personal and social needs	Co-workers, book clubs
Interest groups	Informal voluntary groups that develop to achieve some mutually beneficial objective	Female managers in a hospital interested in discussing issues of sexual discrimination, housekeeping staff interested in discussing working conditions
Work groups	Formal groups that perform day-to-day nonmanagerial work assignments; may include a supervisor and subordinates or may include individuals from various disciplines	Primary care nursing teams; mental health assessment team; research team
Management teams	Formal groups consisting of senior managers that complete managerial work activities on a daily basis; may also include subordinate managers	Hospital senior management team; multidivisional management team for a multihospital system
Temporary groups or task forces	Groups that are formed to complete a specific task; typically disbanded once task is completed	Strategic planning team, program development team, computer conversion team
Intermittent groups	Groups that are composed of people who do not work together but meet regularly to exchange work-related information or to coordinate different work groups	Hospital board of directors, community advisory boards, interorganizational teams
Standing committees	Representatives from an organization's work groups and management teams who meet periodically to coordinate work among different groups	Medical staff committees, quality improvement committee, infection control committee, human resources committee

From John A. Wagner, III/John R. Hollenbeck, MANAGEMENT OF ORGANIZATIONAL BEHAVIOR, © 1992, p. 369. Reprinted by permission of Prentice Hall, Englewood Cliffs, New Jersey.

terests or backgrounds. Many informal groups form in organizations and usually exist to meet individuals' personal, social, or professional needs. By definition, informal groups are generally not formally sanctioned by management and range from individuals who socialize together, to groups formed to discuss particular professional interests, to groups formed to achieve some work-related goal, such as improved working conditions. Such groups may form along occupational lines but may also cut across hierarchical and occupational groups.

Informal groups can have high motivational value for individuals. A simple though valid example of an informal group is a car pool. Car pools meet individual needs by economizing on commuting costs and creating an opportunity for social interaction. They are also viewed positively by the organization in that they may lead to decreased absenteeism and lateness as well as higher employee morale.

There are a number of circumstances under which informal groups can have a negative influence on an organization. In some instances, they may become exclusionary and lead to interpersonal conflict. In other cases, informal groups can undermine the formal authority structure of the organization. Consider Etzioni's classic description of the role of informal groups in factories.

The workers constituted a cohesive group which had a well-developed normative system of its own. The norms specified, among other things, that a worker was not to work too hard, lest he become a "rate-buster;" nor was he to work too slowly, lest he become a "chiseler" who exploited the group (part of the wages were based on group performance). Under no condition was he to inform or "squeal." By means of informal social control, the group was able to direct the pace of work, the amount of daily and weekly production, the amount of work-stoppage, and allocation of work among members.[6]

In this instance, informal groups of employees were able to maintain social control within the factory through the imposition of informal, though well-enforced, rules of behavior.

Finally, informal groups can assume the role of change agent. Informal groups are often responsible for facilitating improvements in working conditions; such informal groups sometimes evolve into formal groups. The most common example of this is the evolution of employee associations and unions. These often begin with a grassroots, informal group, that eventually evolves to an association or union of employees. Informal groups may also emerge to deal with a particular organizational problem or to work towards change in organizational policy. Such groups may, for example, initiate action against a corrupt manager or supervisor.

Informal groups may be further categorized into *friendship* and *interest* groups. Friendship groups emerge simply for social reasons. The former tend to exist merely because people enjoy each other's company. Interest groups, which may also be referred to as coalitions, often form when a group of employees seeks redress on a set of grievances. Informal groups may be formed around such issues as improving wages or working conditions. They may, of course, eventually become more formal and longstanding, such as unions or employee associations.

In sum, informal groups play a special role in organizations. To the extent possible, managers should be aware of informal groups in the organization and what roles they play. Where they play a positive role, they may be encouraged by management; when they appear deleterious, managers might consider a variety of alternative options. Negatively-oriented informal groups may be a sign of dissatisfaction among employees.

Formal groups are established to serve specific organizational purposes and are the focus of this chapter. *Work groups* are organized around specific tasks and responsibilities and are relatively permanent. Operating room nurses, mental health treatment teams, and multidisciplinary cancer treatment teams are all work groups. Work groups have the following characteristics:[7,8]

- The group is perceived as such by both members and nonmembers. It is a defined entity with boundaries, and it is possible to distinguish members from nonmembers.
- Members are dependent upon each other to achieve some shared purpose.
- Members assume different roles. There is agreement among members about how individuals are to behave and the ways in which the group does its work. There exists a collective responsibility for the products or services produced by the group.
- The group operates in an organizational context, managing relationships with other groups or their representatives. These other groups may be within the organization or may be external groups or organizations.

Another type of formal group is a *management team*. Management team members may be separated by significant physical distance and may interact with each other infrequently.[9] The chief executive officer of a Veterans Affairs hospital will be part of larger regional and national teams, but the type and frequency of interaction with fellow team members will be quite different from that found in an inpatient mental health treatment team.

A *temporary group* is a group formed to work on a specific assignment or project. These are extremely important in health services organizations and in many ways are the most difficult type of group to manage. The composition of temporary groups is fluid by nature. Valuable time is often lost in these groups because of the need to establish group goals and procedures. Continuous quality improvement groups, which focus on a specific organizational process, are best characterized as temporary groups because they bring together individuals for a relatively short period of time. Each new process investigated typically requires different members and new group objectives. Temporary groups are sometimes referred to as *task forces*.

A final type of group is known as an *intermittent group*. Individuals are assembled in these groups periodically to exchange information or make decisions. Hospital governing boards and community advisory boards are common examples of intermittent groups. *Standing committees* consist of representatives of different groups and management teams who meet to exchange information and coordinate the work of individuals and groups. Committees of a hospital medical staff, quality improvement committees, and infection control committees are all standing committees. While the membership on these groups is somewhat fluid, standing committees are relatively stable with respect to roles and procedures.

In summary, there exist a variety of formal and informal groups in organizations. Our focus here, of course, is on increasing the performance of formal groups. An understanding of the different types of formal groups is important because management strategies vary depending upon the type of group. The role of the leader itself varies depending upon the type of group under discussion.

A MODEL OF WORK GROUP PERFORMANCE

Why do groups that appear to be similar often vary so much in effectiveness? What can leaders do to help groups be more productive and satisfying? To address these questions, we adopt a model of group performance that takes into consideration factors at the group

and organizational level.[10] At the group level, we include the following group characteristics: composition and size, norms, role relationships, group role clarity, group cohesiveness, and status differences. Also considered in this model are group processes, including leadership, communication, decision making and stages of group development. Taken together, these factors should provide an understanding of the variety of factors that affect the performance of a work group as summarized in Figure 6.1.

A multidimensional model is necessary because group performance is not a simple phenomenon and is influenced by factors at the individual, group, organizational, and at times, interorganizational level. While we cannot always control these factors, an understanding of their potential impact on group performance should provide group leaders with appropriate strategies for group management.

Before embarking on a discussion of these factors, several points are in order. First, our purpose in adopting a particular model of group performance is to provide a framework for organizing a large amount of research spanning several decades. Many other models are available, with varying strengths and draw-

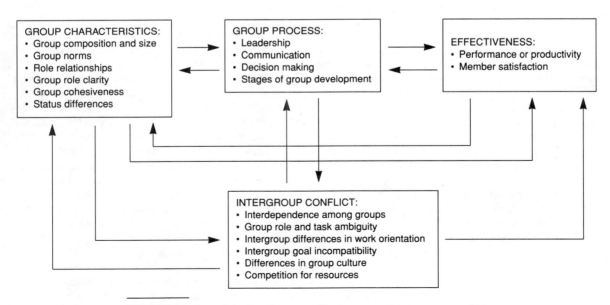

FIGURE 6.1. A model of work group effectiveness and intergroup conflict.

backs.[11-15] The model selected for our framework includes most of the variables considered in other models; further, the variables contained in this model have been subjected to empirical testing with a large sample of work groups. The second point concerns the nature of research that has led to our conclusions about group performance. Work group effectiveness research is frequently inconclusive, due in part to problems with generalizability, small sample sizes, as well as the general problems encountered in testing complex multivariate models. Conclusions and recommendations, therefore, are based on empirical research as well as the qualitative and cumulative experiences of managers.

Group Effectiveness

A good place to begin thinking about groups is the definition of group effectiveness. What is an effective group? By what measures do we assess group effectiveness? Figure 6.1 lists two general factors, performance or productivity and member satisfaction. These are inadequate, however, to capture the complexity of group effectiveness and the variety of methods available to assess effectiveness.

Group effectiveness is often confused with "good" group processes, such as communication, morale, and cohesiveness. We distinguish, however, between process factors (which may or may not be related to performance) and performance outcomes. In a very large study which examined the relationship between group cohesiveness and productivity, for example, it was found that cohesiveness is as often related to low productivity as to high productivity.[16] Thus, we do not view group process as an end in itself but as an intermediate step on the way towards effective group performance. This view is consistent with Hackman's[14] distinction between intermediate indicators of effectiveness, such as the quality of group interaction, and ultimate indicators, such as group outputs and member satisfaction.[17]

As is the case with organizations as a whole, there is no universal way to define group effectiveness. Depending on the purpose of the group, effectiveness can be defined in a number of ways. A group can be assessed by measuring its *productivity* or efficiency, which is essentially the amount of work produced with a given set of resources, such as time, people, money,

and expertise. Steiner includes group process in the definition of productivity by defining group productivity as a group's potential productivity minus losses due to faulty group processes.[18] Another method of assessing group effectiveness is suggested by the sociotechnical approach, which defines effective groups as those that not only fulfill the task requirements imposed on them by the organization but also the social needs and goals of group members.[19-21]

Assessing the quality of a group's work is even more difficult than assessing productivity. Shea and Guzzo suggest that effectiveness should be defined situationally; a group is effective to the extent that it fulfills its mission.[22] Like an organization, a group can be effective in achieving its mission but may do so in a highly inefficient manner. Sometimes, of course, efficiency and quality are inseparable. A strategic planning team may eventually produce a well-developed plan but may take so long to complete the process that it is no longer of use to the organization. Alternatively, a group may be very efficient in its work but produce poor decisions. In other situations, a group may be highly productive yet alienate members in the process and perhaps reduce its productivity in the future. Thus, group member satisfaction can have a substantial impact on current and future group functioning. When we consider group effectiveness, therefore, we usually consider issues involving productivity, quality of work, group member satisfaction, and the capacity of the group for continued cooperation.[23]

GROUP STRUCTURE

Groups are more than a collection of individuals. Every group has structural characteristics that define the way individuals interact with each other. These characteristics include group composition and size, group norms, role relationships, groups role clarity, group cohesiveness, and status differences. The manner in which these are understood and managed are factors in the effectiveness of a group.

Group Composition and Size

Group membership is an important factor in understanding group performance. For certain types of groups, of course, it is easier to control group membership than in others. The chair of a hospital board can select board members to sit on particular committees, while the director of nursing may be highly constrained in the nurses deployed on a particular nursing service. In the latter situation, the director of nursing may be limited by the pool of nurses in the hospital or by the supply of nurses in the labor market. However, an awareness of possible problems related to membership helps, at least, to identify potential problems. In our examination of *group composition,* we consider the following diagnostic questions:[24]

- Is the group well staffed? Is the mix of members appropriate?
- Do members have the expertise required to perform group tasks well?
- Are there signs that members are so similar that there is little for them to learn from one another? Or are there signs that they are so heterogeneous that they risk having difficulty communicating and coordinating with one another?

Most research on group composition concludes that heterogeneity of group members, in terms of traits, abilities, and attitudes, is desirable when task requirements are diverse.[25] Given the multidisciplinary nature of health care, heterogeneous groups are very common in health services organizations, and they present unique management challenges. Oncology treatment teams, for example, may include a variety of physician specialists (medical oncologists, radiation oncologists, surgical oncologists, pediatric oncologists, pathologists, surgeons, psychiatrists, hematologists, gynecologists, radiologists), physicists, nurses, social workers, psychologists, pharmacists, and nutritionists.[26] Many would suggest that the patient and/or family member should be considered a part of the team. While these types of teams tend to be fluid—that is, not all team members will be involved in all cases—the multidisciplinary nature of the team raises questions about leadership, *status differences,* and the manner in which decisions are made. A nurse who is present at all meetings may be the formal leader, but in all likelihood decisional power will reside with the physician most directly involved in treating the patient. The role of formal leadership may be reduced to that of coordinator rather than decision maker.

Status differences have a profound effect on the functioning of multidisciplinary teams. This is particularly true in health care, where status differences among the professions are well-entrenched. In many cases, an individual from a lower status group may be intimidated or ignored by higher status group members. As a result, the group may not benefit from this person's expertise. In well-managed multidisciplinary groups, a lower status individual may feel elevated by being part of a high-profile group.

Multidisciplinary groups may also be less likely to fall prone to the *groupthink* phenomena.[27] Groupthink occurs when members strive towards harmony and unanimity at the expense of making carefully reasoned decisions. Multidisciplinary groups tend to bring out divergent views on subjects, which theoretically should minimize the likelihood that important details are overlooked. Groupthink is discussed in more detail later in this chapter.

Perhaps no other aspect of group and organizational functioning has been studied as much as group size. In general, it is believed that smaller groups are more productive than larger groups. Smaller groups are less cumbersome and there is less opportunity for members to get in each other's way. Social distractions are also decreased in small groups; with a smaller number of individuals, members are less likely to be distracted from the work of the group. Where larger groups have substantial administrative coordination requirements, smaller groups tend to spend less time and energy on coordination and more on task-related concerns. Finally, smaller groups decrease the incidence of *behavioral masking,* also known as "free riding" or "social loafing."[28,29] Individuals in large groups are able to maintain a sense of anonymity and gain from the work of the group without making a suitable contribution to the work of the group.

More often than not, group size is out of the control of the manager, particularly when democratic representational norms pervade an organization. In these situations, constituencies may demand to be represented and the leader may need to design strategies to make the group more manageable (e.g., forming subcommittees). Otherwise, groups may be overstaffed. Overstaffed groups may tend to perform work in a perfunctory, lackadaisical manner. Large size may also lead to competition and jealousy among group members, with individuals guarding their particular domain. Some members may remain aloof from group efforts and be less willing to help others improve their performance.[30] Breaking a group into subgroups (e.g., subcommittees) has its own set of problems. When large groups are divided into smaller groups, each subgroup may become cliquish, and while cohesive within themselves, they may become isolated from the rest of the group.[31]

There are also consequences for groups that are understaffed. These groups are likely to be more willing than other groups to carry out difficult, important, and varied tasks and may adopt a martyr syndrome. Because of the perception of being overworked, members of these groups tend to feel important and highly responsible for their work.

Empirical research on the relationship between size and effectiveness is less definitive than many of our theories predict.[32] In managing groups and teams, however, it is useful to keep in mind the potential problems and benefits that may emerge as a result of group size.

Group Norms

A norm is defined as a standard that is shared by group members and that regulates member behavior. *Behavior norms* are rules that standardize how people act at work on a day-to-day basis, while *performance norms* are rules that standardize employee output. Behavioral norms in groups are far-reaching and may vary substantially from one group to another in the same organization. Norms may govern how much participation is required by each individual, how humor is to be used, the use of formal group procedures (e.g., Robert's Rules of Order), and rules related to absence and lateness. In their study of operating room nurses, Denison and Sutton describe their surprise at the behavioral norms present in the operating room.

At first we were surprised by the norms of emotional expression in the operating rooms. The first time we entered the room where a coronary bypass operation was being done, for example, we were surprised by the loud rock music blaring from the speakers, the smiles on the faces of the surgical team, and the constant joking. Denison observed one surgeon who joked and told a series of funny stories as he performed the complicated task of cutting the veins out of a patient's leg—veins that would be used to bypass

clogged coronary arteries. Similarly, one reason that Sutton almost passed out during a tonsillectomy was that he became very upset when the surgeon laughed, joked, and talked about "what was on the tube last night" while blood from an unconscious child splattered about.[33]

Performance norms, on the other hand, govern the amount and quality of work required of individuals, as well as the amount of time individuals are expected to work. Some performance norms require that workers not work "too hard" so that standards for the group as a whole are kept at a given level. "Rate busters" are subject to serious sanctions by other group members. Researchers have in fact documented the practice of binging, a practice in which workers periodically punched suspected rate busters in the arm until they reduced their level of effort.[34]

Norms are powerful influences in organizations and groups, and the existence of norms is necessary for effective group functioning. Hackman suggests that norms have the following characteristics:[35]

- Norms summarize and simplify group influence processes. They denote the processes by which groups regulate member behavior.
- Norms apply only to behavior, not to private thoughts and feelings. Private acceptance of norms is *not necessary,* only public compliance.
- Norms are generally developed only for behaviors that are viewed as important by most group members.
- Norms usually develop gradually, but members can quicken the process. Norms usually are developed by group members when the occasion arises, such as when a situation occurs that requires new ground rules for members in order to protect group integrity.
- All norms do not apply to all group members. Some norms only apply to newer members, while others may be applied to individuals based on seniority, sex, race, economic status, or profession.

Role Relationships

For groups to function effectively, groups differentiate the work activities of their members. This specialization of work activities is called *role differentiation.*

TABLE 6.2. Functional Roles of Group Members

Category	Role Name	Description
Task-oriented roles: Behaviors directed towards accomplishing the group's objectives, primarily through contributing to the problem-solving process	Initiator	Proposes tasks, goals, or actions; defines group problems; suggests work procedures
	Informer	Offers facts, gives expression of feelings, gives opinions
	Information seeker	Asks for opinions, facts, or interpretations
	Clarifier	Interprets ideas or suggestions; defines terms; clarifies issues before the group
	Summarizer or coordinator	Pulls together related ideas; restates suggestions; offers a decision or conclusion for group to consider
	Reality tester	Makes a critical analysis of an idea; tests an idea against some data to see if the idea will work
	Procedural technician	Records suggestions; distributes materials
	Energizer	Attempts to increase the quality and quantity of task behavior
	Elaborator	Expands on suggestions; offers examples; restates positions; offers rationales
	Consensus tester	Asks to see if a group is nearing a decision; sends up a trial balloon to test a possible conclusion
Building and maintenance roles: Social-emotional behaviors aimed at helping the interpersonal functioning of group. Like the maintenance required to keep a car in good running condition, these behaviors are necessary to keep group members feeling good about the group and interacting effectively with one another.	Harmonizer	Attempts to reconcile disagreements; reduces tension; gets people to explore differences
	Gatekeeper	Helps keep communication channels open; facilitates participation of others; suggests procedures that permit sharing remarks
	Encourager	Friendly, warm, and responsive to others; indicates by facial expression or remark the acceptance of others' contributions
	Compromiser	When own idea or status is involved in a conflict offers a compromise that yields status; admits error; modifies an interest of group cohesion or growth

Individuals assume both formal and informal roles in groups. Formal roles include that of leader as well as specific task-oriented functions, such as chairs and participants of subcommittees. However, individuals also assume informal roles that may positively or negatively affect work group productivity and effectiveness. A group leader should be cognizant of the existence of these roles and how they are carried out in the group setting. Benne and Sheats provide a clear distinction among these informal roles, distinguishing among *task-oriented roles,* which help accomplish group goals; *building and maintenance roles,* which help establish and maintain good relationships among group members; and *personal roles,* or self-centered roles, which serve to satisfy individual needs unrelated to the group's goals or its maintenance (see Table 6.2).[36]

Several points are in order with respect to these roles. First, members may simultaneously assume several roles in a particular group setting. Second, individual roles are not static; depending upon the group, an individual may assume different roles. Roles may even vary from one meeting of a group to another. Finally, emphasis should be placed on the fact that these are

Category	Role Name	Description
Personal roles: Intended to satisfy individual needs rather than contribute to goals or maintenance of group. Although some personal role behaviors do contribute to group's effectiveness, roles characteristic of this category are irrelevant to goals of group and not conducive to its functioning.	Observer or commentator	Comments on and interprets group's internal process
	Follower	Serves as audience; passively goes along with ideas of others
	Aggressor	Deflates others' status; attacks the group or its values; jokes in a barbed or semiconcealed way
	Blocker	Disagrees and opposes beyond reason; resists stubbornly the group's wishes for personal reasons; uses hidden agenda to thwart movement of group
	Dominator	Asserts authority or superiority to manipulate group or certain group members; interrupts contributions of others; controls by means of flattery or other forms of patronizing behavior
	Prince or Princess	Makes a display of own lack of involvement; "abandons" the group while remaining with it physically; seeks recognition in ways not relevant to group task
	Evader	Pursues special interests not related to tasks; stays off subject to avoid commitment; prevents group from facing up to controversy
	Help seeker	Uses group to gain sympathy and solve personal problems unrelated to group's goal
	Recognition seeker	Calls attention to self by boasting and referring to personal achievements; acts in appropriate ways to gain attention
	Special-interest pleader	Speaks on behalf of represented group (e.g., labor, minorities, management) in order to cloak own prejudices or biases in a stereotype that fits own personal needs rather than goals of the current group

Adapted from Benne K, Sheats P. Functional roles of group members. *Journal of Social Issues.* Reprinted by permission of the Society for the Psychological Study of Social Issues. 1948;2:42–47.

informal roles that are not easily changed. Oftentimes individuals assume roles because of their informal power within an organization. For example, a physician who dominates a strategic planning team may assume this role as a result of his status and power outside the group.

Group Role Clarity

Many groups fail to achieve their mission simply because their roles were not clearly established. The output expected of a group may not be clear, which may lead to misunderstood expectations and decreased member morale and motivation. Similarly, the power or influence of a group may be misunderstood. A continuous quality improvement (CQI) group, for example, may assume that its recommendations will be fully implemented when in fact they are only advisory. This too can deflate the enthusiasm of group members. Managers can decrease the likelihood of these problems by clarifying the purpose of the group, the role of the group within the larger organization, and the authority of the group.

Group Cohesiveness

Group cohesiveness is defined as the extent to which individual group members are motivated to remain in a group. Members of highly cohesive groups "are more energetic in group activities, they are less likely to be absent from group meetings, they are happy when the group succeeds, and sad when it fails . . . whereas members of less cohesive groups are less concerned about the group's activities."[37]

A high level of group cohesiveness is not always desirable. The nature of the groups' work determines in large part the level of cohesion to which managers should strive.

> The manager must decide what type of group is wanted. If cooperation, teamwork, and synergy really matter, then one aims for high task interdependence. One structures the jobs of group members so that they have to interact frequently . . . to get their jobs done. . . . If frenzied, independent activity is the goal, then one aims for low task interdependence and large rewards are distributed competitively and unequally.[21]

In our various group memberships, we have an innate ability to evaluate a group on its cohesiveness. Highly cohesive groups have a high degree of camaraderie, group spirit, and sense of oneness. What causes certain groups to be cohesive? Several factors contribute to the development of cohesiveness.[38]

- Motive base of members. To the extent that a group meets the individual needs of group members, it will become attractive to group members (see also the discussion of motivation in Chapter 3).
- Incentive properties of the group. Cooperative group rewards that encourage interaction can stimulate cohesiveness, particularly when members perform interdependent tasks.
- Expectancies about outcomes. Individuals will be more attracted to groups when they feel that group membership will in fact lead to the achievement of personal goals.
- Comparison level. According to equity theory, individuals perform an implicit cost-benefit ratio

of membership and involvement in one group against alternative paths to goal achievement.[39] This factor is particularly salient for voluntary groups.
- External threat. External threats to a group's well-being can strengthen the group's cohesiveness by providing a common enemy. Intergroup conflict (discussed later in this chapter and in Chapter 5) often promotes intragroup cohesion.
- Attitudes of group members. A central tenet of social psychological theory is that individuals are attracted to others with similar attitudes. It follows, therefore, that homogeneous groups should be more cohesive than heterogeneous groups. Although there have been relatively few empirical tests of this proposition, the longitudinal study of student groups by Terborg et al. confirmed this relationship.[40]

Group cohesiveness can have important implications for productivity and effectiveness. First, cohesiveness has been associated with higher levels of satisfaction among group members, lower levels of absenteeism among group members, and greater stability among group members.[40–43] Second, group cohesiveness can promote better enforcement of group norms and general control over group members.

Many managers attempt to develop highly cohesive work groups believing that cohesiveness will lead to higher levels of performance. The relationship between cohesiveness and performance, however, is mediated by performance norms; there are circumstances under which high levels of cohesiveness can lead to lower levels of productivity.[44] If a group's norms favor low productivity, then having a highly cohesive group will likely lead to lower, not higher productivity. Similarly, a highly cohesive group may work against a manager's efforts to involve new members in a group or to have the group interact with other groups. Cohesiveness, therefore, should be viewed in context; in most situations, it is a positive force, while in others, it can reinforce counterproductive norms and practices.[45,46]

To complicate matters even more, another body of literature suggests that conflict may be beneficial to group performance, particularly when a group is dealing with complex problem-solving tasks.[47–49] In this sense, multidisciplinary groups and groups composed of culturally diverse individuals, while likely to exhibit higher levels of conflict, may also be more creative and innovative in their approach to problem solving.[50]

Status Differences

Earlier we discussed the role of status differences in multidisciplinary groups. Status is the measure of worth conferred on an individual by a group. Status differences are seen throughout organizations and serve many useful purposes. Differences in status motivate people, provide them with a means of identification, and may be a force for stability in the organization.[51] In groups, status differences can be a source of difficulty. Many groups develop democratic norms which may run counter to the formal or informal status of individual group members. Within a CQI group, for example, a physician may be highly very influential. Within the group, however, the physician is expected to serve as an equal to analyze problems and suggest solutions. This discrepancy between outside status and inside status may make management of these groups difficult.

In other situations, multidisciplinary teams are idealistically expected to operate as a company of equals, yet the reality of the situation makes this impossible. In a study of end-stage renal disease teams, while the equal participation ideology was accepted by most team participants, it was clear that the physicians, who had higher professional status than other groups, had greater involvement in the actual decision-making process.[52] The mismatch between expectations and reality made many team members, particularly staff nurses, feel a sense of role deprivation with accompanying implications for morale and job satisfaction.

GROUP PROCESSES

Group processes refer to the manner in which a group is managed. We discuss here issues related to group leadership, communications, decision making, and stages of group development.

Leadership

Groups generally have multiple leaders. There may be a *formal leader* as well as several *informal leaders*. Examples of formal leaders are head nurses, depart-

ment managers, project leaders, and board committee chairs. Formal leaders have legitimate authority over the group; that is, the organization has granted these individuals power along with some ability to use formal rewards and sanctions to support that authority. The formal leader may not be the most influential person in the group, however. The extent to which group members will accept the formal leader's wishes is in large part determined by the reaction of the informal leader(s) to those wishes.

Note that there is a difference between ad hoc groups, such as task forces, and formal work groups. In a task force, an informal leader may be selected as the group's formal leader. This is the rationale for appointing high profile individuals to chair important task forces or to serve as honorary chairs of committees. In work groups, however, there is no opportunity for choice. It may be that the formal leader is not the person on whom the group itself confers highest status. It is the "informal leader who embodies the values of the group, aids it in accomplishing its objectives, facilitates group maintenance and individual need satisfaction, and usually serves as group spokesperson."[53]

In deciding upon a leadership style, therefore, group leaders need to consider in realistic terms their formal and informal authority within the group. Use of a coercive or forceful style may backfire when the individual does not have the moral authority to back up decisions. Such a leader may find that the informal leader is able to veto, modify, or sabotage demands of the formal leader. It is best, therefore, for the formal leader to not only consider the views of informal leaders but to collaborate with them if possible. Related issues of leadership are discussed further in Chapter 4.

Communication

A group cannot function effectively as a team unless members can exchange information. It is incumbent upon group leaders to manage communications within a group and between the group and external groups. Consider the case of a nurse in a neonatal intensive care unit who has just met with a patient's physician and must pass on vital information to the nurse on the next shift as well as to the parents who will visit during the next shift. How does information get conveyed?

Without a viable *communication structure,* important information may be lost or inaccurately communicated. In fact, the evaluation and design of communication structures is an important component of many quality improvement projects.

Communication speed and accuracy in a group are influenced both by the nature of the group's communication network and by the complexity of the group's task. When a task is simple and communication networks are centralized, both speed and accuracy are higher. When tasks are relatively complex, centralized communication networks lower both speed and accuracy because people serving as network hubs (e.g., information disseminators) may suffer from information overload. In this situation, communication networks are best decentralized, relieving a manager from the need to filter (and possibly distort) information before it is passed on. In the example of the neonatal intensive care unit, it would be highly undesirable for the nurse on the earlier shift to first communicate the needed information to a head nurse and then have that individual pass it on to the next shift's nurse. Notwithstanding the need for the head nurse to find out about the information, timeliness and accuracy are likely to suffer if the information must first pass through the head nurse en route to the next shift's nurse. It is obviously much more desirable to build a communication structure that encourages direct communication between nurses on sequential shifts.

Managers, of course, need to be comfortable with decentralized communication structures. Many managers fear being left out of the communications loop, that is, being bypassed and not informed. They can overcome this fear by working with group members to design a workable communication structure. Related issues of communication and coordination are also discussed in Chapter 8.

Decision Making

Two aspects of group decision making are worthy of consideration by managers: the distinction between decision making and problem solving and the processes by which decision-making groups make decisions.

Most teams are at some point involved in making decisions. However, not all team members are involved in actually making all decisions. For a particular decision, a hospital president may ask for the opinions of senior management but retain the right to make the final decision. Similarly, a physician may obtain input from a variety of professionals but make the final determination on treatment. Managers can decrease the probability of misunderstandings by clarifying the role of the group and the role of each member of the group. Group members can generally deal with limitations on their influence as long as the boundaries of their influence are clear.

Group leaders also need to clarify the difference between problem solving and decision making. Some groups, such as many CQI teams, are established to solve problems or to seek methods for improving a particular organizational process. They may not be given authority to implement decisions, however, particularly when substantial resources are required.

The second area of decision making regards the process by which information is exchanged and decisions made. Groups naturally attempt to make correct decisions, applying all available information to the problem at hand. One common problem that prevents complete sharing of information among members of a group is that of the free rider. The term "free rider" refers to a member of a group who obtains the benefits of group membership but does not accept a proportional share of the costs of committee membership. "Cheap rider" is a more accurate term for such a group member because receiving benefits from group membership typically involves some minimal cost.[54] Free rider, however, is the more generally used term.[55] The free rider is seen as someone who promotes self-interest—the personal acquisition of benefits—rather than the public interest—the need to contribute to the activity that produces those benefits. It is often observed that the larger the group, the greater the free rider effect.[56]

What can managers do to minimize free riding? Albanese and Van Fleet offer the following suggestions:

> Through effective use of power, design of organizations (including the size of the organizational units), and control of access to rewards and punishment, management influences the incentive system of group members. At a routine level, this influence may be achieved by offering financial incentives or special forms of recognition to particular group members.[61]

In the longer run, it is also important for managers to deal with the free rider problem by attempting to broaden the individual's concept of self-interest and by creating, communicating, and maintaining a group culture that values effort expended on group processes.

Another group process that may inhibit the effective use of information is polarization. When groups become highly cohesive over an issue, polarization occurs. There are two commonly accepted explanations for polarization.[58] The social comparison explanation argues that, as individuals compare their position on a matter with those of others in the group, pressures emerge toward accepting one position or another as the group position. In the persuasive argument explanation, it is argued that groups coalesce around a more forcefully argued alternative when initial discussion reveals no clearly favored argument. Managers should be aware that group polarization does take place and that it often leads to groupthink.[59] This concept emerged from Janis' studies of high level policy decisions by government leaders including decisions about Vietnam, the Bay of Pigs, and the Korean War.

Groupthink occurs whenever the desire for harmony and consensus overrides members' efforts to appraise group judgments realistically. In other words, groupthink occurs when maintaining the pleasant atmosphere of the group becomes more important to members than coming up with good decisions. Signs that groupthink may be present include:

- The illusion of invulnerability. Group members may reassure themselves about obvious dangers and become overly optimistic and willing to take extraordinary risks.
- Collective rationalization. Victims of groupthink may overlook blind spots in their plans. When confronted with conflicting information, group members may spend considerable time and energy refuting the information and rationalizing a decision.
- Belief in the inherent morality of the group. Highly cohesive groups may develop a sense of self-righteousness about their role that makes them insensitive to the consequences of decisions.

- Stereotyping others. Victims of groupthink hold biased, highly negative views of competing groups. They assume that they are unable to negotiate with other groups and thus rule out compromise.
- Pressures to conform. Group members face severe pressures to conform to group norms and to group decisions. Dissent is considered abnormal and may lead to formal or informal punishment.
- The use of mindguards. Mindguards are members who protect the group from dissonant information that might interfere with the group's view of a problem. They may withhold or discount contrary information.
- Self-censorship. Groups subject to groupthink pressure members to remain silent about possible misgivings and to minimize self-doubts about a decision.
- Illusion of unanimity. A sense of unanimity emerges when members assume that silence and lack of protest signifies agreement and consensus.

The consequences of groupthink are clear. Groups may limit themselves, often prematurely, to one or two possible solutions and fail to conduct a comprehensive analysis of a problem. When groupthink is well entrenched, members may fail to review their decisions in light of new information or changing events. The group becomes blinded to new information. Groups may also fail to consult adequately with experts within or outside the organization and fail to develop contingency plans in the event that the decision turns out to be wrong.

Group leaders can avoid groupthink through a number of strategies. First, leaders can reduce groupthink by encouraging members to critically evaluate proposals and solutions. Where a leader is particularly powerful and influential yet still wants to get unbiased views from group members, the leader may refrain from stating his own position until later in the decision-making process. Another strategy is to assign the same problem to two separate work groups. Most importantly, groupthink can be avoided by establishing norms of critical appraisal of ideas and solutions and understanding the warning signs of groupthink. Managers might also consider alternative systematic methods of decision making that emphasize member participation. *Nominal group technique* and *Delphi technique* elicit group members' opinions prior to judgments about those opinions.[60,61] Through these and other approaches, alternative ideas get to the table and the chances for objective debate are enhanced.

Stages of Group Development

Recall the case at the beginning of this chapter when the first meeting of the advisory committee seemed highly productive while the second meeting ended in some disarray and conflict. This led to considerable frustration and confusion for the leader of the group. What she was unaware of was that groups go through stages of development and that each stage is characterized by different group behaviors. Just as knowing the age of a child helps to explain behavior and clarify our expectations of what a child should be able to accomplish, it is important to understand the group's stage of development.

While it is not possible to predict with certainty how a group will proceed through its various stages, the following stages have been found to occur in many different types of groups:[62]

- *Forming*. During the first stage of group development, members begin the process of testing the group environment and developing relationships. Members attempt to discover those behaviors that are acceptable and unacceptable. This early stage is characterized by polite interactions, frequent silence, and tentative interactions.
- *Storming*. At this stage, group members tend to feel more comfortable with each other and attempt to develop a place for themselves within the group. They also may attempt to influence the development of group norms, roles, and procedures. This stage has high potential for conflict.
- *Norming*. During this stage, the group grows more cohesive. There emerges agreement on rules and processes of decision making. There is increased supportiveness among members and a sense of unity of purpose.

- *Performing*. Once group members agree on the purpose and norms of the group, they are able to move forward to the task of defining separate roles and establishing work plans. If a group reaches this stage, decision making occurs more easily and with less emotion, and there is a group focus on achievement.
- *Adjourning*. For temporary groups, the adjournment stage is characterized by a sense of task accomplishment, regret, and increased emotionality.

Several points are in order about these stages. First, not all groups pass through all stages. Some groups may begin at a norming or performing stage, while some may never move beyond the conflictual storming stage. Second, groups can revert to earlier stages of development. Regression can occur as a result of new tasks or responsibilities given the group, a change in formal or informal leadership, the addition of a new member, or the loss of a member. Managers should consider the stage of group development in establishing expectations for the group.

INTERGROUP RELATIONSHIPS

Attention thus far has focused on management issues relevant to the individual group. Effective group performance, however, may not translate into organizational effectiveness unless groups are able to interact with each other in a productive manner. What happens when groups have to work together? What are the factors responsible for effective and ineffective intergroup relationships? How can intergroup relationships be improved?

To begin to address these questions, the importance of intergroup, or lateral, relationships must be emphasized. As health care organizations have moved away from rigid hierarchical structures, and as they have become more specialized, there is increased need for coordination mechanisms. *Intergroup conflict* is inevitable and unavoidable. It is virtually impossible for work processes to be designed such that the work of some groups meshes perfectly with the work of other groups. When conflicts or disagreements occur among organizations, conflict resolution strategies must be employed. In the best case, the interfaces among groups need to be fine tuned; in the worst situations, work processes need to be wholly overhauled in order to make intergroup relationships work. These cross-cutting sets of issues are also addressed in Chapters 5, 7, 8, and 10. In this section, attention focuses on causes of intergroup conflict, consequences of intergroup conflict, and strategies for managing intergroup conflict.

Causes of Intergroup Conflict

While intergroup conflict can occasionally result from interpersonal differences or animosities, most conflict emerges because of factors related to the interdependence among work groups. Blake and Mouton stress that intergroup conflict cannot be addressed in the same manner as conflict between individuals.

> While obviously influenced by a variety of factors, individuals may choose to think or act in a given way simply because they want to or feel a need to. When differences or conflicts arise with another person, then an individual is free to react and to change his or her mind on the basis of new evidence and to give or withhold cooperation in keeping with personal desires.
>
> A group member is not free in the same sense as is an individual acting alone. Rules and standards of behavior—norms—are developed within the group that regulate the behavior of members through sometimes subtle but potent pressures . . . Members who think or act differently are either punished, persuaded, or rejected. Seeking to solve interface disputes at the group level as though they were personal disputes between two individuals not only disregards these important dynamics but also may create new tensions that may provide short-term solutions and at the same time disrupt internal group cohesion, producing new and more serious problems in the future.[63]

Thus, conflict between groups cannot usually be addressed at an individual level: one member of a group can rarely resolve an intergroup conflict in a unilateral manner. If intergroup conflict is viewed as resulting from problems in the interface between groups, then the analysis of the causes of conflict should examine the nature of intergroup relationships. Figure 6.1 summarizes the factors likely to be related to intergroup conflict.

Taking this perspective, conflict is most likely to occur when two groups are dependent upon each other to do their work. Consider the example of a medical group practice that needs to have laboratory results reported in a timely manner. Conflicts can easily result when the system of information transfer proves ineffective or otherwise lacking. Cases of such interface conflict are pervasive in health care organizations.

Intergroup conflict is also more likely to occur when there is ambiguity about groups' respective responsibilities or roles. This situation in large part explains conflicts that occur between psychologists and psychiatrists, who often have overlapping areas of jurisdiction. Role ambiguity is also common between groups located in different organizations, where there may be a lack of consensus over the domains of different organizations. Finally, task ambiguity may lead to important job duties "falling between the cracks"; each group may be upset with the other for what it perceives to be the other's shortcomings.[64] Task ambiguity may also be common in organizations undergoing rapid growth or change. In these situations, changes may be understood differently among work groups.

A third source of intergroup conflict is related to differences in group's work orientation. In many organizations, groups have different perspectives on time. This difference in time orientation was identified and managed when strategic planning was attempted with a group of family physicians.

> By its nature, the activity of planning is at odds with the role orientation of most physicians. Planning is a long-term process in which the results of strategic decisions appear over time. The outcomes of planning are often intangible in the short term. By contrast, physicians are trained to be action oriented.
>
> It was discovered early in the planning process that physician attendance at meetings decreased when the pace of work lagged. Therefore, whenever possible, the pace of work was increased to a level more acceptable to physicians. A work plan with specific deadlines was followed.[65]

Differences in work orientation may also be reflected in different goals among work groups. The finance department of a managed care organization, for example, may have a very different set of priorities from that unit of the organization concerned with quality assurance or quality improvement. Conflicts may emerge as each group works toward different, sometimes conflicting goals.

Differences in culture or interpersonal orientation among groups may also lead to conflict. Researchers, for example, may place great value on informality in dealing with colleagues. However, a principal investigator on a large research grant may need to interact with a highly formalized human resources department to deal with employee issues such as recruitment, hiring, and compensation. The researcher, accustomed to informality, may resist attempts by the human resources department to engage in formal interviews with job applicants or to write detailed job descriptions. Such conflicts are difficult to resolve unless there is at least a recognition of the differences in work orientation as a primary cause of conflict.

Organizations under financial stress are more likely to exhibit intergroup conflict simply because groups may be competing for scarce organizational resources. Groups may find themselves competing for money, use of common support services, or the use of specialized organizational resources. In fact, the movement towards product or program management in hospitals would tend to increase the likelihood of intergroup conflict as product line teams develop internal competitive thrusts. In such systems, teams may also be on some form of incentive system related to team perfor-mance. This raises the issue of whether traditional modes of compensation that reward individuals and not teams are appropriate in the team-centered environment, an issue raised in Debate Time 6.1. Where teams compete with each other for scarce resources, the program manager must be able to compete with other programs and at times defend the relevance of the program.

> A product manager should be a combination of Lee Iacocca, Alexander Haig, Henry Kissinger, and Rodney Dangerfield. The product manager needs to champion the product or service for which he or she is responsible. In so doing, the "persona" of that product will become identified with the attitude and enthusiasm of the manager.[66]

In sum, we would expect intergroup conflict to increase because of resource scarcity in the health care field. Organizational responses to resource scarcity will likely exacerbate tensions between groups.

Consequences of Intergroup Conflict

Through the years researchers have observed the changes that occur within groups when faced with conflict with other groups (see Sherif and Sherif's clas-

DEBATE TIME 6.1: WHAT DO YOU THINK?

Traditional methods of compensation reward individuals for individual performance. Theories of motivation focus on linking rewards to performance, facilitating individual performance through coaching and training, and setting challenging yet realistic goals. While there are some exceptions to this individualistic approach to rewards, such as gainsharing plans where employees are rewarded for overall increased productivity, generations of managers have been inculcated with the need to reward individuals based on the merits of individual performance.

We are now in an era where groups and teams are becoming increasingly important. Teams are expected to work together to solve problems, care for patients, and engage in planning activities. Continuous quality improvement efforts, in fact, are based on effective team functioning. However, our reward systems are still almost entirely focused on the individual. Efforts to implement group reward systems are often met with hostility and suspicion. Many people fear the free rider syndrome, where some members of the group do not perform up to standard yet receive the same reward as productive group members for group performance. Other people worry that group rewards dilute the motivational potential in rewards. With financial resources growing increasingly scarce, managers want to ensure that the impact of merit pay is maximized. There is therefore a reluctance to deviate from traditional merit pay systems. Finally, where employees are organized, formally rewarding employees for group performance may be viewed as a breech of contract.

Is it possible to combine merit pay systems with group reward systems? If efforts continue to implement group rewards, will we eventually see a deterioration in individual motivation and commitment?

sic 1953 study of these changes.)[67] Most important, when groups are faced with external threats, there is almost always a sense of increased group cohesiveness. Loyalty to the group becomes more important, and there is increased emphasis given to the accomplishment of group tasks. Members tend to be less concerned with individual need satisfaction and may be more accepting of autocratic leadership (which often accompanies external threats). As loyalty to the group increases, work processes may become more rigid.

When intergroup conflict emerges, changes also occur in group members' perceptions. One's own group tends to look increasingly, and perhaps unrealistically positive, and weaknesses may be denied. The perception of other groups and their accomplishments are likely to grow increasingly negative and become distorted.

As a result of the hostility that develops between groups, intergroup communication decreases. Decreased interaction only increases the prevalence of negative stereotyping. Negative attitudes between groups leads to breakdowns in communication. Whatever communication that occurs tends to be colored by a we-versus-them perspective. Each group acts on its assumptions about the other, automatically accepting the correctness of its own opinions and perceptions. They are likely to disregard contradictory facts or to reinterpret discrepancies to make them fit prevailing assumptions. The other group may be perceived as poorly managed, incompetent, devious, and inferior. These conditions do not enhance the probability of successful relationships.[68]

In addition, as conflict emerges between groups, cooperative relationships are replaced by a win-lose mentality in which victory becomes more important than solving the problem that may have caused the conflict in the first place.

Strategies for Managing Intergroup Conflict

There are two sets of approaches for dealing with intergroup conflict. The tactical approach focuses on specific strategies and managerial behaviors for dealing with conflict once it has emerged. Arnold and Feldman,

TABLE 6.3. Conflict Management Strategies

Conflict Resolution Strategy	Type of Strategy	Appropriate Situations
Ignoring the conflict	Avoidance	When the issue is trivial; when the issue is symptomatic of more basic, pressing problems
Imposing a solution	Avoidance	When quick, decisive action is needed; when unpopular decisions need to be made and consensus among the groups appears very unlikely
Smoothing	Defusion	As a stop-gap measure to let people cool down and regain perspective; when the conflict is over nonwork issues
Appealing to superordinate goals	Defusion	When there is a mutually important goal that neither group can achieve without the cooperation of the other; when the survival or success of the overall organization is in jeopardy
Bargaining	Containment	When the two parties are of relatively equal power; when there are several acceptable, alternative solutions that both parties would be willing to consider
Structuring the interaction	Containment	When previous attempts to openly discuss conflict issues led to conflict escalation rather than to problem solution; when a respected third party is available to provide some structure and could serve as a mediator
Integrative problem solving	Confrontation	When there is a minimum level of trust between groups and there is no time pressure for a quick solution; when the organization can benefit from merging the differing perspectives and insights of the groups in making key decisions
Redesigning the organization	Confrontation	When the sources of conflict come from the coordination of work; When the work can be easily divided into clear project responsibilities (self-contained work groups); when activities require a lot of interdepartmental coordination over time (lateral relations)

From Arnold HJ, Feldman DC. *Organizational Behavior*. New York, NY: McGraw-Hill; 1986.

MANAGERIAL GUIDELINES

1. To increase the performance of a group, it is important for managers to ensure that the reward structure of the organization rewards group accomplishments as well as individual performance.

2. The manager should identify those group norms that are dysfunctional or obsolete and take steps to eliminate those norms.

3. The assignment of tasks among interdependent work groups should be clarified to avoid misunderstandings and conflict.

4. Managers should be cognizant of their own conflict management tendencies and seek to broaden their repertoire of conflict management strategies.

5. Managers should be aware of how group members communicate with each other both inside and outside the group environment.

6. Managers should be aware of status differences among group members and how these differences affect individual participation, group decision making, and productivity.

7. Managers should be able to apply a variety of structured group decision-making techniques, such as nominal group technique, brainstorming, and the Delphi technique, and understand when each is most appropriate.

8. Managers should be clear that group members understand the purpose and authority of the group, the role of the group in the organization, and the specific contributions expected of each individual.

9. Managers should be conscious of the symptoms of groupthink and develop strategies for moving groups out of this syndrome.

10. Managers should be aware of the stage of group development and manage the group according to its stage. Group leaders should also try to move groups forward to more mature stages.

11. In managing meetings, group leaders should be aware of the following principles:[72]
   a. At the beginning of the meeting, review the progress made to date and establish the task facing the group.
   b. Help group members feel comfortable with one another.
   c. Establish ground rules governing group discussions.
   d. As early in a meeting as possible, get a report from each member who has been preassigned a task.
   e. Sustain the flow of the meeting by using informational displays.
   f. Manage the discussion to achieve equitable participation.
   g. Close the meeting by summarizing what has been accomplished and reviewing assignments.

for example, identify eight conflict management styles.[69] These range from avoidance strategies, such as ignoring the conflict or imposing a solution, to confrontational strategies. Table 6.3 lists these strategies and the circumstances under which each is appropriate. Particularly useful is the idea that managers should be well-equipped to employ each of these strategies. The unique circumstances of each situation determine the appropriateness of one strategy over another. These are also discussed further in Chapter 5.

Another tactical approach to conflict management involves restructuring the relationship between groups around superordinate goals. The emergence of concession bargaining in which labor unions participate in "give-backs" is an example of using a superordinate goal—that is survival of a company or industry—to overcome well-entrenched intergroup conflicts. Other strategies involve the use of buffer devices between potentially conflicting groups. In labor management negotiations, the mediator assumes this role; in fact, we see increasing use of mediators outside of the union-management arena to help parties manage their relationships.

An alternative to tactical methods of conflict management are strategic approaches which attempt to identify the underlying causes of conflict. Blake and Mouton caution against behavioral strategies because of their inability to have long-lasting effects.[70] Their Interface Conflict-Solving Model attempts to build trust and cooperation among groups by examining the interfaces between groups. An interface is defined as any point of contact between groups at which interchanges are necessary to achieve a desired result. Their conflict-solving model is highly structured and focuses on inter-face problems. They have had success with this model in a variety of situations including union-management disputes, parent organization-subsidiary conflicts, and mergers. Specifically, this model of managing interface problems requires the participation of those individuals responsible for and capable of making the decisions necessary to bring about change. Participants in problem solving sessions should also be familiar with the history of the relationship, current norms, and operating practices.

Perhaps the most innovative strategic approach to intergroup conflict is the establishment of self-contained groups. These are regroupings of conflicting groups into new groups that perform their work independently of other groups. These arrangements minimize coordination problems, since the individuals relevant to a particular task are grouped together. These groups are in some respects variants of matrix arrangements, except that self-contained groups are more permanent in nature.

There are also a number of organizational development interventions that attempt to deal with intergroup conflict. These interventions include such methods as third-party peacemaking, intergroup mirroring, and intergroup team building. Like the Interface Conflict-Solving Model, these approaches attempt to identify structural conditions between groups that lead to conflict.

Finally one of the most important tasks for most managers is to coordinate the efforts of groups of people. Groups can become dysfunctional for many reasons and it is important for managers to anticipate the potential causes of problems in group and intergroup functioning and implement strategies to prevent or eliminate those causes. The successful manager will be rewarded with an effective work team that is not only meeting the needs of the organization, but is rewarding and supportive of its members as well. McGregor's[71] description of the characteristics of an effective work team, first published over thirty years ago, still stands as a useful statement of what managers should strive to achieve (see Table 6.4).

These characteristics are valid whether the group in question is a handful of people or a large division with hundreds of workers. As this chapter has tried to show, the manager's task is not only to foster a meaningful sense of group identity, but to control it

TABLE 6.4. McGregor's Characteristics of an Effective Work Team

1. The "atmosphere" tends to be informal, comfortable, relaxed . . . It is a working atmosphere in which people are involved and interested . . .
2. There is a lot of discussion in which virtually everyone participates, but it remains pertinent to the task of the group . . .
3. The task or the objective of the group is well understood and accepted by its members. There will have been free discussion of the objective at some point, until it was formulated in such a way that the members of the group could commit themselves to it.
4. The members listen to each other . . . Every idea is given a hearing . . .
5. There is disagreement. The group is comfortable with this and shows no signs of having to avoid conflict or to keep everything on the plane of sweetness and light . . .
6. Most decisions are reached by a kind of consensus in which it is clear that everybody is in general agreement and willing to go along. However, there is little tendency for individuals who oppose action to keep their opposition private and thus let an apparent consensus mask real disagreement . . .
7. Criticism is frequent, frank, and relatively comfortable . . .
8. People are free in expressing their feelings as well as their ideas both on the problem and on the group's operation . . .
9. When action is taken, clear assignments are made and accepted.
10. The chairman of the group does not dominate it, nor on the contrary, does the group defer unduly to him or her . . . [T]he leadership shifts from time to time, depending on the circumstances . . . The issue is not who controls, but how to get the job done.
11. The group is self-conscious about its own operations. Frequently, it will stop to examine how well it is doing or what may be interfering with its operation . . .

From McGregor D. *The Human Side of Enterprise.* New York, NY: McGraw-Hill; 1960:232–235. Reproduced with permission of McGraw-Hill, Inc.

so that it stays in perspective. This can be accomplished by an approach to group management that recognizes both group structure and group process as important determinants of organizational effectiveness. A group is obviously made up of individuals, but each group has an existence apart from its individual members and a personality all its own. The job of managers is to get things done not only through other people, but through groups of other people. Managers who learn well the techniques described in this chapter will help promote both greater organizational effectiveness and their own careers.

KEY CONCEPTS

Behavior and Performance Norms
Behavioral Masking
Building and Maintenance Roles
Communication Structure
Formal and Informal Leadership
Formal Groups
Friendship Groups
Group Cohesiveness
Group Composition
Group Productivity
Group Role Clarity
Groupthink
Informal Groups
Interest Groups
Intergroup Conflict
Intermittent Group
Management Teams
Membership Groups
Personal Roles
Productivity
Reference Groups
Role Differentiation
Stages of Group Development
Standing Committees
Status Differences
Task Forces
Task-Oriented Roles
Temporary Group
Work Groups

Discussion Questions

1. The recently hired director of a new ambulatory care center in a hospital has been instructed to begin holding weekly management team meetings. The management team is to consist of several physicians, nurses, physician assistants, and a social worker. What advice would you give the director to help promote the team's effectiveness?

2. An interorganizational community task force has been formed to identify obstacles facing the elderly in obtaining needed health and social services. Given the large number of agencies involved in providing services to the elderly and the need for consumer representation, how would you balance the need for full representation with the need to keep group size at a manageable level?

3. Under what circumstances are uncohesive groups more productive than cohesive groups? What strategies can a group leader employ to increase the probability that a cohesive group will be productive?

4. What strategies can a group leader use to increase the commitment of group members? How does a group leader know if group members are motivated and committed to the group?

REFERENCES

1. Fargason CA, Haddock CC. Cross-functional, integrative team decision making: Essential for effective QI in health care. *Quality Review Bulletin.* 1992;7:157–163.
2. Roethlisberger FJ, Dickson WJ. *Management and the Worker.* Cambridge, Mass: Harvard University Press; 1939.
3. Porter LW, Lawler III EE, Hackman JR. *Behavior in Organizations.* New York, NY: McGraw-Hill; 1975.
4. Hasenfeld Y. *Human Service Organizations.* Englewood Cliffs, NJ: Prentice Hall; 1983.
5. Jewell LS, Reitz HJ. *Group Effectiveness in Organizations.* Glenview, Ill: Scott, Foresman; 1981.
6. Etzioni A. *A Comparative Analysis of Complex Organizations.* New York, NY: Free Press; 1961:114.
7. Alderfer CP. An empirical test of a new theory of human needs. *Organizational Behavior and Human Performance.* 1969;4:142–175.
8. Walton RE, Hackman JR. Groups under contrasting management strategies. In: Goodman PS and Associates. *Designing Effective Work Groups.* San Francisco, Ca: Jossey-Bass; 1990.
9. Wagner JA, Hollenbeck JR. *Management of Organizational Behavior.* Englewood Cliffs, NJ: Prentice Hall; 1992.
10. Gladstein DL. Groups in context: A model of task group effectiveness. *Administrative Science Quarterly.* 1984;29:499–517.
11. Nieva VF, Fleishman EA, Rieck A. Team dimensions: Their identity, their measurement, and their relationships. Final technical report for Contract DAHC19-78-C-0001. Washington, DC: Advanced Research Resources Organizations; 1978.
12. Trist E, Bamforth K. Some social and psychological consequences of the Longwall method of goal-setting. *Human Relations.* 1951;4:1–38.
13. Kolodny H, Kiggundu M. Towards the development of a sociotechnical systems model in Woodlands Mechanical Harvesting. *Human Relations.* 1980;33:623–645.
14. Hackman JR. A set of methods for research on work teams. Technical report 1, School of Organization and Management, Yale University; 1982.
15. Steiner ID. *Group Process and Productivity.* Orlando, Fla: Academic Press; 1972.
16. Seashore S. *Group Cohesiveness in the Industrial Work Group.* Ann Arbor, Mich: Institute for Social Research, University of Michigan; 1954.
17. Hackman, op. cit.
18. Steiner, op. cit.
19. Guzzo RA. Group decision making and group effectiveness in organizations. In: Goodman PS and Associates. *Designing Effective Work Groups.* San Francisco, Ca: Jossey-Bass; 1990.
20. Trist E. *The Evolution of Socio-Technical Systems: A Conceptual Framework and an Action Researh Program.* Toronto, Canada; Ontario Quality of Working Life Centre; 1981:18.
21. Cummings T. Self-regulating work groups: A socio-technical synthesis. *Academy of Management Review.* 1978;3:625–634.
22. Shea GP, Guzzo RA. Group effectiveness: What really matters? *Sloan Management Review.* Spring 1987:25–31.
23. Nadler DA, Hackman JR, Lawler III EE. *Managing Organizational Behavior.* Boston, Mass: Little, Brown; 1979.
24. Hackman JR. Introduction: Work teams in organizations, An orienting framework. In: Hackman JR, ed., *Groups That Work (And Those That Don't): Creating Conditions for Effectiveness Teamwork.* San Francisco, Ca: Jossey-Bass; 1990.
25. Nieva, Fleishman, Rieck, op. cit.
26. Fried B, Nelson W. Strategic planning with family physicians. *Canadian Family Physician.* 1987; 33:1309–1312.
27. Janis IL. *Groupthink.* Boston, Mass: Houghton Mifflin; 1982.
28. Fleishman J. Collective action as helping behavior: Effects of responsibility diffusion on contributions to a public good. *Journal of Personality and Social Psychology.* 1980;38:629–637.
29. Jones GR. Task visibility, freeriding, and shirking: Explaining the effect of structure and technology on employee behavior. *Academy of Management Review.* 1984;9:684–695.
30. Wicker AW. *An Introduction to Ecological Psychology.* Monterey, Ca: Brooks/Cole; 1979.
31. Festinger L, Schacter S, Back K. *Social Pressures in Informal Groups.* Stanford, Ca: Stanford University Press; 1950.
32. Gooding RZ, Wagner III JA. A meta-analytic review of the relationship between size and performance: The productivity and efficiency of organizations and their subunits. *Administrative Science Quarterly.* 1985;30:462–481.
33. Denison DR, Sutton RI. Operating room nurses. In: Hackman JR, ed. *Groups That Work (And Those That Don't): Creating Conditions for Effective Teamwork.* San Francisco, Ca: Jossey-Bass; 1990.
34. Wagner, Hollenbeck, op. cit.
35. Hackman JR. Work design. In: Hackman JR, Suttle JL. *Improving Life at Work.* Santa Monica, Ca: Goodyear; 1976.
36. Benne K, Sheats P. Functional roles of group members. *Journal of Social Issues.* 1948;2:42–47.
37. Shaw ME. *Group Dynamics: The Psychology of Small*

Group Behavior. New York, NY: McGraw-Hill; 1981.

38. Cartwright D, Zander A. *Group Dynamics: Research and Theory.* 3rd ed. New York, NY: Harper & Row; 1968.

39. Adams JS. Injustice in social exchange. In: Berkowitz L, ed. *Advances in Experimental Social Psychology.* Vol 2. New York, NY: Academic Press; 1965.

40. Terborg JR, Castore C, DeNinno JA. A longitudinal field investigation of the impact of group composition on group performance and cohesion. *Journal of Personality and Social Psychology.* 1976;34:782–790.

41. Cartwright, Zander, op. cit.

42. Lott AJ, Lott BE. Group cohesiveness and interpersonal attraction: A review of relationships with antecedent and consequent variables. *Psychological Bulletin.* 1965;64:259–302.

43. Stogdill RM. Group productivity, drive, and cohesiveness. *Organizational Behavior and Human Performance.* 1972;8:26–43.

44. Nieva, Fleishman, Rieck, op. cit.

45. McGrath JE. *Groups: Interaction and Performance.* San Francisco, Ca: Jossey-Bass; 1984.

46. Cartwright, Zander, op. cit.

47. Cosier RA. Dialectical inquiry in strategic planning: A case of premature acceptance? *Academy of Management Review.* 1981;6:643–648.

48. Janis IL. *Victims of Groupthink.* Boston, Mass: Houghton-Mifflin; 1972.

49. Schwenk CR. Laboratory research on ill-structured decision aids: The case of dialectical inquiry. *Decision Sciences.* 1983;14:140–144.

50. Jackson SE. Team composition in organizational settings: Issues in managing an increasingly diverse work force. In: Worchel S, Wood W, Simpson JA. *Group Process and Productivity.* Newbury Park, Ca: Sage; 1992.

51. Scott WG. *Organization Theory.* Homewood, Ill: Richard D. Irwin, Inc., 1967.

52. Deber RB, Leatt P. The multidisciplinary renal team: Who makes the decisions? *Health Matrix.* 1986;4(3):3–9.

53. Hunsaker PL, Cook CW. *Managing Organizational Behavior.* Reading, Mass: Addison-Wesley; 1986.

54. Stigler GJ. Free riders and collective action: An appendix to theories of economic regulation. *Bell Journal of Economics and Management Science.* 1974;5:359–365.

55. Albanese R, Van Fleet DD. Rational behavior in groups: The free riding tendency. *Academy of Management Review.* 1985;10:244–255.

56. Roberts KH, Hunt DM. *Organizational Behavior.* Boston, Mass: PWS-Kent Publishing Co; 1991.

57. Albanese, Van Fleet, op. cit.

58. Janis, 1972, op. cit.

59. Fleishman, op. cit.

60. Delbecq A, Van de Ven A, Gustafson D. *Group Techniques for Program Planning.* Glenview, Ill: Scott, Foresman; 1975.

61. Dalkey N. *The Delphi Method: An Experimental Study of Group Opinion.* Santa Monica, Ca: The Rand Corporation; 1969.

62. Forsyth DR. *An Introduction to Group Dynamics.* Pacific Grove, Ca: Wadsworth; 1983.

63. Blake RR, Mouton JS. *Solving Costly Organizational Conflicts.* San Francisco, Ca: Jossey-Bass; 1984.

64. Arnold HJ, Feldman DC. *Organizational Behavior.* New York, NY: McGraw-Hill; 1986.

65. Fried B, Nelson W. Strategic planning with family physicians. *Canadian Family Physician.* 1987;33:1309–1312.

66. Folger JC, Gee EP. *Product Line Management: Organizing for Productivity.* Chicago, Ill: American Hospital Publishing; 1987.

67. Sherif M, Sherif CW. *Groups in Harmony and Tension.* New York, NY: Harper; 1953.

68. Fried, Nelson, op. cit.

69. Arnold HJ, Feldman DC. *Organizational Behavior.* New York, NY: McGraw-Hill; 1986.

70. Blake, Mouton, op. cit.

71. McGregor D. *The Human Side of Enterprise.* New York, NY: McGraw-Hill; 1960.

72. Huber G. *Managerial Decision Making.* Glenview, Ill: Scott, Foresman; 1980.

CHAPTER

7

WORK DESIGN

Martin P. Charns, D.B.A.
Director

Carol Ann Lockhart, Ph.D.
President

LEARNING OBJECTIVES

After completing this chapter, the reader should be able to

1. identify the range of approaches to work design, including the psychological and task inventory approaches
2. understand the relationships between work design and individuals' motivation and productivity
3. discuss the differences between work and working
4. identify components of work, their characteristics and their performance requirements
5. analyze the interconnectedness of components of work among individuals and among work groups
6. understand how to approach the design of individual jobs and of work units

CHAPTER PURPOSE

The differences between the effectively functioning 2-South and the chaotic 5B are seen by many administrators and health care professionals as arising from differences in the leadership of the units. Others attribute the differences to the clustering of nurses on 2-South into three groups, allowing them, unlike the 5B nurses, to identify with a small and cohesive group. Still other observers believe that the differences between the two units are most directly related to the competence of the staff or to their motivation. Rarely mentioned is the design of the jobs of the nurses and other staff on the two units. The purpose of this chapter is to provide a framework for the design of individual jobs and organizational work groups, such as Units 2-South and 5B, and to describe the relationships between work design and

IN THE REAL WORLD

A TALE OF TWO NURSING UNITS

Unit 5B, a small pediatrics unit in a major eastern teaching hospital, is characterized by high dissatisfaction among the nursing staff and is the target of frequent complaints from residents and attending physicians. Absenteeism among members of the nursing staff is high, requiring that the unit be staffed with nurses from a float pool.

The administration views the unit as its major trouble spot in the hospital. The unit generally appears to be in a state of chaos. Parents of patients on 5B often wander around the unit asking physicians, nurses, and other staff for information about their children. Parents frequently complain that they receive conflicting information from the medical and nursing staffs. The largest number of patient complaints received by the administration concern 5B.

The organization of the hospital is similar to that of most major teaching facilities, with the major organizational units representing professional (nursing, social service, dietary) and non-

professional (housekeeping, security, transportation) departments. Responsibilities are delineated in detail by function. Nursing staff members are assigned to units, each geographically located on a wing of one floor. Unit 5B is small. It has 16 beds, 12 of which are usually occupied, and a full-time nursing staff of 17 registered nurses (RNs). The unit offers primary nursing care, an approach to care delivery where each RN is responsible for the total nursing needs of a number of patients. When the primary nurse is not at work, other members of the unit's nursing staff perform the nursing activities for those patients. The nursing staff is responsible to a head nurse, who has administrative responsibility for several patient care units. She is located on another floor, separated from 5B activities. Social workers, dietitians, and therapists provide services for patients throughout the hospital; none spends a majority of his time on 5B.

Unit 2-South is also a pediatrics unit but in a different eastern teaching hospital. It is seen by the nursing and medical staffs and the hospital administration as an exemplary unit. It has the reputation for quality care and responsiveness to both patients and their families. Nurses and other staff express high satisfaction about their work and the hospital and frequently take advantage of the organization's liberal educational benefits to attend courses to increase their professional skills. In general, the unit runs smoothly and responds well to routine situations as well as emergency and unusual cases.

Unit 2-South is also a small unit with 21 beds, 14 RNs, a head nurse, and three multiskilled employees. It uses primary nursing but differs organizationally from 5B in several ways. First, the nurses are organized into three groups. When a primary nurse is not at work, a member of her group assumes the role of associate and takes responsibility for providing nursing care and implementing the care plan. Each group has responsibility for the patients of one team of house staff and attending physicians. An assignment board, located at the entrance of the unit, indicates for each nursing group the corresponding house staff team, the patients, the primary nurse assignments, and the nurses covering for off-duty primary nurses. On a daily basis, primary nurses participate with their corresponding physician group in patient rounds. The head nurse's major responsibilities are managerial—development of nursing staff, orientation of house staff who are beginning their six-week rotation on the unit, coordination with house staff and attending physicians, coordination of nursing staff, and liaison with other parts of the nursing department and hospital. Her office is centrally located on 2-South. In rare instances she serves as an associate to a primary nurse and is directly involved in patient care. One multiskilled employee is responsible for a broad range of environmental support and maintenance tasks including the work of traditional housekeeping, transport, and patient care assistance. Two other multiskilled workers are cross-trained and assist and feed patients, stock supplies, draw blood, and perform EKGs and other technical tasks.

individuals' motivation and productivity. Approaches to job design are discussed along with their inherent assumptions, strengths, and limitations. An integration of the concepts and a framework for their managerial application are then presented.

Work design concepts can be applied at several levels in an organization. In fact, they can be applied to analyze and design the work of two or more related organizations, such as multi-institutional systems, or an organization and its suppliers, or referral networks. In this chapter, the concepts are applied in a single organization. Attention is directed to the design of work contained within single jobs (i.e., job design) and the design of work within organizational units consisting of several jobs (i.e., work unit design).

The individual job is the basic element of any organization. As such, job design has been a focus of attention in the literatures of organizational behavior and health management. Contrasting approaches to job design, however, are found both in the literature and in practice. In many health care organizations, jobs that reflect these differing perspectives exist side by side. For example, professionals (e.g., physicians, nurses, social workers) generally determine for themselves both what work to do and how to do it. Technicians' jobs, however, are often highly engineered and their activities specified. Yet problems of low productivity, low morale, and dysfunctional individual behaviors, such as alcoholism and drug abuse, exist among both professional and nonprofessional workers. To solve such problems it is necessary to consider both the needs of the organization and the individual. Since a job is the interface between the organization and the individual, it is a critical area for managerial attention.

APPROACHES TO JOB DESIGN
Task Inventory Approaches

There are two major approaches to job design. Each focuses almost exclusively on either job activities or the psychological aspects of workers. Several related approaches are aggregated here under the task inventory label.

The task inventory approach is based in the scientific management school of thought developed by Taylor and Gilbreth. Scientific management had its genesis in manufacturing organizations and led to the development of industrial engineering.[1,2] Through examination of job activities in time-and-motion studies, industrial engineers design jobs to most efficiently utilize technology and to minimize wasted human effort. Within a technologically driven work setting, workers most suitable to the jobs are selected and trained. Through experience, workers become more proficient at their jobs, and thus specialization and routinization of work activities attempt to take advantage of the individual's learning curve. Since an objective of this approach is elimination of extraneous activities, its success depends on ensuring that people perform the job as designed.

This approach has made important contributions to management, especially in heavy industries such as the U.S. automobile industry. Scientific management approaches have gone beyond manufacturing settings, however, and can be found in both inpatient and ambulatory health care settings.

The routine nature of many jobs in support services in hospitals and other care settings, such as transport, laboratory, laundry, and radiology, allows job activities to be studied from an industrial engineering perspective. However, systems designed in this manner are tailored to meet specific conditions and are inherently unresponsive to change or uncertainty. Since patient needs and emergencies are not always subject to specification, employees at *all* levels of a health care organization are frequently required to use their own judgment, which limits the usefulness of scientific management principles.

There are three assumptions underlying activity-focused approaches to job design in any setting. These assumptions suggest that:

1. The work can be divided into repetitive routine elements.
2. Workers can be trained and motivated to perform dependably.
3. Workers' motivation derives primarily from

economic rewards which can be associated with their reliably performing their work.

Although these assumptions have face validity in many situations, they are also inherently limiting. Often the work cannot be divided into elements that can be repetitively performed. In addition, workers frequently seek more than economic rewards from their work and react to routine, repetitive jobs by not performing dependably or by quitting the job. From a purely economic perspective, the cost of repeated recruiting and training often exceeds the benefits believed to be gained from technological efficiency. In human terms, the inefficiency and potential for errors which might harm patients is increased.

Another more flexible approach to job activities analysis is the *task inventory* methodology, often used in studies of jobs of health professionals, especially nurses, physicians, and physician assistants. In the mid-1960s, a shortage of health workers was predicted in the United States. In response, the task inventory methodology was developed in order to categorize job activities and determine whether parts of a professional's job might be performed by other workers.[3–5] Kane and Jacoby, for example, demonstrated the feasibility of using physician assistants (Medex) for job activities not requiring a fully trained physician.[6] The same methodology is currently the basis for studies seeking to determine the costs of nursing and other care activities in response to hospital prospective payments, managed care, and continuing changes in health care financing.

In this tradition Gilpatrick, for example, conducted the Health Services Mobility Study, identifying and analyzing tasks of health care workers and determining skills and knowledge needed to perform each task.[7] This approach specified the required skills and knowledge of health care workers, thereby providing a basis for defining their educational needs. Common educational needs for various jobs and career ladders were developed by which individuals could advance not only upward but also across traditional disciplines. Curricula in many schools of allied health have been modified to produce multicompetent health professionals to work in health care settings.[8–11]

In applying the task inventory approach, it is helpful to develop a table similar to that in Figure 7.1. Elements of work, or tasks, are listed in the first column. Then

(1) Task	(2) Who now performs task	(3) Knowledge and skills required	(4) Alternative performers and their training needs
1.			
2.			
3.			
4.			
5.			

Continue as needed.

FIGURE 7.1. Task Inventory.

for each task, who currently performs the task is (are) listed in column 2, the knowledge and skills required are listed in column 3, and other individuals who perform the task or other jobs in which the task could be incorporated are listed in column 4. Additionally, the training required for the individuals is noted in column 4.

Psychological Approaches

In contrast to the task inventory approach is the *psychological approach* rooted in psychology and organizational behavior. Focusing on worker psychology and motivation, this approach assumes that, when individuals perform work that meets their needs for growth and jobs themselves are intrinsically rewarding, substantial motivation results (also see Chapter 3). Professional jobs, in which there generally is a strong relationship between an individual's self-concept and her work, are examples. On the other hand, routine, repetitive jobs that encompass only a small portion of a larger task or jobs that are strictly and narrowly delineated are difficult for anyone to identify with. Such jobs limit the extent of an individual's involvement in the work

and the motivation to perform well; therefore, productivity suffers.

Sometimes, however, when individuals have total discretion over the way they do their work and what work they perform, their motivation may be directed toward other than organizational goals. In fact, they may work against the organization's goals. The assumption that motivation will result in organizationally desirable productivity does not necessarily hold. Even so, professional workers are often given complete discretion over what they do and how they do it. This, in fact, is one of the attributes of a profession. In medicine, generally regarded as the prime example of a profession, professional work is typically off limits to organizational job design analysis.

The autonomy of health care professionals, however, is being challenged. The issues of cost control, quality, competition, and responsiveness to customers have come to dominate the health care system of the 1990s. Health care managers have responded to these issues and to the challenges of a market-driven health care system by moving to make their organizations more price sensitive; cost effective; and patient, family, and client centered.

Work arrangements that made half-hearted attempts at efficiency in the fee-for-service health care system are no longer viable. Coordination and the management of care have become primary tools for controlling health care costs. The caregiver—physician, nurse, or other provider—cannot choose the course of treatment, or the equipment or supplies used to provide that treatment without considering the cost implications of these decisions on the patient, themselves, or their related organization. Where once a provider's convenience in scheduling a procedure was dominant, patient centered services in today's leading organizations often dictate care be given at a time and location preferred by the patient and the insurer. No longer do we assume without question that providers always know or do what is "right" for their patients. Patients, health care organizations, and the benefits provided a patient through their insurance are limiting the discretion of physicians and other providers.

The force of the changes occurring in the health care system is reflected in shifts in power between physicians and managers (also see Chapter 9). There has been a relative increase in power and control exercised by management and a relative decrease in the power of physicians. These changes have been fueled by a surplus of physicians and a lessening of demand for their services as managed patient care, health maintenance organizations (HMOs), and other prepaid arrangements constrain the volume of services used. Prepaid arrangements have also given administrators increased influence over physicians' incomes. Previously, managers had limited means by which to control practitioners in their institutions or organizations. Now, however, they can decide whether the productivity and practice style of these practitioners is consistent with the economic survival of the organization. If it is not, physicians and others are being denied contracts, receiving reduced payments from HMOs and preferred provider organizations (PPOs), and facing an array of sanctions never before encountered. The impact of such controls has only begun to be felt.

Through direct efforts, such as utilization management and tying financial considerations to patient care practices, as well as more indirect efforts, such as creating a cost conscious culture for the organization, managers are influencing physician decision making. The combination of organizational pressures and national efforts to define practice guidelines and outcomes of care are working together to force change. Although it is difficult for physicians to change practice styles developed over many years, to varying degrees they are changing their behavior. Whether the changes will improve or reduce the quality of care or the risk associated with it is still uncertain, but it is a question that will accompany the health care system over the next decade and help drive the quest for quality improvement, as further discussed in Chapter 13.

Like physicians, nurses are facing challenges to their practice. In the 1980s health care organizations experienced a severe shortage of nurses and other health professionals. This was caused by many factors including increased acuity of hospitalized patients, increased numbers of jobs in ambulatory settings and case review for insurance approval, women's increased professional opportunities outside of health care, and the drop in the number of nurses needing to work when other family income earners are doing well in a strong economy. The shortage led many hospitals to rethink the design of professional and nonprofessional jobs both to match the availability of lower skilled workers in the labor force and to create more stimulating jobs that workers would not leave. In addition, some organizations used this as an opportunity to redesign their patient care delivery systems to emphasize the patient as the *raison d'etre.* Even though the nursing shortage ameliorated with the downturn in the world economy in the late 1980s, many organizations continued their redesign efforts.[12-14] Many rural hospitals, characterized by a highly variable census, have found multiskilled workers and cross-training staff to be effective ways to meet their highly fluctuating demand. It has become a critical element to their survival and is increasingly seen as important in the efforts to efficiently manage larger urban hospitals.[15]

Given the opportunity to influence professionals and nonprofessionals in their decision making, rewards, satisfaction, and motivation, as well as the quality and cost of health care, it is more important than ever for managers to recognize the importance of examining work design. How a health care manager chooses to do this is influenced by the range of approaches to work design and their conflicting underlying assumptions. While managers frequently become believers in one or another approach to job design, they limit their effectiveness and the opportunity to integrate a variety of approaches for maximum advantage by doing so. In the multifaceted health care system of today, no one approach can guarantee success.

ANALYSIS OF WORK

Work and Working

One of the prime reasons for poor management and less than optimal performance in health care and other organizations is that managers confuse "work" and "working."[16,17] They also inappropriately manage the relationship between work and working. *Work* is objective and impersonal. It is energy directed at organizational goals, identifiable separately from the person who does it. It is analyzable. *Working,* on the other hand, is a worker's affective response to work. Far from totally analyzable, it is an individual's personal and subjective reaction. Work affects working, and working affects work.

Writers and managers who follow scientific management and related job activity analysis focus on work and largely ignore working. The workers' affective responses are seen as extraneous elements to be controlled so that they do not interfere with work. In contrast, management of professionals is often based almost exclusively upon attention to working. The re-

sult is that work is directed at the goals chosen by the professional, which may or may not be organizational goals. Similarly, managerial efforts to improve working conditions or to humanize work are often pursued with working in mind and with insufficient and inappropriate consideration for the work requirements. Both work and working are important elements in efforts to manage patient care in a cost effective and efficient manner.

Types of Work

An analysis of work recognizes that all organizations perform three different types of work: direct work, management work, and support work. *Direct work* is effort that directly contributes to the accomplishment of an organization's goals. In health care organizations, clinical work performed by doctors, nurses, and other care providers is direct work. In organizations that have multiple goals, such as teaching hospitals, there is a set of direct work activities for each goal (e.g., teaching, research, and patient care). Although an individual may perform more than one type of direct work, the work itself is identifiable and analyzable separate from the person performing it.[18,19]

Management work includes providing the resources and context within which direct work can be

---

DEBATE TIME 7.1: WHAT DO YOU THINK?

The task inventory and psychological approaches to work design were developed by different groups of scholars based on different sets of premises. When applied to the design of any particular job, the two approaches yield very different outcomes.

The scientific management school as one task inventory approach prescribes breaking work down into discrete, repetitive components, and training workers to be expert in their narrow areas of responsibility. Proponents of this approach argue that simplifying work allows development of expertise, and through repetition of tasks, workers become highly proficient. Developed through this form of job engineering, highly skilled workers contribute to organizational productivity.

The psychological school argues that people should be provided with work that represents whole tasks with which they can identify. This provides the opportunity for people to feel that their work is meaningful, and they are more highly motivated to do it well. Workers' high motivation, in turn, is critical to organizational productivity. From the perspective of the psychological school, repetitive tasks are not rewarding to individuals. Without interest in their work, workers' motivation is low and so is productivity.

How do you reconcile these different perspectives? What different assumptions form the underpinnings of the two different approaches? What situational factors have to be considered in applying the different theories?

performed effectively and maintaining an alignment between an organization and its external environment. Management work is decision making about the organizational context within which other work is performed.[20] For example, it includes determining what services to provide, what services to develop or reduce, what resources to make available to whom, and what systems will perform various functions. Since the primary method of influencing decision making is to influence its premises—the information that is considered in making a decision—management work affects all other work because it influences the premises on which other decisions are made.[21]

Support work does not directly result in achievement of an organizational goal, but it is needed for effective accomplishment of other work. For example, support work for clinical work includes such things as maintaining medical records, transporting patients, maintaining the physical surroundings in which care is delivered, and performing laboratory tests. Support work for management work includes providing legal counsel, clerical assistance, data on both internal operations and the external environment, planning and analytical assistance, as well as personnel support.

Recognizing these three major types of work provides the basis for determining the requirements of work. To consider both work and working effectively, a more detailed analysis is needed, one that considers the components of each type of work and their interrelationships. Analysis consists of answering four separate but related questions.[22]

- What are the component parts of work and the characteristics and requirements of each?
- How do the component parts inherently fit together?
- What resources are needed to do the work?
- What controls are needed to determine and evaluate the performance of the work?

Determining Components of Work

The best approach to identifying the components of work involves assessing the natural boundaries in work that occur along the dimensions of time, technology, and territory.[23] When different work is or can be performed at different points in time, such as on different days or at different times of the day, distinct work components can be identified. For example, patient care given during one office visit is distinguishable from that given during another visit, as is patient care delivered to a patient during different hospital admissions. Similarly, discrete components of work can often be identified by the fact that they are performed in different places (territories), such as in hospital, ambulatory, and home care settings. Finally, components of work can be identified by the technology involved.

> Technology should be considered broadly to include not only hardware, but also skills and training, personality characteristics and interpersonal orientations and different practices associated with performing different work. Such different practices may result from tradition, from regulation of government, licensing agencies, or accrediting bodies, or from professional norms of accepted practice. Thus, for example, the work performed by different professional groups is a natural place to look for inherent boundaries.[24]

In doing so, however, analysis must determine whether differences are real and inherent in the work or are maintained only by tradition.

By taking a broad perspective of technology, we can also ask what differences in work are associated with different parts of an organization's environment. For example, do different patients represent different types of work? Do treating different diseases, preventing illness in contrast to treating it, or interacting with people from different ethnic or socioeconomic backgrounds represent the use of different technologies and therefore different work? Often differences in technology overlap with differences in time or territory, but together they help identify discrete components of work.

The task inventory method discussed earlier provides a helpful approach to identifying components of work. When using this method, it is important not to overlook significant but difficult to observe aspects of work. Furthermore, this approach starts with a description of the status quo. To the extent that either an array of jobs or the task inventory does not include important aspects of work which should be present, the analysis will be incomplete.

Galbraith has provided a set of categories for determining the behaviors required for effective task performance.[25] These can be applied to each element of work as well as to the aggregate of elements that comprise a single job. Galbraith's five categories in cumulative order are

1. decisions to join and remain in an organization
2. dependable role performance
3. effort above minimum levels
4. spontaneous and innovative behavior
5. cooperative behavior

In general, all jobs require the first two categories of behavior. Organizations require that people join and remain employed in their jobs and that they perform dependably. These two minimum levels of behavior, however, are often not completely met. Where the work itself or the working conditions do not provide a worker with an acceptable level of rewards—including satisfaction—turnover and absenteeism result. Dependable role performance also does not occur when people do not know what is expected of them or they feel that the work that is expected of them is not equitably balanced with the rewards of the job.

When jobs require more than the first two minimum categories of behavior, the design of the job itself becomes a greater concern. When all elements of the work cannot be anticipated, spontaneous and innovative behavior is required. This requirement can be distinguished from behavior above minimum levels by the frequency with which unanticipated events occur and the degree of innovative behavior required. It is characterized by an individual needing to recognize that spontaneous and innovative behavior is required and having the skills and willingness to act. When, in addition, the work requires an individual to recognize and be willing and able to work with others to achieve the desired outcome, it requires cooperative behavior.

The five categories of behavior are cumulative and form a scale directly related to the inherent uncertainty of the work. Thus, work that is highly certain and predictable generally requires only the first two categories of behavior. Work that is highly uncertain and unpredictable requires cooperative behavior in addition to all four other categories of behavior.

It is important to identify discrete components of work activities to determine their unique requirements. But before using such an analysis to design jobs or units of an organization, it is also necessary to examine the way in which the components must fit together.

Interconnectedness of Work

Once the elements of work are identified by the various methodologies, it is necessary to determine how they fit together to form a coherent whole: to determine for each element of work the other elements essential to its effective performance. At one extreme are elements that can be performed independently of each other. For example, feeding one patient and performing laboratory tests on a specimen from another patient are independent elements of work. In contrast, successful performance of other types of work requires that different work elements occur in sequence or that one element affects a second element which, in turn, acts upon the first element. For example, in medical diagnosis, initial diagnosis determines what laboratory and radiologic procedures are required. The results of those studies refine the original diagnosis. At the most complex level, elements of work affect each other simultaneously. Van de Ven et al. have called this "team interdependence," exemplified by the administration of anesthesia and the performance of surgery on a patient.[26]

The concept of *interconnectedness of work* is critical to effective work design. When interconnected elements of work are performed by different people, components must be coordinated to ensure effective performance. Coordination requires resources from the organization, such as development and use of plans and protocols, supervision of people responsible for interconnected elements, or discussion among those people. Where possible, therefore, it is most effective to design jobs to minimize spreading interconnected elements over several people. Realistically, this model is not always feasible because elements are often too numerous for a one person assignment; because elements are so different from one another that no one individual has the skills, training, desire, or inclination to do them all; or because technological advantages outweigh costs of coordination. When the interconnections cannot reside within one single job, it is best to organize work to contain the interconnected elements within a single work group.[27,28]

It is often the interconnectedness of work that health care organizations fail to address as they attempt to respond to the pressures of a competitive health care system. Efforts to improve institutional responsiveness through reorganization, continuous quality improvement, and other measures must address how the elements of work fit together and how they influence job design and performance.

DESIGNING INDIVIDUAL JOBS

Underlying the design of any job are assumptions about individuals and the relationship between individuals and their work. These assumptions may be formally stated (as in a labor contract) or not, and they may be recognized by managers or not. The job design literature is based upon the general assumptions that people work to satisfy a broad range of needs and that how a job is designed affects the person's ability to meet those needs. Two perspectives can be taken to consider in greater detail the relationship between job design and motivation.

First, consider that people are motivated by unfulfilled needs and that they exert effort to satisfy those needs. If opportunities for meeting a person's needs are provided by the work itself, the person will be motivated to perform the work. Where work itself does not provide opportunities to satisfy individual needs, the person will seek other outlets and may not be motivated to perform the work. Thus, it is important to match people and their needs to jobs and their inherent work requirements. For example, if work requires an individual only to join and remain in the organization and to perform dependably, these behaviors can often be obtained by matching the job to people with economic needs and rewarding them monetarily. When such jobs are held instead by people whose needs are for achievement or other forms of personal growth, the individuals most likely will not respond to only monetary rewards and will direct their efforts away from the dependable role performance required by the organization.[29] These people are better matched to jobs that require spontaneous and innovative behavior.

A second perspective on individual motivation is based upon the assumption that people evaluate courses of action for the purpose of choosing among them. The expectancy model of motivation posits that individuals exhibit behavior that they perceive will result in outcomes that yield valued rewards.[30,31] In its simplest form, the model indicates that people subjectively evaluate possible behaviors in terms of three elements: the probability that a behavior will yield a desired outcome, the probability that the outcome will yield rewards, and the value of those rewards to the individual. These three elements combine multiplicatively in a person's assessment so that, if any one element is low, it is unlikely that the person will choose the associated behavior. Where that behavior is required to perform work effectively, we must ask how the elements in the model are affected by the job.

When work is intrinsically rewarding to individuals—that is, when effectively performing the work itself is inherently rewarding—we can see that there is a direct connection between behavior and rewards. This is likely to occur with the following psychological conditions:[32]

- Experienced meaningfulness. The job is seen as important, valuable, and worthwhile.
- Experienced responsibility. Individuals feel personally responsible and accountable for the results of their efforts.
- Knowledge of results. Individuals understand how effectively they are performing the job.

These three aspects of working have a major impact on a person's motivation and are themselves affected both by characteristics of the individual and by the content of the work itself.

Three characteristics of a job contribute to its experienced meaningfulness: skill variety, task identity, and task significance. Skill variety refers to the variety of different skills and talents required of an individual in performing a job. A job that has task identity represents an identifiable piece of work that an individual can perform from beginning to end and that has a visible outcome. Task significance refers to the impact a job has on the lives of other people. In general, because health care organizations perform work that directly affects other people, great potential exists for designing jobs with high task significance. Yet by designing isolated jobs in which people cannot see how their work is an important part of a whole effort that helps other people, one can create jobs low in all three core dimensions.

Experienced responsibility for work outcomes is directly affected by the degree of autonomy in a job. The components of autonomy are freedom and discretion in scheduling work and in determining procedures to be used in performing it. A considerable degree of autonomy is present in jobs falling into Galbraith's categories of "effort above minimum levels," "spontaneous and innovative behavior," and "cooperative behavior."[33]

Feedback on work performance provides an individual with the third psychological dimension, knowledge of results. The most direct feedback is from the work itself, available primarily in situations in which an individual has responsibility for a whole and identifiable element of work. Where job design itself cannot provide direct feedback, it is important to obtain feedback from supervisors or peers.

An additional potential source of feedback is an organization's performance evaluation system. In some organizations performance evaluation is based solely on the subjective appraisal of an employee's supervisor. In others, however, it is based upon achievement of measurable goals. To the extent the goals for assessment of an individual align with the organization's goals, the individual's efforts can be directed at achievement of the organization's goals, in addition to serving as a feedback mechanism. In some organizations the goals used for performance evaluation are goals of the program or department for which the individual has a major share of responsibility.[34]

To some degree, skill variety, task identity, and task significance can substitute for one another, as they all contribute additively to experienced meaningfulness. Together they combine multiplicatively with autonomy (experienced responsibility) and feedback (knowledge of results) in contributing to the overall motivating potential of a job. A job's motivating potential score (MPS) can be expressed as follows[35]

$$\text{MPS} = \tfrac{1}{3}(\text{Skill variety} + \text{Task identity} + \text{Task significance}) \times \text{Autonomy} \times \text{Feedback}$$

Whether a job with a high MPS will actually result in high individual motivation depends upon the characteristics of the jobholder. People with high growth needs—strong needs for achievement, self-actualization, and personal development—will be most motivated by jobs with high motivating potential. It is also possible for people who do not have high growth needs to find their growth needs stimulated by jobs with a high MPS. On the other hand, not all people react positively to challenging jobs, and the autonomy and challenge may result instead in anxiety and low performance.

When people successfully accomplish work that satisfies their needs, job satisfaction is experienced. This in turn contributes to the expectation that future performance will result in satisfaction, and high levels of motivation generally result. Satisfaction, however, can result from meeting other needs, either within or outside of the work place, that will not contribute to motivation or to job performance. For example, social needs may be satisfied in the work setting, but this may be unrelated to work performance or motivation. Thus high motivation resulting in effective work performance will result in satisfaction, but satisfaction in itself will not necessarily result in future high motivation or performance.

COORDINATING INTERCONNECTED WORK WITHIN ORGANIZATIONAL UNITS

Interconnected elements of work are best placed within an individual job. The next best work design places the interconnected elements within a single organizational unit.[36,37] This design allows for members to identify with the work of the unit and most easily to coordinate the interconnected elements within that single unit. How to achieve that coordination is the subject of this section. Additional aspects of coordination are considered in Chapter 8.

Coordination of work has been the subject of considerable research. A consistent finding is that the most effective way of coordinating varies with the characteristics of the work performed. Duncan, for example, provided one of the first empirical studies of variation in coordination within work units, finding that work units change their patterns of interaction in response to differing levels of task uncertainty.[38] Building upon the theoretical work of March and Simon, Van de Ven et al. found variations in patterns of coordination among units facing different levels of task uncertainty.[39,40] Several authors have found relationships between coordination and organization performance. Knaus et al. found that variations in mortality in critical care units were related to the level of coordination in the units.[41] With the development of more refined measurement tools, this line of work continues to be advanced.[42]

Charns et al. extended the findings of Van de Ven et al. and the theoretical writings of Mintzberg to suggest that work groups use a combination of six approaches to coordination and that the use of these approaches is related to the effectiveness of patient care units.[43–45] Charns and Strayer replicated these findings in a residential school for severely emotionally disturbed children.[46] The six approaches fall into two categories: programming methods and feedback methods. The set of programming approaches includes three ways of standardizing the performance of work that are most effective when the work is well understood and programmable.

- Standardization of work processes is the use of rules, regulations, schedules, plans, procedures, policies, and protocols to specify the activities to be performed. Included are care plans and multidisciplinary clinical critical paths, which specify for a particular patient condition the interventions required and anticipated results at various times.
- Standardization of skills is the specification of the training or skills required to perform work. Often this is achieved through specification of minimum levels and types of education, certification as evidence of meeting minimum qualifications, or on-the-job training.
- Standardization of output specifies the form of intermediate outcomes of work as they are passed from one job to another.

In situations of high uncertainty, programming approaches alone cannot provide the needed coordination. Exchange of information and feedback are needed. Feedback mechanisms, which facilitate the transfer of information in unfamiliar situations, include the following:

- Supervision is the basis for coordination through an organization's hierarchy. It is the exchange of information between two people, one of whom is responsible for the work of the other.
- Mutual adjustment is the exchange of information about work performance between two people who are not in a hierarchical relationship, such as between two nurses or between a physician and a nurse.
- Group coordination is the exchange of information among more than two people, such as through meetings, rounds, and conferences.

Feedback approaches to coordination are more time consuming and require more effort than programming approaches. However, they are needed in situations characterized by high levels of uncertainty. There is some indication that higher performing patient care units in teaching hospitals differ from lower performing units in their greater use of all six types of coordinating approaches.[47] High performing units utilize plans, rules, procedures, and protocols not as constraints and organizational red tape but as guidelines for routine work. Contrary to previous research findings, effective use of programming approaches actually allows staff—especially nurses—greater discretion in their work. In addition, when faced with unfamiliar situations, the higher performing units increase their use of feedback approaches to a greater extent than the lower performing ones.

In applying this framework, it should be noted that, first, what is familiar to one person may not be familiar to another. For example, people with greater experience in a particular job will encounter fewer unfamiliar situations than people with less experience. The people with less experience, therefore, need to use feedback approaches to coordination to a greater extent than do highly experienced people. This is typically reflected in their greater reliance on discussions with their manager or peers. Second, the profile of coordinating approaches that can be used effectively depends upon the nature of the work of the unit. Greater advantage can be taken of programming approaches when the work of the unit is limited in scope and uncertainty. Finally, feedback approaches require trust and understanding among people, which requires consistency in working together. Such relationships are not often achieved in health care organizations. Physicians, nurses, and other health care providers in a hospital, ambulatory, or home care setting must coordinate their efforts. Nursing staff turnover and rotation, house staff rotation, and limited physicians' and other professionals' involvement in a unit or a remote care setting greatly hinder the development of such relationships and prevent full use of feedback approaches to coordination.

When coordination is not fully achieved, work performance is hindered. In addition to having a negative effect on patient care, this precludes people who perform the work from attaining the levels of achievement or obtaining the sense of competence that would satisfy their needs. Professionals often do feel that they are prevented from effectively carrying out their professional work by the ineffective way their organization functions. Where organizational factors hinder work accomplishment, people come to believe that hard work will not result in the desired outcome of good patient care. Using the expectancy model of motivation, the probability that effort will result in the desired outcome is low and thus the motivation to work hard is reduced.

Effective work design requires taking multiple perspectives based upon the analysis of work itself. In designing jobs, the work requirements should be matched to individual workers' needs. To the extent possible, interconnected elements of work should be combined into individual jobs that possess high levels of skill variety, task identity, task significance, autonomy, and feedback. The design of individual jobs must be done within a framework that considers other related jobs, including that of the supervisor.

The failures of job redesign too often have been caused by taking too narrow and restrictive a focus. Such an error can be avoided by taking a variety of approaches, including careful identification of the requirements and interconnections of the elements of work, which provide the basis for considering job design and coordination requirements.

APPLYING THE FRAMEWORK

The work design concepts provide a framework for analyzing Units 5B and 2-South (described at the beginning of the chapter) and determining options for change. Both units changed from a functional nursing organization to primary nursing. In the functional organization, each nurse performed one or at most a few related functions, such as administering medications, providing physical care, or taking vital signs, to a large number of patients. Following the traditions of scien-

DEBATE TIME 7.2: WHAT DO YOU THINK?

In applying the work design concepts to the redesign of patient care delivery systems, two conflicting perspectives typically are raised. On the one hand, heads of existing support departments such as dietary, environmental services, and patient transport argue that staff efficiency can be maximized when staff performing similar activities are organized into separate functional departments. The staff can then be assigned to different patient care units in response to the varying needs of those units. This provides both the most efficient utilization of staff and responsiveness to fluctuations in need for services among patient care units. In addition, when organized in this manner, staff can best maintain proficiency in their particular skill area, thereby assuring the quality of their services.

On the other hand, nurse managers and directors of clinical units argue that multiskilled employees, cross-trained in several functional areas, should be permanently assigned to individual units. Having a broad range of skills reduces fragmentation of delivery of care and allows for flexibility in meeting the varying needs of each unit. By working consistently with the same group of other employees, the multiskilled workers can become part of the patient care team and be most responsive to the unique needs of their units.

Which of these perspectives is correct? If you choose to implement one of these approaches, how do you address the needs expressed by proponents of the other approach? Can you incorporate both perspectives in another creative work design? If so, how?

tific management, this approach attempts to use the personnel efficiently and in line with their education.

Primary nursing, used on both units, provides staff more responsibility and broader professional roles. Jobs of primary nurses inherently have greater skill variety, task identity, autonomy, and feedback than functional nursing and, therefore, have higher motivating potential. While a primary nurse is at work, most of the interconnected elements of nursing work reside within individual jobs. These benefits often outweigh the costs of having highly skilled nurses do routine tasks.

Using Coordinating Mechanisms

Components of patient care work performed by different staff on a unit are highly interconnected. In different ways and with different success, both units used coordinating mechanisms to address these interconnections. Both utilized patient care protocols, although on 2-South they were used to a greater extent and were developed through greater involvement of the medical staff than on 5B. Both units also relied upon standardization of skills by hiring well-trained personnel and providing inservice education. Unit 5B, however, had high absenteeism. Nurses assigned to fill in from the float pool had little experience with the unit, thus limiting their ability to use protocols and other standardized approaches to coordination.

On 5B the administration thought that, since primary nurses had total responsibility for their patients, supervision could be reduced. Thus, the head nurse's responsibilities were expanded to cover several units. Physically removed from the unit, the head nurse gave insufficient attention to professional development of new and junior staff. The head nurse did not effectively orient new nursing and medical staff to the unit's routines, and standardized approaches to coordination broke down.

It was expected that primary nurses would coordinate their work with other members of the nursing and medical staffs, but 5B's organizational arrangements hindered that coordination. Nursing assignments were arranged almost randomly, so that there did not develop a consistent pattern of interactions among staff members that would encourage strong working relationships. This hindered use of personal approaches to coordination among nurses. It also made it difficult for a nurse providing care for another's patient to be involved or to identify with the patient, thereby limiting the motivating potential inherent in those efforts. Interactions with house staff also did not follow any consistent pattern, and each house officer had patients cared for by many different primary nurses. Whereas before implementation of primary nursing many house officers depended upon the head nurse to function as the coordinating link between themselves and the staff nurses caring for their patients, under the new arrangement they had to seek out several different primary nurses. Usually they did not bother to do so. Over time the trust between the nursing and medical staff members on Unit 5B deteriorated.

On 2-South the internal organization of nursing into three groups provided a basis for facilitating coordination both among nurses and between nurses and physicians. The small size of each nursing group and the arrangement for associates to cover for primary nurses within their group allowed nurses to identify with their group's patients. This contributed to the motivating potential of their jobs. Furthermore, the work interconnections among nurses were contained within each group. This facilitated management of these interconnections and contributed to development of trust needed among nursing staff for effective personal coordination. Each group included a mix of experienced and less experienced nurses, and together with the head nurse, the formally designated group leader had responsibility for staff development. Finally, by aligning teams of house staff with the nursing groups, the organization facilitated coordination.

The use of the assignment board further clarified responsibilities and contributed to the ease of locating staff members. As physicians and nurses worked together in a modified joint practice arrangement, trust between groups developed, adding to their ability to use mutual adjustment to coordinate their efforts. Both groups experienced a greater sense of accomplishment, contributing to their satisfaction and motivation. Because of the closeness and commitment of the personnel to other members of their group, they felt a sense of responsibility for the unit. Absenteeism was therefore low, and the more stable staffing in turn contributed to the unit's smooth functioning. The head nurse considered house staff orientation to be a critical responsibility, and this further contributed to the unit's ability to coordinate its work.

Multiskilled Employees

In the late 1980s, 2-South introduced multiskilled employees to perform routine work that had been done by staff from several departments. To utilize these staff efficiently, they cared for patients of all three teams, which did not allow them to be fully integrated into the teams. By being assigned to a single unit, however, they did feel a part of that unit. Performing many tasks for each patient, the multiskilled employees were responsive to patient needs. They saw the results of their efforts and gained much greater satisfaction from their work than had been the case when many people from different departments did those tasks. Multiskilled workers also contributed to patient satisfaction by reducing the number of staff going into each patient's room. Overall, 2-South organizationally addressed its work requirements more effectively than 5B.

As the examples demonstrate, several factors must be considered to design productive work units consisting of inherently motivating and rewarding jobs.[48] The basis for this design is analysis of the work itself. The content of individual jobs, the organization of work units, and the coordination of work both within and between units can be designed effectively only when the work requirements are understood. Just as the framework presented in this chapter can be used to analyze the jobs of health professionals on two different patient care units, it can be used to design work in other settings.

MANAGERIAL GUIDELINES

1. Scientific management and engineering of jobs are concepts applied most effectively to work characterized by low inherent uncertainty. They focus primarily on work and do not consider aspects of working.
2. Psychological approaches, which focus more on working, can be applied most effectively to situations of moderate to high uncertainty.
3. Work should be designed so that the most highly interconnected elements are contained within individual jobs to the extent that is possible, given considerations of size, limitations imposed by technology, and separation of job elements in time and space. Interconnected work elements that cannot be self-contained within single jobs should to the extent possible be placed within single work groups.
4. To enhance motivation, individual jobs should be designed to provide opportunities to satisfy the needs of the person performing a given job. People with high growth needs are more highly motivated by jobs providing experienced meaningfulness, experienced responsibility, and knowledge of results.
5. Coordination of interconnected work elements that are not contained within a single job directly affects work performance. This coordination generally can be facilitated most effectively through a combination of programming (standardization) and feedback (personal) approaches.

KEY CONCEPTS

Analyzing Work
Approaches to Job Design
Coordinating Mechanisms
Coordination among Nurses
Coordination between Physicians and Nurses
Designing Individual Jobs
Designing Work Groups to Address Coordination
  Needs
Determining Components of Work
Direct Work
Interconnectedness of Work
Job Skill and Knowledge Requirements
Management Work
Motivating Potential of Jobs
Multiskilled Employees
Psychological Approach to Work Design
Scientific Management
Standardized Approaches to Coordination
Support Work
Task Inventory Approach to Work Design
Types of Work
Uncertainty Inherent in Work
Work Requirements

Discussion Questions

1. Under what conditions does a job with a high motivating potential lead to high jobholder motivation? To high satisfaction? To frustration?
2. What are the potential pitfalls in job redesign?
3. Give examples of highly motivated people who do not contribute greatly to organizational productivity.
4. What is the relationship among individual motivation and satisfaction and an organization's ability to coordinate work?
5. Give examples of situations in which dependable role performance is required in a job but effort above minimum levels is not. What happens when individuals in such jobs innovate? Give examples of jobs requiring cooperative behavior. What happens when people in such jobs are willing to give only dependable role performance?
6. Under what conditions are standardized approaches to coordination constraints to effective performance? Under what conditions are they facilitating? When are personal approaches to coordination inappropriate?

REFERENCES

1. Taylor FW. *The Principles of Scientific Management.* New York, NY: Harper & Row; 1911.
2. Gilbreth FB. *Motion Study.* New York, NY: Van Nostrand; 1911.
3. *The Utilization of Man Power in Ambulatory Care: Development of a Study Methodology.* Bureau of Health Manpower Education, 1975. Report of a Cooperative Study.
4. Nelson E, Jacobs A, Breer D. A study of the validity of the task inventory method of job analysis. *Medical Care.* 1975;13(2):104–113.
5. Braun JA, Howard DR, Pond LR. The physician's associate: A task analysis. *Physician's Associate.* 1972;2(3):77–82.
6. Kane R, Jacoby I. Alterations in tasks in the physicians office as a result of adding a Medex. Presented at American Public Health Associates Meeting, November, 1973; San Francisco, Ca.
7. Gilpatrick E. *The Health Services Mobility Study.* Springfield, Va; 1977; National Technical Information Service.
8. Hedrick HL. Closing in on cross-training. *Journal of Allied Health.* August 1987:265–275.
9. Beachey II W. Multi-competent health professionals: Needs, combinations, and curriculum development. *Journal of Allied Health.* November 1988:319–329.
10. Russell DD, Richardson RF, Escamilla B. Multi-competency education in radiologic education. *Journal of Allied Health.* Spring 1989:281–289.
11. Blayney KD, Wilson BR, Bamberg R, Vaughn D. The multiskilled health practitioner movement: Where are we and how did we get here? *Journal of Allied Health.* Winter 1989:215–226.
12. Strengthening hospital nursing: A program to improve patient care—gaining momentum: A progress report. St. Petersburg, Fla; 1992; National Program Office of the Strengthening Hospital Nursing Program.
13. Tonges MC. Redesigning hospital nursing practice: The professionally advanced care team (ProACT) model, Part 1. *Journal of Nursing Administration.* 1989;19(7):31–38.
14. Donnelly L. NME's caregiver system: 21st century patient care delivery. *Healthcare Executive.* March/April 1989;4(2):25–27.
15. Brider P. The move to patient-focused care. *American Journal of Nursing.* 1992;9:26–33.
16. Drucker PF. *Management: Tasks Responsibilities Practices.* New York, NY: Harper & Row; 1973.
17. Charns MP, Schaefer MJ. *Health Care Organizations: A Model for Management.* Englewood Cliffs, NJ: Prentice-Hall; 1983.
18. Ibid.
19. Stoelwinder JU, Charns MP. A task field model of organization design and analysis. *Human Relations.* 1981;34(9):743–762.
20. Charns, Schaefer, op. cit.
21. Simon HA. *Administrative Behavior.* 3rd ed. New York, NY: Free Press; 1976.
22. Charns, Schaefer, op. cit.
23. Miller EJ. Technology, territory and time: The internal differentiation of complex production systems. *Human Relations.* 1959;12(3):243–272.
24. Charns, Schaefer, op. cit.
25. Galbraith JR. *Organization Design.* Reading, Mass: Addison-Wesley; 1977.
26. Van de Ven AH, Delhecq AL, Koenig Jr R. Determinants of coordination modes within organizations. *American Sociological Review.* 1976;41:322–338.
27. Charns, Schaefer, op. cit.
28. Thompson JD. *Organizations in Action.* New York, NY: McGraw-Hill; 1967.
29. McClelland DC. *The Achievement Motive.* 2nd ed. New York, NY: Halsted Press; 1975.
30. Vroom VH. *Work and Motivation.* New York, NY: John Wiley & Sons; 1961.
31. Porter LW, Lawler III EE. *Managerial Attitudes and Performance.* Homewood, Ill: Irwin-Dolsey; 1968.
32. Hackman JR, Janson R, Oldham GR, Purdy K. A new strategy for job enrichment. *California Management Review.* 1975;17(4):57–71.
33. Galbraith, op. cit.
34. Kotch JB, Burr C, Toal S, Brown W, Abrantes A, Kaluzny A. A performance-based management system to reduce prematurity and low birth weight. *Journal of Medical Systems.* 1986;10(4):375–390.
35. Hackman, et al., op. cit.
36. Thompson, op. cit.
37. Charns, Schaefer, op. cit.
38. Duncan RB. Multiple decision-making structures in adapting to environmental uncertainty: The impact on organizational effectiveness. *Human Relations.* 1973;26(3):273–291.
39. March JG, Simon HA. *Organizations.* New York, NY: John Wiley & Sons; 1958.
40. Van de Ven, et al., op. cit.
41. Knaus WA, Draper EA, Wagner DP, Zimmerman JE. An evaluation of outcome from intensive care in major medical centers. *Annals of Internal Medicine.* 1986;104:416–418.
42. Shortell SM, Rousseau DM, Gillies RR, Devers KJ, Simons TL. Organizational assessment in intensive care units (ICUs): Construct development, reliability, and validity of the ICU nurse-physician questionnaire. *Medical Care.* 1991;29(8):709–727.
43. Charns, Schaefer, op. cit.

44. Charns MP, Stoelwinder JU, Miller RA, Schaefer MJ. Coordination and patient unit effectiveness. Presented at the Academy of Management Annual Meetings; August 1981; San Diego, Ca.

45. Mintzberg H. *The Structuring of Organizations.* Englewood Cliffs, NJ: Prentice-Hall; 1979.

46. Charns MP, Strayer RG. A socio-structural approach to organization development. Presented at the Academy of Management Annual Meetings; August 1981; San Diego, Ca.

47. Charns, Stoelwinder, et al., op. cit.

48. Charns MP, Tewksbury LS. *Collaborative Management in Health Care: Implementing the Integrative Organization.* San Francisco, Ca: Jossey-Bass, 1993.

CHAPTER

COORDINATION AND COMMUNICATION

Beaufort B. Longest, Jr., Ph.D.
Professor

James M. Klingensmith, Sc.D.
Assistant Professor

CHAPTER TOPICS

Interdependence
Coordination
Communication

LEARNING OBJECTIVES

After completing this chapter, the reader should be able to

1. differentiate between pooled, sequential, and reciprocal interdependence
2. differentiate between intraorganizational coordination and interorganizational coordination
3. discuss a variety of coordination mechanisms used in intraorganizational settings
4. consider the application of the intraorganizational coordinating mechanisms to a given situation using the contingency approach
5. discuss the three major types of transactions used in interorganizational coordination
6. discuss the management of interorganizational linkages
7. describe the elements of effective communication
8. discuss the technical mechanism of communication
9. discuss the barriers to communication
10. describe the flow of intraorganizational communication
11. describe the flow of interorganizational communication
12. discuss the special case of communication between units of a system

CHAPTER PURPOSE

Coordination and *communication* are two closely related strategies through which managers link together the various people and units within their organizations and link their organizations to other organizations and agencies. Because health care organizations have become increasingly complex internally and have established a wide variety of external relationships, the establishment and maintenance of effective linkages is a significant managerial challenge. If linkages are not effective, organizations may become fragmented, fractioned, and isolated with concomitant declines in performance.

Central to understanding the critical importance of communication and coordination strategies is an appreciation of the high level of interdependence exhibited by health care organizations. This interdependence exists in both their internal structure and external relationships.

The purpose of this chapter is to explore the managerial challenges associated with coordination and communication and to examine effective strategies for meeting these challenges. This is done in the context of the high level of interdependence generally found within health care organizations and between them and their external stakeholders.

IN THE REAL WORLD

THE SEARCH FOR A NEW PRESIDENT

The chairperson of the ad hoc search committee called the meeting to order at 7:30 P.M. She noted that the purpose of the meeting was to establish the criteria the committee would use in selecting a new president for Memorial Hospital. The committee, comprised of members of the governing board and two members of the medical staff, had been appointed upon the announcement by the present chief executive officer (CEO) that he had accepted another position.

Memorial Hospital is a prestigious teaching hospital located in a large eastern city. The 600-bed institution is nationally prominent in cardiac services and is the primary teaching hospital for the medical school located in the same city, although it is organizationally separate from the medical school. Memorial is considered by most members of the health care industry in its region to be the most influential trendsetter in the city. However, another large general hospital nearby has enjoyed very favorable response to its recent efforts to build a vertically-integrated system in the region.

One of the more aggressive members of the committee spoke first. "It is not all clear to me what kind of person we ought to seek to be our next president. Obviously, we need someone who can manage this organization. Some things are a mess internally. But I am even more concerned that we appear to be isolated from the rest of the health care system, especially in comparison to our main competitor."

After considerable discussion, it became clear that this latter concern was shared by all members of the committee. One member, an attorney, expressed his view that health care services would increasingly be provided through vertically-integrated systems of care. Most members nodded their concurrence.

Another member, while concerned about the isolation problem, pointed out how important she thought it was to find a president who could manage the day-to-day operations of a major teaching hospital with all the complexities that entailed. "I'm not at all certain that any one person can effectively manage the internal affairs of this hospital and its relationship to the rest of the world. Maybe we need two people for this position."

Sensing that this dichotomy was going to be troublesome for the committee, but recognizing

that Memorial Hospital could only have one president, the chairperson asked the members of the committee to begin thinking about the skills and attributes they thought the next president should possess. After a reflective pause, a member spoke. "Clearly, the person we select will have to be able to link together in an effective way all the various people and units that make up Memorial Hospital and, at the same time, link our hospital to other external organizations and stakeholders."

The chairperson turned to the chalkboard in the conference room and, condensing what had been said, wrote:

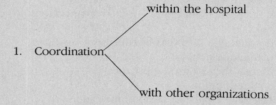

SKILLS NEEDED BY THE NEXT PRESIDENT

within the hospital

1. Coordination

with other organizations

The meeting went on for another hour. During that time, 15 skills were listed, but coordination remained at the top of the list. The committee adjourned, satisfied that they knew what kind of person the next president should be.

INTERDEPENDENCE

Interdependence among the individuals and units within an organization or among organizations, while extant in all organizations, varies with the structural complexity and goals of organizations. Thompson, for example, has identified three forms of interdependence: pooled, sequential, and reciprocal.[1]

Pooled interdependence occurs when individuals and units are related but do not bear a close connection; they simply contribute separately in some way to the larger whole. For example, a group of geographically dispersed nursing homes owned by a single corporation may be viewed as linked largely in the sense that each contributes to the overall success of the cor-

poration, but they have very little direct interdependence. Their activities are pooled to make the corporation more effective.

Sequential interdependence occurs when individuals and units bear a close but sequential connection. For example, a patient admitted to an acute care hospital becomes the focal point for an extended chain of sequentially interdependent activities. The admitting office checks him in, schedules him in the operating room, notifies the dietary department of special needs, notifies the laboratory of the need for tests, and so on. Most of what is done for the patient until he is discharged occurs in a sequential manner.

Reciprocal interdependence occurs when individuals and units bear a close relationship and the interdependence goes in both directions. For example, a vertically-integrated health care system with acute care and long-term care capacity exhibits reciprocal interdependence. The long-term care beds are occupied by patients referred from the acute care beds; the acute care unit depends upon the long-term care unit as a place to which to discharge certain patients. The acute care unit suffers if the long-term care unit cannot accept a patient. Conversely, the long-term care unit suffers if patients are not discharged to it from the acute unit. Further, the long-term care unit may need to transfer patients back to the hospital when acute episodes of illness occur. The interdependence between these units is reciprocal.

Bolman and Deal have pointed out that the level of interdependence intensifies as its form moves from pooled to sequential to reciprocal.[2] The higher the level of interdependence, the greater the need for managerial attention to effective linkages. Health care organizations generally exhibit very high levels of interdependence among their component parts, usually of the sequential or reciprocal forms. Thus, the need for effective coordination and communication is usually very great in these organizations. Charns and Schaefer note that "in health care organizations, coordination among different groups of providers and between providers and support services encompass critical interconnections in the delivery of care. How well these are addressed contributes directly to organizational performance."[3] Similarly, the importance of effective communication has been noted by Rakich et al. in that, if "communication is adequate, the work gets done more effectively and problems are solved more efficiently. In any organized effort, communication is essential for people to work together because it permits them to influence and react to one another."[4] Clearly, in highly interdependent health care organizations, coordination and communication are critical tasks for managers. These tasks are examined in depth below.

COORDINATION

Coordination, as a means of effectively linking together the various parts of an organization or of linking together organizations and dealing with interdependence, is one of the most important functions of management. Kraut et al. found that "coordinating interde-

pendent groups" was rated highly important by middle managers and executives and increased in importance as one moved into higher management positions.[5] Conceptually and historically coordination has been defined as the conscious activity of assembling and synchronizing differentiated work efforts so that they function harmoniously in attainment of organization objectives.[6] Some authors use the term "integration" for this concept. Lawrence and Lorsch define integration as "the process of achieving unity of effort among the various subsystems in the accomplishment of the organization's tasks."[7] Obviously, the two terms have similar meaning.

The classical definition provided above pertains to coordination within an organization, an *intraorganizational* perspective. Increasingly important today, with the elaboration of a wide variety of multiorganizational arrangements, is the issue of coordination among and between organizations, an *interorganizational* perspective (also see Chapter 11). While much of what is known about intraorganizational coordination applies to interorganizational coordination, there are basic differences and these will be examined below. It is important here, however, to extend the definition of coordination to encompass both inter- and intraorganizational situations. Thus, coordination is conscious activity aimed at achieving unity and harmony of effort in pursuit of shared objectives within an organization or among a set of organizations participating in a multiorganizational arrangement of some kind.

Intraorganizational Coordination

The mechanisms of coordination—the activities managers use to achieve coordination—are diverse and achieve different levels of success depending upon characteristics of specific situations. This contingency view of coordination is very important for the reader to keep in mind; clearly, no single coordinating mechanism is best for all situations. A contingency approach to intraorganizational coordination requires that managers match the most appropriate coordinating mechanism to a given situation, recognizing that often a combination of coordinating mechanisms will be needed.

In addition to the impact that the level of interdependence has on the need for coordination, as previously discussed, two other factors require special consideration in selecting coordination mechanisms within health care organizations. They are the distinctive structural arrangements that have evolved for health professionals and the unique manner in which differentiated units and activities must combine within health care organizations if effective performance is to be achieved.

A contingency approach to coordination in health care organizations is necessary, in large measure, because of the predominance of professionals within these organizations. Scott points out that, because the activities of health professionals are seen as being complex, uncertain, and of great social importance, three distinctive structural arrangements have evolved to support the autonomy of these professions.[8] The *autonomous arrangement* is present when an organization delegates to a professional group goal setting, implementation, and evaluation of performance, and the administration manages the support staff. Historically hospitals have had such arrangements with their medical staffs. The *heteronomous arrangement* occurs when professionals are subordinated to the administrative structure with specific responsibilities delegated to various professional groups. Nursing and social service, for instance, traditionally have had such a relationship with hospitals. A third relationship, the *conjoint arrangement*, occurs when the professionals and administration are equal in power. This arrangement is growing in importance as hospitals and physicians recognize the need to further integrate their activities in response to environmental forces. Clearly, the type of structural arrangement affects the coordinating mechanisms employed.

In the same way that there are diverse mechanisms for coordination available to the manager, there are different levels of need for coordination within organizations. The activities required for organizational performance are separated through vertical and horizontal differentiation. Differentiation, in this context, is defined as "the state of segmentation of the organizational system into subsystems, each of which tends to develop particular attributes in relation to the requirements posed by its relevant environment."[9] Vertical differentiation establishes the hierarchy and number of levels in the organization.[10] Horizontal differentiation is used to separate activities so that they may be performed more effectively and efficiently. This usually results in

formation of departments within the organization. For instance, in a hospital horizontal differentiation accounts for radiology, pharmacy, and pathology. Vertical differentiation accounts for a CEO, a second managerial level composed of vice presidents, and a third level composed of department heads.

Once the organization's activities have been differentiated, they must be coordinated. In some organizations, it is possible to separate activities in such a way as to minimize the degree of coordination needed. In other organizations, particularly those functionally departmentalized such as most health care organizations, a high degree of coordination is essential. It is necessary to recognize the interaction between the need to specialize activities and requirements for coordination. The greater the differentiation of activities and specialization of labor, the greater will be the need for coordination. This culminates most distinctively where the patient is the focal point, such as on a patient care unit.

Intraorganizational Mechanisms of Coordination

Organizations typically establish several mechanisms to achieve intraorganizational coordination including through the hierarchy, the administrative system, and voluntary activities.[11] In *hierarchical coordination* the various activities are linked by placing them under a central authority. In a simple organization, this form of coordination might be sufficient. However, in complex health care organizations that have many levels and many specialized departments, hierarchical coordination becomes more difficult. Although the CEO is a focal point of authority, it would be impossible for one person to cope with all the coordinating problems that might arise in the hierarchy. Therefore, coordination through the hierarchical structure must be supplemented.

The *administrative system*, emphasizing formal procedures, provides a second mechanism for coordinating activities.[12] Many work procedures, such as memoranda with routing slips, help coordinate efforts of different operating units. To the extent that these procedures can be programmed or routinized, it is not necessary to establish specific means for coordination.

For nonroutine and nonprogrammable events, administrative mechanisms such as committees may be required to provide integration.

A third type of coordination is through *voluntary action* in which individuals or groups see a need for coordination, develop a method, and implement it.[13] Much of the coordination may depend upon the willingness and ability of individuals or groups to voluntarily find ways to integrate their activities with other organizational participants.

Achieving voluntary coordination is one of the most important yet difficult problems for the manager. Voluntary coordination requires that individuals have suf-

ficient knowledge of organizational objectives, adequate information concerning specific problems of coordination, and the motivation to do something. Fortunately, in health care organizations, voluntary coordination is often facilitated by the high degree of professionalism extant in many participants. One of the primary forces ensuring voluntary coordination is the overall value system supportive of the patient's welfare, which is developed through the training and professionalization of many participants in health care organizations.

Mintzberg identifies the following five coordinating mechanisms which are also illustrated in Figure 8.1.[14]

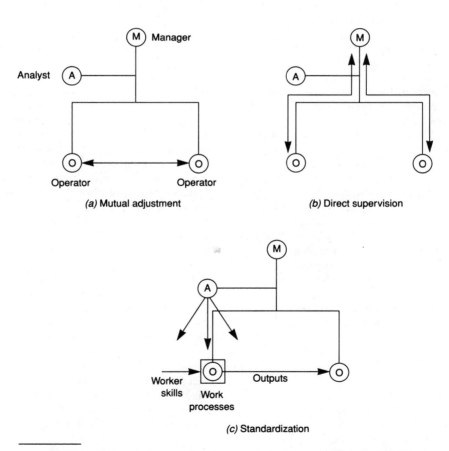

FIGURE 8.1. Mintzberg's five coordinating mechanisms. SOURCE: Mintzberg H. *Structure in Fives: Designing Effective Organizations.* Englewood Cliffs, NJ: Prentice-Hall; 1983:5. Reprinted by permission.

- *Mutual adjustment* provides coordination by informal communications among those whose work must be coordinated. Like the voluntary actions noted above, work is coordinated by those performing it.
- *Direct supervision,* similar to hierarchical coordination, is a way of coordinating work that occurs when someone takes responsibility for the work of others, including issuing instructions and monitoring actions.
- *Standardization of work processes* is an alternative coordinating mechanism that programs or specifies the contents of work. Health care organizations standardize work processes when possible, such as standard admission and discharge procedures or standard methods of performing laboratory tests.
- *Standardization of outputs* specifies the product or expected performance, with the process of how to perform the work left to the worker.
- *Standardization of worker skills* occurs when neither work processes nor output can be standardized. If standardization is to occur in such situations, it must be through worker training. This form is often found in health care organizations where the complexity of much of the work does not allow standardization of work processes or outputs. In such situations, standardization of worker skills and knowledge is an excellent coordinating mechanism. "When an anesthesiologist and a surgeon meet in the operating room to remove an appendix, they need hardly communicate; by virtue of their respective training, they know exactly what to expect of each other. Their standardized skills take care of most of the coordination."[15]

Hage offers a third perspective by describing four kinds of coordination mechanisms for health care organizations: programming, planning, customs, and feedback.[16,17] In general, this framework builds on the early work of others and, with the exception of customs, is similar to those of Van de Ven et al.[18–21]

In *programming* organizations develop explicit rules and prescriptions, called programs, that define the job of each person in the organization and the sequence of activities for all jobs within a department and, beyond that, for the organization as a whole. With programs, everyone can learn his job and execute it. The purpose of programming is to reduce the need for communication except for questions about interpretation of a particular rule. The programming of an organization is accomplished with rules, manuals, job descriptions, personnel procedures, promotion policies, and so on. This category is quite similar to use of the adminsitrative system described above and to Mintzberg's standardization of work, process, and skills. Health care organizations often rely heavily on programming as a means of coordination.

Planning differs from programming in that a plan is usually a set of objectives that the organization hopes to achieve and the means by which it expects to achieve them. Planning and programming can, of course, be combined. Plans are the objectives and means for achieving them, whereas programs are the concrete specification of the means used to achieve the objectives. The usefulness of planning as an intraorganizational coordination mechanism can be seen in the need to think of planning in one unit of a health care organization as part of a larger whole.[22] For example, the expansion plans of a health maintenance organization (HMO) must take into account the unit responsible for physician recruitment and retention. No subunit plan should be made that does not contribute to the objectives set out in the plans of the organization. It is the responsibility of top level management in the organization to ensure that all managers understand the objectives of the organization. It is the joint duty of all managers to determine whether their plans are compatible with all other plans in the organization. To the extent this is done, coordination will be facilitated.

Many managers rely heavily upon the *customs* developed in their organizations as coordination mechanisms. For example, it may be customary in a particular nursing home to use the holiday season as an occasion to invite the families of residents into the facility for a meal and social interaction. Knowing this custom permits the various departments to begin their preparations for this event well in advance and facilitates the coordination of their various contributions to its success. While programming is a rational attempt to spell out specific norms of human behavior in organizations, customs are norms developed over time that specify behavior of different participants in an organization's social system. In this sense, customs may be more rational than programming rules because customs, based on a history of trial and error, represent a distillation of good practice, whereas programming can result from a manager's ideal sense rather than lessons learned from reality. Customs can be an important coordinating mechanism; but in complex health care organizations they are not, in and of themselves, sufficient to meet the coordination challenge.

Feedback can indicate when the organization is not functioning well or when problems of conflict or inefficiency arise. Not all forms of communication represent feedback, but some, such as routine operating reports that serve to provide needed interunit information, represent attempts on the part of the organization to coordinate through feedback.

Another approach to coordinating activities is through *committees*. Often committees are made up of members from a number of departments or functional areas and are concerned with problems requiring coordination. Using committees for purposes of coordination is a well-established approach in health care organizations. Of course, committees serve other purposes besides coordination; they may act in a service, advisory, informational, or decision-making capacity.

In contrast to committees, the coordinating mechanism may be a single person. For example, Lawrence and Lorsch found that well-coordinated organizations often rely upon individuals, whom they term *integrators,* to achieve coordination.[23] Successfully playing an integrator role depends more on having professional competence than occupying a particular formal position. People are successful integrators because of specialized knowledge and because they represent a central source of information. Examples of effective integrators are found among all health professionals. In most health care organizations, individual nurses—regardless of formal position—often function as integrators linking physicians to the organization's formal administrative structure. These integrators often provide significant coordination among various departments and subunits, particularly as they relate to patient care. The integrator role is also played by people chosen to be project, program, or product line managers in matrix structures.

Coordination may be especially difficult in managing large scale projects that require skills of people in different departments or that incorporate multidisciplinary approaches to patient care. For example, the decision by a health care organization to organize services into a comprehensive home health care program for the chronically ill would benefit from a team organized around the focus of the program—home services for the chronically ill. Team members would be drawn from nursing, social services, respiratory therapy, occupational therapy, pharmacy, and physicians specializing in chronic disease. To market the program and to handle finance and reimbursement issues expertise would be provided by team members drawn from the organization's administration. A project manager would be named. *Project management* is a structural means for coordinating a large amount of talent and resources for a given period on a specific project.[24] The project team of various specialists is assembled under the direction of the project manager who is responsible for coordinating their efforts. In this situation, project organization permits flexibility and facilitates coordination.

Health care organizations can easily use the project organization design by superimposing it on the existing functional departmental design. This can be done in a few areas, such as the home care program noted earlier, or for the whole organization. As discussed in Chapter 10, when the entire organization is structured in this way, it is called a *matrix design*. The reader may wish to refer to Figure 10.6 which is a matrix design for a psychiatric hospital in which functional managers head departments and program or product line managers head major clinical programs or product lines. Notice that the individual worker depicted is a member of nursing *and* the Alzheimer program. This coordination mechanism can be very important as health care organizations continue to move toward a product line management orientation.

Other structural forms have been recommended to help with problems of coordination. One mechanism for achieving integration is to have people serve as *linking pins* between various units in the organization.[25] Horizontally, there are certain organizational participants who are members of two separate groups and serve as coordinating agents between them. On the vertical axis, individuals serve as linking pins between their level and those above and below. Through this system of linking pins, a multiple overlapping group structure in the organization is formed, and the coordination necessary to make the dynamic system operate effectively is achieved. Likert notes:

> To perform the intended coordination well, a fundamental requirement must be met. The entire organization must consist of a multiple, overlapping group structure with every work group using group decision-making processes skillfully. This requirement applies to the functional, product, and service departments. An organization meeting this requirement will have an effective interaction-influence system through which the relevant communications flow readily, the required influence is exerted laterally, upward, and downward, and the motivational forces needed for coordination are created.[26]

Other coordination mechanisms such as quality circles and cross-functional quality improvement teams also exist. They rely on nominal group process, multicriteria decision making, cause and effect diagrams, and related problem-identification and problem-solving tools to improve communication, coordination, and ultimately the quality of work.

Interorganizational Coordination

Interdependence is not limited to situations *within* organizations. Increasingly, health care organizations experience interdependencies with other health care organizations, as in systems or other multiorganiza-tional arrangements, or with other elements in their external environments such as various levels of government, suppliers, third party payors, and so on. These interdependencies may be pooled (a group of nursing homes under a single ownership), sequential (provider organization and fiscal intermediary), or reciprocal (vertically-integrated health care system). Whatever the form of interdependence, it requires management. That is, the focal organization must coordinate and communicate with other organizations or agencies with which it is interdependent if these relationships are to be effectively managed.

While their choices arise from the circumstances of a particular situation, managers typically have a number of strategies for managing their interorganizational interdependencies. These range from straightforward buying and selling of goods and services between organizations to the buying and selling of organizations themselves. In between are a number of more subtle strategies for managing interorganizational interdependencies. For example, Thompson developed a categorization of interorganizational linkages including contracting, coopting, and coalescing.[27] Pointer, Begun, and Luke have applied the concept of the quasifirm to the health care sector.[28] Zuckerman and Kaluzny have examined interorganizational linkages from the construct of strategic alliances.[29] Longest incorporates many of these categorizations into a typology of three general classes as summarized below.[30]

DEBATE TIME 8.1: WHAT DO YOU THINK?

As we have seen, there are a number of intraorganizational coordination mechanisms including: administrative system, committees, cross-functional teams, customs, feedback, hierarchy, integrators, linking pins, matrix organization, planning, programming, project management through task forces or teams, quality circles, or voluntary action. Utilizing a contingency approach, managers in health care organizations use various combinations of these mechanisms to achieve coordination; usually a number of them are used concurrently. Depending upon situations, various packages of these mechanisms might be appropriate.

Assume that you are the president of a large teaching hospital and that you are concerned about how the responsibilities, roles, and performance of the departments in the hospital are coordinated. Choose the five coordination mechanisms that have been discussed thus far that you would emphasize in ensuring good coordination among the departments in your hospital.

Now, assume that you are the vice president for nursing services in the same hospital and that you have become concerned about the level of coordination *within* nursing services. Again, choose the five coordination mechanisms that have been discussed thus far that you would emphasize in ensuring good coordination within nursing services.

Market Transactions

Market transactions involve the focal organization and other organizations entering into relationships in order to obtain operational resources or product markets. This is perhaps the simplest form of linkage between organizations. It may entail nothing more than establishing an acceptable contract to purchase some needed supply or service or to provide defined services to a defined population as in an agreement with an HMO. At the more complex level, contracts permit a health care organization to establish stable and predictable (albeit interdependent) relationships with the federal government for reimbursement for Medicare patients, state governments for reimbursement for Medicaid patients, and with commercial insurers for their subscribers. Contracts are, in essence, formal agreements, usually negotiated, which define parameters of exchanges between two or more parties. Thus, they are widely used as a mechanism of coordination in a great variety of interorganizational relationships. Negotiation ability as discussed in Chapter 5 is the most important managerial skill for market transactions.

Voluntary Interorganizational Relationship Transactions

A second category of interorganizational linkages is distinguished by the voluntary dimension of the transactions. Horizontal and vertical systems, joint ventures, partnerships, various affiliations, consortia, and confederations are examples of voluntary interorganizational relationships. They can be further categorized as follows.

Coopting involves the absorption of leadership elements from other organizations into the focal organizations. In the healthcare industry, this coordination mechanism often takes one of two forms: management contracts and the placing of representatives of interdependent organizations on the focal organization's governing body.

Management contracts, labeled by Starkweather as an example of coopting, permit one organization to supply day-to-day management to another by agreement.[31] Management includes at least the CEO, who reports to the governing body of the managed organization and to the managing organization. This

is in contrast to the practice prevalent in many health care organizations of using outside contractors to manage individual departments and programs such as housekeeping, food service, or respiratory therapy.

A second coopting mechanism is the appointment of significant representatives from external organizations to positions in the focal organization, usually the governing body. For example, a hospital system interested in access to capital may find considerable advantage in placing a banker on its governing body. Similarly, an HMO may find it advantageous to place members of its medical group on its board.

Coalescing includes such forms as joint ventures, partnerships, consortia, and federations. It occurs when two or more organizations *partially* pool resources to pursue defined goals. This is often referred to as "loose coupling" and is characterized by interorganizational relationships in which interdependent and mutually responsive organizations are linked while preserving their legal identities and autonomies and most of their functional autonomies.[32] Such linkages are stronger than those in market transactions but less binding and less extensive than in ownership.

Joint ventures, increasingly common among health care organizations, "can be predicted by considerations of resource interdependence, competitive uncertainty, and conditions that make various forms of interdependence more or less problematic."[33] Shortell et al. have described primary care group practices sponsored jointly by hospitals and physicians as one form of joint venture activity.[34] Major health care networks, such as the Voluntary Hospitals of America and the American Health Care System, explore joint venture relationships with health insurance providers to develope a range of new alternative delivery system products.

A particularly prevalent form of loosely coupled or coalesced structure in the health care industry is represented by trade associations. For example, the American Hospital Association has over 5,000 member organizations and has developed a sophisticated political or lobbying activity on behalf of its member hospitals. Similarly, there are regional and state hospital associations that base affiliation on a geographical or state community of interests. As states have become increasingly involved in regulation of the health care sector and in its reform, state hospital associations have increasingly undertaken important lobbying efforts. Associations also serve other functions which help member organizations deal with their interdependencies; centralized information, research, and product definition are examples.

The *quasifirm,* defined as "a loosely coupled, enduring set of interorganizational relationships that are designed to achieve purposes of substantial importance to the viability of participating members," lies between market transactions and ownership arrangements.[35] Quasifirms are similar to a true firm in relation to shared goals, mutual dependency, task subdivision and specialization, bureaucratic structures, and formal coordinating and control mechanisms. However, they are critically distinguished by their absence of ownership linkages.

An example of a quasifirm configuration would be the collaboration of an acute care general hospital, a large multispecialty group practice, a skilled nursing facility, and an insurance carrier for the purpose of designing, producing, and marketing a managed care product. This arrangement may be strategically important to the survival of the participants, but allows each to independently pursue other objectives.[36]

Ownership is another category of interorganizational relationships. Critical to this category is the voluntary nature of the ownership transaction. Although hostile acquisitions and takeovers are possible and foreseeable in the future for the health care sector, most ownership transactions to date have been voluntary. An example may be the joint creation and ownership by multiple organizations of a new organizational entity which has a designated purpose. An organization may also choose to voluntarily merge with, acquire, or be acquired by another organization with which it is interdependent.

One form of ownership transaction is to create a new organization, sometimes called an umbrella organization, to span but not to replace those organizations forming it. Starkweather describes two important subtypes of the umbrella corporation in regard to hospitals.[37] One subtype gives the umbrella corporation limited authority within which its decisions are final. In the other, the umbrella corporation has more general authority that is usually exercised through unified management, policy, and fiscal control.

An extreme organizational response to interdependence is to absorb or consume it, as in a merger or consolidation. Consolidation is a formal combination of two or more organizations into a single new legal entity that has an identity separate from any of the pre-existing institutions. Merger is a formal combination of two or more institutions into a single new legal entity that has the identity of one of the pre-existing organizations. Both forms of consumption, as interorganizational coordinating mechanisms, involve an essential restructuring of organizational interdependence. The restructuring can be in the form of vertical integration (a nursing home merges with a hospital in which the hospital gains the ability to discharge patients to a less intensive level of care and the nursing home gains a source of referrals); horizontal expansion (two hospitals merge with a resulting larger capacity); or diversification (a hospital absorbs a retail pharmacy chain, gaining a new source of revenue).

Involuntary Interorganizational Transactions

Market transactions and voluntary interorganizational transactions are not sufficient to manage all organizational interdependencies found in the health care sector. Examples include relationships with regulatory agencies, fiscal intermediaries, and utilization management companies. Regulated organizations have an interdependent relationship with the organizations that regulate them. Such interdependence cannot be legally managed through market transactions, which by definition involve economic exchanges. Furthermore, the nature of the interdependent relationship between a regulated health care organization and its regulator means that the relationship is not subject to the voluntary types of interorganizational transactions described above.

These involuntary relationships lead to unique ways of managing interdependence. Many ingenious strategies have evolved.[38] Several of the most common ones are presented below. It should be noted that these strategies are specific to an individual organization's interactions with regulatory bodies, but they can be modified for use in other involuntary interorganizational transactions. Perhaps the most common approach—at least it is always available to organizations in dealing with their regulators—is litigation. Most regulatory decisions can be appealed in the courts which are sensitive to procedural errors or infringement of due process rights. Regulators who overlook requirements for notice, public hearings, or the opportunity for full consideration of issues invite litigation.

While distasteful to many, another strategy organizations use to deal with their regulators involves cultivating supportive relationships with the executive and legislative branches and with state and federal regulatory agencies. Such political intervention strategies can afford effective protection against overly enthusiastic or even dutiful regulators. It is no accident that hospitals routinely place prominent public officials and politically connected private citizens on their governing bodies, that physicians are among the most generous political campaign contributors, or that well-connected consultants flourish in and around Washington, D.C., and state capitals.

Other strategies, unethical or illegal though they may be, are sometimes used by regulated organizations to attempt to manage relationships with their regulators. For example, one advantage regulated organizations often have over their regulators is their technical expertise and the ability to assemble and manipulate large volumes of data. When challenged, regulated organizations may flood their regulators with technical data seeking to justify their position or simply obscure the issues as part of a data overload strategy intended to foster ambiguity. Although it is clearly illegal and unethical, outright deception is possible in relationships between organizations and their regulatory stakeholders. The cost and scope of projects can be understated; pertinent data can be fabricated or falsified; projects or protocols can be altered after approval. The complexity of projects, long lead times, turnover of regulatory staff, and the difficulty government agencies have in coordinating their programs can prevent close scrutiny of regulated organizations and encourage cheating.

Managing Interorganizational Linkages

As with intraorganizational coordination, it is important for a manager to use a contingency approach

MANAGERIAL GUIDELINES

1. Within health care organizations, managers must be aware of the relationship between functional specialization and the need for coordination. Whereas the establishment of additional organizational units may improve the coordination *within* such units, the added units may make it more difficult to coordinate activities *among* all units within the organization or within a multi-organizational system.

2. Managers should recognize the need for developing overlapping forms of coordination within their organizations, including
   a. structural relationships such as committees, project management teams, and quality circles
   b. administrative systems such as planning, programming, and feedback processes
   c. organizational culture or customs

3. In relationships with other interdependent organizations, health care managers should choose from a variety of interorganizational mechanisms for coordination. In making their selection, managers should carefully consider the relative benefits and costs inherent in available mechanisms.

when establishing and maintaining relationships with interdependent organizations. The manager must do this both in terms of selecting the interdependent organizations with which linkages are needed and determining the most appropriate linkage from those available. Chapter 11 elaborates on this process. However, it is important to note here that interorganizational coordination is not achieved without costs. The obvious ones are time, personnel, and money needed to support the various forms of linkages described above. The less obvious, but very important, costs include what Porter has termed the cost of compromise and the cost of inflexibility.[39] The cost of compromise arises when effectively coordinating across organizational boundaries requires that an activity be performed in a consistent way that may not be optimal for any of the participants in the interorganizational relationship. From the manager's perspective, the cost of compromise can be reduced if an activity is designed for sharing. For example, two merger participants may find that a new management information system designed to accommodate the needs of the new organization is better than applying that of either of the previously existing organizations or of simply linking together and "fixing" gaps in two separate management information systems.

The cost of inflexibility is not an ongoing cost of interorganizational coordination mechanisms but arises with the need for flexibility, usually in the form of potential difficulty in responding to a competitor's move or to a new market opportunity. It is simply a matter that linkages developed to manage interorganizational interdependencies involve added complexity and, often, greater inflexibility.

COMMUNICATION*

As we noted earlier, coordination and communication share the characteristic that both are important challenges for managers as they seek to establish linkages within and outside their organizations to effectively manage interdependencies. As with coordination, communication becomes more important as interdependence moves from pooled to sequential to reciprocal forms. Communication, especially in the feedback form and in programming and plans, is an important coordination mechanism itself. Yet it fulfills other functions besides coordination. When managers communicate, one of four major functions or some combination of them is served: information transmission, motivation, control, and emotive expression.[40]

Communication provides information people need to make decisions. People need information about operating activities, resources, alternatives, and the plans and activities of others in the organization if they are to make good decisions. Managers must also provide a great deal of information to external stakeholders,

especially potential customers, third-party payors, and regulators, if their organizations are to function effectively within their environments.

While motivation is a process internal to the person experiencing it (see Chapter 3), managers can effect motivation in others by informing them about rewards that will result from their performance, by giving them information that builds commitment to the organization and its objectives, and by using communication skills to help people understand and fulfill their personal needs. Managers also communicate with external stakeholders to influence them to act in ways that benefit the health care organization such as selecting the organization as a provider of medical services, offering favorable reimbursement levels for services, or establishing favorable regulatory policies. To the extent communication provides a path by which managers can influence behavior, it serves a motivation function.

Many kinds of communications control the performance of health care organizations and those who work in them; activity reports, policies to establish standard operating procedures, budgets, and face-to-face directives are examples. Such communications enhance control when they clarify duties, authorities, and responsibilities.

A final function of communication results from the fact that it is people who communicate, even though they may speak on behalf of the organization. Without exception, they have emotions and feelings such as satisfaction, happiness, sadness, anger, and the like which must often be expressed. Communication permits this necessary venting to occur among people within the organization. Emotive communication also permits the health care organization to increase acceptance of the organization and its actions both internally and with external stakeholders.

Communication, from the manager's perspective, has intraorganizational and interorganizational dimensions. Intraorganizational communication depends on formal establishment of channels and networks within the organization. Interorganizational communication occurs between organizations or between organizations and constituencies outside them. Both intra- and interorganizational communication can be defined as the creation or exchange of understanding between sender(s) and receiver(s). This definition does not restrict communication to words alone; it includes all

* Adapted with permission from Rakich JS, Longest Jr BB, Darr K. *Managing Health Services Organizations,* 3rd ed. Baltimore, Md: Health Professions Press; 1992: chap 15.

methods (verbal and nonverbal) through which meaning is conveyed to others. Even silence can convey meaning and must be considered part of communicating. A central component of this definition is "understanding." A sender will want the receiver to understand what was sent; this means the sender wants the receiver to interpret the message exactly as it is intended. Unfortunately, communication seldom results in complete understanding because there are so many environmental and personal barriers to effective communication. It is important for the manager to realize that information can be easily transmitted to others but this does not ensure that they will understand it.

Elements of Effective Communication

Shortell identified several key elements to effective communication in a model developed for physicians and hospitals to improve their communication abilities.[41] The following summarizes these and Figure 8.2 illustrates their interrelationships.

• An effective communicator must have a desire to communicate which is influenced both by one's personal values and the expectation that the communication will be received in a meaningful way.

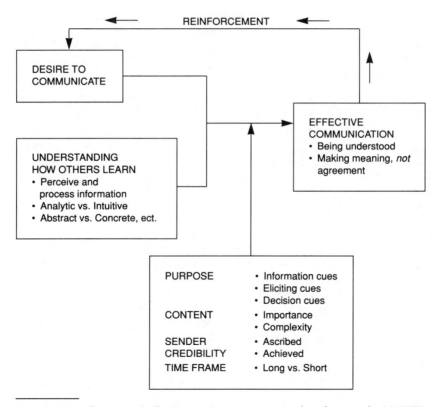

FIGURE 8.2. Elements of effective communication: A guiding framework. SOURCE: Shortell SM. *Effective Hospital-Physician Relationships.* Ann Arbor, Mich: Health Administration Press; 1991:87.

- An effective communicator must have an understanding of how others learn that includes consideration of differences in how others perceive and process information (e.g., analytic vs. intuitive, abstract vs. concrete, verbal vs. written)
- The receiver of the message should be cued as to the purpose of the message—that is, whether the message is to provide information, elicit a response or reaction, or arrive at a decision.
- The content, importance, and complexity of the message should be considered in determining the manner in which the message is communicated.
- The achieved or ascribed credibility of the sender effects how the message will be received, with "trust" (an achieved credibility) being most significant.
- The time frame associated with the content of the message (long vs. short) needs to be considered in choosing the manner in which the message is communicated. That is, more precise cues are needed with shorter time frames.

The Technical Mechanism of Communication: A Model

Figure 8.3 models the basic mechanism of communication. The reader should note the feedback loop in this model. In intraorganizational communication, where interdependencies among individuals and units are significant, the feedback loop has special importance. Similarly, interorganizational communication such as marketing or lobbying is greatly improved if receivers provide feedback to senders, who can then adjust the message if it isn't received as intended. When a sender encodes and transmits a message to a receiver who decodes the message and indicates understanding by giving feedback, effective two-way communication occurs.

In this *communication process model,* the *sender* has ideas, intentions, information, and a purpose for communicating. Senders can be individuals, departments or units of the organization, or the organization itself. The sender uses words and symbols to *encode* ideas and information. Because words have different meanings for people, care must be taken to communicate in words that are easily understood. These must

also be augmented with other symbols if communication is to be effective.

In health care organizations, many kinds of symbols have a role in communication. These symbols can be physical things, pictures, or actions. For example, different uniforms permit quick identification of people in the organization. Nurses wear white uniforms, nurse aides may wear yellow, and physicians wear long white coats. These physical symbols communicate identifying information. Pictures or visual representations are another type of symbol. They can be quite efficient and helpful in communicating and increase understanding in many situations. Consider how many words would be needed to explain a hospital's organizational structure in lieu of an organization chart. Or imagine the difficulty of communicating all the information in a PET scan using only words. Finally, action is a symbol that communicates. A smile or a pat on the back has meaning. A promotion or pay increase conveys a great deal to the recipient and to others. Furthermore, lack of action can have symbolic meaning. Davis and Newstrom note:

> Failure to act is an important way of communicating. A manager who fails to praise an employee for a job well done or fails to provide promised resources is sending a message to that person. Since we send messages both by action and inaction, we communicate almost all the time at work, regardless of our intentions.[42]

The *message* that results from the encoding process can be verbal or nonverbal. Managers seek to serve various purposes with their messages, "such as to have others understand their ideas, to understand the ideas of others, to gain acceptance of themselves or their ideas, or to produce action."[43] Messages can be for intraorganizational audiences or for interorganizational audiences.

The *channels* or methods of communication are the means by which messages are transmitted. Channels include face-to-face or telephone conversations involving individual or groups of senders or receivers, facsimile messages, letters, memos, policy statements, operating room schedules, reports, electronic message boards, video teleconferences, newspapers, television and radio commercial spots, and newsletters for internal or external distribution. The selection of channels is an important part of the communication process. Effective communication often involves using multiple

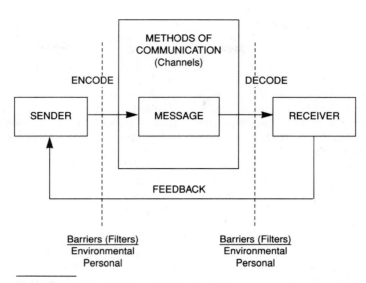

FIGURE 8.3. The basic mechanism of communication. SOURCE: Rakich JS, Longest Jr BB, Darr K. *Managing Health Services Organizations.* 3rd ed. Baltimore, Md: Health Professions Press, Inc.; 1992:562.

channels to transmit a message. For example, a major change in an organization's personnel policy such as changing the benefit package might be announced in a letter from the vice president for human resources to all employees, graphically illustrated by posters in key locations, and then reinforced in group meetings where managers explain the policy and answer questions. A decision to lobby the legislature for more generous Medicaid reimbursement might result in messages transmitted through letters to legislators, direct contact between the organization's managers and trustees and legislators, and newspaper advertisements stating the organization's position. If other organizations would benefit from the legislation, they might participate—perhaps through an association—to produce and distribute television commercials or use other channels to increase support for their position.

Messages transmitted over any channel must be *decoded* by the *receiver*. Decoding means interpreting the words and symbols in the message. Since decoding is done by the receivers of messages, it is affected by their prior experiences and frames of reference. Decoding becomes the receiver's perceptual assessment of both the content of the message *and* the sender

and the context in which the message is transmitted. The fact that messages must be decoded (interpreted) by the receiver raises the possibility that the message the sender intends is not the message the receiver gets. The closer the decoded message is to the one intended by the sender the more effective the communication. The best way to determine if messages are received as intended is through *feedback.* "Without feedback, you have a one-way communication process. Feedback makes possible a two-way process, reversing the sender and receiver roles so that information can be shared, recycled, and fine-tuned to achieve an unambiguous mutual understanding."[44]

Barriers to Communication

Another important element of the model in Figure 8.3 are the barriers to effective communication. *Environmental barriers* are characteristic of the organization and its environmental setting; *personal barriers* arise from the nature of individuals and their interaction with others. These environmental and personal barriers, typically present in any setting, can block, filter, or distort the message as it is encoded and sent, as well as when it is decoded and received.

Environmental Barriers

Two common examples are competition for attention and time. These barriers apply to intra- and interorganizational communication. Multiple and simultaneous demands on the sender may cause the message to be packaged inappropriately; such demands may also cause the message to be incorrectly decoded. In such situations the receiver may hear the message without comprehending it because it is not getting complete attention—the receiver is not really "listening." Time may be a barrier to effective communication by giving the sender little opportunity to think through and structure the message to be conveyed and by giving the receiver too little time to determine its meaning.

Other environmental barriers that can filter, distort, or block a message include the organization's managerial philosophy, multiplicity of hierarchical levels, and power or status relationships between senders and receivers. Managerial philosophy can directly inhibit as well as promote effective communication. As a rule, managers who are not interested in promoting intraorganizational communication upward or disseminating information downward will establish procedural and organizational blockages. Requiring that all communication "flow through channels," inaccessibility, lack of interest in employees' frustrations, complaints, or feelings, and insufficient time allotted to receiving information are symptoms of a philosophy that retards communication flow. Further, failing to act on complaints, ideas, and problems is a signal to those wishing to communicate upward that the effort is unlikely to have much effect and will discourage information flow.

Managerial philosophy also has a significant impact on interorganizational communications with external stakeholders. Differences in philosophy could lead two health care organizations to react differently in communicating with external stakeholders in a crisis. For example, knowledge that patients might have been exposed to a dangerous infection while hospitalized in their institutions could lead some managers to cover up the incident. Other managers would make wide use of the public media hoping that everyone who might have been exposed would come forth to be

tested. Varying reactions to similar events reflect different managerial philosophies about communicating.

Multiple levels in an organization hierarchy, and especially among organizations in a multiorganizational arrangement, tend to cause message distortion. As the message is transmitted up or down through people at many levels, it is likely that each will interpret the message according to a personal frame of reference and vantage point. When multiple links exist in the communication chain, information can be filtered, dropped, or added, and emphasis can be rearranged as it is retransmitted. As a result, a message sent through many levels is likely to be distorted or even totally blocked. For example, very often a message sent from the CEO to employees through several layers of the organization is received in quite a different form than that originally sent, or a report prepared for the CEO that passes through the hierarchy may not reach its destination because it is lying on a desk and is, in essence, blocked.

Power or status relationships can also distort or inhibit transmission of a message. A discordant superior-subordinate relationship can dampen the flow and content of information. Furthermore, an employee's past experiences may inhibit communicating because of fear of reprisal, negative sanctions, or ridicule. For example, it is not unusual to find that, as a result of poor superior-subordinate rapport, the subordinate does not inform the superior that something is wrong or that a plan will not work. Power or status communication barriers are prevalent in health care organizations where many professionals interact and status relationships create a complex situation. How often does the head nurse with 20 years of experience tell a new resident that a procedure or treatment thought to be appropriate and about to be ordered is not efficacious? How is the nurse's message encoded—bluntly or obliquely? Status and role conflicts, particularly among professionals, can be a major barrier to effective communication.

A final environmental barrier that may cause a breakdown in communication occurs when messages require the use of specific terminology unfamiliar to the receiver or when messages are especially complex. Each profession has its own jargon. Managers in a health care organization may use very different terminology than those responsible for direct care. Both may use terminology unfamiliar to external stakeholders. Communications between people who use different terminology can be ineffective simply because people attribute different meanings to the same words. When a message is both complex and contains terminology unfamiliar to the receiver, it is especially likely that misunderstanding will occur.

Personal Barriers

Another set of potential barriers—personal barriers—exists when people communicate. These barriers arise from the nature of people, especially in their interaction with others. When people encode and send messages or decode and receive them, they tend to do so according to their frames of reference or beliefs. They may also consciously or unconsciously engage in selective perception or be influenced by fear or jealousy.

The sum of socioeconomic background and previous experiences that represent an individual's frame of reference shapes how messages are encoded and decoded, or even whether communication is attempted. For example, someone whose cultural background is "don't speak unless spoken to" or "never question elders" may be inhibited in communicating. Naive people accept all communication at face value without filtering out erroneous information or bragging. By contrast, aggressiveness in disseminating self-edifying information can result in transmitting a message that is distorted for personal gain. Furthermore, unless one has had the same experiences as others, it is difficult to completely understand their message. The wealthy may have difficulty understanding the concerns of people without health insurance. Those who have never experienced pain or childbirth or witnessed death may be unable to fully understand messages about these experiences.

Closely related to one's frame of reference are beliefs, values, and prejudices. They can cause messages to be distorted or blocked in either transmission or reception. This occurs because people and their personalities and backgrounds differ; they have preconceived opinions and prejudices in areas such as politics, ethics, religion, union vs. management, sex, race, and life style. These biases, beliefs, and values filter and distort communication.

Selective perception is one of the most difficult personal barriers to overcome, both for the sender and receiver. People tend to screen derogatory information and amplify words, actions, and meanings that flatter them—there is a tendency to filter out the "bad" of a message and retain the "good." Selective perception can be conscious or unconscious. When it is conscious—often because one fears the consequences of the truth—intentional distortion results. For example, supervisors whose units have high turnover may fear the consequences of this fact if their superiors notice it. They might amplify the argument that turnover is due to low wages over which they have no control (or responsibility) or delete, alter, or minimize the importance of this information in reports to their superiors.

Sometimes jealousy, especially when coupled with selective perception, may result in conscious efforts to filter and distort incoming information, transmit misinformation, or both. For example, the manager with an extremely able assistant who routinely makes the manager look good may tend to block or distort information that would reveal the situation to superiors. Sometimes nothing more than petty personality differences, the feeling of professional incompetence or inferiority, or raw greed can lead to jealousy resulting in communication distortion.

Two other potential personal barriers to communication arise because people receiving messages have a tendency to evaluate the source (the sender) and because people often prefer to maintain the status quo. Both of these personal barriers to effective communication are common in health care organizations. Receivers often evaluate the source to decide whether to filter out or discount some of the message. However, this can lead to bias on the parts of communicators. For example, a hostile union-management atmosphere may cause employees to ignore messages from management, or managers may ignore messages from physicians with whom they frequently disagree. Source evaluation may be necessary to cope with the barrage of communication received by people in typical health care organizations, but one must recognize the hazard that legitimate messages will be misunderstood.

The status quo barrier results from a conscious effort by the sender or receiver to filter out information either in sending, receiving, or retransmitting that

MANAGERIAL GUIDELINES

1. Environmental and personal barriers are reduced if receivers and senders ensure that attention is given to their messages and feedback and that adequate time is devoted to listening to what is being communicated. Personal barriers to effective communication are reduced by conscious efforts of sender and receiver to understand each other's frame of reference, values, and beliefs.

2. A management philosophy that encourages open and free flow of communications is constructive. Reducing the number of links (levels in the hierarchy or steps between the health care organization as a sender and external stakeholders as receivers) through which messages pass reduces opportunities for distortion.

3. The power or status barrier is difficult to eliminate because it is affected by interpersonal and interprofessional relationships. However, consciously tailoring words and symbols so messages are understandable and reinforcing words with actions significantly improves communications among different power or status levels.

4. Using multiple channels to reinforce complex messages decreases the likelihood of misunderstanding.

5. Recognizing that people engage in selective perception and are prone to jealousy and fear is a first step toward eliminating or at least diminishing these barriers. Empathy with those to whom messages are directed may be the surest way to increase the likelihood that the messages will be received and understood as intended.

external stakeholders and react by transmitting messages that are explicitly designed to protect the status quo.

A final personal barrier to effective communication is a lack of empathy on the part of communicators. Having empathy means being sensitive to the frames of reference or emotional states of other people in the communication relationship. Such sensitivity promotes understanding. Empathy helps the sender decide how to encode a message for maximum understanding and helps the receiver interpret its meaning. For example, subordinates who empathize with their superiors may discount an angry message because they are aware that extreme pressure and frustration can cause such messages to be sent even when they are not warranted.

Similarly, a sender who is sensitive to the receiver's circumstance may decide how best to encode a message or that it is better left unsent. If, for example, the receiver is having a "bad day," a reprimand may be interpreted as stronger than it is. Or if a receiver has just emerged from a traumatic experience such as family illness or financial setback, the empathetic sender might decide to delay bad news until later, if possible. Managers who are concerned about a health care organization's community image might delay announcing a generous across-the-board wage increase or a large price increase just after a major local employer announces a plant closing because of a bad economy.

Flows of Intraorganizational Communications

Intraorganizational communication flows downward, upward, horizontally, and diagonally. Typically, downward flow is communication between superiors and subordinates; upward communication uses the same channels but in the opposite direction. Horizontal flow is manager to manager or worker to worker. Diagonal flow cuts across functions and levels; this violates the chain of command but is permitted if speed and efficiency of communication are particularly important.

Downward Flow

Downward communication flow primarily involves passing information from superiors to subordinates. It commonly consists of information, verbal orders, or

would upset the present situation. Internally, conditions that promote "fear of sending bad news" or a lack of candor among participants can lead to the erection of this barrier. This barrier to effective communication may also exist when communicators in an organization do not want to upset the status quo with important instructions from manager to subordinate on a one-to-one basis. It may also include speeches to groups of employees or meetings. The myriad written methods such as handbooks, procedure manuals, newsletters, bulletin boards, and the ubiquitous memorandum are also channels of downward communication. Computerized information systems contribute greatly to downward flow in many health care organizations.

Upward Flow

Objectives of *upward communication flow* include providing managers with decision-making information, revealing problem areas, providing data for performance evaluation, indicating the status of morale, and generally underscoring the thinking of subordinates. Upward flow becomes more important with increased organizational complexity and scale. Managers rely on effective upward communication and encourage it by creating a climate of trust and respect as integral parts of the organizational culture.[45]

Upward communication flow helps employees satisfy personal needs. It permits those in positions of lesser authority to express opinions and perceptions to those with higher authority; as a result they feel a greater sense of participation. The hierarchical structure (chain of command) is the main channel for upward communication in health care organizations, but this may be supplemented by grievance procedures, open door policies, counseling, employee questionnaires, exit interviews, participative decision-making techniques, and the use of ombudsmen.[46]

Horizontal and Diagonal Flows

Unhindered downward and upward communication flows are insufficient for effective organizational performance. In complex health care organizations, especially those subject to abrupt demands for action and reaction, *horizontal flow* must also occur. For example, the work of interdependent patient care units must be coordinated. The concept of an acute care hospital as a matrix organization, as described in Chapter 10, illustrates the value of horizontal communication and coordination in these organizations. Committees, task forces, and cross-functional project teams are all useful mechanisms of horizontal communication.

The least used channel of communication in health care organizations are *diagonal flows*. Diagonal flows, however, are growing in importance. For example, diagonal communication occurs when the director of a hospital pharmacy alerts a nurse in medical intensive care about a potential adverse reaction between two medications ordered for a patient. Diagonal flows violate the usual pattern of upward and downward communication flows by cutting across departments, and they violate the usual pattern of horizontal communication because the communicators are at different levels in the organization. Yet such communication is important in health care organizations. Committees, task forces, and cross-functional project teams made up of members from different levels of the organization can each serve as useful mechanisms of diagonal communication.

Communication Networks

Downward, upward, horizontal, and diagonal communication can be combined into patterns called *communication networks*. A communication network is "system of decision centers interconnected by communication channels."[47] Figure 8.4 illustrates the five common networks: chain, Y, wheel, circle, and all-channel.

The *chain network* is the standard format for communicating upward and downward and follows line authority relationships. An example is a staff nurse who reports to a head nurse, who reports to a nursing supervisor, who reports to the vice president for nursing, who reports to the health care organization's president.

The *Y pattern* (turned upside down) shows two people reporting to a superior who reports to two others. An example is two staff pharmacists who report to the pharmacy director, who reports to the vice president for professional affairs, who reports to the president.

The *wheel pattern* shows a situation where four subordinates report to one superior. There is no interaction among subordinates, and all communications are channeled through the manager at the center of the wheel. This pattern is rare in health care organizations although elements of it can be found in a situation where four vice presidents report to a president if the vice presidents have little interaction among themselves. Even though this network pattern is not used

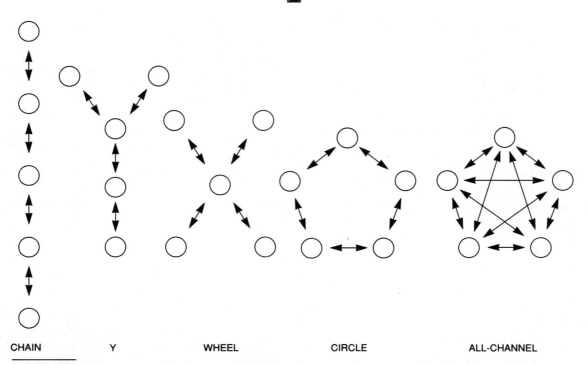

CHAIN   Y   WHEEL   CIRCLE   ALL-CHANNEL

FIGURE 8.4. Common communication networks. SOURCE: Rakich JS, Longest Jr BB, Darr K. *Managing Health Services Organizations.* 3rd ed. Baltimore, Md: Health Professions Press, Inc.; 1992:568.

routinely, it may be used in circumstances where urgency or secrecy are required. For example, the president with an emergency might communicate with vice presidents in a wheel pattern because time does not permit using other modes. Similarly, if secrecy is important, such as during an investigation of possible embezzlement, the president may require that all relevant communication with the vice presidents be kept confidential for a period of time.

The *circle pattern* allows communicators in the network to communicate directly with only two others, but since each communicates with another communicator in the network, the effect is that everyone communicates with everyone and there is no central authority or leader. The *all-channel network* is a circle pattern except that each communicator may interact with every other communicator in the network.

Communication networks vary along several dimensions and none is best in all situations. The wheel and all-channel networks tend to be fast and accurate compared with the chain or Y-pattern networks, but the chain or Y-patterns promote clear-cut lines of authority and responsibility. The circle and all-channel networks enhance morale among those in the networks better than other patterns because everyone is equal in the communication activity, but these patterns result in relatively slow communication. This is a serious problem if an immediate decision is needed or an action must be taken quickly. Managers must choose networks to fit the various communication situations they face.

Informal Communication

Coexisting with formal communication flows and networks in health care organizations are *informal communication flows,* which have their own networks. Informal flows and networks result from the interpersonal relationships of organization members. The common name for informal communication is *grapevine,* a term that arose during the Civil War, when telegraph lines were strung between trees much like a grapevine.[48] Messages transmitted over those flimsy lines were often garbled. As a result, any rumor was said to come from the grapevine.

By definition, the grapevine or informal flow of communication consists of channels that result from the interpersonal relationships of organization participants. Informal communication flows in an organization are as natural as the patterns of social interaction that develop in all organizations. Like the informal organization itself, informal communication flows coexist with the formal patterns established by management. There is no doubt that informal communication channels can be and routinely are misused in organizations, especially in transmitting rumors. Yet, properly managed informal communication flows can be useful. Downward flows move through the grapevine much faster than through formal channels. In many health care organizations, much of the coordination among units occurs through informal give-and-take in informal horizontal and diagonal flows. In the case of upward flow, informal communication can be a rich source of information about performance, ideas, feelings, and attitudes. Because of its potential usefulness

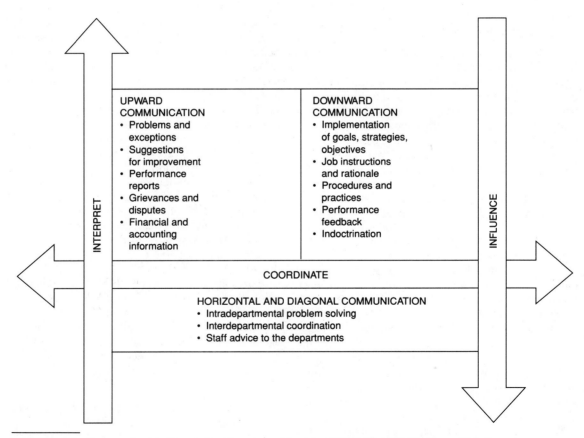

FIGURE 8.5. Communication flows in health care organizations. SOURCE: Daft RL, Steers RM. *Organizations: A Micro-Macro Approach.* Copyright © 1986 by Scott, Foresman and Company. Reprinted by permission of HarperCollins Publishers.

and pervasiveness, managers should try to understand informal communication flows and use them to advantage.

The multidirectional communication flows and the networks they form within health care organizations each have a purpose, and each is an important tool for managers. To the extent these flows are planned and designed into the organization, they are formal communication channels and networks. To the extent they are natural communication between and among people, they are informal communication channels and networks. Figure 8.5 summarizes the key uses of downward, upward, horizontal, and diagonal communication flows in health care organizations.

Flow of Interorganizational Communication

Health care organizations enter into a variety of linkages to manage their interdependencies with other organizations and agencies. In doing so, they must develop communication flows to and from those with whom they are interdependent. This means that health care organizations typically maintain relationships with a large and diverse set of external stakeholders. The sheer number and variety of external stakeholders complicates *interorganizational communication* for managers of health care organizations. Another complication is the nature of relationships. Positive relations between an organization and its external stakeholders make it easier to manage the relationships, and communication flows are more effective than when relations are negative.

Figure 8.6 uses a large hospital as an example and illustrates the extraordinary diversity of interorganizational relationships that must be maintained by such institutions. The figure also suggests the difficulty of maintaining these relationships when many are negative or neutral at best. It is important to note that the arrows connecting the hospital with stakeholders go in both directions. Managers in health care organizations must be concerned about communication flows to external stakeholders *and* about flows from these stakeholders.

Conceptually, the interdependence between the hospital in Figure 8.6 and its stakeholders can be managed in one of two ways: the hospital can adapt to fit the requirements and expectations of interdependent others or it can alter the interdependent others so that they fit its capabilities and preferences. In practice both occur and both depend on effective communication. Unless what is expected from interdependent others is known and understood, effective adaptation is impossible. Conversely, changing interdependent others requires effective communication from the health care organization to the stakeholder, although on occasion the organization can enlist others in attempts to change external stakeholders. For example, it is likely that the hospital in Figure 8.6 belongs to a state hospital association and to the American Hospital Association. These associations represent many hospitals and lobby government to alter policies in favor of hospitals or to create more favorable environmental contexts for them. Lobbying is, at its heart, communication.

Boundary spanning is the process through which health care organizations develop the means of communicating with external stakeholders, and boundary spanners are the people who carry out this process. They obtain critical information from external stakeholders that can be used for decision making as the organization adapts to their preferences and demands. The strategic planning and marketing departments or functions in health care organizations are good examples of boundary spanning. Since information is the object of these boundary spanning activities, communication is critical to their success. Boundary spanners also represent the organization to external stakeholders. This activity takes many forms, including marketing, public relations, guest or patient relations, government relations, or community relations. The common thread in these activities is information. If the health care organization is to be effectively represented to its external stakeholders, communication is key. Boundary spanning activities are not limited to a few departments or managers. Table 8.1 shows that many managers in health care organizations are involved in spanning the boundaries between the organization and its external stakeholders.

The Special Case of Communicating Among Units of Systems

Like many other health care organizations, the hospital in Figure 8.6 belongs to a system. The sys-

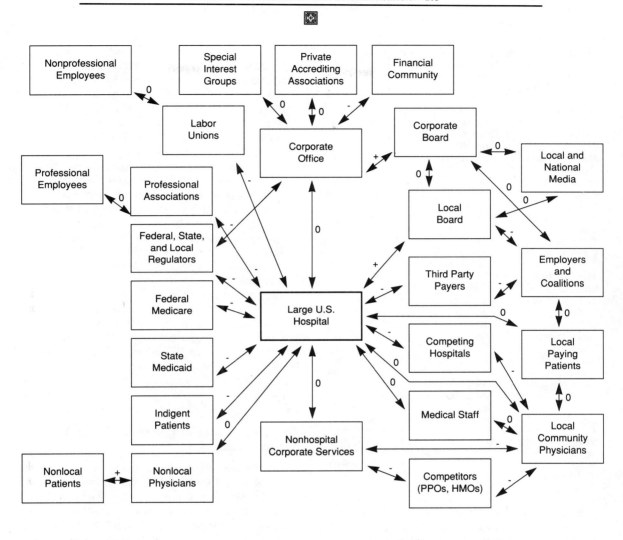

FIGURE 8.6. Stakeholders in a large hospital. SOURCE: Fottler MD, Blair JD, Whitehead CJ, Laus MD, Savage GT. Assessing Key Stakeholders: Who Matters to Hospitals and Why? *Hospital and Health Services Administration.* Winter 1989; 34:530. Copyright 1989, Foundation of the American College of Healthcare Executives.

tem has a corporate board and the hospital has a local board. This hospital faces the added challenge of communicating effectively with the other organizations in a multiunit system. Systems of health care organizations have become common through corpo-

rate restructuring (creating several entities to perform medical and nonmedical functions previously done by one corporation) and through active programs of merger and consolidation in the health care industry.

TABLE 8.1. Hospital Executives Responsible for Particular Key Stakeholders

Key Stakeholders	Responsible Managers
Medical staff	CEO, COO, associate administrator, medical staff director
Patients	Director of marketing, director of guest relations
Hospital department managers	COO, associate administrator, assistant administrator, product or service line manager
Professional staff	CEO, COO, associate administrator, human resources director
Board of trustees	CEO, COO, associate administrator
Federal government	Depends on issue
Corporate office	CEO, COO
Nonprofessional staff	Human resources director
Third party payers	VP for finance, reimbursement manager
Elected public officials	CEO, director of government relations, director of public relations
Political pressure groups	CEO, director of government relations, director of public relations, director of community relations
Local business/ industry	CEO
Accrediting/licensing agencies	VP for risk management, director of quality assurance, appropriate department head
Other hospitals	CEO, COO
Media	Director of public relations, director of marketing
Labor unions	Director of human resources

SOURCE: Fottler MD, Blair JD, Whitehead CJ, Laus MD, Savage GT. Assessing Key Stakeholders: Who Matters to Hospitals and Why? *Hospital and Health Services Administration.* Winter 1989:34:542. Copyright 1989, Foundation of the American College of Healthcare Executives.

Effectively communicating among units in a system is a demanding management task. Adapting Porter's approach to achieving effective linkages among business units in a diversified corporation suggests ways to manage the task of communication in a system.[49]

- Horizontal structure: Using devices that cross unit lines, such as partial centralization and interunit task forces or committees, facilitates communication.
- Horizontal systems: Using management systems tailored for the purpose and with a cross-unit dimension in areas such as planning, control, incentives, capital budgeting, and management information systems enhances communication.

- Horizontal human resource practices: Using human resource practices that facilitate unit cooperation, such as cross-unit job rotation, management forums, and training, increase the likelihood that managers in one part of the system will understand their counterparts elsewhere in the system and that they will communicate more effectively.
- Horizontal conflict resolution processes: Using management processes that resolve conflicts among units enhance communication. Such processes are different from horizontal structure and systems and relate more to the style of managing a multiunit system. The key is that corporate management installs and operates a system that fairly settles interunit disputes. Equitable settlement of disputes facilitates effective communication.

Multiunit systems such as that shown in Figure 8.6 can enhance communication through interlocking boards, which are usually defined as boards with overlapping membership. Interlocking boards provide a stable structure of coordinated activity and communication flow.

The Special Case of Communicating When Things Go Badly

Occasionally, things go very badly even in the most well-managed health care organization. A hospital might lose its accreditation status or state certification because of code violations; serious clinical errors occur, perhaps causing a patient's death; infections break out; or serious financial difficulties occur, perhaps threatening the organization's existence or raising the specter of major layoffs or closure. As in other large, complex organizations things can—and do—go wrong in health care organizations. When they do, communication with internal and external stakeholders takes on intensified importance. How managers communicate in such circumstances is significant in resolving the problems and in the perception of the organization held by its stakeholders after the problems are resolved.

For example, a hospital suddenly has a situation wherein a diabetic patient being treated for complications of that disease dies unexpectedly. Results of blood tests on a sample taken six hours before his death show insulin levels 200 times too high. There are several possible explanations, but few are good. The possibilities include a fatal overdose of insulin given by accident or on purpose in a criminal act committed by any of several people. How should the hospital handle this situation? Whose interests are to be protected? What information is to be communicated? To whom? By whom?

There are few hard-and-fast rules to guide managers in communicating with stakeholders under circumstances such as these. However, actions in response to a serious problem and communications made about the actions, can be characterized along a continuum of reactive to proactive.[50,51] At one end of the continuum, reactive responses include concealing the problem—do and say nothing. Less extreme, but highly reactive is to admit that a problem may exist (perhaps in response to a reporter alerted by someone) but deny any wrongdoing and take no action to find the cause of the problem or resolve it. An obstructionist position could be taken by the health care organization's managers regarding further communication about the problem.

A similar reaction is one best labeled defensive. The organization's managers and spokespersons act and communicate about the problem in a way that complies with the letter of the law. These actions and communications are intended to minimize legal liability and are a common response. This reaction partly reflects how expensive responsibility for serious problems involv-

ing human health and life can be. However, even when the issues are layoffs, mergers, closures, or problems that do not involve potential lawsuits, a defensive position is commonly taken in communicating with stakeholders who have a legitimate interest in the issue.

Figure 8.7 illustrates these reactive responses and two that are more proactive: accommodation and prevention. Accommodation involves accepting responsibility for the problem and taking aggressive actions to resolve it. In this type of response, the actions and communications about them are proactive. Communications are characterized by openness and candor about the problem, its causes, and the actions being taken to resolve it. Prevention is further along the continuum and focuses on aggressive and concerted actions to prevent problems from occurring. Continuous quality improvement (see Chapter 13) is an important approach in prevention, as are risk management and traditional quality assessment and improvement programs. Communications are characterized by openness and candor as in accommodation, but they focus on the existence and probabilities of potential problems and the steps that have been taken to prevent them.

Health care organizations are far better served in managing difficult situations by actions and communications that are proactive rather than reactive. Reactive responses imply crisis management and invite the scrutiny of stakeholders. Technically, managers who choose accommodation are reacting to a problem, too, but their response is positive and proactive in that they take responsibility, aggressively seek to resolve the problem, and communicate openly and candidly about

REACTIVE   PROACTIVE

CONCEALMENT	OBSTRUCTION	DEFENSE POSITION	ACCOMMODATION	PREVENTION
(Hide the existence of the problem; no communication)	(Resist communication; disavow any wrongdoing)	(Comply with letter of the law; communicate only favorable, factual information)	(Accept responsibility for the problem; take aggressive actions to resolve it; communicate openly and candidly about the problem and its resolution)	(Take aggressive actions to prevent problems from occurring; communicate openly about potential problems and steps to prevent them)

FIGURE 8.7. Continuum of actions and communications to stakeholders in difficult times. SOURCE: Rakich JS, Longest Jr BB, Darr K. *Managing Health Services Organizations.* 3rd ed. Baltimore, Md.: Health Professions Press; 1992:575.

MANAGERIAL GUIDELINES

1. A key to assigning the proper managerial priority to coordination and communication efforts is the degree to which interdependence exists between or among people, units, and entire organizations. Assessing the degree and nature of interdependence is the first step toward effective coordination and communication strategies.

2. Managers should pay careful attention to selecting and implementing compatible and, whenever possible, mutually reinforcing mechanisms of coordination and communication if they are to successfully link together the people and units within their organizations and link their organizations to others.

3. The predominance of professionals in health care organizations both facilitates and complicates coordination and communication. Their presence facilitates because professional education prepares these people to link their efforts with those of others as part of the normal course of their work. But their presence also requires careful attention to maintaining collegial and consultative relationships, which in turn should guide managers' choices about coordination and communication.

4. Coordination and communication, while treated separately in this chapter for ease of presentation, are in fact highly interrelated and interactive phenomena. Managers should always consider the communication implications and opportunities when seeking to coordinate and vice versa.

the problem and their actions regarding it. Prevention involves aggressive action to avoid problems. Here, managers communicate to stakeholders that problems might occur, but that actions have been taken to prevent them and minimize their impact. No level of effort will prevent all problems from occurring in health care organizations, but many can be prevented by careful actions and their consequences can be managed far more effectively if managers have laid a foundation of understanding and trust with stakeholders by communicating about potential problems and their actions to prevent them or prepare for them.

KEY CONCEPTS

Administrative System
All-Channel Network
Autonomous Arrangement
Boundary Spanning
Chain Network
Channels
Circle Pattern
Coalescing
Committees
Communication
Communication Networks
Communication Process Model
Conjoint Arrangement
Coopting
Coordination
Customs
Data Overload
Deception
Decode
Direct Supervision
Encode
Environmental Barriers to Communication
Feedback
Flows of Interorganizational Communication
Flows of Intraorganizational Communication
   (downward, upward, horizontal, and diagonal)
Grapevine
Heteronomous Arrangement
Hierarchical Coordination
Informal Communication
Integrators
Interdependence (pooled, sequential, reciprocal)
Integrators
Interorganizational Communication
Interorganizational Coordination
Intraorganizational Communication
Intraorganizational Coordination
Linking Pins
Litigation
Market Transactions
Matrix Design
Message
Mutual Adjustment
Ownership
Personal Barriers to Communication
Planning

Political Intervention
Programming
Project Management
Quasifirm
Receiver
Sender
Standardization of Work Processes
Standardization of Outputs
Standardization of Worker Skills
Voluntary Action
Wheel Pattern
Y Pattern

Discussion Questions

1. Distinguish between intra- and interorganizational coordination in health care organizations. What are the key mechanisms available to managers to achieve each type of coordination?
2. Define communication and draw a model of the basic technical process. How can managers overcome the barriers to effective communication?
3. You have just been appointed manager of a joint venture between the hospital where you work and some members of its medical staff to operate an ambulatory surgery facility. One of your initial concerns is the establishment of effective linkages to the hospital. Drawing upon the material in this chapter, develop your approach to this task and indicate the reasons for your plan.
4. Think of a situation in which a health care organization receives bad press. How might the organization respond along the reactive-proactive continuum? How should it respond?

REFERENCES

1. Thompson JD. *Organizations in Action.* New York, NY: McGraw-Hill; 1967.
2. Bolman LG, Deal TE. *Modern Approaches to Understanding and Managing Organizations.* San Francisco, Ca: Jossey Bass; 1984.
3. Charns MP, Schaefer MJ. *Health Care Organizations: A Model for Management.* Englewood Cliffs, NJ: Prentice-Hall; 1983:144.
4. Rakich JS, Longest Jr BB, Darr K. *Managing Health Services Organizations.* 3rd ed. Baltimore, Md: Health Professions Press, Inc.; 1992:557.
5. Kraut AI, Pedigo PR, McKenna DD, Dunnette MD. The role of manager: What's really important in different management jobs. *The Academy of Management Executive.* 1989;3(4):286–293.
6. Haimann T, Scott WG. *Management in the Modern Organization.* 2nd ed. Boston, Mass: Houghton-Mifflin; 1974:126.
7. Lawrence PR, Lorsch JW. Differentiation and integration in complex organizations. *Administration Science Quarterly.* 1967;11(3):1–47.
8. Scott WR. Managing professional work: Three models of control for health organizations. *Health Services Research.* 1982;17(3):213–240.
9. Ibid.
10. Kast FE, Rosenzweig JE. *Organization and Management: A Systems Approach.* 2nd ed. New York, NY: McGraw-Hill; 1974:214.
11. Litterer JA. *The Analysis of Organizations.* New York, NY: John Wiley & Sons; 1965:223–232.
12. Ibid., 230.
13. Ibid., 223.
14. Mintzberg H. *Structure in Fives: Designing Effective Organizations.* Englewood Cliffs, NJ: Prentice-Hall; 1983.
15. Mintzberg H. *The Structuring of Organizations.* Englewood Cliffs, NJ: Prentice-Hall; 1979:6–7.
16. Hage J. *Theories of Organizations: Forms, Processes, and Transformations.* New York, NY: Wiley-Interscience; 1980.
17. Hage J. Communication and coordination, in Shortell SM, Kaluzny AD. eds. *Health Care Management: A Text in Organization Theory and Behavior.* 1st ed. New York, NY: John Wiley & Sons; 1983:241–243.
18. March J, Simon H. *Organizations,* New York, NY: John Wiley & Sons; 1958.
19. Thompson, op. cit.
20. Perrow C. A framework for the comparative analysis of organization. *American Sociological Review.* 1967;32:194–208.
21. Van de Ven A, Delbecq A, Koenig Jr R. Determinants of coordination modes within organizations. *American Sociological Review.* 1976;41:322–338.
22. Longest Jr BB. *Management Practices for the Health Professional.* 4th ed. East Norwalk, Ct: Appleton & Lange; 1990.
23. Lawrence, Lorsch, op. cit., 1–47.
24. Cleland DI, King WR. *Systems Analysis and Project Management.* 3rd ed. New York, NY: McGraw-Hill; 1983.
25. Likert R. *The Human Organization.* New York, NY: McGraw-Hill; 1967:156.
26. Ibid., 167.
27. Thompson, op. cit.
28. Pointer, DD, Begun JW, Luke RD. Managing interorganizational dependencies in the new health care marketplace. *Hospital and Health Service Administration.* 1988;33(2):167–177.
29. Zuckerman HS, Kaluzny AD. Strategic alliances in health care: The challenges of cooperation. *Frontiers of Health Services Management.* 1991;7(3):3–23.
30. Longest Jr BB. Interorganizational linkages in the health sector. *Health Care Management Review.* 1990;15(1):17–28.
31. Starkweather DB. *Hospital Mergers in the Making.* Ann Arbor, Mich: Health Administration Press; 1981.
32. Weick K. Educational organizations as loosely coupled systems. *Administrative Science Quarterly.* 1976;21(1):1–19.
33. Pfeffer J, Salanick GR. *The External Control of Organizations: A Resource Dependence Perspective.* New York, NY: Harper & Row; 1978:161.
34. Shortell SM, Wickizer TM, Wheeler JRC. *Hospital-Physician Joint Ventures.* Ann Arbor, Mich: Health Administration Press; 1984:327.
35. Luke RD, Begun JW, Pointer DD. Quasi firms: Strategic interorganizational forms in the health care industry. *The Academy of Management Review.* 1989;14(1):13.
36. Pointer DD, Begun JW, Luke RD. Managing interorganizational dependencies in the new health care marketplace. *Hospital and Health Services.* 1988;33:171.
37. Starkweather, op. cit., 37–38.
38. Altman D, Greene R, Sapolsky HM. *Health Planning and Regulation: The Decision-Making Process.* Ann Arbor, Mich: Association of University Programs in Health Administration Press; 1981.
39. Porter ME. *Competitive Advantage: Creating and Sustaining Superior Performance.* New York, NY: Free Press; 1985.
40. Scott WG, Mitchell TR. *Organization Theory: A Structural Behavioral Analysis.* Homewood, Ill: Richard D. Irwin, Inc.; 1979:3.
41. Shortell SM. *Effective Hospital-Physician Relationships.* Ann Arbor, Mich: Health Administration Press; 1991:70–92.

42. Davis K, Newstrom JW. *Human Behavior at Work: Human Relations and Organizational Behavior.* 8th ed. New York, NY: McGraw-Hill; 1989:89.

43. Gibson JL, Ivancevich JM, Donnelly Jr JH. *Organizations: Behavior, Structure, Process.* 7th ed. Homewood, Ill: Richard D. Irwin, Inc.; 1991:540.

44. Holt DH. *Management: Principles and Practices.* 2nd ed. Englewood Cliffs, NJ: Prentice-Hall; 1990:483.

45. Robbins SP. *Management.* 3rd ed. Englewood Cliffs, NJ: Prentice-Hall; 1991.

46. Luthans F. *Organizational Behavior: A Modern Behavioral Approach to Management.* New York, NY: McGraw-Hill; 1973:253.

47. Scott WG. *Organization Theory.* Homewood, Ill: Richard D. Irwin, Inc.; 1967:165.

48. Davis, Newstrom, op. cit., 370.

49. Porter, op. cit., 394.

50. Carroll AB. A three-dimensional conceptual model of corporate performance. *Academy of Management Review.* 1979;4:497–505.

51. Holt, op. cit., 69–71.

CHAPTER

POWER AND POLITICS IN HEALTH SERVICES ORGANIZATIONS

Jeffrey A. Alexander, Ph.D.
Professor

Laura L. Morlock, Ph.D.
Professor

CHAPTER TOPICS

LEARNING OBJECTIVES

After completing this chapter, the reader should be able to

1. distinguish between rational and political models of organization and their appropriateness to health services organizations
2. know the practical, managerial implications of the effective use of power in health services organizations
3. identify the conditions that promote the use of power, politics, and informal influence in health services organizations
4. understand the range of political strategies and tactics employed by members of health services organizations
5. understand the sources of power in health services organizations
6. know the key approaches for consolidating and developing power by managers, physicians, and other groups in health services organizations

CHAPTER PURPOSE

Whether at hospitals, health maintenance organizations (HMOs), group practices, or preferred provider organizations (PPOs), the conflicts presented at Suburban General Medical Center are not unique. Managers of health care organizations are continually required to balance the rational, or task-oriented, with the social reality of organizational life.[1-4] This chapter will discuss the means by which power distributions in health care organizations can be identified, the conditions under which conflict between groups may result, the use of power to resolve conflict, and the strategies and tactics that are commonly employed in the effective use of power.

IN THE REAL WORLD

TURF BATTLES AMONG THE MEDICAL STAFF

Terry Johnson leaned back in her chair feeling overwhelmed by the stacks of memos and reports piled on the desk before her. As the new administrative resident at Suburban General Medical Center, she had been delighted when Sandy Shulman, the chief operating officer, suggested that Terry assist her and the finance director to prepare for a series of meetings with clinical chiefs that would help develop the next three-year capital budget.

Sandy had handed over a thick folder filled with budget requests and then explained that Terry's role would be to help track down any additional patient volume and market area data that could help determine both the need for and the desirability of each of the major proposals for equipment or renovations. Delight had quickly faded into dismay, however, as Terry wondered

what types of information could possibly be helpful to senior management and the governing board as they tried to evaluate the array of proposals with their competing priorities and sometimes contradictory assumptions.

A good example was the proposal from the Department of Surgery for renovation funds and equipment to create their own capability within the department for performing cardiac catheterizations, angiographies, and angioplasties. Currently these procedures were performed in laboratories within the Department of Radiology, but according to the Surgery Department proposal, the limited space and equipment available could no longer accommodate the growing demand for these procedures. Terry noted that the budget request from the Department of Radiology included funds to purchase an additional image intensifier as well as other equipment needed to increase the capacity of radiology for performing catheterizations and angiographies.

At Sandy's suggestion, Terry had met with the manager in Radiology responsible for scheduling these procedures. It appeared that afternoon time slots were almost always available without a long waiting period for an appointment. Competition was severe, however, among physicians trying to schedule patients in the early morning, particularly during the 7 A.M.-9 A.M. periods. In addition, during the past few months a number of complaints had resulted from emergency cases "bumping" patients undergoing elective procedures from the schedule. Perhaps additional capacity was needed, but in which department?

There also seemed to be several other duplicate proposals with requests for similar equipment purchases. It appeared, for example, that both the Department of Radiology and the Obstetrics and Gynecology Service were planning to double their capacity to perform pelvic ultrasounds and mammography. Terry was aware that a large freestanding diagnostic imaging center recently had opened nearby and wondered whether the utilization projections of either proposal would be likely to materialize.

In a subsequent meeting with Sandy to go over detailed population projections by gender and age group for their market area, Terry voiced her confusion regarding the duplication in requests for new equipment. Could it be cost effective for the same types of procedures to be performed by multiple specialties in different clinical services within the hospital?

Sandy commented that this question was being pondered in similar hospitals throughout the country as technological advances continued to create important new devices and techniques that are not clearly the domain of any one specialty. In a number of large hospitals, for example, cardiologists, cardiovascular surgeons, vascular surgeons, and interventional radiologists all claimed to have relevant credentials for performing certain types of angioplasties, procedures that involved the surgical repair of blood vessels.

Similarly, in some hospitals general surgeons and gastroenterologists argued over who should be credentialed to perform laparoscopic cholecystectomies—a surgical procedure that allows a patient's gallbladder to be removed through small incisions in the abdomen. In other medical centers, disputes waged over whether obstetricians-gynecologists or radiologists were better trained to perform and interpret pelvic ultrasounds and mammograms, whether radiologists or gastroenterologists should perform gastrointestinal endoscopy, and whether general surgeons or otolaryngologists were better trained to conduct head and neck surgery.

Sandy emphasized that such "turf disputes" were only likely to intensify as technological advances continued to outstrip the development of medical standards and guidelines for designating the credentials appropriate for performing specific procedures and utilizing specialized medical equipment in hospitals. Terry realized that these controversies were likely to have important economic consequences as physicians attempted to retain and further expand their patient bases. But how, she wondered, could these types of conflicts be resolved?

SOURCE: *Adapted by permission from Stephanie Lin Bloom, "Hospital Turf Battles: The Manager's Role,"* Hospital and Health Services Administration *36:4 (Winter 1991):590–599. Health Administration Press, © 1991, Foundation of the American College of Healthcare Executives.*

THE ROLE OF POWER AND POLITICS IN HEALTH SERVICES ORGANIZATIONS

Health care managers continually strive to improve efficiencies and productivity in the delivery of clinical care as well as meeting established organizational goals. Yet the reality is that these goals are not easily defined or universally accepted by organizational members. As we see at Suburban General Medical Center, interests within a given organization vary widely across departments, occupational groups, and individuals; and the role of management is to achieve a sense of balance. Success requires that managers must be cognizant of the distribution of power in their organization, the circumstances under which power is utilized, and tactics and strategies associated with the effective use of such power.[5,6]

If asked, most health services managers would acknowledge the existence and importance of informal power and politics as central forces in their organizations. However, these same managers are often reluctant to legitimize power and politics as acceptable bases of the management process.[7] Official de-emphasis of the use of informal power in organizations stems from a number of sources. First, such power is viewed as illegitimate by many managers because it often operates outside the formal authority system of the organization.[8,9] Any casual examination of the organization chart of a large tertiary hospital would reveal a complex system of reporting relationships and authority channels. This official system of accountabilities, control, and influence, however, does not fully represent what transpires between managers, physicians, and other groups of health care providers.[10] What gets done, how it gets done, and even the establishment of organizational goals themselves may be determined largely through a process of coalition building and influence that operates outside of, and sometimes in spite of, the formal authority structure expressed on the organizational chart.[11,12]

Secondly, many view the use of informal power as leading to subversion of organizational goals. Anything that occurs outside the formal authority structure of the organization is potentially motivated by self-serving interests on the part of individuals or groups. Such behavior is often assumed to run counter to the attainment of officially sanctioned organizational goals.[13]

Jeffrey Pfeffer, for example, has recently argued that this is a short-sighted view of the use of power and politics in organizations and that informal power can be used within the framework of organizational goals and objectives.[14,15] His argument rests on the premise that making decisions is a relatively easy job for managers. It is the implementation of these decisions that brings into play various constituencies, interests, and potential resistance. The use of power provides a means through which good managers can manage the consequences of their decisions.

The importance of power and its use is reinforced if one considers that, in most health care organizations, ambiguity and uncertainty surround both the establishment of organizational goals and the means to achieve these goals. The pervasiveness of ambiguity and uncertainty in health delivery organizations suggests that problems, particularly important problems, are typically not solved exclusively by logical analysis and sound reasoning. The existence of disagreements about what organizational goals should be, how they should be measured, how they should be prioritized, and the means by which they should be achieved, creates situations where different perspectives and interests come into play.[16–18] Managerial success in organizations is frequently a matter of working with and through other people.[19] Organizational success is often a function of how well individuals can coordinate their activities.[20,21] These functions are often a direct outcome of the effective use of power by managers. Informal power, although frequently operating outside the boundaries of the formal authority system of health care organizations, is not necessarily antithetical to the achievement of organizational goals. To acknowledge power and its utility in organizations is simply to acknowledge the diversity of interests and goals within the organization, the existence and normalcy of conflict, and that organizational results may stem from the political behavior of participants with different preferences.[22] Power can be analyzed systematically so as to make management more effective. An underlying theme is that politics is a means to resolve disagreements and that an appropriate role for politics is to resolve conflicts in order to achieve ends that benefit the organization.

POWER, INFLUENCE, AND POLITICS—DEFINITIONS

Power has been a notoriously elusive term to define and identify within organizations.[23,24] One cannot see it, it is not wholly captured in formal organizational charts, and it is not well operationalized or researched in the organizational literature. Indeed, terms like power, influence, and authority have been used in a variety of ways in the literature on organizations and management. To facilitate our discussion we will define power as the ability (or potential) to exert actions that either directly or indirectly cause a change in the behavior and/or attitudes of another individual or group. Put another way, power may be defined as the probability that one actor within a social relationship will be in a position to carry out his own will despite resistance, regardless of the basis on which this probability rests.[25] The term *influence* has been used most often to indicate actions that, either directly or indirectly, cause a change in the behavior and/or attitudes of another individual or group. Influence might be thought of as power translated into action.[26,27] Finally, *politics* is a domain of activity in which participants attempt to influence organizational decisions and activities in ways that are not sanctioned by either the formal authority system of the organization, its accepted ideology, or certified expertise.[28]

WHY SYSTEMS OF POWER AND POLITICS ARISE

Most writers agree that the use of power and politics in organizations occurs most frequently in situations in which goals are in conflict, where power is decentralized or diffused throughout the organization, where information is ambiguous, and where cause and effect relationships between actions and outcomes are uncertain or unknown (high task or strategic uncertainty).[28–33] Although health services organizations are far too varied to claim that they all meet these conditions, one could easily see how, for certain decisions and domains of activity, these characteristics might easily apply to organizations as diverse as hospitals, HMOs, nursing homes, and group practice organizations. It is often the case, for example, that governing boards and senior management have difficulty expressing clear,

unconflicting goals and objectives capable of being operationalized by the formal structure and control systems of the organization.[34,35] Many argue that political activity and informal influence systems arise because of inherent failings in the formal system of authority. This logic is based on the notion that an important function of the formal control system is to articulate and operationalize organizational goals and to direct the behavior of organizational members toward the achievement of those goals.[36,37] In many organizations, particularly health care organizations, this is at best an imperfect process since many goals are operationalized quite imperfectly, and some, such as the quality of medical care and service, are difficult to operationalize at all. In addition, most health services organizations have multiple goals such as providing high quality and accessible care and maintaining financial viability. However, organizational participants are rarely provided with the means to weigh the importance of different goals in order to direct their activities.

The ambiguity and uncertainty in how to operationalize and prioritize organizational objectives creates an arena for potential conflict among even the most dedicated, well-intentioned participants.[38] As the opening example illustrates, this situation may be reinforced by the complex division of labor and differentiation that occurs in many health care organizations. This pattern may be due to the assignment of different tasks and sometimes different organizational goals to different units or occupational groups. The tendency is for each unit or subgroup to emphasize the importance of its own activities and sometimes to treat its own tasks as ends in themselves rather than focusing on larger organizational goals.[39,40] Such differentiation creates group pressures that promote solidarity within the group and mistrust or misunderstanding of other groups—a we-they relationship.[41,42] Table 9.1, for example, illustrates the differences in principal orientations of managers and physicians that often foster conflict between the two groups.

Together, these types of organizational factors generate attempts to influence decisions and activities outside of the formal system of authority in organizations. Of primary importance here is that such systems of power and influence outside the formal authority system are naturally occurring phenomena in organizations and must be acknowledged and used by managers

TABLE 9.1. Cultural Differences Between Health Care Executives and Physicians

Attribute	Health Care Executives	Physicians
Basis of knowledge	Primarily social and management sciences	Primarily biomedical sciences
Exposure to relevant others while in training	Relatively little exposure to physicians, nurses, other health care professionals, or patients	Great deal of exposure to nurses, other health care professionals, and patients; little exposure to broader business or economic world of health care
Patient focus	Broad: all patients in the organization and the larger community	Narrow: one's individual patients
Time frame of action	Middle to long run; emphasis on positioning the organization for the future	Generally short run; meet immediate needs of patients
View of resources	Always limited; challenge lies in allocating scarce resources efficiently and effectively	More limited view emphasizing resources needed for one's own patients; resources should be available to maximize the quality of care
Professional identity	Less cohesive; less well-developed	More cohesive; highly developed

SOURCE: From S. Shortell, *Effective Hospital-Physician Relationships.* Ann Arbor, MI: Health Administration Press, 1992. Reprinted with permission from the Hospital Research and Educational Trust.

to effectively render some decisions and to implement those decisions in such a way as to benefit the organization as a whole.

RATIONAL VS. POLITICAL PERSPECTIVES ON MANAGEMENT

The acknowledgment and effective use of power, influence, and politics in organizations requires a fundamentally different outlook on organizational life than that prescribed in many graduate programs of health administration. The key differences between the *rational* and *political* perspectives on organizations are displayed in Table 9.2. Rational models imply that the managers of health care organizations are orchestrat-

ing the activities of a team whose members all subscribe to a common set of goals and objectives. Organizational members—whether physicians, nurses, ancillary care personnel, or others—are expected to perform the roles for which they have been appointed. Their behavior should be consistent with the achievement of commonly agreed upon organizational goals. Conflict in this context is seen as a source of trouble and an unwanted intrusion. Formal authority or professional expertise are the only legitimate sources of power, and all others are viewed as antithetical to the attainment of organizational goals.

By contrast, managers who acknowledge the existence of power and influence other than that vested in the formal authority system or professional expertise

TABLE 9.2. Rational vs Political Models of Organizations.

Organizational Characteristic	Rational Model	Political Model
Goals, preferences	Consistent across members	Inconsistent, pluralistic within the organization
Power and control	Centralized	Diffuse, shifting coalitions and interest groups
Decision process	Logical, orderly, sequential	Disorderly, give and take of competing interests
Information	Extensive, systematic, accurate	Ambiguous, selectively available, used as a power resource
Cause-effect relationships	Predictable	Uncertain
Decisions	Based on outcome maximizing choice	Results from bargaining and interplay among interests
Ideology	Efficiency and effectiveness	Struggle, conflict, winners and losers

Reprinted by permission from page 405 of *Organization Theory and Design,* 4th edition by Richard L. Daft; Copyright © 1992 by West Publishing Company. All rights reserved.

have a fundamentally different view of organizational life. These managers recognize that individuals and groups have different *interests,* aims, and objectives and that organizational membership is often a platform for pursuing their own ends. The central task of management is to balance and coordinate the various interests of organizational members so that concerted effort can be achieved to work within the constraints set by the organization's formal goals. Perhaps most importantly, the power-oriented manager often uses uncomfortable situations involving disagreements and conflicts and turns them into positive aspects of organizational life. Conflict, for example, can energize an organization, keep it from becoming lethargic, stale, and subject to inertia.[43] Conflict can form the basis for self evaluation that challenges conventional wisdom and theories in use.[44] Indeed, organizations themselves are viewed from this perspective not as unified systems but as loosely coupled systems where semiautonomous parts strive to maintain a degree of independence while working under the same name and framework provided by the organization. To be successful, managers must have the ability to read developing situations, analyze the interests that affect or are affected by these situations, understand conflicts, and explore power relations.

To put these claims in perspective, consider the various means by which things get done in health services organizations. The most commonly considered mechanism through which decisions are implemented and action is developed is through the hierarchical authority system, reflected in the organizational chart. But as an effective means for accomplishing organizational goals or implementing decisions, the formal authority structure suffers from several shortcomings. First, it is somewhat out of fashion in an era in which cooperation, teamwork, and cross-disciplinary integration is emphasized. Second, in most health services organizations, to accomplish objectives requires the cooperation of others outside the formal chain of command. Finally, the use of the hierarchical authority system assumes that those decision makers at the apex of this system are infallible, or at least most knowledgeable, in their judgments. It does not allow for poor judgment or bad decisions on the part of top level managers.[45,46]

A second means for marshaling concerted action to meet organizational goals is through a shared vision or organizational culture. Whereas this perspective has been gaining wide currency recently, it also suffers from several shortcomings. First, it takes considerable time and effort to fashion an effective organizational culture that is consistent with the overarching vision or mission of the organization. Second, the culture, once established, tends to be relatively impervious to new ideas or paradigms and thus may become a significant obstacle to organizational change.[47,48]

This leaves power and influence as a primary means by which change is accomplished in organizations. Here the emphasis is not so much on the structure established by hierarchical authority or the system of norms and values subsumed under the organization's culture but on the methods by which political support and resources are marshaled to get things done.[49,50]

Although important, power is not used indiscriminately in health services organizations, nor can it be used as the only means by which organizational change is achieved. This is true largely because converting power into influence requires expenditure of time, energy, or other limited resources and may also demand utilization of interpersonal or political skills which are not equally distributed among organizational members. One might think of power itself as a finite resource which must be selectively utilized to preserve that resource.[51,52]

POWER USE CONDITIONS

To effectively use power, it is important to recognize the conditions under which it is most appropriately used. First, because power is a finite resource, organizational members are more apt to employ it for decisions they consider to be important such as those made at higher organizational levels and those that involve crucial issues like reorganization and budget allocations.[53] Second, power is more likely to be a factor for those domains of activity in which performance is more difficult to assess (e.g., staff activity rather than line production) and in situations in which there are likely to be uncertainties and disagreement (e.g., goals, priorities, and the means to achieve them).[54,55] Such conditions are apparent in the case of improving cardiac care, described below.

IN THE REAL WORLD
THE ECG DEPARTMENT

Even a seemingly simple goal such as improving cardiac care services is subject to different perspectives and interests. For the ECG department, it may mean new types of tests or longer hours of staffing. For the radiology department, it may mean new imaging equipment. For the lab, it may mean developing the capability to do new types of tests. For surgery, it may mean adding a new heart team. For the CCU, it may mean new monitoring equipment or hiring a clinical specialist. Given financial constraints, not every one of these departments will get all it wishes, nor will it be obvious which single perspective or combination of perspectives will provide the most improvement in patient outcomes or in the financial status of the hospital.

It is interesting to note that *all* of these conditions are evident in the description of turf battles among medical staff members at Suburban General Medical Center. The decisions to be made involve critical resource allocations across departments that will determine what major equipment purchases and renovations will be made during the next three years. These decisions are likely to have important economic consequences for the departments involved as well as for individual physicians. Moreover, the major disagreements described are in new areas of activity in which performance is difficult to assess due to the lag time involved in developing medical standards, including appropriate certification and credentialing requirements for innovative diagnostic and therapeutic procedures. The situation is also characterized by disagreements regarding which specialties are more competent to perform specific procedures and who should have priority in scheduling patients and accessing equipment and support staff. In addition, there are uncertainties regarding future demand for the new technologies and the likely impact of increased competition in the market area. These circumstances in combination are highly likely to stimulate attempts to influence decisions and events through the exercise of political power.

The conditions described above are created by *interdependencies* among organizational members or units. Interdependence exists whenever one actor does not entirely control all the conditions necessary for the achievement of an action or for obtaining the outcomes desired from the action. When interdependence exists, our ability to get things done requires us to develop power and the capacity to influence those on whom we depend.[56,57] The development and use of power is particularly important when the people or groups with whom we are interdependent differ in their point of view from ours and thus cannot be relied upon to do what we would want. Even where there is clear agreement on these goals, different perspectives have a way of presenting problems. Consider the challenges facing a multispecialty group practice.

Given the multifaceted and reciprocal nature of patient care activity, there is often a high need for interdepartmental coordination. Further, there tends to be higher degrees of interdependence at higher levels of the organization, where tasks are less likely to be either simple or self-contained (e.g., strategic planning, restructuring).

It is important to note, however, that *very* high degrees of interdependence do not promote political or power activity because failure to cooperate under such conditions would assuredly mean the demise of the organization or the organizational unit. For example, very little political maneuvering occurs in the operating room or in intensive care units where interdependence is extremely high and where strong incentives to work together and coordinate activities are tantamount to organizational success. Taking the opposite perspective, we would expect power and political activity to be relatively low in those organizational settings that are characterized by simple or self-contained tasks.[58] In the hospital setting, for example, housekeeping and security might be examples of functional units that

THE GROUP PRACTICE

In a medium-sized midwestern city, a multi-specialty group practice wanted to recruit a new board-certified cardiologist. The group presently had only one cardiologist, and several of the primary care physicians felt the patients they referred to the cardiologist were not being seen on a timely basis. The cardiologist who was currently a member of the group was extremely busy, and due to the contractual mechanisms by which she was compensated, quite satisfied with her income. However, being the only board-certified cardiologist in the group gave her considerable influence in decisions such as capital acquisition and in her contract negotiations. Thus she was not in favor of recruiting a new cardiologist and was able to stall the process. This resulted in some of the primary care physicians losing patients who went to see cardiologists associated with other group practices. Eventually, the group practice threatened to risk terminating the cardiologist's contract and recruit two new cardiologists rather than lose patients.

reflect a low degree of interdependence and, thus, limited political activity. These ideas are easy to illustrate with respect to medical staff turf battles. For example, conflict can be decreased and the resulting political activity dampened if resources are plentiful enough to decrease departmental interdependence by providing duplicate equipment, space, and support staff. Bloom describes a university hospital where an intense dispute arose between radiologists and cardiologists regarding the most effective size for the lens on an image intensifier—a piece of equipment used during catheterizations and angiographies. Although both groups of specialists performed the same procedures and used the same type of equipment, the radiologists preferred a 14-inch lens, while the cardiologists had a strong preference for a 9-inch lens. To satisfy both groups, hospital management purchased image intensifiers with lenses of each size and established separate catheterization and angiography laboratories with their own distinct support staffs. If patient volumes and financial resources are not adequate to support such duplication, however, it is likely that conflicts of this type will be resolved through the political process.

The degree of interdependence in organizations is, in part, determined by the amount of resources available to the organization.[59] Slack resources reduce interdependence while scarcity increases it. When resources are plentiful, individual and departmental interests are more easily satisfied.[60] Organizational members and units tend to depend less on each other

for the achievement of their personal or subunit interests, and thus interdependence is decreased. However, when resources are scarce, interdependencies are increased. The allocation of scarce resources means that some organizational units will benefit while others will lose.

Interdependence as a catalyst for the use of power and politics in organizations is only applicable if the players in the interdependent situation possess different points of view. If everyone has the same goals and shares the same assumptions about how to achieve those goals, there will be minimal conflict and thus little room for power and influence. Such differences in points of view are more likely to emerge where there is a higher degree of task specialization or differentiation in the organization.[61] Simply put, when work is divided into different specialties and units, it is more likely that these units will be staffed by people with different backgrounds and training which will cause them to take different views of similar situations. Table 9.1, for example, illustrates some of the fundamental differences in orientations between managers and physicians that may promote different perspectives on organizational goals, "best practices," and legitimate authority.

It is important to note that, even if the above conditions are met, power and influence will not be used indiscriminately. As mentioned previously, power is a valuable resource and it is typically conserved for important issues. Thus, power is more likely to be exerted in situations involving major capital outlays, budget allocations, or strategic change as opposed to decisions on dress codes or changes in reporting forms. However, even minor decisions can sometimes hold significant symbolic importance in their ability to convey the appearance of power. For example, decisions regarding the relative location of the offices or parking spaces of the vice president for planning and marketing and the vice president for finance may be bitterly disputed since locations are often symbolic of an individual's or department's power within the organization.[62]

SOURCES OF POWER

Understanding the conditions under which power is used can help health care managers determine when power and influence are appropriate as methods for achieving organizational objectives. However, effectively using power in these domains assumes that one has the requisite amount of power to influence the outcomes of organizational decisions. Thus, understanding the *sources of power* is an important step in acquiring such power. Although some power is derived from personal attributes such as sensitivity, articulateness, self-confidence, and aggressiveness, an alternative perspective suggests that structural sources of power are more important.[63–66] From this perspective, power is derived from where individuals stand in the division of labor and the communications system of the organization. One's placement in these structures fosters power from a control over resources, the ties one has to other influentials in the organization, the formal authority system of the organization, or the ability to deal with important uncertainties or contingencies that face the organization.

Jurisdiction over resources is an important source of power within the structural framework but only to the extent that one actually controls the resource and its use. Further, resources that serve as a basis of power must be critical for the organization. That is, the resource must be essential to the functioning of the organization; in short supply, or concentrated in terms of the number of people who possess it, and nonsubstitutable. These three attributes make the resource critical and thus create organizational dependency on those individuals or groups who control its availability and

use. Power is created by the dependence of others, and that dependence is a function of how much others need what we control, as well as how many alternative sources for that resource there are.[67–69] For example, many physicians in health services organizations will emphasize the revenue-generating capabilities of their clinical departments as the basis for further capital acquisition or the purchase of new medical technology. One hospital physician noted, "Of course, our argument about our financial contribution to the hospital is primarily useful with the administration and the board. It should also have some meaning to other physicians, however, if our work conditions become so intolerable that we are unable to continue to generate revenue for the hospital, and we are unable to continue maintaining our quality of service, there will be financial ramifications for everyone associated with the hospital."[70] Access to and control over critical resources can occur at lower as well as higher levels in health services organizations.[71] For instance, a purchasing agent often has considerable latitude regarding negotiating contracts for equipment and supplies. She can seriously inconvenience a surgical suite by dragging her feet on ordering replacement equipment or by refusing to expedite a request without approval from a department's administrator.

The acquisition of power through access to and discretionary control over resources is often accomplished through the formation of *alliances* and *coalitions*.[72,73] The literature attaches considerable significance to the importance of finding others with common interests and building long-term relationships with them. Such coalitions differ from ad hoc arrangements insofar as they imply future as well as present commitment. Alliances and coalitions are developed through several different mechanisms, including helping people to obtain positions of power through appointments and promotions and doing favors for those whose support is needed.[74] Although both these strategies would appear to some to be decidedly antirational, and even illegitimate, they are often necessary in complex, interdependent systems with many actors and points of view. In health service organizations, alliances often emerge among the chiefs of clinical services in their requests for capital improvements. For example, the chief of radiology and the chief of orthopedic surgery may support each other in their respective requests for a portable fluoroscope and for renovations to departmental facilities. Frequently, such alliances may be used to mount a campaign against capital requests by other services or service chiefs.

A second major strategy for acquiring and developing new sources of power is control over or access to information. Power accrues as a function of one's position in the network of communications and social relations within organizations.[75-77] How central one is in this network is dependent on one's location within the communication pathways that link individuals within the organization, the number of others with whom one has contact, and the distance between one's own location and all other individuals in the communication network.

A second source of power based on access to information derives from claims to special knowledge or skills that are critical to the organization. The primary power base of the hospital medical staff, for example, is usually perceived to be its control over a specialized body of knowledge and technical skills used to diagnose and treat patients.[78-80] Because patients are vital to the hospital's continued viability and survival, physicians' expertise gives them a strong power base within the organization. However, it has recently been recognized that the expertise required to deal effectively with increasing financial and legal complexities of health care organizations has accrued to management and that that expertise has increased the power of management in their relationships with physicians over the past several decades.[81]

The third and most obvious source of power in organizations is that which is vested by formal authority, often expressed in the role or position of an individual in the organizational hierarchy.[82,83] When observing an organizational chart, such as that depicted in Figure 9.1, it is relatively easy to discern what positions have *authority* over others and what positions are subordinate to higher positions. The *formal authority system* of the organization is usually defined in terms of rights and obligations which create a field of influence within which an individual or department can legitimately operate with the formal support of those with whom one works. In other words, the organizational structure codifies official control over resources, information, and interaction with potential sources of uncertainty.

Typically, those in higher positions are vested with the power to direct and influence those in lower positions. However, this should not be taken as a given by managers. Power vested in the formal authority structure of the organization holds only so long as those who are subject to this kind of authority respect and accept the nature of that authority. If formal power is not legitimated by those who fall under its purview, the source of power itself will be weakened. This sometimes occurs in situations where a tyrannical boss will so alienate the workers of an organization that they will refuse to further acknowledge his authority and will delegitimate his power by refusing to carry out his orders or by quitting the organization.

The ability to cope with uncertainties that influence the day to day operations of an organization is yet another source of power for individuals and groups.[84-87] Much organizational *uncertainty* stems from interdependencies that occur within organizations—expressed by: relationships between departments, occupational groups, or subunits—interdependencies that are defined in terms of the organizations' relationship to external organizations or actors upon which the focal organization depends for critical resources. With respect to the latter, the ability to deal with the vagaries of markets, sources of raw materials, or financing and capital can provide opportunities for those with the skills to tackle these critical elements and minimize their effects on the organization as a whole. Thus, managers in health care organizations who are equipped with the skills to deal with regulatory, accrediting, and legal forces affecting the viability of their organizations are in a position to cope with the critical uncertainties that these external forces create.[88-90] From an internal uncertainty perspective, it may be argued that physicians are particularly skilled at dealing with the complex and uncertain situations presented by certain types of patients. Indeed, some have argued that the use of professionals in organizational settings is an administrative mechanism to deal with critical uncertainties that would be too costly to handle through the use of bureaucratic means.[91] It should be noted, finally, that the power derived from an individual's or group's ability to deal with organizational uncertainties is directly related to the centrality of their functions to the organization and inversely related to the degree to which their skills are substitut-

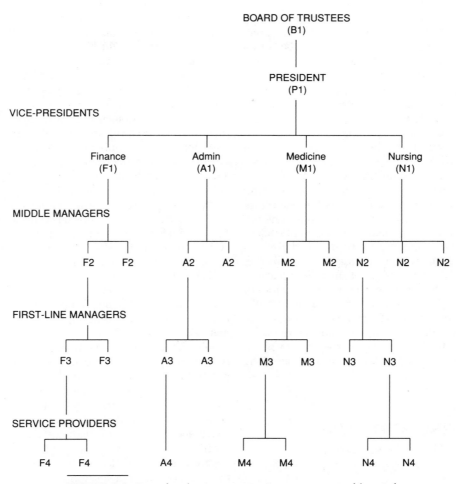

FIGURE 9.1. Formal authority structure: Acute care general hospital.

able. For example, a political analyst in the health care organization whose responsibility is to interface with state regulatory agencies may lose some of his power if such functions can be performed equally well by a member of the hospital's marketing department. In health services organizations, physicians are viewed as a central source of unpredictability vis-a-vis the organization's production of patient care services. Physicians admit patients, diagnose them, order tests and procedures, decide on levels of care, and make the discharge decision. Through their exclusive control over patient care, physicians control three of health services organi-

zations critical resources: admissions, length of stay, and demand for ancillary services.[92] The centrality of physicians to the organization is a major source of power to this occupational group. However, this power is increased by virtue of monopolistic control over a specialized body of knowledge. Physicians' monopoly over technical expertise frees them from most supervisory controls by hospital management and further weakens any attempts to reduce the unpredictability of patient care in most health services organizations. Finally, physicians maximize their control over the uncertainties in health care production through implicit or explicit threats to send their patients to other hospitals or facilities.[93,94] The use of these and other strategies are illustrative of the use of present power advantages by an occupational group to insure and expand their prerogatives in the future.

Health services managers, despite having to deal with the uncertainties created by physician control over the production of health care delivery, are not without their own sources of power. The first of these are represented in procedural checks upon hospital activities imposed by external agencies such as certificate of need programs, PPOs, prospective payment systems, utilization review, and others. Such programs represent yet another source of uncertainty for health care organizations which managers are well-positioned to deal with. Also reducing the power base of physicians are changes in the numbers and employment patterns of other physicians within the organization's market or region. This has the effect of diluting explicit or implicit threats to deprive health care organizations of critical resources (e.g., patients, admissions). Finally, new competitive pressures facing health services organizations often compel trustees to take a more proactive stance toward limiting the prerogatives of physicians so as to increase the competitive viability of the organizations they govern.

DEVELOPING AND USING POWER—DOMAINS OF POLITICAL ACTIVITY

Power is a latent force until the possessor of such power chooses to utilize it in the form of influence or political action. In general, the use of influence and political tactics to reach decisions or to assist in the implementation of decisions is highest under conditions of high uncertainty. In its most extreme form, some view organizations themselves as consisting of nothing more than a variety of political interests or coalitions that disagree about goals and have poor information about alternatives for action (see Table 9.2). Because of the existence of groups that have separate interests, goals, and values, disagreement and conflict are normal and expected, and the exercise of power through influence and political processes are needed

to reach and to implement decisions. It is unlikely that most health care organizations are as totally politicized as these models would suggest. However, there are certainly conditions within many health care organizations that promote the use of power and politics as a means for accomplishing the ends of certain groups or coalitions.

There are four domains of activity, in particular, that tend to be linked most strongly with the use of power and politics in organizations. These are structural change, interdepartmental coordination, management succession, and resource allocation and budgeting. Structural change is important because it potentially reallocates formal authority on the organizational chart. If, for example, a hospital is considering shifting from a functional to a divisional design, change in responsibility and tasks attendant to such design changes will also affect the underlying power base of various departments and individuals within the organization. Because of the potential effect on increasing and decreasing power among certain groups or individuals, political activity is often needed to initiate and implement such a change.[95]

One of the primary conditions for the use of power is interdependencies between different groups or departments within organizations. Such interdependencies often compel coordination among departments with different goals, strategies, and cognitive orientations. Because formal rules, policies, and procedures with respect to conducting tasks are often department-specific, there are few rules to guide the way in which departments should deal with one another. Perhaps more important, coordination often has implications for the responsibility and prerogatives of departments involved in a particular task. Hence, it is often the case that political processes and influence help define respective authority and task boundaries.[96] For instance, in some institutions medical staff turf battles have resulted in the clear delineation of practice domains. To cite one example, it may be determined that radiology should have the authority to control cardiac catheterization laboratories with their associated technology, technicians, and policies, while other specialists may request use of the facilities. Task boundaries also may be established and turf battles reduced through a negotiation process in which strict performance-based credentialing criteria are determined which must be met by any medical staff members seeking to expand their scope of practice.

In many health care organizations today, there is a great deal of instability in the ranks of mid-level and top-level management. Whether succession involves hiring new executives, promoting individuals from within, or transferring management to other units within a hospital or multi-institutional system, such changes may bring with them considerable change in the power structure of an organization. A new manager often brings a new set of alliances or values which can upset existing alliances and working relationships, as well as previous agreements among organizational personnel. From another perspective, managerial hiring or promotion can be used as a strategy to enhance one's political position if the new manager has allegiances or values consistent with those of particular coalitions in the organization.[97,98] Politically-based promotions are often apparent when "unobvious" choices are picked for advancement. This means that the candidate may be chosen for promotion not based on his skills, expertise, or experience but on his loyalty or similarity to the dominant political coalition in the organization.

On the surface, resource allocation should be made on the basis of rational considerations such as allocating funds to those activities or units most central to the achievement of key organizational or strategic goals. However, the value of resources within organizations is so high that survival of various individuals and departments often depends on obtaining adequate resources. Resource allocation and budgeting become, in effect, the battlegrounds over which organizational priorities are debated.[99] The allocation of resources, the budgeting process, and political influence in setting the organization's agendas are inextricably interrelated. Such political action becomes particularly important in periods of resource decline. If resources are plentiful, all departments potentially receive an allocation that permits them to pursue their own goals and interests. However, as the pie gets smaller, a zero-sum game mentality sets in such that resources allocated to one department are viewed as resources denied another. As illustrated below, this sets the stage for considerable political activity within organizations.[100]

CONSOLIDATION OF POWER

The distribution of power in organizations is not a fixed but a dynamic phenomenon that requires constant monitoring and adaptation on the part of managers and others who would effectively use it. Opportunities to gain power and use influence shift with changes in resource availability, contingencies that must be addressed, and the effects of others to gain control over resources, decision premises, and information. Several strategies are available to consolidate or expand power bases by groups or individuals to insure that their power is maintained.

- The use of organizational structure to build one's own power or stall the acquisition of power on the part of others in the organization. Plans for organizational differentiation and integration, designs for centralization and decentralization, and the tensions that can arise in matrix organizations often entail hidden agendas related to power, autonomy, or interdependence among departments and individuals. For example,

IN THE REAL WORLD

POWER SHIFTS AND ORGANIZATIONAL CHANGE

A hospital negotiated a new prospective payment contract with a large local HMO. The contract could be very beneficial for the hospital, if costs could be kept under control. The chief financial officer developed a financial assessment of the contract, using pessimistic assumptions to show that a number of cuts would need to be made for the contract to be profitable. He then developed an organizational chart that would cut several outreach programs and the administrator in charge of them—a long time rival—in order to meet the cost figures he projected.

fragmenting opponents' power bases by adopting a functional structure is a common tactic that sometimes has no basis in rational organizational design. Viewed from the opposite perspective, the rigidity and inertia of organizational structures sometimes reflect the tendency to preserve existing structures in order to protect the power that individuals or groups derive from them. Resisting revisions in job descriptions or organizational designs or the adoption of certain new technologies or programs are examples of inertial reactions based on preservation of power or authority in the organization.[101] An illustration of this tendency is evident in resistance to the implementation of Total Quality Management (TQM) among middle managers who do not have a clear role in quality improvement efforts and who may feel threatened by new relationships that result from program activities (see In the Real World).

- Expansion of organizational boundaries or domains of activity. An HMO marketing department, for example, may choose to expand its power by taking on the function of strategic planning, which some view as a natural extension of the marketing function. A move into strategic planning would clearly give marketers access to key information and enable them to influence top

level decision makers of the organization, thereby increasing their power. In health services organizations, the dynamics of power, acquisition, development, and use are often expressed in the relations between different occupational groups and their attempt to improve their professional position and status through expanding their domains of activity and responsibility. Nurses, for example, are becoming more highly trained and seek to increase their prestige vis-a-vis physicians. At the same time, nurses must fend off encroachments to their professional domain by medical technicians. Technicians, in turn, seek to establish their power through enhancing their professional legitimacy within the organizational hierarchy, often at the expense of nurses.

- The principle of *cooptation*. To diffuse the influence of rivals or to gain support from important groups, managers will often appoint influential members of these groups to special committees or task forces that are controlled by the manager. By giving them legitimate roles in a context supportive of the goals and interests of the organization, members of competing factions are coopted into accepting these goals and/or the legitimacy of the current authority structure.[102] In health services organizations, some managers maintain that appointing physicians to the board

IN THE REAL WORLD
IMPLEMENTING TOTAL QUALITY MANAGEMENT

The Johns Hopkins Health System began its efforts to implement Total Quality Management in the fall of 1988. One of the first steps was to select and study four Fortune 500 companies well known for their quality improvement initiatives in order to benefit from lessons learned regarding possible pathways to success and pitfalls to avoid. All four of these companies reported that one of their greatest mistakes was failure to sufficiently involve middle management in the planning and implementation process.

Discussions of TQM are likely to focus on the

critical role of top level commitment, as well as the formation of quality improvement teams whose members are deeply involved in front line operations. There is little emphasis on the role that middle managers might play in the process. These Fortune 500 companies found, however, that failure to involve this level of management resulted in threatened individuals who could—and did—slow program implementation. In an effort to avoid this problem, many of the efforts at Johns Hopkins during the first 18 months focused on getting middle managers "on board."

of trustees is a way to coopt them into accepting official organizational goals as well as to reduce conflict and tension based on disparate interests between medical staff and the organization.

THE STRUCTURE OF POLITICAL ACTIVITY IN ORGANIZATIONS

Power may be converted into political influence within the organization. The exercise of such influence is often described as a set of "games," each with its own structure and rules that are played outside the legitimate system of authority.[103-105] Mintzberg has described these games as structured in the sense that they have established positions, paths through which individuals gain access to positions, and rules that could constrict the range of decisions and actions that are acceptable.[106] The most common *political games* and the reasons they are played are listed in Table 9.3.

The insurgency games are usually played to resist authority, or as a means to affect or prevent change in the organization. Frequently they are played at the point where decisions made at the upper levels of the authority hierarchy have to be implemented. They may be played by lower level participants who attempt to circumvent, sabotage, or manipulate elements of the authority system and are often played by managers who distort or limit the amount of information sent to superiors in the authority structure. They can be played subtly by individuals or small groups or aggressively by a large number of participants willing to take unified visible action.

The insurgency games are sometimes met by attempting to increase authority, that is, by tightening personnel and bureaucratic controls and by administering sanctions. They also may be countered in a retrospective or prospective fashion by the counterinsurgency games. The most frequent are limiting the amount of information available to subordinates, fostering competition among subordinates to maintain control and various forms of cooptation.

There are a variety of political games played to build power bases. Sponsorship games have simple rules: The individual attaches himself or herself to a rising star—or one already in place—and professes loyalty in return for a piece of the action. The alliance-building game is played by individuals or groups who negotiate with their peers implicit contracts of support for each other. The empire-building game is played by individuals to enlarge their power base by collecting subunits or loyal subordinates. In her study *Men and Women of the Corporation*, Kanter found that individuals who wanted to have significant influence on the organization had to play at least one of these three games: "people without sponsors, without peer connections, or without promising subordinates remained in the situation of bureaucratic dependency."[107]

Budgeting games are used to acquire more resources for the positions or units the individual already has under his or her control. They are the best known of the political games, probably because they are the most visible and have the most well-defined rules. With respect to operating budgets, a variety of strategies are used to gain the largest possible allocation (e.g., always requesting more than required in the knowledge that a given percentage will be cut in the final negotiations). In the case of capital budgets, methods are typically found to underestimate costs and overestimate benefits (see Table 9.4).

TABLE 9.3. Political Games

Games to resist authority	Insurgency games
Games to counter the resistance to authority	Counterinsurgency games
Games to build power bases	Sponsorship games (with superiors)
	Alliance-building games (with peers)
	Empire-building games (with subordinates)
	Budgeting games (with resources)
	Expertise games (with knowledge and skills)
	Lording games (with authority)
Games to defeat rivals	Line vs. staff games
	Rival camps games
Games to effect organizational change	Strategic candidates games
	Whistle-blowing games
	Young Turks games

Adapted from Henry Mintzberg, *Power in and Around Organizations,* copyright © 1983, p. 188. Reprinted by permission of Prentice-Hall, Inc., Englewood Cliffs, New Jersey.

TABLE 9.4. Budgeting Games

Strategy	Description
Games to Obtain Funding for New Programs or Equipment	
Foot in the Door	Initially request funding for a modest program. Conceal its actual magnitude until it has gotten underway and built a vocal constituency.
Keeping Up with the Joneses	Base the budget request for new program funding on the rationale that the organization must stay abreast of the competition (whether or not there is a demonstrated need for the new program).
Keeping Up to Date	The rationale is based on the argument that the organization must be a leader and therefore must adopt the latest technology. An actual "Jones" need not be found and cited.
Call It a Rose	Utilize appealing (but misleading) labels. A classic example is the strategy used to obtain additional space by the National Institutes of Health in the early 1960s. During this time period it was impossible to obtain budget approval for new building construction, but it was possible to get funding to build "annexes." It is probably not surprising that at least one "annex" is more than double the size of the original building.
Games to Maintain Programs at Their Current Levels and to Resist Budget Cuts	
Sprinkling	Increase budget estimates by only a few percent, either across-the-board or in areas difficult to detect. Frequently this is done in anticipation that arbitrary cuts will be made. The goal is to attain a final budget allocation that is at the level it would have been without "sprinkling" or arbitrary reductions.
Create a Public Outcry	When budget reductions are ordered, decrease or eliminate a popular program in an effort to elicit client support and divert attention away from less popular program areas where cuts might indeed be feasible. A common example is the reduction of firefighter and police force positions that big city mayors often make when asked to reduce their budgets. The action is often taken in an effort to elicit popular support for budget restorations.
Witches and Goblins	Make the assertion that, if the budget request is not approved, dire consequences will follow. Appeals are based on emotion, not evidence.
We are the Experts	Assert that the proposed budget must be approved because it reflects expert knowledge that "mere managers" cannot hope to understand. This strategy is frequently used by professionals of all types, including scientists, military officers, professors, and physicians.

SOURCE: Adapted from Robert Anthony and Regina Herzlinger, *Management Control in Nonprofit Organizations* 3rd edition, (Irwin, 1980), pp. 344–353.

Professionals may play a variety of games in which their expertise is exploited as a political means of influence. These games are played offensively by emphasizing the uniqueness and importance of their skills and knowledge and defensively by both limiting the access of others to their expertise and discouraging attempts on the part of managers and others to rationalize or routinize it (i.e., to disaggregate it into easily learned steps). The lording games involve the utilization of legitimate authority or certified expertise for illegitimate, usually personal reasons.

Games to defeat rivals, such as the line vs. staff or rival camp games, are zero sum struggles for control over organizational resources, decisions, and/or activities by weakening or sometimes eliminating competitors.

The strategic candidates game is the most common of the games played to effect organizational change. An individual or group seeks a strategic change by promoting through the legitimate systems of influence its own project, proposal, or person as a "strategic candidate." The decision-making process involving strategic decisions often is relatively unstructured, thus encouraging political influence attempts. Furthermore, power within the organization is frequently redistributed during periods of strategic change, usually in favor of those who initially proposed and fought for it. Although strategic candidates in this game are promoted through the legitimate channels of influence, it is important to note that they are supported, at least in part, for nonlegitimate reasons (e.g., in order to defeat rivals or to facilitate empire building).

The whistle-blowing game is usually played by an individual at a relatively low level in the hierarchy of authority who questions the legitimacy of actions by superiors and appeals to powerful individuals outside the organization for support. In the young Turks game, a small group, often with a significant power base, uses political means in attempts to effect fundamental changes in the organization's mission or in the systems of authority, expertise, or ideology. For example, in one religiously-sponsored multi-institutional system, a group of newly hired M.B.A. graduates working at the corporate level engaged in a campaign to shift the emphasis of the system toward a bottom-line orientation and away from a traditional, mission-driven orientation.

Most health care organizations must coordinate the activities of a diverse group of highly trained professionals. The traditional system of formal authority tends to be relatively weak in these organizations. Specifically, there is often ambiguity in how to operationalize or prioritize organizational goals, particularly with respect to the curing, caring, and rehabilitation functions of health services organizations. In addition, because of the difficulties involved in measuring outcomes of professional performance, when goals are imposed on professionals by a managerial hierarchy, they are often easy to deflect. Second, among highly trained professionals, identification with a discipline and professional society may well be stronger than with the organization. When many types of professionals are present, intergroup conflict is likely as factions develop along lines of varying professional interests, orientations to patient care, or status distinctions among such groups. Third, highly skilled professionals have a tendency to invert means and ends—to focus on maintenance and further development of their own skills rather than broader organizational objectives. Further, although the skills themselves may be well defined, the situations to which they may be most appropriately applied often are not. As the opening case illustrates, this situation may lead to territorial disputes over patients, clients, and activities among different disciplines and specialties within health services organizations. Finally, professionals traditionally have been expected to give the highest priority to the needs of their own individual patients or clients—an expectation likely to generate conflicts both with other professionals serving as patient or client advocates and with managers espousing organization-wide objectives. This combination of weak formal authority and highly developed systems of expertise creates strong catalysts for the use of politics as a means for achieving organizational goals or implementing major decisions.

The ambiguities and conflicts generated by strong expertise and weak authority systems are most likely to give rise to those political games in which peers compete with each other for the allocation of resources. Alliance and empire building, budgeting, rival camps, and strategic candidates games tend to be particularly important. It is also important for managers to note that they can often exercise considerable influence in health services organizations not by relying on the formal system of authority but by their centrality in the organization and a willingness to engage in the political process. When conflict resolution emerges as a critical organizational function, managers may attain influence commensurate with their skills in mediation and negotiation.

POWER STRATEGIES AND TACTICS

The actual use of power to affect organizational decisions or to implement those decisions is, in practice, a subtle, artful process. Power is most effectively used when it is employed as unobtrusively as possible.[108] For example, implicit threats by physicians to withdraw their patients or to send them to other institutions are most effective when such threats remain unspoken and not expressed overtly or presented as an ultimatum. A second principle related to the use of power is that attempts to influence are most effective if they are cloaked in an aura of legitimacy and rational purpose. That is, although personal or subunit preferences may drive the exercise of power toward a certain decision, outcome, or implementation process, the outward arguments presented for such outcomes or processes must be based ostensibly on achieving legitimation of actions or decisions. A third type of power strategy involves increasing support from other powerful actors in the organization for a particular decision or action.

The first two strategies, unobtrusive use of power and legitimation of decisions or actions, can be accomplished through a variety of means. One of the most common is to advocate the use of criteria which favor one's own position. This is a particularly common tactic in situations where multiple measures for assessing alternatives are available. Physicians operating in a high

MANAGERIAL GUIDELINES

1. Recognize different sources of power. In the majority of health care organizations, power is derived from multiple sources—formal authority, control over critical resources, expertise, and to a lesser extent, individual charisma. Effective health care managers must be able to distinguish among different types of power, be sensitive to the source of their own power, and be careful to keep their actions consistent with others' expectations.

2. Use power selectively. Effective health care managers must understand the costs, risks, and benefits of using each type of power and must be able to recognize which to draw on in different situations and with different people.

3. Power and influence are not inexhaustable. Influence in health services organizations should be considered a finite rather than an unlimited resource. Managers should direct their influence attempts toward those issues of highest priority or where the greatest benefits are likely to result and be willing to defer in other areas.

4. Position yourself centrally in communications networks. The highly complex and professional nature of most health services organizations usually results in multiple power centers. Managers can often exercise considerable influence not by relying on the formal system of authority but rather by establishing themselves in a central position vis-a-vis other power holders and being willing to engage in the political process.

5. Use negotiation and mediation skills to control conflict. The diffuse power arrangements and multiple goals of health services organizations may lead to recurring conflicts among individuals and groups. When conflict resolution emerges as a critical function, managers who have developed negotiation and mediation skills may attain considerable influence.

6. Develop power by controlling strategic contingencies and resources. Be aware of less visible but important power relations that occur outside the formal system of authority in organizations. Increase individual and departmental power by effectively dealing with strategic contingencies that face the organization.

7. Political behavior and conflict are normal aspects of organizational change. Regard political behavior and conflict as expected, normal aspects of organizational life. To be an effective agent for change, use power through building coalitions, cooptation of influential members of the organization or external stakeholder groups, and the control of decision-making premises.

8. Use politics under conditions of ambiguity and uncertainty. Employ principles of the rational model of organizations when goals are well defined and easily measured, when alternatives are clear, and when the relationship between means and outcomes is unambiguous. When these conditions are not present, consider using the political process to achieve desired ends.

cost, technology-intensive cardiac care facility may advocate the use of quality-related criteria for budget allocation decisions rather than efficiency-related measures. The key point here is that by politically advocating that a certain set of standards or criteria be applied to a rational process, the use of power becomes legitimated through a standard organizational practice such as budgeting. A related strategy frequently employed in health services organizations is the use of outside experts or consultants. Such consultants can permit power to be used to affect decisions in a less visible way as well as lend to the decision-making process an aura of legitimacy fostered by the expertise of the consultant. At the same time, however, consultants may be carefully chosen to represent certain positions advocated by particular groups or interests within the health care organization. For example, a manager interested in adopting a diversification strategy in his hospital may hire consultants known for their expertise in this area.

The third major strategy, coalition building, reflects the processes through which power and support is developed for political contests within organizations. Somewhat ironically, it is the interdependencies that exist within organizations that promote coalition building just as these interdependencies promote the conflict that leads to political action and influence attempts in organizational settings. In health services organizations, the formation of coalitions or alliances between groups and individuals is particularly central to the implementation of organizational decisions because power itself tends to be widely diffused in these types of organizations. The diffusion of power suggests that it is unlikely that any one individual or group will have the requisite degree of power or influence to effectively push the organization toward change or to implement an important strategic decision. For example, to effectively implement a decision to diversify into long-term care, hospital management may be required to build coalitions among key groups of physicians, nurses, and ancillary personnel who share an interest in this arena and who can help to defend this decision and overcome resistance by those groups who are more oriented toward acute inpatient care. The facts that multiple groups are affected by such decisions and that power is diffused so broadly among different subunits and occupational groups within the hospital suggest that coalition building is a necessary strategy for decision implementation, particularly for far-reaching and important decisions.

A frequently overlooked aspect of coalition building in health care organizations is that such coalitions may be externally as well as internally based. Many health care organizations are highly dependent upon important actors and organizations in their environment such as regulatory bodies, major purchasers of health care, key community leaders, and members of the board of directors. Thus, many subgroups in health care organizations often attempt to develop relationships with external stakeholder groups as a way of enhancing their power within the organization and as a means of gaining support for their positions in organizational decisions. Medical staff members of a hospital may, for example, attempt to develop friendships with key members of the hospital's governing board in order to exercise influence over the purchase of a new piece of medical technology or, in some cases, express displeasure over the behavior of the hospital CEO. The hospital CEO may attempt to develop a relationship with key local purchasers of health care who would support him in key decisions affecting the strategic direction of the hospital. In developing any external alliance, managers must be prepared to weigh the trade-offs between the utility of these alliances and the potential influence exercised by external actors versus the cost that cultivating external sources of support might be construed as a disloyal act by others in the organization.

POWER, POLITICS, AND ORGANIZATIONAL PERFORMANCE

This chapter began with the claim that many managers view the use of power and politics in their organizations as dysfunctional for the attainment of organizational goals and positive organizational performance. Recent writings, in contrast, have maintained that the use of power and politics in organizational settings can serve to facilitate the implementation of important decisions in these organizations. In all likelihood, the truth probably lies somewhere between these two extremes. There is no doubt that influence attempts can be expensive and time consuming. Engaging in political activity, for example, may dissipate the energies and focus of management in health care organizations, restrict the flow of important information to decision makers and distort perceptions about the opinions of others in the decision-making process. Indeed, in organizations that appear to be operating effectively and efficiently, the use of politics and informal influence is likely to make the organization more inefficient. Managers of successful health services organizations who desire to reduce inefficiencies stemming from political activity in their organizations might choose several approaches.

- If possible, increase the level of slack resources in their organizations to reduce conflict and to allow subunits to attain their own goals.

- Reduce differentiation and heterogeneity among organizational members and units so as to promote consensus in organizational goals, common views of means to achieve these goals, and a common culture to bind organizational members together.
- Divide organizational rewards more evenly so that nothing substantial is to be gained from attempts at political influence.

Such strategies for reducing the level of influence and politics in organizations are also appropriate for managers who simply do not feel comfortable or have the skills associated with using power in organizational settings.

However, in the current health care environment, few organizations can be successful without adapting, often in significant ways, to the changing demands imposed by stakeholders, regulators, or competitors.

In situations where major changes in strategy, technology, approach to the market, and management of the work force are required, power and influence processes may be useful and even necessary to achieve such transformations. Over time, power may become institutionalized in health services organizations, that is, imbedded strongly in certain individuals, occupational groups, or departments. This is likely to result in a situation characterized by status quo orientation and inertia. Those in power will strive to keep that power by advocating positions that maintain the structures, strategies, and activities that brought them to power in the first place. As illustrated below, change and adaptation typically come only after great internal political struggle. Thus, to effect change which will ultimately benefit the organization, managers must be prepared to utilize power in a fashion to overcome inertia, resolve turf battles, and channel the diverse interests of organizational members and stakeholders.

DEBATE TIME 9.1: WHAT DO YOU THINK?

Trauma services in "Bay State" are coordinated by the state's Institute for Emergency Medical Services, a broad network that includes the State Shock-Trauma Center, other trauma centers strategically located in hospitals across the state, and the ambulance and helicopter personnel who transport patients. Since its founding a quarter of a century ago, the 130-bed shock-trauma facility has been reserved for the most critical trauma patients, many of whom are flown in from all regions of the state with life-threatening injuries due to auto accidents. The Shock-Trauma Center also performs medical triage for the statewide Emergency Medical Services (EMS) system.

For some years the Shock-Trauma Center shared facilities with the state's major University Hospital. Although they were both governed by the same not-for-profit corporation, the Shock-Trauma Center operated with considerable autonomy. In 1984 the state granted approval for a new $35 million separate facility for the Shock-Trauma Center. Part of the agreement included the decision to transfer all trauma care provided in the University Hospital Emergency Department, including patients with knife and gunshot wounds, to the Shock-Trauma Center which would be located only a few

blocks away. The rationale for this decision was to conserve resources by not duplicating trauma care personnel and equipment.

Although the move to the new building was completed in 1989, Shock-Trauma physicians resisted treating a category of patients that they perceived as diluting the center's main mission. In 1992 a new director for the Shock-Trauma Center was hired by the not-for-profit corporation that governed both that facility and the University Hospital. The Shock-Trauma Center was ordered by top managers of the corporation to begin treating all trauma injuries that would in the past have been seen in the University Hospital Emergency Department. Three prominent Shock-Trauma physicians who resisted these changes were fired. At a well-attended news conference defending these changes, the new director, Dr. Bradley, explained that in an era of dwindling resources and soaring health care costs, it was important to end duplication and to move the Shock-Trauma Center into a closer collaboration with the adjacent university medical center.

Since the initial organization of the state's EMS system, the Shock-Trauma Center had assumed responsibility for medical triage, including directing the personnel transporting trauma victims to the most appropriate facility with available resources. The proposal to tighten the relationship between Shock-Trauma and University Hospital generated considerable concerns among other trauma system members regarding whether "patients would continue to be sent to where they could get the best treatment." Separate news conferences were called by a group of physicians representing other hospitals with trauma centers and by the state's volunteer firefighters responsible for the transport of trauma patients. The firefighters complained that they had not been consulted about recent changes in the EMS system. In addition, in separate statements to the press, conflicting positions on these issues were adopted by the governor who supported the new Shock-Trauma director, and several key legislators who sided with the fired surgeons in their belief that broadening the center's focus would dilute its quality.

At this point in the conflict, the state's largest newspaper published an article comparing Dr. Bradley to the original founder of the Shock-Trauma Center, Dr. Gordon, who "was a one-man wrecking crew if someone got in his way." According to the newspaper, Dr. Gordon:

> . . . did not suffer fools or foes for very long. As he told colleagues, "Only a dog needs to be loved." The results, not his popularity, were all that mattered.
>
> And he succeeded brilliantly. Over the vehement opposition of other hospitals, jealous physicians, possessive bureaucrats and busy-body legislators, he carved out a new field of medicine—emergency medical services.
>
> Employing innovative techniques, he declared war on behalf of critically injured accident victims. By getting patients into the operating room in that first "golden hour," and by throwing teams of surgeons into

the battle, he performed miracles. More often than not, he won the war. Thousands of lives were saved.

Along the way, he collected enemies. It didn't faze him. He was smart enough to win the loyalty of a governor, key legislators, firefighters, and paramedics. Only when he was slowing down, when his own Shock-Trauma doctors turned against him in 1989 for creating "general chaos," did he step down. He died last fall.

Now some of the same doctors are seeking another scalp: Dr. Bradley's. Their complaint is ironic: they don't want Shock-Trauma to change. Yet this is an institution created out of change—a dramatic rethinking of how to treat critically injured accident victims. Dr. Gordon's whole life at the Shock-Trauma Center was about change. He kept the place in constant turmoil.

Time, especially in today's high-tech medical world, does not stand still. This is an era of severe government deficits, a time when the public is demanding accountability. Yet Shock-Trauma had been notorious for its lack of accountability and its free-spending ways. It insisted on total independence. That is now changing. Interdependence is the key word. And there is a strong effort to depoliticize what are essentially medical matters.

Dr. Gordon was superb at getting what he wanted from the politicians and winning public acclaim. At this stage, Dr. Bradley lacks the political skills that served Dr. Gordon so well. The circus at Shock-Trauma is likely to continue. Dr. Bradley's foes will see to that. But, what the heck. As Dr. Gordon used to say, "You can tell the pioneers by the arrows in their backs."

Fortunately, most political conflict in organizations does not reach the level of intensity displayed in this example. It does provide a vivid illustration, however, of the types of conflicts that may be encountered in determining organizational goals, as well as the fragility of the balance of influence in many multi-institutional arrangements.

Adapted by permission from Barry Rascovar, "Shock and Trauma at the Shock-Trauma Center," The Baltimore *Sun August 9, 1992.*

KEY CONCEPTS

Alliances
Authority
Coalitions
Cooptation
Cope with Uncertainties
Formal Authority System
Influence
Influence Systems
Interdependency
Interests
Political Games
Political Model of Organizations
Politics
Power
Rational Model of Organizations
Sources of Power
Uncertainty

Discussion Questions

1. Using concepts from the chapter, can you identify the various political strategies used by Dr. Gordon and Dr. Bradley?

2. As illustrated in Debate Time 9.1, what are some of the functions and some of the possible dysfunctions of using political strategies to effect change in organizations?

3. Do you agree that a strong effort should be made to "depoliticize what are essentially medical matters?"

4. Do you agree with Dr. Gordon's statement, "You can tell the pioneers by the arrows in their backs?" Is this type of outcome inevitable for change agents? (You may want to base your reasoning on concepts from this chapter as well as Chapter 12, Organizational Innovation and Change.)

REFERENCES

1. Cyert RM, March JG. *A Behavioral Theory of the Firm.* Englewood Cliffs, NJ: Prentice-Hall, 1963.
2. Buck VE. A model for viewing an organization as a system of constraints. In: Thompson JD, ed. *Approaches to Organizational Design.* Pittsburgh, Pa: University of Pittsburgh Press, 1966.
3. MacMillan IC. *Strategy Formulation: Political Concepts.* St. Paul, Minn: West, 1978.
4. March JG, Olsen JP. *Ambiguity and Choice in Organizations.* Bergen, Norway: Universitetsforlaget, 1976.
5. Pfeffer J. *Power in Organizations.* Marshfield, Mass: Pitman Publishing, 1981.
6. Pfeffer J. *Managing With Power: Politics and Influence in Organizations.* Boston, Mass: Harvard Business School Press, 1992.
7. Ibid.
8. Kanter RM. Power failure in management circuits. *Harvard Business Review.* 1979; 57(4):65–75.
9. Kotter JP. *Power and Influence: Beyond Formal Authority.* New York, NY: Free Press, 1985.
10. Young DW, Saltman RB. *The Hospital Power Equilibrium: Physician Behavior and Cost Control.* Baltimore, Md: The Johns Hopkins University Press, 1985.
11. Perrow C. The analysis of goals in complex organizations. *American Sociological Review.* 1961:854–866.
12. Perrow C. Goals and power structures: A historical case study. In Freidson E, ed. *The Hospital in Modern Society.* New York, NY: Macmillan, 1963.
13. Pfeffer, 1992, op. cit.
14. Pfeffer, 1981, op. cit.
15. Pfeffer, 1992, op. cit.
16. Kotter JP. Power, dependence and effective management. *Harvard Business Review.* 1977;55(4):135–136.
17. Kouzes JM, Posner BZ. *The Leadership Challenge: How to Get Extraordinary Things Done in Organizations.* San Francisco, Ca: Jossey-Bass, 1988.
18. Salancik GR, Pfeffer J. Who gets power—and how they hold on to it: A strategic contingency model of power. *Organizational Dynamics.* 1977;5:3–21.
19. Pfeffer, 1992, op. cit.
20. Bennis W, Nanus B. *Leaders: The Strategies for Taking Charge.* New York, NY: Harper and Row; 1985.
21. Kotter JP. Power, success, and organizational effectiveness. *Organizational Dynamics.* 1978; 6(3):27–40.
22. Morgan G. *Images of Organization.* Beverly Hills, Ca: Sage, 1986.
23. Bacharach SB. *Power and Politics in Organizations.* San Francisco, Ca: Jossey-Bass; 1980.
24. Mintzberg H. *Power In and Around Organizations.* Englewood Cliffs, NJ: Prentice-Hall; 1983.
25. Morgan, op. cit.
26. Mintzberg, op. cit.
27. Cialdini RB. *Influence: Science and Practice.* 2nd ed. Glenview, Ill: Scott, Foresman; 1984.
28. March, Olsen, op. cit.
29. Pfeffer, 1981, op. cit.
30. Perrow, 1961, op. cit.
31. Perrow, 1963, op. cit.
32. Morgan, op. cit.
33. Mintzberg, op. cit.
34. Young, Saltman, op. cit.
35. Crozier M. *The Bureaucratic Phenomenon.* Chicago, Ill: University of Chicago Press; 1964.
36. Mintzberg, op. cit.
37. O'Donnell C. The source of managerial authority. *Political Science Quarterly.* 1952; 67:573–588.
38. Morgan, op. cit.
39. Perrow C. Departmental power and perspectives in industrial firms. In: Zald MN, ed. *Power in Organizations.* Nashville, Tenn: Vanderbilt University Press, 1970:58–59.
40. Lourenco SV, Glidewell JC. A dialectical analysis of organizational conflict. *Administrative Science Quarterly.* 1975:489–508.
41. Pfeffer, 1992, op. cit.
42. Morgan, op. cit.
43. Hannan MT, Freeman J. Structural inertia and organizational change. *American Sociological Review.* 1984;49:149–164.
44. Tushman ML, Newman WH, Romanelli E. Convergence and upheaval: Managing the unsteady pace of organizational evolution. *California Management Review.* 1986;29:29–44.
45. Pfeffer, 1981, op. cit.
46. Pfeffer, 1992, op. cit.
47. Pfeffer, 1981, op. cit.
48. Pfeffer, 1992, op. cit.
49. Pfeffer, 1981, op. cit.
50. Pfeffer, 1992, op. cit.
51. Morgan, op. cit.
52. Mintzberg, op. cit.
53. Pfeffer J, Salancik GR. Organizational decision making as a political process: The case of a university budget. *Administrative Science Quarterly.* 1974;19:135–151.
54. MacMillan, op. cit.
55. Salancik GR, Pfeffer J. The bases and use of power in organizational decision making: The case of a university. *Administrative Science Quarterly.* 1974;19:453–473.
56. Pfeffer, 1981, op. cit.
57. Pfeffer, 1992, op. cit.

58. Hinings CR, Hickson DJ, Pennings JM, Schneck RE. Structural conditions of intraorganizational power. *Administrative Science Quarterly.* 1974;19:22–44.
59. Pfeffer J, Salancik GR. *The External Control of Organizations: A Resource Dependence Perspective.* New York, NY: Harper and Row; 1978.
60. Pfeffer, 1992, op. cit.
61. Hinings, et al., op. cit.
62. Edelman M. *The Symbolic Uses of Politics.* Urbana, Ill: University of Illinois Press, 1964.
63. Pfeffer, 1992, op. cit.
64. Mechanic D. Sources of power of lower participants in complex organizations. *Administrative Science Quarterly.* 1962;7:349–364.
65. Brass DJ. Being in the right place: A structural analysis of individual influence in an organization. *Administrative Science Quarterly.* 1984;29:518–539.
66. Hickson DJ, et al. A strategic contingencies' theory of intraorganizational power. *Administrative Science Quarterly.* 1971;16:216–229.
67. Jacobs D. Dependency and vulnerability: An exchange approach to the control of organizations. *Administrative Science Quarterly.* 1974:45–59.
68. Blau PM. *Exchange and Power in Social Life.* New York, NY: John Wiley, 1964.
69. Pfeffer J, Davis-Blake A. Understanding organizational wage structures: A resource dependence approach. *Academy of Management Journal.* 1987;30:437–455.
70. Young, Saltman, op. cit., 60.
71. Mechanic, op. cit.
72. McNeil K. Understanding organizational power: Building on the Weberian legacy. *Administrative Science Quarterly.* 1978:65–90.
73. Gamson WA. A theory of coalition formation. *American Sociological Review.* 1961:373–382.
74. Pfeffer, 1992, op. cit.
75. Ibid.
76. Izraeli DN. The middle manager and the tactics of power expansion: A case study. *Sloan Management Review.* 1975:57–70.
77. Hackman JD. Power and centrality in the allocation of resources in colleges and universities. *Administrative Science Quarterly.* 1985;30:61–77.
78. Burns LR, Andersen RM, Shortell SM. The impact of corporate structures on physician inclusion and participation. *Medical Care.* 1989:27(10):967–982.
79. Shortell SM. *Effective Hospital Physician Relationships.* Ann Arbor, Mich: Health Administration Press, 1992.
80. Scott WR. Managing professional work: Three models of control for health organizations. *Health Services Research.* 1982;17:213–240.
81. Moore T, Wood D. Power and the hospital executive. *Hospital and Health Services Administration.* 1979; 24:30–41.

82. Weber M. *The Theory of Social and Economic Organization.* New York, NY: Free Press, 1947.
83. Tannenbaum AS. *Control in Organizations.* Englewood Cliffs, NJ: Prentice-Hall, 1968.
84. Pfeffer, 1992, op. cit.
85. Brass, op. cit.
86. Hickson, et al., op. cit.
87. Fligstein N. The intraorganizational power struggle: Rise of finance personnel to top leadership in large corporations, 1919–1979. *American Sociological Review.* 1987;52:44–58.
88. Alexander JA, Morrisey MA, Shortell SM. The effects of competition, regulation and corporatization on hospital-physician relationships. *Journal Health and Social Behavior.* 1986;27:220–235.
89. Glandon GL, Morrisey MA. Redefining the hospital-physician relationship under prospective payment. *Inquiry.* 1986;23:175–186.
90. Roemer MI, Friedman JW. *Doctors in Hospitals.* Baltimore, Md: Johns Hopkins University Press, 1971.
91. Scott, op. cit.
92. Young, Saltman, op. cit.
93. Burns, et al., op. cit.
94. Heydebrand WV. Autonomy, complexity, and nonbureaucratic coordination in professional organizations. In: Heydebrand, W, ed. *Comparative Organizations.* Englewood Cliffs, NJ: Prentice-Hall; 1973:158–189.
95. Eisenhardt M, Bourgeois LJ. Politics of strategic decision making in high-velocity environments: Toward a midrange theory. *Academy of Management Journal.* 1988;31:737–770.
96. Morgan, op. cit.
97. Pfeffer, 1981, op. cit.
98. Pfeffer, 1992, op. cit.
99. Davis OA, Dempster MAH, Wildavsky A. A theory of the budgeting process. *American Political Science Review.* 1966;60:529–547.
100. Hills FS, Mahoney TA. University budgets and organizational decision making. *Administrative Science Quarterly.* 1978;23:454–465.
101. Hannan and Freeman *op. cit.*
102. Pfeffer, 1992, op. cit.
103. Mintzberg, op. cit.
104. Maccoby M. *The Gamesman.* New York, NY: Simon & Schuster; 1976.
105. Allen RW, et al. Organizational politics: Tactics and characteristics of its actors. *California Management Review.* 1979;22:66–83.
106. Mintzberg, op. cit.
107. Kanter RM. *Men and Women of the Corporation.* New York, NY: Basic Books, 1977.
108. Pfeffer, 1992, op. cit.

THE NATURE OF ORGANIZATIONS: FRAMEWORK FOR THE TEXT

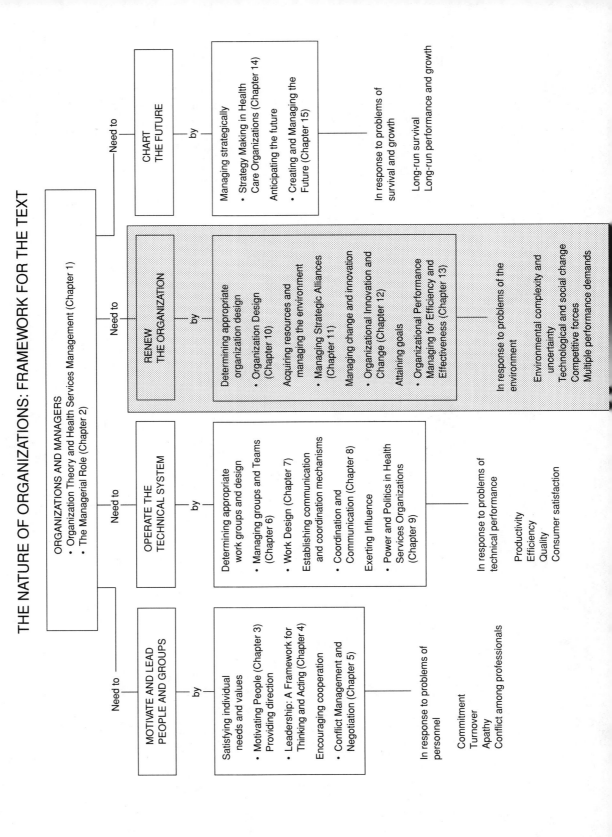

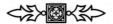

PART FOUR

RENEWING THE ORGANIZATION

Organizations operate within a complex and dynamic environment. Health care executives thus manage the environment as well as the operations within their own organization. The four chapters in this section highlight the nature of the managerial role in terms of understanding and developing strategies for effective intervention.

Chapter 10, Organizational Design, focuses on fundamental principles, evolution, and alternative designs in terms of their strengths and limitations. The chapter addresses the following questions:

- What is organization design? What is the role of management in the design and redesign of organizations?
- What are the components and characteristics of design?
- What designs are available, and what are their strengths and weaknesses relative to different environments?

Chapter 11, Managing Strategic Alliances, deals with the emergence and operations of such alliances. The chapter focuses on the following questions:

- What are the types and forms of alliance structures?
- What are the processes and dimensions which distinguish these structures?
- What are the stages or processes involved in the development of an alliance?

Chapter 12, Organizational Innovation and Change, presents an analysis of the change process and the various types of changes involved in health services organizations. Among the questions it addresses are the following:

- What are the stages of the change process, and what factors facilitate or inhibit that process?
- What are the different types of changes that may occur, and what strategies are appropriate to assure successful implementation and institutionalization?

Chapter 13, Organizational Performance: Managing for Efficiency and Effectiveness, provides an overview of the various dimensions of performance and the issues that face health care managers and their organizations. Among the questions addressed are the following:

- What is organizational performance?
- What criteria are appropriate to differential performance?
- What can managers do to improve quality?

Upon completing these four chapters, readers should understand the fundamental design of organizations, their relationship to other organizations, and how this relationship affects organizational performance and change.

CHAPTER

10

ORGANIZATION DESIGN

Peggy Leatt, Ph.D.
Professor

Stephen M. Shortell, Ph.D.
Professor

John R. Kimberly, Ph.D.
Professor

CHAPTER TOPICS

The Meaning of Organization Design
Levels of Organization Design
Systematic Assessment before Design
Designs for a Variety of Health Services
    Organizations
New Evolving Designs
Influences on Future Organization Designs

LEARNING OBJECTIVES

After completing this chapter, the reader should be able to

1. understand the principles of organization design
2. have an awareness of the evolution of organization design
3. use a framework for understanding organization design considerations
4. analyze common organization designs in terms of their applicability, strengths, and limitations
5. consider guidelines for changing organization designs

CHAPTER PURPOSE

The purpose of this chapter is to explore ways in which organizations, especially health services organizations, make decisions about redesigning organizational structures. Given the complex nature of the external environment in which organizations must operate in order to survive, managers must actively decide who has responsibility for making which decisions at various levels. In other words, who will have power in the organization and for what purposes? The focus of the chapter is on

IN THE REAL WORLD
TO DECENTRALIZE OR NOT TO DECENTRALIZE?

- Does the decentralization and restructuring of work into patient-centered multidisciplinary teams lead to better outcomes of care?
- Does *patient-centered care* result in different costs? That is, how much will it cost to integrate care through patient-centered multidisciplinary teams? To what extent will the increased efficiency and cost effectiveness achieved through such approaches outweigh the added costs of implementing these programs?
- What is the impact of patient-centered care on the satisfaction, recruitment, and retention of physicians, nurses, and other clinical staff?
- Based on observations of the skills and knowledge required of clinical and technical staff in a patient-centered system, what recommendations can be made for the future education and training of physicians, nurses, and other clinicians?

In the pursuit of providing more cost-effective care, many health services organizations are asking themselves the above questions. One such organization is the New England Medical Center (NEMC): a 516-bed hospital, affiliated with the Tufts Medical School in Boston. NEMC has been a leader in experimentation and innovation in

health care delivery. Its overarching goal is to improve the quality of life, functioning, and satisfaction of patients, the center's affiliated institutions, and staff. NEMC is guided by three fundamental values

- to be patient-centered, not task- or location-centered, taking into account the patients' role in managing their health and medical care
- to be outcome driven, broadening the definition and measurement of outcomes to include not just traditional clinical indicators but also patient functional status and the satisfaction of both patients and clinicians
- to continuously improve performance with particular focus on improving quality, empowering staff, and aligning reward and recognition systems with the institution's overall goals and mission

Consistent with their mission, in the early 1990s NEMC undertook a series of interrelated changes designed to promote more patient-centered care. The objective was to organize care on the basis of an entire episode of illness as viewed from the patient's perspective. Components of this redesign included

- restructuring clinical jobs and roles
- decentralizing support and technical functions
- creating multidisciplinary teams that could function across professional, technical, and geographic boundaries
- developing clinical care protocols to assist teams in the provision of care across the episode of illness
- using patient satisfaction and, where possible, clinical outcome data to continuously improve performance

These changes were to be implemented initially in the adult and pediatric hematology-oncology units and the cardiology-cardiovascular surgery unit. The above represented a substantial change in organizational design with significant structural and behavioral implications. Fortunately, NEMC has three strong traditions upon which to build

- a long-standing commitment to clinical excellence and a track record of innovation in the pursuit of such excellence
- a matrix management system involving collaboration among physicians, nurses, and managers centered around a collaborative practice model that uses a case management approach
- the involvement of clinical and operating staff

in the design, development, and implementation of innovative programs

Operating within such a culture of change and innovation, NEMC is successfully dealing with numerous issues associated with the organizational redesign. These have included

- dealing with the very different processes associated with inpatient care versus ambulatory and home care
- dealing with the threat to people's traditional roles
- dealing with historical differences among the involved departments
- gaining cooperation from departments not directly involved in the change
- contending with naturally occurring staff turnover

Two keys to NEMC's success have been customizing its approach to the different units affected by the redesign (using a group process with the pediatric unit and an individual process with the cardiology-cardiovascular unit) and providing a common visible set of information to all parties involved regarding the status of everyone's efforts. In addition, the entire process has been overseen by an adept project director with sufficient support resources to deal with contingencies as they occur.

SOURCE: *Evaluation of the New England Medical Center project to restructure work in support of patient centered outcome-driven care models. Evanston, Ill: Center for Health Services and Policy Research and JL Kellogg Graduate School of Management, Northwestern University. Funded by the PEW Charitable Trusts, January 1, 1990 through October, 1993.*

exploring a variety of organization designs which are typical of health services organizations and analyzing where the designs seem to work best. Given the changing environment of health care, designs which will help organizations maintain high performance during times of transition are highlighted.

THE MEANING OF ORGANIZATION DESIGN

Design is Dynamic

Organization design refers to the way in which the building blocks of organization—authority, responsibility, accountability, information, and rewards—are arranged or rearranged to improve effectiveness and adaptive capacity. Organization design and redesign are dynamic, being simultaneously *both outcome* and *process*. As outcome, organization design can be represented by the boxes and lines on an organization chart. These represent how the building blocks are arranged. As many organizations face increasingly uncertain and rapidly changing environments, new ways of representing organization are emerging, replacing boxes and lines. Intersecting circles, inverted triangles, and lattices are alternative ways of describing the outcomes of design and redesign.

Design outcomes, however, are generally transitory. Top management of most organizations is always searching for more effective ways to carry out their mission; and as external circumstances change, redesign may well be indicated. In effect, then, design and redesign constitute a process whereby current arrangements are evaluated and new ones are introduced, in some cases almost continuously.

Although we might like to think of organizational design as a rational, deliberate, and planned series of activities in which men and women of vision create organizational arrangements supportive of mission and strategy and performance-enhancing, in reality—particularly in a sector as volatile as health care—the design process reflects the realities of change. Changes in leadership, changes in goals and strategies, and pure accident are all reasons why a change in design may occur on other than a perfectly "rational" basis.[1]

Management's Role in Organization Design

Management's primary task is to maintain and improve performance in the organization. In fact, management texts refer to organization design as one of management's most critical functions.[2-4] Usually, the activities of design are seen as the responsibilities of senior management; however, the most successful designs appear to be those that have been built with input from a broad range of organizational members, including key external and internal stakeholders and persons at all levels within the organization. Outside consultants are sometimes brought in to provide technical advice on the range of designs that might be considered.

Often organization design has been thought of as a "once and for all event" parallel to an architect or engineer designing and constructing a new building. In our view, when a new organization is formed, a new design will be created; however, the redesign of the organization is an ongoing process in which the design needs will change as the organization's needs change. The idea that designing organizations may be a recurring activity is most important for managers who may not only have responsibility for redesigning their organizations but also for ensuring that the design is implemented.[5]

The design process is not carried out in isolation from other management activities. In fact, ideas about the type of design that might be appropriate should be derived from the organization's mission and strategic planning process.[6] For example, if an organization such as a hospital decides to diversify its product lines and expand to new patient programs, it may be necessary to rearrange the division of labor within the organization. Alternatively, if a long-term care facility decides to close down a geriatric day program, it may be necessary to regroup ongoing services within the organization.

The way in which an organization is designed also has considerable importance for the nature and content of the information system needed by the organization. Since an organization design specifies who has power to make which decisions, it also indicates which positions need what types of information and at what times. Organization design also has implications for how performance will be evaluated and especially for the degree to which the reward system of the organization matches achievement or performance. Finally, the knowledge gathered from performance indicators will be fed back to subsequently influence the organization's mission. The relationships of organization design to these other management activities can be seen in Figure 10.1.

When Should an Organization's Design be Rethought?

There are a number of circumstances that would suggest a manager should be reconsidering the appropriateness of an organization's design. Some examples of triggers or indicators that the best design may not be in place include:

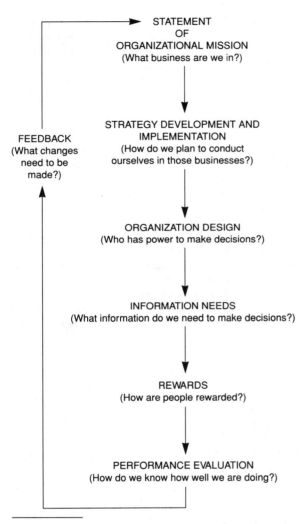

STATEMENT
OF
ORGANIZATIONAL MISSION
(What business are we in?)

STRATEGY DEVELOPMENT AND
IMPLEMENTATION
(How do we plan to conduct
ourselves in those businesses?)

FEEDBACK
(What changes
need to be
made?)

ORGANIZATION DESIGN
(Who has power to make decisions?)

INFORMATION NEEDS
(What information do we need to make decisions?)

REWARDS
(How are people rewarded?)

PERFORMANCE EVALUATION
(How do we know how well we are doing?)

FIGURE 10.1. Organization design in relation to other management activities.

- The organization is experiencing severe problems. Indicators of inadequate performance may be presented to the manager from external reviews such as accreditation processes and customer satisfaction surveys or from internal reviews such as financial statements and clinical audits. These problems may be identified at varying levels within the organization, for example, for a particular position, a work group, a department, or a total organization.

- There is a change in the environment which directly influences internal policies. In some circumstances there may be major changes in the environment, such as prospective payment for hospital services, capitation payment for all health services received by a given population, or new policies regulating pharmaceuticals. These changes may require a redesign and refocusing of key organizational groups.

- New programs or product lines are developed. When an organization recognizes certain markets or product lines as high priority, an organization design change may be necessary to infuse resources into the new areas. Conversely, when old programs are to be dropped, new structural arrangements may be necessary.

- There is a change in leadership. New leadership may provide considerable opportunity to rethink the way in which the organization has been designed. New leadership tends to view the organization from a different perspective and may bring innovative ideas to the reorganization.

LEVELS OF ORGANIZATION DESIGN

Several aspects of an organization can be redesigned or changed. For example, decisions can be made to change the overall size of the organization, the number and types of units or departments within, and how these units may be grouped. We can also decide to change the span of control of individual managers, reorganize tasks, specify rules and procedures in a formalized or standardized way, reallocate decision-making authority, alter communication channels, change mechanisms of control and reward, and determine how coordination will be achieved.

We typically think of design being achieved for a whole organization, such as a nursing home, a hospital, or a public health unit; however, design may take place for a particular group of departments, for an individual unit or department, or for a specific position (also see Chapter 7). Mintzberg has pointed out that the design of individual positions forms the basic building blocks on which the design of a whole organization is developed.[7] On a wider scale than a single organization, we may also create a design for a network of organizations in a given community or for a system of organizations (also see Chapter 11). These interlocking *levels of organization design* are illustrated in Table 10.1.

Designing a Position

In terms of designing individual positions in the organization, there may be hundreds to choose from, depending upon the organization's size and complexity. For example, a new manager might be hired into a health services organization as an executive assistant to the president. If you were in this position, you would likely be excited about the possibilities and ask the

TABLE 10.1. Levels of Design in Health Services Organizations

Renewing the Organization	
Levels	Some Illustrations
Individual positions	Managers
	Staff positions
	Health professionals
	Other workers
Work groups	Task forces and committees
	Teams
	Units and departments
Clusters of work groups	Division of two or more units
	Medical staff organization
Total organizations	Hospitals
	Primary care centers
	Public health units
	Long-term care facilities
	Health maintenance organizations (HMOs)
	Multispecialty group practices
Network of organizations	Organizations providing services for geriatric patients
	Organizations providing services for oncology patients
	Preferred provider organizations (PPOs)
	Affiliated groups of hospitals
Systems	A chain of hospitals under single ownership
	All home health services in a state
	A national system of health services

president for a copy of your job description. The president, being amused, might inform you that your first task is to prepare a draft of your own position description for management's approval.

In designing an individual job or position for any level within an organization, it is necessary to identify the breadth and scope of tasks that can be performed and the extent to which the work can be standardized.[8] Both of these factors have implications for the skills and training that will be necessary for the persons filling the job.[9] Some of the basic parameters that should be identified include the major responsibilities and roles inherent in the position, to whom the position is accountable, for whose work the position is accountable, and the relationship of other peer positions to it. One technique which has been successfully used in clarifying responsibilities of individual positions is responsibility accounting. With this method the perceptions of members of the relevant role set are obtained to identify who is responsible for which decisions in the organization and who they believe should be responsible.[10] Additional suggestions are discussed in Chapter 7.

Designing a Work Group

Often managers are placed in the position of creating a task force or team to solve a complex problem in a short time frame. For example, a health services manager may be interested in identifying approaches that could be used to examine work processes which could improve the speed with which the results of blood tests are reported. A continuous quality improvement (CQI) or total quality management (TQM) group could be formed for this task. The manager should clarify the specific purpose of the work group, the time frame for completion of the problem solving, and the boundaries of the group's authority.[11] Depending upon the complexity of the problem at hand, the manager should make decisions about the skills and knowledge necessary to complete the task. For example, to investigate the CQI-TQM issue with the results of blood tests, it may be appropriate to use a multidisciplinary approach which includes a nurse, a physician, a laboratory technician, a hematologist, an orderly, or other health workers.[12] The appointment of a leader for the group is also a critical design decision. A similar design approach may be used for deciding upon more permanent work groups such as clinical units, strategic business units, departments, or other groups.[13] These issues are further discussed in Chapters 6 and 7.

Designing a Cluster of Work Groups

In some circumstances it may be necessary to redesign a cluster of departments or units within an organization to form a division. One of the most important design decisions to be made in clustering work groups involves the most appropriate grouping of units to achieve coordination within the division. Grouping of units implies that the units will share a common manager, common resources, and common performance measures.[14] To illustrate the various ways in which units may be grouped, we use the example of the medical staff organization in a general hospital.[15–17] Units may be grouped by knowledge and skill. For example, physicians may be grouped to form divisions by specialty and subspecialty (such as all medical specialities and all surgical specialities). Physicians may also be grouped by work process, for instance, by placing the operating rooms, emergency departments, and radiology under the same management, where they have a common patient flow. Ambulatory care clinic physicians may be grouped by time because they tend to hold clinics in the same time frame. Physicians may be grouped by commonality of clients or patients, for example, cardiovascular surgery and cardiology. Finally, physicians may be grouped because they are geographically located in the same hospital. Mintzberg points out that in large organizations such as hospitals, which employ many professionals, a number of these bases for grouping may be used simultaneously.[18] In addition to the decisions about grouping in designing a division, all the other variables mentioned for designing a work group must be considered. Chapters 6–8 provide further discussion of these issues.

Designing and Redesigning a Total Organization

The parameters of design decisions at this level of analysis have already been mentioned. The challenge at this level is enormous, and the amount of investment necessary to manage the redesign process is extensive.

Perhaps most important, the process has to unfold in such a way that behaviors, not just formal structures, change. And, as Paul Allaire, the chief executive officer (CEO) of Xerox and the principal architect of the redesign of that company, said, "If you talk about change but don't change the reward and recognition system, nothing changes."[19]

Designing a Network

A network of organizations comprises those organizations that exist in a particular community or environment, which may be loosely or closely connected to achieve a common purpose or serve a common clientele.[20] An example is the network of health and social services that may exist in a community to provide services to geriatric patients. Types of organizations within the network may include an acute hospital, a psychiatric hospital, a nursing home, home health services, day care services, meals on wheels, housing and transport services, and so on. The objective in the design of the network is to ensure coordination of services and smoothness of client flow between organizations to maximize effectiveness. One of the key tasks in designing a network involves the identification of the target population to be served by the network. The main demographic and health characteristics of the specific target population must be identified including age, sex, cultural group, language, morbidity and mortality rates by specific diseases, and so on. At the network level, the design process is relatively complex because it involves examining the nature of the relationships among the organizations in the network. Design decisions may include analyzing the interorganizational relationships in terms of deciding which organizations should have the most power, which resource transactions may take place, and how innovations will be diffused.[21] These issues are also considered in Chapter 11.

Designing a System

At the system level, design decisions are even more complex, depending upon the purpose(s) of the system and the heterogeneity of the programs provided. One of the most important factors to be analyzed at the system level is concerned with the degree of *cen-*

tralization and decentralization of decision making.[22,23] For example, given a system of hospitals, which may include as many as 80 acute general hospitals, it is essential to clarify which decisions will be made at the corporate level and which decisions will be made at the regional or individual hospital level.[24–27] Such decisions can be further categorized as those involving the setting of policy (e.g., wage and salary guidelines), initiating activities (e.g., hiring new staff), and granting final approval (e.g., capital budgets). Where the majority of decisions are centered at the corporate office, the organization is said to be vertically centralized. In high technology industries such as health care, greater vertical decentralization is expected because of the expertise at lower levels in the organization. As a general rule, decisions should be made at the lowest possible levels, especially when the majority of workers are professionals.[28,29] Horizontal decentralization refers to the extent to which influence and decision making is shared laterally. In the example of the hospital chain, an important design factor may be deciding upon the extent to which individual hospitals can develop their own strategic plans separately from those developed by the corporate office. A major part of the activities at the decentralized level are concerned with the implementation of policies and ensuring quality.

SYSTEMATIC ASSESSMENT BEFORE DESIGN

Earlier in this chapter, the need to match a design with the organization's mission and strategies as well as obtaining participation from major stakeholders was emphasized. A number of models have been suggested as frameworks for categorizing the information needed for a thorough assessment.[30,31] A model or conceptual framework is an essential tool to guide analysis and action. Most people who have been exposed to organizations have an implicit experience-based model; however, organizational theorists and researchers have now developed general models for thinking about organizations as total systems. The major factors that are essential to consider in an organizational *assessment for design* are shown in Figure 10.2. These factors recognize that organization design decisions should not be made in a vacuum; they need to be made in

the context of a broad managerial framework in which several factors are assessed simultaneously.

The Mission

One of the first and most important considerations in beginning an organization design strategy is to identify the mission of the organization. The mission may have been established through a strategic planning process in which a wide range of stakeholders worked together to provide a clear statement of the vision for the organization. Usually a mission statement identifies "what business the organization is in" and what business it is not in. It may also include statements about the values and ideology of the organization in terms of client services and management. A mission statement usually outlines some more specific formal goals for the organization. Gellerman quotes the American architect Louis Sullivan, writing in 1890, who said, "Form follows function." Gellerman reaffirms that this principle also applies when designing organizations—they should be designed for a specific purpose or function, hence the importance of the mission statement.[32]

Environmental Assessment

Understanding the relationships between organizations and their environments has progressed rapidly since Terreberry suggested that organizational change is increasingly induced by external factors and that organizational adaptability is a result of key members making accommodations to changes in the environment.[33]

Environmental complexity, as defined by Lawrence and Lorsch, assumes that both instabilities in the environment and the heterogeneity of components of the environment create uncertainties which result in different organization designs.[34] It has been assumed that environmental uncertainty affects the degree of formality of structure, the nature of interpersonal relationships, and the time orientation (short- vs. long-run of employees). As uncertainty increases—that is, as environmental conditions become less stable—organizations may divide into specialized subunits along functional lines. As a consequence, the subunits may develop varying priorities and have different time horizons. To ensure expected levels of effectiveness,

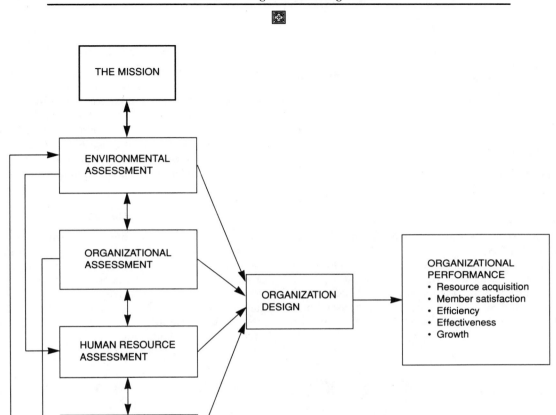

FIGURE 10.2. Overall framework for organization design considerations.

managers must design a variety of mechanisms to achieve integration across subunits. Absence of such mechanisms may lead to conflict and diminished performance.

What design options are available to the manager faced with the consequences of increasing environmental uncertainty? Lawrence and Lorsch advocate the creation of lateral relations such as direct managerial contact across functions, interfunctional teams (either permanent or temporary), liaison roles, and integrating departments.[35] Such design strategies have the ultimate effect of decentralizing decision making so that it takes place at the level of the organization where the neces-

sary information exists. As we discuss later in this chapter, Stein and Kanter have suggested a parallel organizational design as one mechanism for integrating persons from all levels in the organization in the decision-making process.[36] And as Robert Howard's interview with Paul Allaire, the CEO of Xerox, indicates, increasing environmental volatility calls for an organization design which pushes responsibility, resources, and accountability as close to the market as possible.[37]

It has also been recognized that organization design may be contingent upon the technology of the organization. Perrow indicated that in many human service organizations where technology is more likely to be nonroutine, the structure will be less bureaucratized—there will be less programming of tasks, fewer rules and regulations, fewer levels in the hierarchy, greater coordination by feedback, greater decentralization in decision making, and a tendency to employ more professionals.[38]

Organizational Assessment

An important stage in preparing to redesign an organization is to identify the strengths and limitations of the organization. Since every organization is different, this assessment can be carried out in a number of ways.[39] A frequently used approach is to conduct focus group discussions of the most important strengths and weaknesses of the organizations. Most organizations will try to build on their strengths. Focus groups for this kind of task are usually multidisciplinary and are made up of key stakeholders of the organization.

Human Resources Assessment

Organizations are made up of people who give life to the organizations. The availability of individuals with appropriate knowledge and skills to carry out the mission of the organization is critical. It may not be possible, under some circumstances, for an organization to obtain highly specialized expertise at the exact time it needs it. Accordingly, organization designs are influenced by the availability of critical human resources.

Political Process Assessment

All organizations have informal organizations as well as a formal one. It is important that managers understand the nature of the informal organizations that exist, who the key leaders are, and how this network can influence changes in organization design. For example, key leaders can facilitate or create barriers to the implementation of a new organization design; therefore, it is essential for managers to be aware

IN THE REAL WORLD

THE VISITING NURSE AGENCY, A CHANGING ENVIRONMENT

The Visiting Nurse Agency (VNA) was founded over 40 years ago by Jennie Johnson. Johnson's mother and grandmother before her had been known in their local community as persons who had always been called by neighbors to help deliver babies or provide support when family members were sick. Johnson saw VNA as an opportunity to carry on the family tradition by providing expert nursing services to those in need of care when sick in their homes.

The VNA was located in a rapidly growing suburb of a large city. During the initial years, VNA concentrated on two goals: first, attracting enough families to provide services to mothers with new babies and elderly persons requiring personal care at home; second, developing a reputation for providing a high quality, caring service. All patients and clients appeared content with the service; and the agency, a private nonprofit organization, was in a financially stable situation.

During the 1980s, VNA's growth slowed. While VNA was perceived to provide good care in the home, there were a number of new nursing services being provided by the local public health unit and a nearby general practitioner's office. The public health unit was providing more extensive home visits for postnatal care in the evenings and on weekends. Nurses from the general practitioner's office were providing extensive nursing services in conjunction with a local nursing home and a home for the aged on an outreach basis. Their services were available 24 hours a day, 7 days a week. The local community general hospital was also experimenting with health promotion clinics where services were being provided at a minimal charge to local residents. The VNA was seen as a very traditional "nursing" agency with rather specialized nursing services in the home and insufficient flexibility to meet the new needs of the community.

The VNA's hours of operation were Monday to Friday, 8:30 A.M. to 4:30 P.M. In 1984, VNA employed 51 registered nurses and 5 nurse-managers. The agency prided itself on the fact that all the nurses were registered nurses and about half of them had a university education. Johnson, however, was becoming increasingly concerned by the decreasing demand for their services.

By 1988, Johnson had begun to replace some of her nurse-managers, hoping to bring in new energy and fresh ideas. She still believed that the agency was respected because of its high quality of nursing services and the good relationships the agency enjoyed with established families in the community. Johnson called in the nurse-managers and stressed the importance of the quality philosophy to them. She emphasized the need for careful supervision of the nurses. She said all nurses must arrive at their house calls on time; punctuality was very important. She stressed the need for all nursing procedures conducted in the home to adhere to predefined standards. She pointed out the importance of the need for regular performance evaluations for the nurses so that they could be given immediate feedback on areas in which they were not following the exact protocol of the agency.

As new nurse-managers gained experience in VNA, they began to propose changes. One nurse-manager suggested that they establish an advisory board to serve as a liaison between the VNA and the local community. The advisory board would be made up of Jennie Johnson and key people from the local area, such as business people, women, minority group members, and senior citizens' group members. The nurse-manager who proposed the idea argued that advisory board members could counsel prospective clients about the nursing services and in general provide a public relations function for VNA.

Another new nurse-manager proposed that the VNA engage in more advertising and marketing strategies. She argued that the agency nurses should become more involved in community groups such as the community center's senior citizen events. She also argued that the VNA should support lobbyists to government entities who were attempting to change legislation to decrease taxation on senior citizen pensions.

As Johnson considered these and other proposals, the government announced approval of funding for a major expansion of the Metropolitan Home Care Program. Home care programs had been successful in other metropolitan areas and had been shown in some cases to be an excellent alternative to inhospital care, especially because a range of community support services could be provided. The new funding seemed to favor the provision of a variety of professional services in the home including nursing, medical, rehabilitation, and several homemaker services.

Jennie Johnson and the nurse-managers were very uncertain about the impact the Home Care Program could have on VNA.

In January 1992, Jennie Johnson felt overwhelmed and wondered whether she was up to managing the VNA. The agency had grown little over the past five years and was receiving fewer and fewer referrals from its long-standing clients. The impact of the expanded Home Care Program was difficult to anticipate, and she was not sure how VNA should respond. Two of the sharpest nurse-managers had been to see her about a change in management structure and approach. They encouraged the creation of several internal committees to study the problems. They also suggested that VNA begin planning the formation of specialized teams, organized around clients' needs and more appropriately able to respond to special interest groups. "The home nursing service industry is becoming more complex and is changing rapidly," one nurse-manager argued, "and if we don't adapt to it we will be left behind." Jennie Johnson thought the best thing might be to retire and get out of the provision of visiting nurse services—so dear to her family tradition.

SOURCE: Adapted from First National City Bank #2. In: Daft RL, Sharfman MP. *Organization Theory: Cases and Applications.* 3rd ed. New York, NY: West Publishing; 1990.

of the informal political processes underpinning the organization's life.

In the framework shown in Figure 10.2, we see the systematic assessment of mission, environment, organization, human resources and political process being necessary in order to tailor an organization design for the specific needs of the organization. With this systematic approach, it is more likely that the design will facilitate the organization to achieve high levels of performance.

The VNA case provides an example of a health services organization which is facing changing times and is thinking about changing its organization design. How should this organization reconsider its mission in relation to the changing environment? What strengths and weaknesses does the organization have? How might the work of the nurse-managers be built upon?

DESIGNS FOR A VARIETY OF HEALTH SERVICES ORGANIZATIONS

Specific design options available for health services managers depend on environmental demands, the organization's strategies, how activities can be grouped, and how decisions will be made. Some examples of common designs seen in health services organizations are functional, divisional, and matrix designs.

Functional Design

A *functional design* exists when labor is divided into departments specialized by functional area.[40] An example is shown in Figure 10.3. This kind of structure is typical of a nursing home, chronic-care facility, or small (less than 100 beds) community general hospital. In Figure 10.3, the basic hospital services are separated from the clinical services. The actual number of functional departments (and departmental manager positions) depends upon the size of the organization. The functional design is most useful when the organization has only a few products or goals. From the management's viewpoint, the functional design enables decisions to be made on a centralized, hierarchical basis. Departmental managers are usually promoted from within the organization and have a depth of technical knowledge in the functional area.

The functional design is most appropriate when an organization is in a relatively simple, stable environment in which there are few changes taking place and there are a limited number of other organizations with which the organization has contact. Clearly, a functional design becomes unsuitable when an organization grows and begins to diversify its services because interdepartmental coordination tends to be poor and decisions pile up at the top. If the environment becomes unstable, the functional design cannot cope because it does not have the facility to handle rapid information input or output and the response time is generally too slow.

Divisional Design

The *divisional design* is often found in large academic medical centers that operate under conditions of high environmental uncertainty exacerbated by relationships with the medical school and high technological complexity because of intensive research activities. It is also frequently found in pharmaceutical companies and health supplier organizations where a large variety of products and markets are involved. It is most appropriate for situations where clear divisions can be made within the organization and semiautonomous units can be created. Traditionally, in teaching hospitals the way of grouping units has been relatively clear cut; units have been grouped according to the accepted medical specialities, such as medicine, surgery, pediatrics, psychiatry, radiology, and pathology. More recently, hospitals are beginning to question the appropriateness of these traditional groupings and are moving towards defining product lines that cross traditional boundaries such as discussed in the opening New England Medical Center case. Examples of "new" product lines are those organized around body organs, such as the heart (grouping cardiology and cardiovascular surgery) and the liver (grouping endocrinology, internal medicine, and surgery), or those grouped around services to specific target groups, such as the elderly or persons with cancer. Similarly, in pharmaceutical companies, divisions are being created among related drugs. Divisionalization decentralizes decision making to the lowest level in the organization where the key expertise is available. Individual divisions have considerable autonomy for the clinical and financial operations. Each

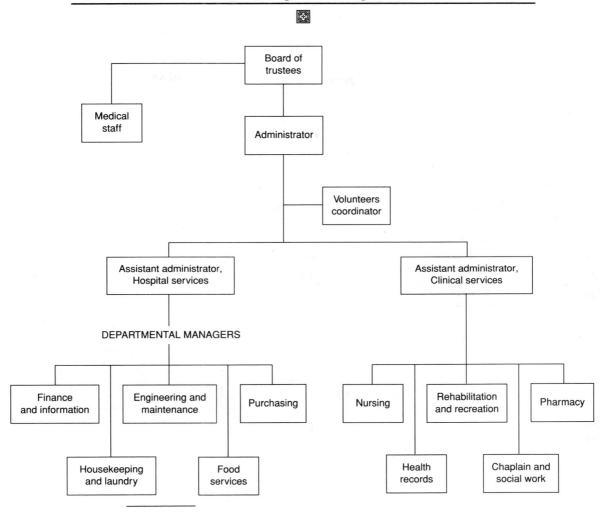

FIGURE 10.3. A functional design: Nursing home or chronic-care facility.

division has its own internal management structure, as illustrated in Figure 10.4.

The model illustrated in Figure 10.4 shows the physician in charge of each clinical service as the person with direct authority over all divisional operations. Each division has a manager of nursing or patient services, a manager of administrative services, and a finance officer. These managers work as a team to direct the division's operations. The managers are also accountable to the vice presidents of their disciplines. In some hospitals, a collaborative model is used to provide leadership of the team at the divisional level; that is, physicians, nurses, and administrators combine their skills to ensure knowledge of both the clinical and financial operations.

This subunit structure enables the specialized units to handle relevant elements of the environment directly, enhancing the organization's capacity to exchange information with the environment and to develop strategies tailored to the product lines. In many instances the divisions "purchase" central services from within the hospital and are provided incentives

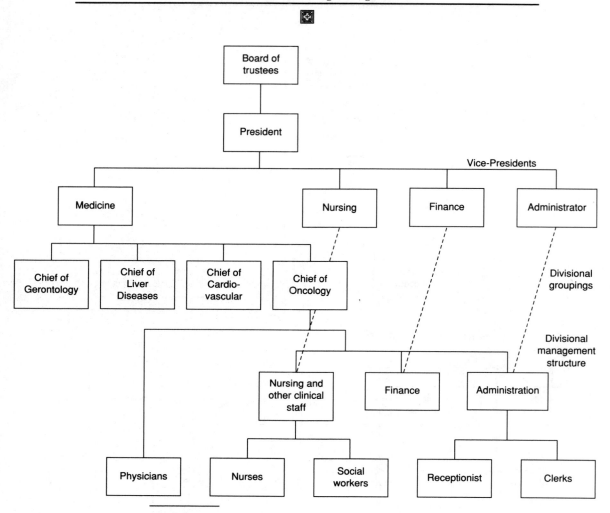

FIGURE 10.4. A divisional design: An academic medical center.

to operate their units cost effectively.[41] At the same time, the central service units are driven to operate efficiently; otherwise, the divisions may choose to purchase services outside the hospital at a better rate.

Difficulties with the divisional design tend to occur in times of resource constraints, when priorities must be set at higher organizational levels. For example, a large teaching hospital may have difficulty arriving at a consensus about which patient programs should be given priority if divisional managers cannot see the perspective of the whole organization. In times of resource constraints, greater sharing of resources between divisions is required, and more effective horizontal integrating mechanisms need to be established.[42,43]

Matrix Design

To overcome some of the problems of the functional and divisional designs, *matrix* or *mixed designs* have evolved to improve mechanisms of lateral coordination and information flow across the organization.[44] An example of a matrix organization for a psychiatric center is provided in Figure 10.5.

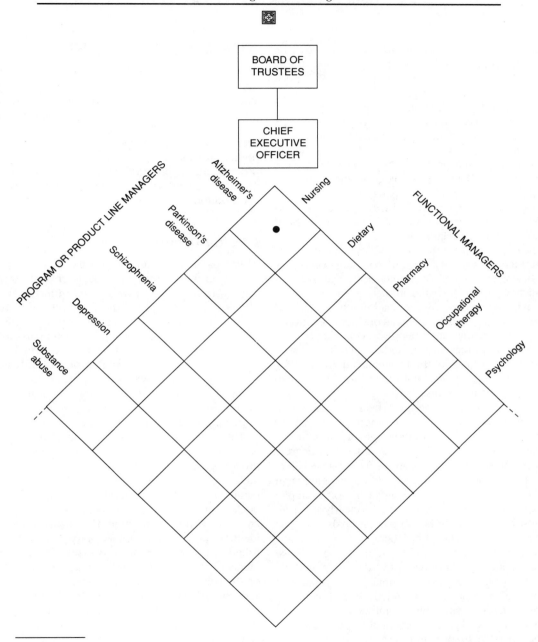

FIGURE 10.5. A matrix design: A psychiatric center. An individual worker in this example is part of the Alzheimer program as well as a member of the nursing department.

The matrix organization, originally developed in the aerospace industry, is characterized by a dual authority system. There are usually functional and program or product line managers, both reporting to a common superior and both exercising authority over workers within the matrix. Typically, a matrix organization is particularly useful in highly specialized technological areas that focus on innovation. The matrix design allows program managers to interact directly with the environment vis-a-vis technological developments. Usually each program requires a multidisciplinary team approach; the matrix structure facilitates the coordination of the team and allows team members to contribute their special expertise.

The matrix design has some disadvantages that stem from the dual authority lines. Individual workers may find having two bosses to be untenable since it creates conflicting expectations and ambiguity. The matrix design may also be expensive in that both functional and program managers may spend a considerable amount of time in meetings attempting to keep everyone informed of program activities. Additional costs may also be incurred because of the frequent requirement for dual accounting, budget, control, performance evaluation, and reward systems.

The use of the matrix design in health services organizations is becoming more common, particularly in organizations in which multidisciplinary approaches to patient care are being encouraged. To some degree, most health services organizations have many characteristics of a matrix organization, although their design may not be formally named as such. For example, multiple authority over patient care is clearly apparent in most hospitals. Most health professionals—such as nurses, psychologists, physiotherapists, pharmacists, occupational therapists, and social workers—have formal reporting relationships to their functional departments but are also accountable to physicians for the quality of care provided. Multidisciplinary teams, which facilitate lateral communication and coordination of work, are an essential feature of almost all health services organizations, including community health, long-term care, home care, and hospitals. As a result, learning to manage matrix structures is particularly important for health services managers.

NEW EVOLVING DESIGNS

Although the functional, divisional, and matrix designs represent the main types of organizational designs for health services organizations, a number of new organizational designs are being introduced which build upon the strengths of the basic designs yet modify them for individual circumstances. Two important modifications are the parallel design and the product line or program design. Both of these types place the patients or clients at the central focus of the organization.

Parallel Design

The parallel structure was originally developed as a mechanism for promoting quality of working life in organizations.[45] The *bureaucratic* or functional *organization* retains responsibility for routine activities in the organization, while the parallel side is responsible for complex problem solving requiring participatory mechanisms. The parallel structure is a means of managing and responding to changing internal and external conditions. It also provides an opportunity for persons occupying positions at various hierarchical levels in the bureaucratic structure and across functional areas to participate in organizational designs.

The *parallel design* is one we commonly see being used by organizations implementing CQI/TQM approaches. CQI/TQM places the clients or patients and their concerns at the center of the organization. The parallel side of the organization is often headed by a quality council made up of members of the bureaucratic side of the organization. The quality council then identifies areas where CQI/TQM teams may be established to investigate work processes where improvements in client services may be made. Representation on the teams is drawn from all levels in the hierarchy and from all departments that are involved in the work process under investigation. An example of a parallel structure for an acute general hospital is shown in Figure 10.6.

Advantages of the parallel structure to individual staff members are perceived to include expansion of their power, opportunities to affect the organization's decisions, the feeling of being involved in organiza-

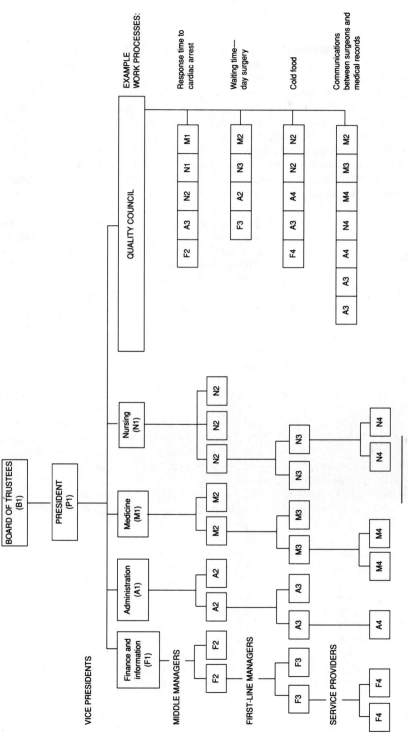

FIGURE 10.6. A parallel design: An acute general hospital.

tional issues, and the potential for individual growth through broadening of the range of work activities. Advantages to the organization are potentially those of increased performance and quality. Some possible disadvantages of the parallel structure are: organization members may spend too much time in meetings, thus increasing costs of operations; the parallel structure may begin to assume responsibilities for routine decisions, consequently overriding the bureaucratic structure; and conflicts over perceived priorities and resource allocation may occur between the bureaucratic and parallel structures.

Product Line or Program Design

Product line management is defined as the placement of a person in charge of all aspects of a given product or group of products.[46,47] The product line is a revenue and cost center, and the person in charge is responsible for all budgetary and financial responsibilities associated with the product. The person is also responsible for coordinating all the functional resources (e.g., planning, marketing, human resources, etc.) required to successfully manage the product line. Product line management can provide important advantages by increasing operational efficiencies and enhancing market share. Operational efficiencies can be gained by analyzing cost and revenues across related product lines so that redundancies will be eliminated and synergies captured. Market share can be enhanced by targeting marketing strategies to the group of products and being able to promote these to different segments of the market as appropriate (e.g., the elderly, women, and children).

The major challenges hospitals face in implementing product line management include educating the board, management, and medical staff to the change; choosing criteria for grouping the products; and selecting and training the product line managers. Hospitals realize that the change requires board and top management support and appropriate involvement and support of key medical staff and hospital-based physician leaders. The physicians must see it as a better way to manage resources, maintain or enhance quality, and increase patient flow.[48–52]

While many criteria can be used for grouping products, the most common are similarity of technology, similarity of markets, similarity in the production process, similarity in the distribution process, and similarity in the use of human resources. By grouping products with these kinds of similarities, economies of scale and synergies ($2 + 1 = 5$ solutions) can be generated. Based on these criteria, for example, a hospital can consider the following product line candidates: women's care, oncology, cardiology, rehabilitation, substance abuse, long-term care, and health promotion.

The selection and training of the product line managers is particularly important. Individuals must be identified who have good technical knowledge of the product line and good analytical and interpersonal skills. In particular, they must be innovative, feel comfortable with ambiguity and complexity, and be able to work with more than one manager. The latter is reflected in Figure 10.7. This chart shows a matrix-type organization in which the product line managers work with both the functional department heads and the product line assistant vice president. Recognizing that many problems and issues cut across the product lines, hospitals may establish a committee to deal with these issues. This committee can be composed of both product line managers and functional department heads and charged with reviewing the overall performance of the product lines and recommending addition, deletion, or modification of existing product lines.

Key success factors for this design include

- a strong management information system that links clinical, financial, and volume data by product
- a strong budgeting-financial system that can disaggregate costs and revenues so that accountability can be appropriately assigned
- reward systems to encourage innovation and risk taking
- relevant clinical involvement of physicians, nurses, and other health professionals to deal with new technology, diagnosis and treatment patterns, quality, and patient convenience issues
- a strong support staff, particularly in the areas of marketing, finance, and planning
- the need to align authority and responsibility

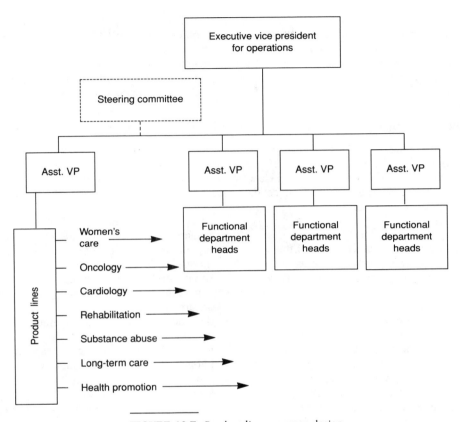

FIGURE 10.7. Product line manager design.

- the need for integrative mechanisms that cut across product lines; hence the development of the steering committee
- the need for a concerted management development program that emphasizes the ability to work with more than one manager, communication skills, conflict management skills, computer literacy, and creativity

INFLUENCES ON FUTURE ORGANIZATION DESIGNS

Based on the previous sections, a number of suggestions can be made about particular factors, somewhat unique to health services organizations, that may influence design decisions. These factors are generic and are likely to vary in importance through time and in various geographic locations. These influences may be classified according to whether they originate from the mission, the environment, the organization itself, human resources, or the political process (see Figure 10.2).

The Mission

The most important factor relating to the mission of health services organizations is concerned with the level of specificity of the mission in determining what will be an appropriate design. As noted previously, health services organizations are beginning to narrow their focus and identify key market driven areas in which they will operate. The move to identify specific target populations where inputs and health outcomes can be measured is a trend towards increasing the accountability of organizations for a social contract with the community.

The Future Environment

The future environment for most health services organizations is predicted to be both complex and dynamic (see Chapters 1 and 15). A variety of pressures will be exerted externally which will, by necessity, influence design decisions. Some of the most important pressures will be

- changing demographic characteristics of the population being served with an increase in the proportion of elderly persons needing services
- greater sophistication of the general public and consumers of health services in terms of their demands on the system
- increasing range of services being provided outside of traditional hospitals including ambulatory care programs, home care, long-term care, hospital without walls, and so on
- increasing competition among health services organizations providing similar services in the same geographic location to maximize their market share
- increasing attempts by governments at all levels to regulate the quantity and quality of services provided
- changing systems of reimbursement to health services organizations to control costs
- expanding private sector involvement in health services organizations to augment services and control costs
- increasing involvement of trustees, physicians, and other health professionals in the strategic planning and management of health services organizations
- increasing attempts by external professional associations and accrediting bodies to set standards for professional conduct in health services organizations

- rapidly developing medical technologies and proliferation of increasing specialized services
- increased information demands, development of real-time information processing systems to relate to the external environment, and growth of artificial intelligence systems

The Organization

Internal to most health services organizations are a series of structural and operating processes which provide opportunities or constraints on design decisions. For example

- greater emphasis on team work
- greater accountability for the governance of the organization in terms of a social contract
- increasing corporatization of the structure of health services organizations
- demands to continuously improve the quality of care
- demands to control costs, operate efficiently, and increase productivity
- increasing need for comprehensive and integrated clinical and financial information systems
- fewer financial resources
- changing working relationships to create more situations with two or more supervisor systems
- increasing need to coordinate activities internally and to manage conflict creatively

Human Resources

The particular characteristics of employees and other service providers available now or in the future may strongly affect the types of design decisions that may be made. For example

- greater emphasis on cross-skill training versus traditional professional training
- greater emphasis on horizontal teams and collaborative practices
- greater numbers of women in managerial positions requiring flexibility such as accessibility of day care, job sharing

- greater ethnic and cultural diversity of the workforce
- greater need to experiment with new work arrangements such as self-managed work teams, and CQI/TQM strategies
- many physicians who historically have had considerable autonomy becoming employees
- increasing attention by physicians to malpractice insurance
- shortages of key health services professionals; for example, pharmacists, physical therapists, and occupational therapists
- increasing need for managers with professional training
- increasing unionization of workers in health services organizations
- closer scrutiny by unions as some health services organizations undergo retrenchment
- increasing need to educate all levels in strategic management and in adopting a marketing orientation
- the need for succession planning, career planning, and management development programs linked more closely to the organization's strategic plan
- escalating pressures to provide continuing education programs to health professionals, especially clinical managers

The Political Process

Because of the uncertainty and ambiguities which may exist in health services organizations and the variety of professional groups involved, the informal network within organizations may be particularly active. Informal leaders may be especially helpful to managers in identifying how a change in organization design might be received. Informal leaders may be useful in communicating ideas about change to the grass-roots level in the organization or in repressing incorrect rumors that could damage the implementation process. Through the informal network, managers can identify which units or departments might be most or least receptive and attempt to involve key players in the redesign process. Additional suggestions are discussed in Chapter 8.

Although these factors are perhaps not comprehensive of all situations or applicable in all circumstances, they are potentially important when considering a new organization design. Most importantly, they emphasize the need for designs that are flexible, designs that can breathe and grow with the organization.

Organizations in Transition

Until now our discussion has focused on the importance of designing organizations in keeping with their mission, environment, information needs, human resources, and politics. However, missions, environment, information needs, human resources, and politics all change. To a certain extent, organizations go through relatively predictable cycles that have different design implications. For example, Starkweather and Kisch suggested four phases through which health services organizations pass.[53] The first is the search phase, which is characterized by newness, innovation, and a sense of ascendency as the organization procures resources and seeks to establish its identity. The organization design of an organization in this phase is typically open and informal. The success phase is characterized by achievement in procuring patients, staff, and financial resources. The design of the organization during this phase becomes somewhat more formalized to manage the usually larger scale of operation. The bureaucratic phase is characterized by a relatively rigid conformity to rules and procedures; the organization is isolated from its clients in that it receives little feedback from them. During this phase the organization may begin to decline because of its inability to respond to changes in the environment or to alter the environment to fit its needs. The succession phase is characterized by the development of new ways of providing services, often through the development of new units within the organization.

Kimberly, Miles, and Quinn raise important questions about organization design issues associated with such stages of the life cycle.[54,55] Given that managers wish to design organizations for optimal performance, it makes sense that different designs are more appropriate at different stages of an organization's development. For example, a functional structure might be appropriate for a new organization during its search phase. As the organization grows, achieves success, and perhaps diversifies, a different design, such as a product line or program design, may be appropriate. During periods of temporary or permanent decline, the organization may need to consider the appropriateness of a parallel design to help generate new ideas and maintain quality of services. These issues are critically important for organizational viability.

The following provides a case study of a *geriatric program in transition*. This case study illustrates the need to continuously examine the appropriateness of organization designs as organizations go through transition periods. It also illustrates some of the complexities in configuring an appropriate design for an organization when the program cuts across traditional hospital boundaries and domains.[56–58]

IN THE REAL WORLD

THE REGIONAL GERIATRIC PROGRAM, A MATURING ORGANIZATION

The growing proportion of elderly in society has created one of the central public policy issues facing many societies. Present health and social policy strategies designed for a young, affluent generation are no longer adequate as demographic shifts result in a much higher proportion of older citizens. In 1987, funding was provided by a government agency to establish regional geriatric services in a health science center in a large metropolitan area. A Regional Geriatric Program (RGP) was defined as a comprehensive, coordinated system of health services for the elderly within a region. The program encompassed a full range of ambulatory and inpatient hospital services provided by a consortium of acute and chronic care hospitals, including

- a geriatric assessment unit with a full range of diagnostic and therapeutic resources
- specialized outpatient clinics
- outreach teams consisting of a geriatrician, nurse, social worker, occupational therapist, and physiotherapist
- a geriatric day hospital to provide a therapeutic environment so that elderly persons can otherwise live independently
- inpatient geriatric services encompassing a multidisciplinary team within the hospital
- a service for the elderly requiring sociopsychological support
- long-term beds incorporating respite care, rehabilitation, and palliative care

At the inception of the RGP, the metropolitan area consisted of three hospital clusters, each providing regional geriatric services. In each service area (north, central, and east), there was an academic health science center, a general hospital, and a center for rehabilitation. The projected population of 65 years and older for the city was 260,000 persons. It was recognized that this program configuration represented a starting phase and that regional services might be developed to serve the southern and western areas of the city at a later time. It was considered essential that the initial three regional geriatric services should be developed simultaneously under the umbrella of a university program in geriatrics if the large numbers of elderly residing within the city were to be served effectively.

Organization Design—Stage 1

It was considered vital that the three regional service areas act in a coordinated manner. The cosponsoring institutions had agreed, therefore, to work as part of a single RGP program. The mission of the program was defined broadly as "providing clinical services to the very old population in an environment supportive to academic activities." The organization design for the program (central office) when it was established is shown in Figure 10.8.

A management council was formed for the RGP, which was comprised of the CEOs of the

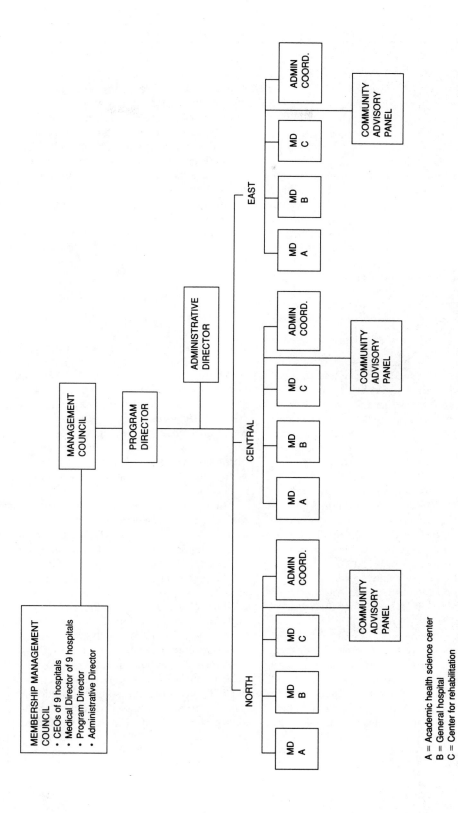

FIGURE 10.8. 1987 organization design.

hospitals, the medical directors of geriatrics from each hospital, a program director-geriatrician, and an administrative director. As each service area developed a community advisory panel, the Chair became a member of management council, adding three community members.

At the service area level (north, central, and east), management was provided by the medical directors of geriatrics from each hospital and an administrative coordinator. Also, a community advisory council made up of local representatives, patients, clients, and families was established.

During the first four years, the management committee acted as the governing body, and the hospital CEOs were extremely active in moving the RGP forward to achieve its mission. During this period of time, some difficulties were identified. For example:

- The hospital CEOs were considered by some geriatricians to be too dominant and to hold the interests of their individual hospitals higher than the interests of the RGP.
- Some of the physicians thought that resources should simply flow through the central office to the hospitals for their allocation and use. One physician asked, "Why is the central office interfering with our funding?"
- Health professionals other than physicians wanted to be part of the decision-making process at the management committee level. Nurses and other important groups such as social workers and rehabilitation therapists felt they were being excluded.
- The program had difficulty recruiting a director (geriatrician) to spearhead the program and provide leadership during its early years of development.

In the third year of operation some stability was brought to the program by the recruitment of a renowned geriatrician to be the program director. An organizational analysis was initiated because frustrations were growing about matters of program governance and management. No one seemed sure how decisions were made, or more often, not made; who was involved, or not in-

volved in making decisions; and, once a decision was made, how difficult it was to make it stick. The roles of management council, the central office, the service area, and the participating hospitals were not clear and at times in conflict. The distinctions between governance and management were blurred. The composition of management council was thought by some to be an impediment to good governance, because it was comprised of stakeholders whose interests were often in conflict with those of the RGP, rather than nonpartisan citizens committed to advancing the mission of the program.

Organization Design—Stage 2

Because of these changing circumstances, a task force was established to assess the organization and reconsider the organization design. Membership of the task force included the RGP program director (geriatrician), three CEOs of hospitals involved with service delivery, the administrative director, a chair of a community advisory panel from a service area, the executive director of a community nursing service agency, the director of a regional planning council, and a university representative. Discussions were held with a broad range of stakeholders and experts in organizational design.

The main design issues being debated related to distinguishing between governance and management and the extent to which decisions should be centralized or decentralized. In particular, what decisions should be made by the corporate office, what decisions could be decentralized to local offices, and who should be involved?

The task force made a number of recommendations based on the principle of decentralization. Management council would be reconstituted as a board of directors, with a strengthened mandate to govern. This would include responsibility for determining the philosophy, mission, and goals of the RGP, determining resource allocation among service areas, and ensuring appropriate fiscal management. Within the broad governing policies set by the board, the program director would be responsible for the management of the RGP;

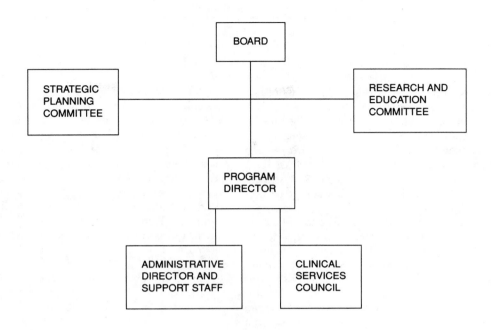

FIGURE 10.9. 1993 Organization design of central office.

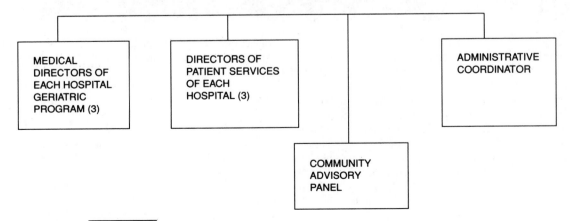

FIGURE 10.10. 1993 Organization design of service area (Example: Eastern area)

namely the ways and means to be used to achieve board goals. Service areas would be responsible for the planning, monitoring, and implementation of services in accordance with board policies. Individual member hospitals would be accountable to contribute to the RGP mission and goals within the framework established by the board, the program director, and service areas. To enhance both the profile and the authority of the RGP, the task force recommended that the program become legally incorporated.

Board membership was revised to strike a balance between broad public accountability and essential knowledge about the individual member hospitals. Each of the hospitals would continue to be represented, but not necessarily by the CEO. The hospital board would be asked to nominate one of its trustees or a member of senior management. The three areas included one representative from each of the participating hospitals (but it could now be a trustee or a member of senior management), the chairs of community advisory panels would remain, three members from the community at large, and one representative of the university would be added. The program director would be an ex-officio member. The new board membership did not provide for inclusion of clinical service directors or other health professionals.

It was recommended that the program director establish a management structure for the RGP and the service areas. A program management committee and a clinical services council serve as the principal mechanisms for horizontal coordination across the RGP. The design for the program central office is shown in Figure 10.9. At each of the geographic service areas (central, north, and east), a decentralized organization design was outlined (see Figure 10.10). The service area management teams (medical directors at each hospital (3), directors of patient services for each hospital (3), and the administrative coordinator) were to be given full authority for the provision of services in their areas. The members of the service area management teams were expected to work collegially and collaboratively. No specific program director was designated for each area. Each area was to continue to be advised by a community advisory panel made up of representatives from the community. There was agreement from all major stakeholders that a plan should be developed for the implementation of the new organization design and to monitor the experiences with it.

SOURCE: Adapted with permission from the proposal and experiences of the University Regional Geriatric Program in metropolitan Toronto, 1987.

DEBATE TIME 10.1: WHAT DO YOU THINK?

The Oriole Women's Shelter is a not-for-profit corporation and registered charity which began its operation in 1984 as a crisis care facility for physically and emotionally abused women and their children. The staff is organized as a feminist collective and works in conjunction with a volunteer board of directors. The collective was founded by a group of women and front line social agency workers concerned about this unmet need within their community. Some had themselves been victims of domestic violence; others came to the group because of feminist social philosophy and commitment to effect change at a grass roots level. The total annual budget for the facility is approximately $1.4 million. The mission statement of the shelter states:

> The Oriole Women's Shelter is committed to reducing the incidence of violence and oppression against women and children. It is an emergency crisis facility for abused women and their children, which provides safety, counselling, information, advocacy, and other assistance in a supportive environment, in times of personal or family crisis.

Community outreach and political action are significant components of the collective's work.

MANAGERIAL GUIDELINES

Design Preparation

1. The organization must have a clear understanding of its mission (i.e., it should be clear to everyone what business the organization is in and what it is not).[59]
2. The external environment of the organization must be assessed in terms of its uncertainty. The social, technological, political, economic, legal, cultural, and ecological characteristics of the environment could have important consequences for the choice of organization design.
3. It is important to understand the strengths and weaknesses of the organization so that the design strategy can accentuate the centers of excellence.
4. Assessment of the human resources available in the organization is essential to the task of organization design. There must be systematic understanding of the human resource capability, especially at the senior management level.[60] It may be necessary to consider both short- and long-term succession planning as part of the preparation for redesign.
5. The informal network inside the organization should be assessed so that key informal leaders can participate in the design process and, therefore, contribute to its success.

Design Process

1. Key organizational leaders must anticipate that the process of organization design may take several weeks or months depending upon the individual circumstances of the organization.
2. Some organizations may find it useful to establish a task force or a team to consider alternative organization designs. Key members of senior management and major stakeholders may be members of this team, recognizing that the task force is advisory to the CEO. It is often helpful to expand the membership of the task force to selected individuals at other levels of the organization. For example, it may be useful to have representation from middle managers, unions, and client groups.[61]
3. An external consultant can also be useful in outlining the design options for the organization. Ultimately the decision on the actual acceptability of the design for the organization rests with the organization.
4. During the design process, it is important to identify the ramifications of any new design.[62] Who will stand to gain or lose from the changes being made?

Design Outcome

1. Once an appropriate organization design has been agreed upon, it is important that a plan be developed for the communication of the design, its implementation, and evaluation.[63,64]
2. The new design must be communicated to everyone inside and outside the organization who is likely to be affected by the changes. Many organizations develop elaborate, staged plans to communicate the changes so that the individuals most affected by the design hear first.
3. Implementation of the new design will vary depending upon how different the new design is from the old one.[65] Implementation may be staged during three to five years in large complex organizations when the new design is radically different and when there is a need for extensive education of individuals to fill new roles. All the principles of implementing change, outlined in Chapter 12, are applicable to implementing new designs.
4. Although not often carried out in the past, it is important to formally monitor the implementation of the design and assess the effect of the design on organizational performance. Recognizing that organization designs exist to help work get done and to achieve the mission of the organization, it is essential that an evaluation process be defined in order to assess the effects on clients, employees, and other relevant stakeholders.[66]

The population served by the shelter is extremely diverse ethnically, and a significant proportion are refugees and new immigrants to the country. Issues which have arisen include the need for increased funding for translation services, ethnic foods, and more staff to accompany residents to legal, immigration, and other interviews. Residents and staff have had to address serious issues surrounding racism in addition to the emotional, mental, and physical stresses of working with clients who have been victims of abuse.

The problem of physical and emotional abuse of women and children by men has become more widely publicized in the years that the shelter has been in operation. This publicity has led to increased success with in-house fundraising, as well as greater ease in obtaining government funding for the work of the shelter. Nevertheless, the slumping economy of the past year has taken a toll on all publicly funded programs and the shelter being no exception.

From its inception, the shelter has rejected the concept of a traditional hierarchical structure which is believed by the founders and staff to reflect a male-dominated social structure that has contributed to power imbalances in society. These imbalances are felt to allow segments of the population to be oppressed and abused. Instead, the staff is structured as a collective, with decisions made on the basis of consensus. The key characteristics of a *collectivist-democratic or-*

TABLE 10.2. Comparisons of Two Ideal Types of Organization

Dimension	Bureaucratic Organization	Collectivist-Democratic Organization
1. Authority	1. Authority resides in individuals by virtue of incumbency in office or expertise; hierarchical organization of offices. Compliance is to universal fixed rules as these are implemented by office incumbents.	1. Authority resides in the collectivity as a whole; delegated, if at all, only temporarily and subject to recall. Compliance is to the consensus of the collective, which is always fluid and open to negotiation.
2. Rules	2. Formalization of fixed and universalistic rules; calculability and appeal of decisions on the basis of correspondence to the formal, written law	2. Minimal stipulated rules; primacy of ad hoc, individuated decisions; some calculability possible on the basis of knowing the substantive ethics involved in the situation
3. Social control	3. Organizational behavior is subject to social control, primarily through direct supervision or standardized rules and sanctions, tertiarily through the selection of homogeneous personnel, especially at top levels.	3. Social controls are primarily based on personalistic or moralistic appeals and the selection of homogeneous personnel.
4. Social relations	4. Ideal of impersonality, relations are to be role-based, segmental, and instrumental.	4. Ideal of community; relations are to be wholistic, personal, of value in themselves.
5. Recruitment and advancement	5a. Employment based on specialized training and formal certification 5b. Employment constitutes a career, advancement based on seniority or achievement	5a. Employment based on friends, social-political values, personality attributes, and informally assessed knowledge and skills 5b. Concept of career advancement not meaningful; no hierarchy of positions
6. Incentive structure	6. Remunerative incentives are primary.	6. Normative and solidarity incentives are primary; material incentives are secondary.
7. Social stratification	7. Isomorphic distribution of prestige, privilege, and power (i.e., differential rewards by office); hierarchy justifies inequality.	7. Egalitarian; reward differentials, if any, are strictly limited by the collectivity.
8. Differentiation	8a. Maximal division of labor: dichotomy between intellectual work and manual work and between administrative tasks and performance tasks 8b. Maximal specialization of jobs and functions; segmental roles. Technical expertise is exclusively held; ideal of the specialist-expert.	8a. Minimal division of labor; administration combined with performance tasks; division between intellectual and manual work reduced 8b. Generalization of jobs and functions; wholistic roles. Demystification of expertise: ideal of the amateur generalist

SOURCE: (67) Rothchild, Joyce, & Whitt, J. Allen. *The Co-operative Workplace. Potentials and dilemmas of organizational democracy and participation.* Cambridge University Press. Cambridge, 1989.

ganization are described in Table 10.2.[67] All staff (11 full-time equivalents) receive the same salary, regardless of prior education, experience, or seniority within the organization. There is no identified manager, no model of supervision; performance reviews are controversial and conducted by the collective in the context of staff meetings. Weekly staff meetings are facilitated (led) in turn by collective members. The meetings tend to be long, emotionally charged, and perceived by some to be inefficient in conducting the business of the collective. Decision making is laborious and in many cases inconsequential.

Staff interactions have become exhausting and time consuming. Staff meetings therefore evoke negative emotional reactions from the collective members. Fears of isolation or appearing to be out of tune with the culture of the organization are regularly expressed, and there is a tendency to see fault as lying elsewhere.

Anyone who assumes a leadership role, proffers skills or competence in certain areas, or expresses a political viewpoint which counters the prevailing attitude is seen as attempting to take control. Having power is seen as negative and abusive and a source of anxiety or fear on the part of those who perceive themselves as not having power. Although there is a strong commitment in principle to the collective process, many staff members believe that an informal hierarchy does exist. This has its basis along lines of seniority, race, personal characteristics, and depth of commitment to the political beliefs of feminism and collectivism.

The board consists of eight professional and business women who could be described as successful in their respective professions. (Men are not accepted as board or staff, and a release regarding this policy has been obtained from the Human Rights Commission).

The personal and corporate culture of members of the board is typically hierarchical, and they are often in conflict with the organizational culture of the shelter. All agree with and support the concepts of feminism and collectivism but have difficulty reconciling the legal and practical requirements for structure with the collective's wish for its values to be supported and honored. Lack of accountability, responsibility, and commitment to task completion are problems identified by the board which relate to the collective structure as it now stands.

During the past three years, there have been increasing difficulties with intrastaff and staff-board communication, perceived staff stress, and anger in the workplace. Serious problems have arisen in the areas of administrative activity and accountability. No single individual willingly accepts responsibility for specific tasks or assignments. Although attempts have been made to address individual issues, no long-term or comprehensive solutions have been achieved.

1. What is the nature of decision making in this organization? What are its strengths and weaknesses?
2. Is designated leadership essential to the operation of an organization? Can power and accountability be shared?
3. What might be the impact of a formal organization design on this organization?
4. What mechanisms might preserve the values or culture of the organization while facilitating decision making?

SOURCE: *Adapted from Zahn C, Quinn B. Lands' End 40. In: Daft RL, Sharfman MP. Organization Theory: Cases and Applications. 3rd ed. New York, NY: West Publishing; 1990.*

KEY CONCEPTS

Assessment for Design
Bureaucratic
  Organization
Collectivist-Democratic
  Organization
Centralization and
  Decentralization
Design Outcome
Design Preparation
Design Process
Divisional Design
Environmental
  Assessment

Functional Design
Human Resources
  Assessment
Levels of Organization
  Design
Matrix Design
Organization Design
Parallel Design
Patient-centered Care
Political Process
  Assessment
Product Line or
  Program Design

Discussion Questions

1. You have been hired as an assistant to a new CEO of an academic medical center. You have been asked to recommend a variety of organization designs for the 300-bed inpatient facility. The academic medical center is fully affiliated with the medical school which is internationally renowned for its work in cardiovascular diseases, neurosciences, and transplant programs. The CEO's main objectives in the reorganization are to decentralize decision making to physicians and other clinicians, to pave the way for more effective information systems for monitoring quality and cost, and to break down traditional barriers between professional hierarchies and groups. What are your recommendations?

2. A not-for-profit home health program has decided it would like to begin to examine mechanisms for the continuous monitoring and improvement of quality of services being provided. The home health program is located in a small rural town with a population of 12,000 persons. The majority of the clients served are 70 years old and above and require a range of nursing and social services as well as homemaker services. Funding for the program is from a wide variety of sources. What process would you recommend for deciding upon an appropriate organization design?

3. As administrator of a home care program in a city of 500,000 persons, you are planning to expand your services. Your program has been in operation for about five years, and until now you have focused on clients with relatively short-term needs. Clients' average length of time in the program is 25 days. The expansion will consist of providing comprehensive services to persons who are chronically ill and who consequently require long-term home care. On the basis of a preliminary survey, you estimate that the size of your program will triple within a year. The chronic-care clients will most likely have problems of the circulatory system, neoplasms, or diseases of the musculoskeletal system. Most clients will need long-term nursing services,

physiotherapy, occupational therapy, homemaking services, and a variety of supplies and equipment. Your organization is currently structured according to function (nursing, physiotherapy, homemaking, administration, finance). You have a staff of over 200, but with the new program you will probably need to double your staff. You are wondering about changing your organization design in preparation for the expansion. What would be the advantages and disadvantages of a divisional structure or a matrix structure for the home care program? On what basis might you group activities and personnel (e.g., by type of clients, by geographic area of the city, or by services)?

4. Consider an organization you are familiar with (preferably one you have worked in). Reflecting on your experience in this organization, define at least one problem in its design. What were the symptoms of the problem? What might be (or should have been) done to solve the problem? Why do you think that nothing was done?

REFERENCES

1. Kimberly JR. The anatomy of organizational design. *Journal of Management.* 1984;10(1):109–126.
2. Daft RL. *Organization Theory and Design.* 4th ed. New York, NY: West Publishing Co.; 1992.
3. Morgan G. *Creative Organization Theory: A Resource Book.* Newbury Park, Ca.: Sage; 1989.
4. Nadler DA, Gerstein MS, Shaw RB and Associates. *Organizational Architecture: Designs for Changing Organizations.* San Francisco, Ca: Jossey-Bass; 1992.
5. Pfeffer J. *Managing with Power: Politics and Influence in Organization.* Boston, Mass: Harvard Business School Press; 1992.
6. Pearce JA. The company mission as a strategic tool. *Sloan Management Review.* Spring 1982;23(3):15–24.
7. Mintzberg H. *Structuring in Fives: Designing Effective Organizations.* Englewood Cliffs, NJ: Prentice-Hall; 1983.
8. Jaques E. *Requisite Organization: The CEOs Guide to Creative Structure and Leadership.* London, England: Cason Hall and Co.; 1989.
9. McCann JE, Gilmore TN. Diagnosing organizational decision making through responsibility charting. *Sloan Management Review.* Winter 1983;24(2):3–15.
10. Ibid.
11. Shipper F, Manz CC. An alternative road to empowerment. *Organizational Dynamics.* 1992;20(3):48–61.
12. Kaluzny AD. Design and management of disciplinary and interdisciplinary work groups in health service organizations: Review and critique. *Medical Care Review.* 1985;42(1):77–112.
13. Fitzgerald L, Stust J. Clinicians into management: On the change agenda or not? *Health Services Management Research.* 1992;5(2):137–147.
14. Pool J. Hospital management: Integrating the dual hierarchy? *International Journal of Health Planning and Management.* 1991;6:193–207.
15. Shortell SM. The future of hospital-physician relationships. *Frontiers of Health Services Management.* 1990;7(1):3–32.
16. Leatt P, O'Rourke K, Fried B, Deber R. Regulatory intensity, hospital size and the formalization of medical staff organization in hospitals. *Health Services Management Research.* 1992;5(2):123–136.
17. Lemieux-Charles L, Leatt P. Hospital-physician integration: Case studies of community hospitals. *Health Services Management Research.* 1992;5(2):82–98.
18. Mintzberg, op. cit.
19. Howard R. The CEO as organizational architect: An interview with Paul Allaire. *Harvard Business Review.* September-October 1992:107–121.
20. Kaluzny AD, Morissey JP, McKinney MM. Emerging organizational networks: The case of the community clinical oncology program. In: Mick SS and Associates, eds. *Innovations in Health Care Delivery: Insights for Organizational Theory.* San Francisco, Ca: Jossey-Bass; 1990:86–115.
21. Aldrich HE, Whetten DA. Organization-sets, action-sets, and networks; Making the most of simplicity. In: Nystrom PC, Starbuck WH, eds. *Handbook of Organizational Design.* Vol. 1. London, England: Oxford University Press; 1981:385–408.
22. Alexander JA. Adaptive change in corporate control practices. *Academy of Management Journal.* 1991;34(1):162–193.
23. Arndt M, Bigelow B. Vertical integration in hospitals: A framework for analysis. *Medical Care Review.* 1992;49(1):93–115
24. Alexander, op. cit.
25. Arndt, Bigelow, op. cit.
26. Perrow C. The bureaucratic paradox: The efficient organization centralizes in order to decentralize. *Organizational Dynamics.* Spring 1977:2–14.
27. Kosnik RD, Shortell SM. Differentiated patterns of centralization in multidivisional organizations: Strategic decision making in multi-hospital systems. Presented at the Annual Meeting of the Academy of Management Association, OMT Division; 1992; Las Vegas, Nev.
28. Lawler EE. Choosing an involvement strategy. *Academy of Management Executive.* 1988;2(3):197–204.
29. Pfeffer J. Organization theory and structural perspectives on management. *Journal of Management.* 1991;17(4):789–803.
30. Nadler, et al., op. cit.
31. Tichy NM. Diagnosis for complex health care delivery systems: A model and case study. *Journal of Applied Behavioural Sciences.* 1978;14(3):305–320.
32. Gellerman SW. In organizations, as in architecture, form follows function. *Organizational Dynamics.* 1990;18(3):57–68.
33. Terreberry S. The evolution of organizational environments. *Administrative Science Quarterly.* 1968;12:590–613.
34. Lawrence P, Lorsch J. The organization and its environment. Cambridge, Mass: Harvard University Press; 1967.
35. Ibid.
36. Stein BA, Kanter RM. Building the parallel organization: Creating mechanisms for permanent quality of work life. *Journal of Applied Behavioural Science.* 1980;16:371–386.
37. Howard, op. cit.

38. Perrow C. *Organizational Analysis: A Sociological View.* Belmont, Ca: Wadsworth Publishing Co. Inc.; 1970.

39. Ginter PM, Duncan WJ, Richardson WD, Swayne LE. Analyzing the healthcare environment: You can't hit what you can't see. *Health Care Management Review.* 1991;16(4):35–48.

40. Duncan R. What is the right organization structure? Decision tree analysis provides the answer. *Organizational Dynamics.* Winter 1979;7(4):59–80.

41. Heyssel RM, et al. Decentralized management in a teaching hospital. *New England Journal of Medicine.* 1984;310:1477–1480.

42. Leatt P, Murray M, Lemieux-Charles L. Decentralization of decision-making in Canada's health system: The Sunnybrook experience. University of Toronto; Department of Health Administration Working Paper; 1992.

43. Smith T, Leatt P, Ellis P, Fried B. Decentralized hospital management: Rationale, potential and two case examples. *Health Matrix.* 1989;7(1):11–17.

44. Griener LE, Schien VE. The paradox of managing a project-oriented matrix: Establishing coherence within chaos. *Sloan Management Review.* Winter 1981;2(2):17–22.

45. Stein, Kanter, op. cit.

46. Stuart N, Sherrard H. Managing hospitals from a program perspective. *Health Management Forum.* Spring 1987:53–61.

47. MacStravic R. Product-line administration in hospitals. *Health Care Management Review.* 1986;41(1):23–32.

48. Alfirevic J, Kroman B, Ruflin P. Informational needs for a product line management system. *Healthcare Financial Management.* 1987;31(3):60–66.

49. Flynn MK. Product-line management: Threat or opportunity for nursing? *Nursing Administration Quarterly.* 1991;15(2):21–32.

50. Nackel JG, Kues IW. Product-line management: Systems and strategies. *Hospital and Health Services Administration.* March/April 1986:109–123.

51. Patterson DJ, Thompson KA. Product line management: Organization makes a difference. *Financial Management.* 1987;41(2):66–72.

52. Monaghan BJ, Alton L, Allen D. Transition to program management. *Leadership.* September/October 1992:33–37.

53. Starkweather D, Kisch A. A model of the life cycle dynamics of health service organizations. In: Arnold M, et al., eds. *Administering Health Systems.* New York, NY: Atherton Press; 1971.

54. Kimberly JR, Miles RH. *The Organization Life Cycle: Issues in the Creation Transformation, and Decline of Organizations.* San Francisco, Ca: Jossey-Bass; 1980.

55. Kimberly JR, Quinn RE. *Managing Organizational Transitions.* Homewood, Ill: Richard D. Irwin, Inc.; 1984.

56. Luke RD, Begun JW, Pointer DD. Quasi firms: Strategic interorganizational forms in the health care industry. *Academy of Management Review.* 1989;14(1):9–19.

57. Thomas JB, Ketchen DJ, Trevino LK, McDaniel RR. Developing interorganizational relationships in the health sector: A multicase study. *Health Care Management Review.* 1992;17(2):7–19.

58. Hirschhorn L, Gilmore T. The new boundaries of the "boundaryless" company. *Harvard Business Review.* May-June 1992:104–114.

59. Bettis RA. Strategic management and the straitjacket: An editorial essay. *Organization Science.* 1991;2(3):315–319.

60. Whetten DA, Cameron KS. *Developing Management Skills.* 2nd ed. New York, NY: HarperCollins Pub.; 1991.

61. Kumar K, Thibodeaux MS. Organizational politics and planned organization change. *Group and Organization Studies.* 1990;15(4):357–365.

62. Isabella LA. Evolving interpretations as a change unfolds: How managers construe key organizational events. *Academy of Management Journal.* 1990;33(1):7–41.

63. Glick WH, Huber GP, Miller CC, Doty DH, Sutcliffe K. Studying changes in organizational design and effectiveness: Retrospective event histories and periodic assessments. *Organizational Science.* 1990;1(3):293–312.

64. Weick KE. Agenda setting in organizational behavior: A theory-focused approach. *Journal of Management Inquiry.* 1987;1(3):171–182.

65. Jaques E. In praise of hierarchy. *Harvard Business Review.* 1990;90(1):127–133.

66. McClintock C. Administrators as applied theorists. *New Directions for Program Evaluation.* Fall 1990;47:19–33.

67. Rothchild J, Whitt JA. The Co-operative Workplace, Potentials and Dilemmas of Organizational Democracy and Participation. Cambridge, England: Cambridge University Press; 1989.

68. Miller D. Organizational configurations: Cohesions, change and predictions. *Human Relations.* 1990;43(8):771–789.

CHAPTER

11

MANAGING STRATEGIC ALLIANCES

Edward J. Zajac, Ph.D.
Professor

Thomas A. D'Aunno, Ph.D.
Associate Professor

LEARNING OBJECTIVES

After completing this chapter, the reader should be able to

1. better understand why strategic alliances are increasing in use, particularly among health care organizations
2. distinguish between different types or forms of strategic alliances, using a number of dimensions
3. classify an alliance both in terms of what it looks like and what it is meant to do
4. understand how alliance motivation is often related to alliance structure and outcomes
5. identify whether your motivations for a strategic alliance are compatible with those of your alliance partner
6. think about strategic alliances in terms of the likely stages of development that alliances often experience and the critical issues that you may face at each stage
7. distinguish between an alliance problem and an alliance symptom and recognize the different implications for managerial intervention
8. understand both the pros and cons of alliances

CHAPTER PURPOSE

There is no doubt that the U.S. health care environment is undergoing major changes that could be characterized as turbulent. The word was originally used to depict highly complex and rapidly changing environments; "turbulence" has been somewhat vaguely used to describe many industry contexts.[2] However, a closer inspection of the Emery and Trist definition reveals that the term applies when two general conditions are met: (1) organizations are highly interconnected with one another, and (2) organizations are highly interdependent with the society in which organizations find themselves.

This emphasis on connectedness and interdependence is an important basis for viewing a specific organization's environment not as some amorphous external force but rather as the set of other organizations that are interconnected or interdependent with it. This organization, in turn, is part of the environment for the other organizations. In other words, when an organization looks out with concern or anticipation at its *turbulent environment,* what it

IN THE REAL WORLD

THE ROCHESTER AREA HOSPITALS CORPORATION

In 1978, all nine hospitals in the Rochester, New York area formed a voluntary alliance, the Rochester Area Hospitals Corporation (RAHC). The alliance has a governing board and an executive director whose responsibility is to provide direction for the alliance; several hospital chief executive officers (CEOs) serve on the RAHC board. In addition, there is a small corporate staff that develops and operates RAHC programs.

Though the alliance has initiated several programs to assist its members, its most important and widely known effort is an experimental hospital payment plan. Under this plan, the member hospitals were paid a fixed amount per year based on operating expenses for 1979. This plan, in effect, created a community-wide budget ceiling. Further, RAHC's members have agreed through-

out the years not to duplicate each other's services. Instead, there is a relatively high degree of specialization—for example, open-heart surgery is performed primarily at one hospital.

The results for cost containment have been impressive. Blue Cross Blue Shield of Rochester reports that the cost of care for its enrollees in Rochester is about one-third less than costs reported in a recent national survey of employers. Indeed, in both 1984 and 1989, Rochester gave back $4.8 million to surprised Medicare officials because RAHC had managed to generate a surplus by keeping its costs below national Medicare rates. It is not surprising that President Clinton cited Rochester as a model for health care reform during the 1992 campaign.

RAHC has not always had smooth sailing.[1] Its

members face constant pressure to control health care costs from two large employers that have headquarters in Rochester: Kodak and Xerox. Several of these corporations' executives serve on the local hospital boards. As board members, they have played a key role in encouraging the hospitals to work cooperatively. This has led some to ask how voluntary the cooperation is in Rochester and whether it can be duplicated elsewhere.

Further, there are concerns that Rochester, because it keeps a tight rein on capital expenditures, might fall behind the nation in access to new technologies and quality of care. Despite these concerns, the alliance has continued for about 15 years and has much success to show for its work.

sees is other organizations looking out at that organization![3]

This conceptualization of organizational environments suggests the need to focus more attention on how specific organizations interact with one another. This chapter emphasizes one such type of interaction; namely, cooperative interorganizational relations. Longest, in discussing what he terms "interorganizational linkages in health care," distinguishes between market transactions, voluntary relationships, and involuntary relationships.[4] We focus most of our attention on those interorganizational relations that are noncoercive and entered into primarily for strategic purposes, that is, that are important to an organization's mission and expected to enhance organizational performance. Such relationships we term *strategic alliances,* which are defined as any formal arrangements between two or more organizations for purposes of mutual gain.

ALLIANCES IN HEALTHCARE

Alliances are often viewed as facing high failure rates; some claim 50% to 80%. For example, some have argued that strategic alliances, by their very nature, are risky endeavors.[5] The cooperative linkages between two or more organizations are viewed as somewhat fragile, exposing each party to the risk that the other party or parties may not continue to cooperate as expected. The business press has also had a penchant for describing, in detail, particular joint ventures or other alliances that failed. (For example, one of the authors was approached several years ago by a reporter who wanted to do a story on the five biggest joint venture failures). The failure of a cooperative alliance between two organizations often involves considerable drama, as interorganizational cooperation turns to conflict.

While it is important to recognize the pros and cons of alliances (see Debate Time 11.1), we believe that the usual fixation on the likely failure and inherent riskiness of alliances may be misguided. Specifically, we contend that any assessment of the *risk of strategic alliances* should be balanced with an assessment of the expected return or benefit of the alliance in terms of improved financial performance, innovation, and organizational learning, and the opportunity cost of not engaging in a strategic alliance. Regarding the first point, while financial performance is an obvious outcome to consider when analyzing the success or failure of a strategic alliance, it is not clear that it should be considered the most important, direct outcome. For example, innovation may be a driving force behind strategic alliances, and more generally, alliances may be viewed as a desirable way for organizations to learn about new markets, services, and ways of doing business.[6] These may actually be negatively correlated with financial performance, at least in the short run.[7] This issue is discussed in greater detail in the section on how strategic intentions drive alliance activity.

In terms of opportunity cost, the relevant question is not Is it risky? but rather, Which is riskier: going it alone, doing nothing, or engaging in an alliance? Riskiness is not necessarily a problem. For example, the virtues of entrepreneurship are often extolled, despite the high risk and high failure rates involved. Strategic alliances may appear risky when the baseline comparison is not made explicit, but when compared with attempting a *de novo* entry into a new market or ignoring the market altogether, the alliance may actually seem like a relatively low risk proposition.[8] In fact, as subsequently discussed, the creation of a strategic

DEBATE TIME 11.1: WHAT DO YOU THINK?

There are a few facts and many more unknowns about strategic alliances. One fact is that we are witnessing a substantial increase in strategic alliances in health care. An unknown, however, is whether this fact reflects a positive or negative development. An interesting recent example of a debate on this issue is found in Duncan, Ginter, and Swayne.[72] In this section, we consider some of the arguments swirling around the use of strategic alliances. Kaluzny and Zuckerman argue on the positive side for alliances, while Begun offers counterarguments on the negative side.[72] The lowing list of issues summarizes their points of disagreement.

Positive

1. Alliances reflect a fundamental shift in how health service organizations do business; namely, a change from thinking in terms of control to thinking in terms of commitment, trust, shared risk, and common purpose.
2. Alliances provide organizations with a way to manage growing complexity and interdependence while maintaining a fair amount of individual organizational autonomy.
3. Alliances enable organizations to transcend the existing organizational inertia that is often created by complexity and vested interests seeking to maintain the status quo.
4. Alliances have been found to be effective in other sectors of our society, and failure to apply these concepts to health services would be a missed opportunity for meeting the challenges in the future.

Negative

1. Alliances distract organizations from their basic goal, which is to clobber your competitors or at least behave as if you have that need. Managers like the thrill of the competitive chase, and competition creates loyalty and team spirit in an organization.
2. Alliances are essentially a fad whose benefits have been exaggerated, similar to Theory Z, the pursuit of excellence, product line management, and total quality management.
3. Alliances can lead to collusion between otherwise competing organizations, can lead to legal problems relating to antitrust challenges, and are attractive only to lazy organizations that are not interested in competition.
4. The process hassles of initiating and managing alliances are tremendous and costly, and these arrangements are quite fragile.
5. Governing an alliance means governing by committee, which we know to be an ineffective way to run a business. In particular, this problem reduces the speed and flexibility of an organization.
6. Cooperative strategy makes sense for large, multinational firms seeking to enter new and unknown markets or share expensive research and development projects but not for health care organizations who face well-known local markets and do not need to finance much research and development.

Which of the above perspectives do you favor? How would you justify your position?

---

alliance is often motivated by an organization's desire to reduce uncertainty.

The issues raised above are particularly relevant for health care organizations, which have seen an explosion of alliance building in the past several years. For example, since the late 1970s more than 15 large hospital alliances have emerged that include over 1,600 members. About 30% of the nation's hospitals are members of alliances.[9] Alliance building is not limited to hospitals.[10,11] There are alliances between hospitals and physician groups, between hospitals and health maintenance organizations (HMOs), and between hospitals, physicians, and agencies of the federal government.[12-14] Nor are alliances limited to providers of care. Alliances known as business coalitions have emerged among buyers of care—that is, employers who band together to increase their effectiveness as purchasers of care for their employees. The variety of possible alliance partners is quite high, given the myriad of interdependencies between organizations in the health sector (see summary in Table 11.1).

The causes for this outburst of activity are not difficult to identify. Perhaps the most important and obvious factor is that health care organizations are experiencing what Meyer has referred to as a series of

TABLE 11.1. Interdependencies between Organizations in the Health Sector

In the health sector, focal organizations have potential interdependencies with organizations such as:

Accrediting agencies
Affiliated organizations
Alternative health systems
Competitors
Confederated organizations
Consortia members
Consumer representatives (public and private)
Employee representatives (unions)
Fiscal intermediaries
Financial organizations (bond rating)
Foundations
Government (all levels)
Health maintenance organizations (HMOs)
Independent practice associations (IPAs)
Insurance companies
Joint venture partners
Media
Physician-Hospital Organizations (PHOs)
Multiinstitutional systems
Other partners
Owners
Political groups
Preferred provider organizations (PPOs)
Suppliers (including capital, consumables, equipment, and human resources)
Third party associations (TPAs)
Trade associations
Utilization management companies

SOURCE: Adapted from Longest B. Interorganizational linkages in the Health Sector. in *Health Care Management Review.* 1990;15:17–28, with permission of Aspen Publishers, Inc., © 1990.

"environmental jolts."[15] These are relatively abrupt, major, and often qualitative changes in an environment that threaten organizational survival. The introduction of the Medicare Prospective Payment System, for example, qualifies as an environmental jolt and has led to massive changes in the strategies of hospitals in recent years.[16,17] Further, a growing number of hospitals have closed. Other jolts include increased competition, a surplus of hospital beds, concern with cost containment, an increase in the number of uninsured patients, an aging population, and the AIDS epidemic.

These jolts create great uncertainty for health care managers. Alliances may reflect the reality that it is sometimes better to face life's uncertainties with partners than to go it alone. Of course, alliances are but one response to the environmental changes described above. There also has been a marked increase in other types of multiorganizational arrangements, particularly multihospital systems.[18] Further, other strategic adaptive responses to environmental change have emerged, including vertical integration and diversification.[19] In short, as Starr argued a decade ago, the landscape of the health care field is itself changing: where there were once many small and independent organizations there are now clusters of organizations, including alliances and other types of multiorganizational arrangements.[20]

TYPES AND FORMS OF ALLIANCES

While the incidence of strategic alliances has increased dramatically in recent years, it would be an exaggeration to say that they are a new phenomenon. Strategic alliances in a wide range of shapes and sizes have been historically observed in many industries, particularly in health care. Given the variety in types of alliances, it is therefore not surprising that early research on alliances devoted considerable initial attention to the categorization of interorganizational relations (often called multi-institutional arrangements) found in the health care industry, much in the way that a botanist might develop an organizing schema for classifying plants. The earliest approaches towards understanding these arrangements were usually interested in establishing a continuum upon which the arrangements could be located for purposes of comparison and contrast.[21-23] DeVries, for example, arrays multi-institutional systems on a continuum of "less commitment, more institutional autonomy" to "more commitment, more system control," in the following order[24]

- formal affiliation
- shared or cooperative services
- consortia for planning or education
- contract management
- lease
- corporate ownership but separate management
- complete ownership

Ownership vs. Control

DeVries and others have arrayed multi-institutional systems on a continuum of more autonomy to more *control.*[25] However, these rankings often really reflect the degree of *ownership,* with complete ownership being equated with the highest form of control. While it seems reasonable to view ownership as related to control, we argue that this can sometimes be misleading.

For example, it is well known that McDonald's Corp. is very interested in maintaining control over its raw materials to ensure that quality is highly consistent. In dealing with its exchange partners who supply these raw materials, one might therefore expect that McDonald's would prefer an interorganizational arrangement that would involve substantial ownership interest in suppliers in order to have greater control. This is not the case, however. Even with no ownership interests, McDonald's simply communicates its quality requirements to the supplier organizations, and the organizations are typically quick to oblige.

How can this be? Two factors seem to be relevant. The first is obvious. McDonald's, by virtue of its size, enjoys substantial relative power in its relationship with suppliers; McDonald's represents a very large portion of a food supplier's business. This obviates, at least in large part, the need for McDonald's to also own some or all of the suppliers' assets. Ownership and control are essentially separated in this case. The second reason has much less to do with the relative power of the organizations involved and more to do with the establishment of a tradition of mutual gain and cooperation. Specifically, McDonald's has made it a policy to

be loyal to high quality suppliers and to use its size to protect the supplier from dramatic swings in sales revenue. In this way, both parties have incentives to ensure a long-term cooperative relationship—with no ownership interests.

This simplified example is not intended to show that ownership and control are usually unrelated, of course. Rather, the example demonstrates that tight control can exist even in cases where there is no ownership interest. The lesson here is twofold: there are many dimensions upon which one can categorize strategic alliances, and one must exercise caution in interpreting what the dimension really represents. The discussion to follow addresses several additional dimensions upon which one can distinguish one type or form of strategic alliance from another.

Number of Members

Alliances vary greatly in size. They can consist of two organizations, but they often consist of many more. For example, Voluntary Hospitals of America (VHA) is a national hospital alliance that has 100 original members. Size makes a substantial difference in several ways. Larger alliances are more difficult to govern because it is more difficult to represent all members on a single board of directors. Larger size may also entail greater diversity among members, which in turn may make it more difficult to find common ground on important issues ranging from alliance strategy (i.e., what are the overall purpose and goals of the alliance) to the management of alliance programs. Further, even when agreements are reached on alliance strategy and operations, larger size makes it difficult to coordinate members' efforts.

On the other hand, size has virtues. It creates power, as noted earlier. Larger alliances typically have more purchasing power because they can buy in larger volume (assuming, of course, that all members can agree on a particular vendor, which is often difficult). Similarly, larger alliances have more clout in lobbying at various levels of government. Further, larger alliances can generate capital easier simply from having a larger number of members' fees to collect.

Nonetheless, the costs and benefits of alliance size are difficult to assess in the abstract. What often matters most in determining an effective size for an alliance is its strategic purpose and particular situation. For example, RAHC has a relatively small number of members compared to other hospital alliances (e.g., VHA). Yet, it has exactly the number of members it needs for its purpose which is to provide the Rochester area with a comprehensive service system. If it had just one less member, RAHC might be too small for its purpose and might not be nearly as effective as it is.

Governance Structure

In the case of an alliance with two members, it is often not necessary to be concerned about establishing a way to govern alliance activities so as to give them direction. But beyond the simple case of a two-party alliance, governance issues can be considerably complex.

The governing bodies of many alliances, especially hospital alliances, tend to include at least one member from each participating organization, often the director or CEO of the member organization. This practice stems largely from important distinguishing features of alliances, that is, that they are a form of organization in which the members are equal and have a great deal of autonomy.

Further, the boards of health care organizations traditionally have been based on what Fennell and Alexander term a philanthropic model which assumes that "bigger is better."[26] In other words, boards were viewed as a key link to the local community and its resources; having more individuals on a board provided a hospital, for example, with greater community support and access to donors. Similarly, we have observed that alliance boards often are large so as to represent various interest groups.

Indeed, as Carman reports, alliance boards often have physician representatives, board members from participating organizations, and community members as well.[27] Moreover, Carman argues persuasively that alliance boards should not consist entirely of CEOs. He points out that there is enough turnover among CEOs so as to create instability for an alliance if its governance rests only with them.[28] In contrast, organizational commitment to the alliance is enhanced if it is represented in alliance governance by leaders other than CEOs.

As just noted however, this means that larger alliances can have boards with dozens of members which, in turn, can make it difficult to achieve consensus and

can slow down decision making. Of course, large alliance boards can, and sometimes do, have executive committees that consist of a smaller subset of elected members who have the authority to make key decisions. Thus, an important choice for larger alliances is whether to represent all or some members on the alliance board and to determine what kinds of individuals (CEOs, physicians, trustees) should be alliance board members.

Mandated vs. Voluntary Participation

Another important dimension on which alliances vary is whether they are voluntary or mandated by an external group with legal or legitimate authority.[29] Most health care alliances are voluntary. These alliances reflect the efforts of individual organizations to strategically adapt to external changes by choosing to band together. But, it is important to recognize that even voluntary alliances may emerge in large part as a result of external pressure from powerful actors such as in the Rochester case.

A central issue to note in comparing mandated and voluntary alliances is the extent to which the former are characterized more by style than substance and by instability than longevity. Scott argues that mandated forms of organization tend to be adopted only superficially and, as a result, also tend to be short-lived.[30] Many international alliances (including the League of Nations and the United Nations) come to mind in this regard. Superficial compliance with a mandate to form an alliance is especially likely to occur when the participating organizations lack other motives for forming a relationship.[31] In general, managers and other organization members chafe under external constraints and regulation, even when such rules have some merit.

Discussion

Existing typologies have been useful in documenting and describing the common and different features of a wide range of interorganizational arrangements in health care. However, it is also important to ask what difference an organization should expect to see if it were to choose one form versus another.

This seemingly simple question is actually quite difficult to answer. More specifically, we believe that gaining an understanding of the various forms of alliances is only part of understanding the fuller picture of strategic alliances. An additional piece of this puzzle lies in asking not only, What do they look like? but also What are they meant to accomplish?

In other words, an exclusive focus on the different types or forms of health care strategic alliances implicitly assumed that certain forms imply certain functions, and even outcomes. Otherwise, if a single form could actually serve multiple functions, there would not be such an interest in discussing the differences among forms. Zajac, in an analysis of contract management arrangements, argues that organizations choosing to engage in a similar type of strategic alliance may have widely varying strategic intentions and that expected performance will vary correspondingly.[32] This suggests that it may not be reasonable to expect a particular form of interorganizational arrangement to translate into a particular performance result.

The form of alliance used may be much less important in suggesting particular performance outcomes than the strategic intentions, as articulated by key decision makers, that motivate that choice of alliance. In other words, the form of the alliance is not necessarily a good predictor of what the alliance can achieve.

WHAT ARE ALLIANCES MEANT TO DO?

Pooling vs. Trading Alliances

Most broadly, one can distinguish between *pooling* alliances that bring together organizations seeking to contribute similar resources and *trading* alliances that bring together organizations seeking to contribute different resources.[33] This distinction is more precise than the often-made statement that organizations generally seek "complementarities" in alliances. The term complementarity suggests differences, but it is important to remember that similarities can often drive alliance activity as well. An example of a pooling or similarity-driven strategic intent for an alliance is one that seeks to gain purchasing power over a supplier or group of suppliers. Such alliances are often seen in health care, in the form of business coalitions (against hospitals) or hospital alliances (against health care supply organizations).

Examples of a trading or difference-driven alliance are a physician group-hospital joint venture, where each party contributes something distinct to the alliance, and a joint venture between two health care supply firms, such as Johnson & Johnson and Merck, where the former is known for its marketing expertise, the latter for its product development skills. These examples also highlight how strategic intent can often drive the form of a strategic alliance. Pooling strategies tend to involve more organizations and take the form of federations, consortia, or coalitions; and trading strategies tend to involve fewer (often only two) organizations and take the form of joint ventures, licensing agreements, and related arrangements.

Cost Reduction vs. Revenue Enhancement

The strategic intent of alliances can also be examined in terms of their expected outcomes. An emphasis on expected alliance outcomes is relevant for several reasons: the success of an alliance will generally be defined by the degree to which the desired outcomes are achieved; some performance outcomes may be largely incompatible with others; and one alliance partner's perception of the expected outcome may not be shared by that of other partners.

The first and most basic expected outcome refers to financial performance and addresses the issue of whether the alliance is primarily conceived for *cost reduction* or *revenue enhancement*. While this is not to say that the two outcomes are mutually exclusive, there are differences in the challenges for success for alliances, in how one gauges success, and in how cost reducing vs. revenue enhancing alliances might be organized.

For example, consider a local alliance of four hospitals with historically complementary specialties (or distinctive competencies) that is seeking to increase the volume of patients to be treated in these specialties. Compare this alliance with a similarly sized and similarly located hospital alliance seeking to share the costs of providing indigent care to the local community. One would not measure success the same way, nor would the interaction between partners be the same in the two alliances. One might expect that the alliance motivated by the desire to increase patient volume would require substantial coordination, given that there is a reciprocal interdependence between the partners. In the case of the cost-sharing alliance, one would likely observe a combining of similar resources requiring relatively less active coordination, given that there is a pooled interdependence among the partners.[34]

Quality, Innovation, and Learning

Another way of classifying the intent of an alliance is the degree to which the alliance seeks to enhance outcomes such as innovation, organizational learning, and quality.[35,36] These outcomes are distinct from those discussed above in that, while they may lead to revenue enhancement or cost reduction, their relationship to such financial performance measures may be difficult to discern, or in a more extreme case, may be negatively related to financially-oriented targets.[37]

For example, Zuckerman and D'Aunno note that hospitals can increase their reputation for quality by joining a strategic alliance that involves other prestigious organizations.[38] Membership in such an alliance may require only a minor contribution of time, effort, or capital. An interesting feature of such an alliance is that one partner's actions can damage the reputation of another by not delivering the expected level of quality. This suggests the need for appropriate screening of partners in terms of their commitment to quality.

There may also be regional differences in the degree to which membership is prestige-enhancing. One of the authors was involved in a research project on multihospital systems in which a voluntary membership affiliation with a large national, for-profit hospital system was viewed by the local community as an asset to the hospital. The name of the hospital system was proudly displayed at the hospital entrance and on hospital stationery. However, another hospital affiliated with that same system—but located in a different part of the country—made every attempt to downplay that affiliation. No signs were posted with the system name, and no trace of the system could be found on hospital stationery. The reason for this very different treatment? In the first example, the region had many for-profit affiliations, and several of the major hospital chains had their headquarters in that region of the country. In the second example, for-profit hospitals were much less common in the region and were viewed somewhat suspiciously by many in that environment. The point to be made is that, before seeking membership in an alliance for purposes of increasing actual or perceived quality, an organization must be aware of the limits of that benefit.

Other motives driving alliance activity, such as innovation and learning, are also conceptually distinct from other more straightforward motives. The payoffs from alliances that are driven by innovation and learning motives are often slow to emerge. This requires a particularly high level of partner commitment and patience. An additional factor to consider is that many organizations underestimate the involvement necessary to realize benefits such as innovation and learning. In these alliances, a more substantial personnel flow between partners can often accelerate the learning and innovation process.

Power Enhancement, Uncertainty Reduction, and Risk Sharing

Power enhancement and *uncertainty reduction* are grouped together because one often has implications for the other. Specifically, alliances can be motivated by an organization's desire to gain influence over (or reduce dependence on) an aspect of the organization's environment. This reduction in dependence may also represent a reduction in uncertainty, although the two are conceptually distinct. An organization might be dependent on another organization, but if the more powerful organization is reliable, then the dependent organization may face little uncertainty.

This perspective can be seen in much of the early literature on interorganizational relations in health care. Longest, for example, views the growth of multiinstitutional systems as the result of an "external dependency relationship" between the hospital and its environment.[39] In doing so, Longest is applying the resource dependence perspective to the health care industry.[40] Longest uses the term "stabilization strategy" to characterize multihospital arrangements, which he explains are "formulated by people for a hospital that exists in relation to an external environment upon which the hospital is highly dependent."[41]

Uncertainty reduction as an alliance motive can also be compared with a similar, yet distinct, motive: risksharing. The difference between the two motives is that the former highlights one organization's attempts to reduce its own uncertainty, whereas the latter emphasizes the joint reduction of uncertainty for both (or more) partners. Not surprisingly, the former is equated more with gaining influence of an exchange partner, while the latter is used more in terms of pooling resources to reduce common risk.

Summary

It is important to note that the above-mentioned strategic intentions that can drive alliance activity are not at all mutually exclusive. For example, a business coalition may be formed because it wants to gain influence over local area hospitals, but it also has as its major objective a reduction in the cost of health care that the coalition members have had to pay. Thus, power and cost reduction motives are both driving alliance formation. Similarly, a joint venture between a hospital and a multispecialty physician group may have as its objective the creation of new innovative services, yet also have the intent of increasing revenues.[42]

Understanding the strategic intent of an alliance can be a critical success factor for the alliance. The understanding has several components, including understanding your own motivation for considering an alliance, expressing this understanding to your alliance partner, eliciting and then listening carefully to your

partners' expression of their strategic intentions, and examining the compatibility (which could be compatibly similar or compatibly different) of your intentions and those of your partners. The lack of an articulated mission statement is often cited as the root of many failures in organizational strategy. The same is equally if not more true for strategic alliances, particularly given the potential for incompatible intentions across partners.

THE ALLIANCE PROCESS: A MULTISTAGE ANALYSIS

Previous studies of alliances have focused primarily on why they emerge, how they are structured, and what they do. Less attention has been given to how alliances evolve and behave over time.[43-47] Thus, we develop models that managers can use to understand how alliances develop as they do and what can be done to improve their chances for success.

Alliances can be considered within the context of a life cycle model (see Table 11.2). This model suggests that organizations often move through predictable stages of growth, with one or more factors triggering such movement. Further, each stage brings distinctive

TABLE 11.2. A Life Cycle Model of Organizational Alliances in Health Care

Stages			
Emergence	Transition	Maturity	Critical Crossroads
Key factors in development at each stage			
Environment poses threat to and uncertainty about valued resources	Motivation to achieve purposes of the alliance	Willingness to put alliance interests first	Increased centralization and dependence on alliance motivates members to seek hierarchy or withdraw from alliance
Organizations share ideologies and similar dependencies	Increased dependence on alliance for valued resources	Members receive benefits from previous investments	
Examples of tasks at each stage			
Define purposes of the alliance	Hire or form a management group	Attain stated objectives	Manage decisions about future of the alliance
Develop membership criteria	Establish mechanisms for coordination and control	Sustain member commitment	

SOURCE: D'Aunno TA, Zuckerman HS. A life cycle model of organization federations: The case of hospitals. *Academy of Management Review.* 1987; 12:534–545.

tasks that alliance leaders and members need to address.

Emergence: Finding Partners

In the first stage, environmental threats, opportunities, and uncertainty lead organizations with similar ideologies and dependencies to seek out each other. Further, this dance often begins when the potential partners relate to each other *symbiotically* as well as *competitively*.[48,49] In other words, alliances may be more likely to emerge when one organization uses some services or products of the other as opposed to the case when two organizations are vying for the same resources. A common example of symbiosis is a rural community hospital that refers cases for tertiary care to an urban teaching hospital.

Interorganizational exchange processes involve distinct stages.[50] For example, in the early stage each organization engages in the process of projecting exchange into the future and constructing net present valuations of alternative exchange relationships on a continuum ranging from markets (i.e., arms-length transactions with another independent organization), through strategic alliances (i.e., a formal cooperative arrangement between organizations, preserving the independent identity of each partner), and finally to hierarchies (i.e., the merging of two or more organizations into one organization).[51] Perceptions of what each exchange partner seeks also emerges more clearly, enabling the more precise identification of similarities and differences that can form the basis for mutually beneficial exchange.

Thus, in the early stage there is preliminary communication and negotiation concerning mutual and individual organizational interests. An organization's behavior in this stage can set a precedent for future exchange and provide information through which a firm can learn about the expected behavior of its partner. During this phase initial relational exchange norms are being forged and commitments tested in small but important ways to determine credibility.[52] To summarize, in this initial stage, the purposes and expectations of the partners are stated, membership criteria are established, and group norms begin to evolve.

Though it is important for expectations to be realistic, it turns out that many young alliances have broadly stated goals that do not necessarily coincide with their activities. This is because goal statements reflect compromises made among members who are, as of yet, not willing to subordinate their interests to those of the group as a whole. Further, broad goal statements may attract other partners, and early members want to have the advantages that popularity typically affords.

Thus, in many cases, the criteria for alliance membership are selective and designed to assure homogeneity among members. This reduces some of the governance and management problems discussed above. Further, many alliances seek to limit overlap in market areas so as to minimize competition among members and avoid antitrust issues.

At this initial stage, most alliances are not likely to form or hire a management group to direct their activities.[53] This is because organizations must initially identify and agree on a set of purposes. Organizations are also reluctant to yield authority and commit resources to a management group. Nonetheless, this is typically what happens in the second stage of alliance development.

Transition

In this stage the alliance establishes mechanisms for coordination, control, and decision making. This often entails forming or hiring a management group, moving the alliance to a form that Provan, D'Aunno, and Zuckerman term a federation.[54,55] The transition may be rocky because, as just noted, organizations are reluctant to grant authority to others or to sacrifice their own autonomy. It is thus critical that alliance managers assure that their efforts and programs are responsive to members' needs. During this stage the governance structure also takes shape. This may also be threatening to members, especially if they are not directly represented on the governing board.

Alliances vary in the extent to which their members are willing to commit resources to initiate and sustain programs and activities. An important weakness of many alliances is their inability to gain adequate commitment of members' resources. For example, there may be free-rider problems in that some members make little commitment but yet can benefit from the investments of others. It is likely that such problems are directly proportional to the value that members perceive in committing resources to the alliance. The more value that members perceive from active participation, the more resources (including autonomy) they are willing to commit to the alliance.

Of course, this leads to a challenging "chicken and egg" dilemma. On the one hand, members increase their commitment in proportion to threats from their environment and the alliance's ability to reduce threats and uncertainty. On the other hand, for the alliance to be effective in meeting members' needs, it may require the investment of valued resources from members as well as their willingness to coordinate efforts with each other. At some point, alliances require an investment of resources that are risked by members who have no certainty of return equal to their investment. At this point, trust becomes particularly important.

Maturity

The third stage of an alliance's life cycle is that of maturity and growth. In this stage it is critical that the alliance begin to achieve its objectives and aid members in coping with external threats. Such success enables an alliance to continue and to grow. It is also central that members be willing to put the interests of the alliance, at least sometimes, ahead of their own interests. This is necessary because alliances cannot meet the needs of all of their members, at least not simultaneously. Members must recognize that they will not necessarily benefit equally from alliance activities; it is essential, however, that they benefit as equitably as possible.

As alliances seek to attain objectives and sustain member commitment, several issues may arise. For example, alliances that add many members may find it impossible to avoid having members with overlapping market areas. If such overlap does occur, what role, if any, should the alliance play in mediating disputes that may arise among members?

Relationships between the members and alliance managers (if there are any) also become more complex. For example, are new programs initiated through the alliance manager's office, individual members, or both? If through the alliance office, what happens to similar programs already developed by individual members? For instance, suppose that a hospital alliance wishes to develop an alliance-wide HMO, but some members already have HMOs. Further, are there or should there be incentives for members to produce innovative programs that can be shared by all alliance members? In the absence of such incentives, how will the alliance develop innovations in management or services?

Zajac and Olsen, in their discussion of the development of interorganizational relationships, note that alliances in this stage of development face some particularly sensitive issues because value is not only created but also claimed and distributed.[56] Surrounding the issue of claiming and distributing value is the question of interorganizational conflict. Explicit or implicit norms for managing the divergence of interest will often arise.[57] To the extent that these norms—defined as "shared and reasoned expectations that may arise from agreement or past acts—emphasize the importance of joint value maximization, this should lead to searches for mutually satisfactory resolutions of conflict situations.[58] On the other hand, if these evolving norms do not develop in this way, the pursuit of individual firm interests would lead to an escalation of conflict that could ultimately be destructive to the strategic alliance. As noted in Chapter 5, the accepted use of conflict resolution systems can limit the potential damage of interorganizational conflict.[59]

The continued development of trust is a key issue in this stage of interorganizational exchange. Trust stems from a growing confidence in a firm's expectations of the future.[60] Schelling also notes that "trust is often achieved simply by the continuity of the relation between parties and the recognition by each that what he might gain by cheating in a given instance is outweighed by the value of the tradition of trust that makes possible a long sequence of future agreement."[61]

Trust and conflict management systems are subsets of other relational norms underlying the process exchange over time. These norms include shared expectations of reciprocity between alliance partners and a growing sense of the value of preserving the relationship.[62,63] These norms set the tone for the continued execution of contracts.

Critical Crossroads

As they evolve into the fourth stage of development, alliances move to what may be a critical crossroads. Up to this point, members became increasingly dependent on each other for needed resources, and there was growing pressure for greater member commitment to the alliance and more centralized decision making. In many ways, however, these developments run counter to the reasons why many organizations join an alliance. That is, alliances are attractive because they provide a relatively low-cost vehicle to reduce resource dependence while maintaining organizational autonomy. Thus, this stage may be a critical crossroads at which some members conclude that the price of belonging to an alliance is too high and withdraw. Indeed, it appears that at least one hospital alliance collapsed precisely on this point.[64] In contrast, others may decide that it is necessary to move toward more hierarchical arrangements to gain the full benefits of collective action.

The underlying issue is whether there is sufficient commitment or "glue" to hold alliances together over time.[65] Though there may be common goals, ideologies, values, and inducements that keep members together, alliances typically remain loose arrangements. Can the degree of commitment required of members be secured in the long run? Will members be willing to sacrifice autonomy to allow for greater discipline in decision making? What coordination mechanisms are most appropriate and under what circumstances?[66,67] To survive, alliances must balance the need for and benefits of collective action with the need for individual members to retain adequate autonomy.

This critical crossroads represents a reconfiguring stage in the developmental process of a strategic alliance.[68] It is usually triggered by reaching the end of the expected duration of the relationship or by changes

---

IN THE REAL WORLD
THE SOUTHEAST HOSPITAL ALLIANCE

The Southeast Hospital Alliance (SHA) was formed by a dozen relatively large teaching hospitals about ten years ago. It began as an alliance founded by the hospital CEOs, and it did not have a management group. Further, members were geographically distant from each other, enough so that their market areas did not overlap. The original members perceived common threats to teaching hospitals, especially from increased competition from community hospitals that were growing in sophistication and tertiary services.

After a few years, it became clear to the founding members that they needed a management group to help them move beyond discussion to develop useful programs. Further, there were several other hospitals that wanted to join the alliance. A well-regarded management consulting firm, led by a very capable individual, was hired to provide leadership and technical expertise to the alliance.

The new management group suggested adding new members, and the alliance tripled in size.

SHA, under the direction of its management group, began to realize large savings from group purchasing of various supplies. The management group, flush with its initial success, continued to develop new programs. There began to develop, however, subtle but increasing discontent among many of the CEOs. Further, beyond the initial programs, it was not clear what overall direction SHA should take. The SHA manager contacted an external consultant to develop a strategic plan for SHA.

The consultants soon discovered some of the causes for the CEOs' discontent. The SHA management group, through its original and main line of business—management consulting—was leasing mobile MRI and CT scan equipment to rural hospitals. The leased equipment effectively helped the rural hospitals to compete with SHA members. Moreover, in an effort to increase its size to support its group purchasing program, SHA had admitted several members whose market areas overlapped with each other.

in the partners' perceived level of the relationship's value. Reconfiguring may imply that an exchange partner will choose to leave, or it may mean that partners will join more tightly together by widening the scope of interorganizational exchange processes. For example, a group of hospitals may move from a shared purchasing arrangement to developing a joint preferred provider network.

With respect to perceived changes in the value of the strategic alliance, such changes may emerge from a new and changing environment or a historical comparison of actual to expected value creation. While this performance gap can lead to a re-evaluation (positive or negative) of the interorganizational relationship itself, it may simply lead to a reassessment of the developmental processes. In other words, the reconfiguring stage may not involve a change in the type of strategic alliance *per se* but only a change in the process of interaction within the existing strategic alliance. These change options suggest that this stage may loop back to either the emergence stage, where value forecasts are respecified and strategic motivations are clarified for a new forecast period, or the transition stage, where the forms of exchange are revised and updated based on the continued experiences of the partners). Thus, the process model of strategic alliance development outlined here does not propose a one-way, deterministic path for alliances; instead, it highlights a sequence of likely phases that many alliances may experience and emphasizes a set of critical issues that health care organizations may face at the various stages of alliance development.

FRAMEWORKS FOR ANALYZING ALLIANCE PROBLEMS

A major difficulty that organizations face in addressing alliance problems is actually their inability to identify the problem correctly! By that we mean that individuals within an organization often don't know or disagree strongly on what the problem is, and this is compounded by differences of opinion between partners in alliance problem identification and diagnosis. These disagreements, we contend, can often lead to false diagnoses and the treatment of *symptoms* rather than the root *problems* facing the alliance. These incorrect interventions subsequently lead to greater friction, gridlock, and ultimately an increased likelihood of alliance failure. The two simple frameworks offered below are intended to lessen the likelihood of such failure.

Locating the Problem

If one were to ask several involved individuals why a particular alliance was in trouble, it is possible that one would get a uniform response. In such cases, locating the problem is simple. We argue, however, that such agreement is the exception rather than the norm. Typically there are a host of possible reasons why an alliance might be facing difficulties. Without some way of organizing these reasons, there may be little hope of remedying the situation. We propose that alliance problems can be viewed as generally falling into the following categories[69]

- environmental problems
- strategy problems
- structure problems
- behavior problems

These categories follow a macro to micro continuum, but more important for purposes of this chapter, they also tend to follow an uncontrollable to controllable continuum. For example, SHA faced controllable problems. The problems first appeared to stem from competitors in the environment. But, closer analysis showed that the SHA management group was fueling the competition for its own members; thus, a change in management's behavior was needed. Further, SHA had a structural problem: members with overlapping market areas. This problem was also under SHA control. We use an interesting non-health care example of an alliance failure to further illustrate this point.

In 1990, a consortium called U.S. Memories was conceived to provide a secure supply of chips for U.S. computer makers who were unhappy with the occasional shortages and price fluctuations brought on by Japanese chip makers, who controlled almost 90% of the DRAM market. This alliance, made up of U.S. chip buyers and a few U.S. chip makers, never got off the ground, as initial players backed out and new players refused to commit resources. Analysts offered several reasons as to why the alliance failed. Some attributed

MANAGERIAL GUIDELINES

1. In assessing the risk of forming or entering an alliance, managers should compare the potential costs and benefits of alliances to doing nothing or to alternative strategies that involve going it alone; alliances may well be less risky than other strategies.

2. The form or structure of alliance should follow from its function, that is, what it is intended to do.

3. Managers should consider their options with respect to several important aspects of alliance structure, including ownership and control, number of members, governance structure, and mandated vs. voluntary participation.

4. Many of the benefits of control in interorganizational relationships can be achieved without ownership; trust, commitment, and even power may be important substitutes for control based on ownership.

5. Increased size brings greater complexity and often more difficulty in coordinating efforts, but larger alliances tend to be more powerful for certain purposes (e.g., lobbying, purchasing in volume).

6. Large alliances often need more complex governance structures, and a key issue is who will be represented on an alliance board. It may be a mistake to have only CEOs or executive directors on alliance boards because the interests of other groups may be neglected; further, turnover among top managers is common and may disrupt the alliance if the board has no other types of members.

7. Mandated participation in an alliance is often less preferable to voluntary participation. Alliances are not likely to succeed if members' only or most important motive for participation is to comply with external demands.

8. Recognize that alliances can be created to achieve one or more of the following objectives: to pool similar resources (e.g., as in joint purchasing arrangements); to trade dissimilar resources (e.g., as in a symbiotic relationship between a hospital and physician group); to reduce costs; to enhance revenues; to promote innovation, learning, or quality of services; to enhance power, reduce uncertainty, or share risks among members.

9. From the above list, it is important to understand your own motives for seeking an alliance and to express these motives to potential or current partners.

10. Similarly, managers need to listen carefully to the intentions of potential or current partners in order to assess compatibility; failure to articulate a shared mission is an important reason for alliance failure.

11. Two kinds of problems are typical when it comes to alliance objectives. First, even

the failure to the fact that, once the temporary chip shortage was over, the alliance had no purpose. Others said it was ill-conceived and that the U.S. could never have competed with the more efficient Japanese chip makers. Some said that not enough players were involved; some said *too many* players were involved; and others said that the deal was not well-structured. Finally, some blamed the leader of the consortium, saying that he was not well-suited for such a position.

What do we make out of this mess? Could this alliance have been salvaged? Basically, we can start by using the framework above to categorize the myriad of alliance problems into environmental ("the market changed"), strategic ("it was a bad idea from the beginning"), structural ("it wasn't organized correctly"), and behavioral ("we had the wrong person at the top") problems. The point here is that, from a managerial perspective, a person responsible for gathering information about the alliance, processing that information, and making a decision on whether or how to intervene,

MANAGERIAL GUIDELINES

though alliance objectives may be shared by members, the objectives may conflict with each other, especially over time. Second, there may be lack of consensus among members concerning alliance objectives. Both problems highlight the need for effective communication.

12. Recognize that alliances often develop in several stages that each bring distinctive threats and opportunities.

13. In the first stage (emergence), it is important to define the purposes of the alliance and select partners accordingly. Clear communication and acknowledgement of interests are critical.

14. After forming an alliance, managers must find ways to coordinate and control activities; this may entail hiring or forming a management group to focus specifically on alliance concerns.

15. As alliances mature, managers are likely to face complex issues about how much individual members must conform to and, indeed, place alliance interests ahead of their own. Further, there may be conflict about how to distribute the benefits (resources) that alliances have generated. Thus, managers need to focus on ways to sustain member commitment through trust, goal attainment, and the use of appropriate mechanisms to resolve conflict.

16. Mature alliances face the task of measuring up to members' original and changing expectations. Such alliances need to rethink their structure and objectives to make sure that they keep pace with members' needs.

17. More specifically, managers can diagnose alliance problems according to whether they are primarily environmental (i.e., stemming from external sources such as shift in market demands); strategic (i.e., concerning the overall purpose and direction of the alliance); structural (i.e., alliance form fits poorly with its purposes); or behavioral (i.e., skills are not adequate for carrying out alliance activities).

18. It is important to match alliance problems with appropriate means to deal with them, ranging from educating members to negotiating with them to coercing them.

19. Alliances can be just a management fad—be careful that you are forming one for the right reasons.

20. Recognize that alliances have their costs for managers in terms of time spent in understanding and negotiating with potential and current partners. In fact, alliances can slow down decision making and make organizations less flexible—precisely what they are designed to avoid.

21. Select partners and develop ways of relating to them so as to avoid charges of collusion and antitrust problems.

22. Don't let alliance arrangements make your organization lazy and lose its interest in continuous improvement.

---

can begin to piece together problems into useful clusters or categories.

Secondly, the categories themselves are useful in assessing the degree to which intervention can be effective. For example, after analyzing the categorized reasons, a manager may believe that the primary problem is environmental, that is, the market conditions no longer support the alliance. This is largely an uncontrollable factor and, therefore, suggests that the alliance is not likely to succeed. On the other hand, the manager may believe the primary problem is structural—that the number or composition of the alliance is not right (as in the SHA example) or that the incentives for participation are inadequate. This is more of a controllable factor and suggests that the alliance can be modified and thus face improved odds for success. In this way, the Environment→Strategy→Structure→Behavior framework can be a useful tool in identifying and diagnosing alliance problems.

Separating the Root from the Symptom

If you had a rash and were to go to a physician, what would be the first thing the physician would do? Treat the rash or first ask a set of questions to discern why you have the rash? Hopefully, the latter approach is the more common. Unfortunately, many organizations involved in strategic alliances take the former approach. There's a problem; let's fix it. This "can do" attitude is laudable in one sense, but potentially reckless (even rash?) in another sense. Specifically, when one observes friction in strategic alliances, we argue that the most important response is to first delve more deeply to understand the source of that friction before attempting to treat the problem.

This advice regarding diagnosis before treatment may seem obvious, but it often is not done in alliances. The reason it is often not done stems from alliance partners' unwillingness or inability to put themselves in their partners' shoes. In the SHA example, it was the management group that was not putting itself in members' shoes. By this we mean that signs of noncooperative behavior from a partner are often viewed with hostility on the part of other partners. The other partners then devise their own response strategy before an analysis or diagnosis is done as to why the partner may appear to be acting noncooperatively. Quite simply, we are stating that the noncooperative behavior is only a symptom of a deeper problem.

The obvious questions then become, What could the deeper problems be, and how do we treat them? We propose that there are at least four categories of problems

- parochial self-interest
- misunderstanding and a lack of trust
- different assessments
- low tolerance for ambiguity

These categories, interestingly, match discussions of problems that exist in managing change.[20] While the categories are not mutually exclusive, they are quite distinct from one another. For example, the first category represents rational, calculative, noncooperative behavior in which one partner knowingly acts in his own interest to the detriment of the other partner. The second type of problem is based less on selfishness than on the absence of accepted and well-developed norms; that is, a trusting relationship between partners has yet to emerge. The third category differs from the first in that, while the first category (i.e., selfish, noncooperative behavior) reflects disagreement on ends and means, the third category reflects agreement on ends but not means. In other words, partners may share the same goal but diverge in their views on how to achieve that goal. Lastly, some alliance partners simply feel uncomfortable with the ambiguity and fluidity of alliances. The absence of full control, as is typical in strategic alliances, may not agree with some reluctant partners.

Identifying different categories of problems is in and of itself useful as a way to move beyond the symptom and towards the problem. Treating the problem is the next step, and we propose a simple principle: the treatment should match the problem. Again, while this seems obvious, we find that all too often in alliances the treatment is either insufficient or too harsh. Both of these situations are unfavorable. There are at least six ways of dealing with alliance problems

- education
- participation
- facilitation
- negotiation
- cooptation
- coercion

Matching this set of treatments with the set of problems identified earlier represents a step towards effective alliance management.[71] Consider the case where a partner faces a particularly calculative, self-interested partner. That partner is not lacking information; she knows what the situation is but does not want what her partner wants. In this case, an approach that emphasizes negotiation or cooptation is likely to be more effective than one that emphasizes participation or education. Contrast such a case with a partner whose actions are based on a misunderstanding. Here, negotiation as a response does not address the root problem; education and participation are more appropriate. We invite the reader to draw further matches between problem and treatment.

In summary, both of the frameworks presented seek to avoid a major problem in alliance management—recognizing the problem and matching the type of problem to an appropriate type of response.

KEY CONCEPTS

Alliance Problems vs.
   Symptoms
Alliance Process
Alliance Risk
Cost Reduction vs.
   Revenue
   Enhancement
Ownership vs. Control

Pooling vs. Trading
   Alliances
Strategic Alliance
Symbiotic vs. Competitive
   Interdependence
Turbulent Environment
Uncertainty reduction

Discussion Questions

1. Under what circumstances would you agree with someone who said that alliances are very risky?
2. What dimensions would you use to classify the various types of strategic alliances? Why those dimensions?
3. Which alliance motivations do you think are the most compatible with each other?
4. What do you consider to be the likely stages of strategic alliance development? Does every alliance have to go through each stage?
5. What is the difference between an alliance problem and an alliance symptom, and what does this difference mean in terms of managerial intervention?

REFERENCES

1. Georgopolous BS, D'Aunno TD, Saavedra R. Hospital-physician relations under hospital prepayment. *Medical Care.* 1987;25(8):781–795.
2. Emery F, Trist E. The casual texture of organizational environments. *Human Relations.* 1965;18:21–32.
3. Shortell SM, Zajac EJ. Health care organizations and the development of the strategic management perspective. In: Mick S, ed. *Innovations in Health Care Delivery: New Insights into Organization Theory.* San Francisco, Cal: Jossey-Bass, 1990:141–180.
4. Longest BB. Interorganizational linkages in the health sector. *Health Care Management Review.* 1990;15:17–28.
5. Harrigan KR. *Managing for Joint Venture Success.* Lexington, Mass: Lexington Books; 1985.
6. Zajac EJ, Golden BR, Shortell SM. New organizational forms for enhancing innovation: The case of internal corporate joint ventures. *Management Science.* 1991;37:170–184.
7. Shortell SM, Zajac EJ. Internal corporate joint ventures: Development processes and performance outcomes. *Strategic Management Journal.* 1988;9:527–542.
8. Ibid.
9. Zuckerman HS, D'Aunno TA. Hospital alliances: Cooperative strategy in a competitive environment. *Health Care Management Review.* 1990;15(2):21–30.
10. Zuckerman H, Kaluzny A. The management of strategic alliances in health services. *Frontiers of Health Services Management.* Spring 1991;7(5):3–23.
11. Alter C, Hage J. *Organizations Working Together.* Beverly Hills, Ca: Sage; 1993.
12. Shortell, Zajac, 1988, op. cit.
13. Shortell, Zajac, 1990, op. cit.
14. Kaluzny A, Morrissey J, McKinney M. Emerging organizational networks: The case of the community clinical oncology program. In Mick S and Associates, eds. *Innovation in Health Care Delivery.* San Francisco, Ca: Jossey-Bass; 1990.
15. Meyer A. Adapting to environmental jolts. *Administrative Science Quarterly.* 1982;27:515–537.
16. Shortell SM, Morrison EM, Friedman B. *Strategic Choices for America's Hospitals: Managing Change in Turbulent Times.* San Francisco, Ca: Jossey-Bass; 1990.
17. Zajac EJ, Shortell SM. Changing generic strategies: Likelihood, direction, and performance implications. *Strategic Management Journal.* 1989;10:413–430.
18. Shortell SM. The evolution of hospital systems: Unfulfilled promises and self-fulfilling prophecies. *Medical Care Review.* 1988;45(2):177–214.
19. Clement JP. Does hospital diversification improve financial outcomes? *Medical Care.* 1987;25:988–1001.
20. Starr P. *The Social Transformation of American Medicine.* New York, NY: Basic Books; 1982.

21. Starkweather DB. Health facility mergers: Some conceptualizations. *Medical Care.* 1971;9:468–478.
22. Brown M, Lewis HL. *Hospital Management Systems: Multi-Unit Organization and Delivery of Health Care.* Germantown, Md: Aspen Systems Corporation; 1976.
23. DeVries RA. Strength in numbers. *Hospitals: Journal of the American Hospital Association.* 1978;55:81–84.
24. Ibid.
25. Ibid.
26. Fennell ML, Alexander TA. Hospital governance and profound organizational change. *Medical Care Review.* 1989;46(2):157–187.
27. Carman JM. *Strategic Alliances among Rural Hospitals.* Berkeley, Ca: Institute of Business and Economic Research, University of California; 1992. 92–003.
28. Alexander TA, Fennell ML, Halpern MT. Leadership instability in hospitals: The influence of board-CEO relations and organizational growth and decline. *Administrative Science Quarterly.* March 1993;74–99.
29. Provan KG. The federation as an interorganizational linkage network. *Academy of Management Review.* 1983;8(1):79–89.
30. Scott WR. The adolescence of institutional theory. *Administrative Science Quarterly.* 1987;32:493–511.
31. Oliver C. Determinants of interorganizational relationships: Integration and future directions. *Academy of Management Review.* 1990;15(2):241–265.
32. Zajac EJ. *Organizations, Environments, and Performance: A Study of Contract Management in Hospitals.* Philadelphia, Pa: University of Pennsylvania; 1986. Dissertation.
33. Nielsen RP. Cooperative strategies. *Planning Review.* 1986;14:16–20.
34. Thompson JT. *Organizations in Action.* New York, NY: McGraw Hill; 1967.
35. Zajac, Golden, Shortell, op. cit.
36. Prahalad CK, Hamel G. The core competence of the corporation. *Harvard Business Review.* May-June 1990; 68(3):79–82.
37. Shortell, Zajac, 1990, op. cit.
38. Zuckerman, D'Aunno, op. cit.
39. Longest, op. cit.
40. Pfeffer J, Salancik GR. *The External Control of Organizations: A Resource Dependence Perspective.* New York, NY: Harper & Row; 1978.
41. Longest, op. cit.
42. Longest, op. cit.
43. D'Aunno TA, Zuckerman HS. The emergence of hospital federations: An integration of perspectives from organizational theory. *Medical Care Review.* 1987;44(2):323–343.
44. Zajac EJ, Olsen CP. From transaction costs to transactional value analysis: Implications for the study

❖

of interorganizational strategies. *Journal of Management Studies.* 1993;30:131–146.

45. Luke RD, Begun JW, Pointer DD. Quasi firms: Strategic interorganizational forms in the health care industry. *Academy of Management Review.* 1989;14(9):19.

46. Provan KG. Interorganizational cooperation and decision making autonomy in a consortium multihospital system. *Academy of Management Review.* 1984;9:494–504.

47. Sofaer S, Myrtle RC. Interorganizational theory and research: Implications for health care management, policy, and research. *Medical Care Review.* 1991;48:371–409.

48. Hawley AH. *Human Ecology: A Theory of Community Structure.* New York, NY: Ronald Press; 1950.

49. Pfeffer, Salancik, op. cit.

50. Zajac, Olsen, op. cit.

51. Macneil IR. Values in contract: Internal and External. *Northwestern University Law Review.* 1983;78:340–418.

52. Ibid.

53. D'Aunno, Zuckerman, *Medical Care Review,* op. cit.

54. Provan, 1983, op. cit.

55. D'Aunno TA, Zuckerman HS. A life cycle model of organizational federations: The case of hospitals. *Academy of Management Review.* 1987;12:534–545.

56. Zajac, Olsen, op. cit.

57. Ibid.

58. Kaufmann PJ. Commercial exchange relationships and the "negotiator's dilemma." *Negotiation Journal.* 1987;3:73–80.

59. Ury WL, Brett JM, Goldberg SB. *Getting Disputes Resolved.* San Francisco, Ca: Jossey-Bass; 1988.

60. Luhmann N. *Trust and Power.* New York, NY: John Wiley and Sons; 1979.

61. Schelling TC. *The Strategy of Conflict.* Cambridge, Mass: Harvard University; 1960.

62. Macneil, 1983, op. cit.

63. Macneil IR. Exchange revisited: Individual utility and social solidarity. *Ethics.* 1986;96:567–593.

64. Ury, et al., op. cit.

65. Zuckerman, Kaluzny, op. cit.

66. Alter, Hage, op. cit.

67. Kaluzny A, Zuckerman H. Strategic alliances: Two perspectives for understanding their effects on health services. *Hospital and Health Services Management.* Winter 1992;37:477-490.

68. Zajac, Olsen, op. cit.

69. Johnson DEL. American Healthcare Systems. *Modern Healthcare.* 1986;16:78–82.

70. Kotter JP, Schlesinger LA. Choosing strategies for change. *Harvard Business Review.* 1979;57:106–114.

71. Ibid.

72. Duncan WJ, Ginter PM, Swayne LE. *Strategic Issues in Health Care Management: Point and Counterpoint.* Boston, Mass: Kent Publishers; 1992.

CHAPTER

12

ORGANIZATIONAL INNOVATION AND CHANGE

S. Robert Hernandez
Professor

Arnold D. Kaluzny
Professor

CHAPTER TOPICS

The Change Process
Types of Change

LEARNING OBJECTIVES

After completing this chapter, the reader should be able to

1. describe the change process that occurs within health services organizations and identify factors which facilitate or inhibit that process
2. identify and understand the types of change associated with technical operations and the methods to manage such change
3. identify and understand the types of change and methods associated with identifying and introducing new services
4. describe the types of change involving administrative, structural, or strategy mechanisms and the approaches that affect such change processes
5. describe human resource changes and identify methods for managing such changes

CHAPTER PURPOSE

Community Hospital of Roanoke like so many health care institutions is involved in change—change which is occurring at an unrelenting pace in an increasingly uncertain environment. The objective of this chapter is to provide an understanding of the change process occurring in health services organizations. First, change is viewed as a process involving a series of stages. Next, four types of change—technical; product or service; administrative, structural, or strategy; and human resource—are defined and briefly discussed. Then, each type of organizational change is described in detail along with the factors which influence the change and the managerial strategies available for managing each type of change. The chapter concludes with a series of managerial guidelines to improve organizational change and innovation.

IN THE REAL WORLD
THE COMMUNITY HOSPITAL OF ROANOKE

By 1984 Community Hospital of Roanoke had just completed the second phase of a three-phase construction project expanding to 400 beds and modernizing and expanding administrative and support services, surgical services, outpatient services, and intensive care services. Things were going well. Operating as a not-for-profit, acute care facility in a Standard Metropolitan Statistical Area (SMSA) of 225,000, Community Hospital of Roanoke maintained a patient mix of slightly more than 50 percent Medicare patient days and a steady 80 percent occupancy rate. Management and professional staff were confident that the hospital was well positioned to meet the future needs and expectations of their community.

The 1985 implementation of the Medicare Prospective Payment System (PPS) challenged the stability if not the very survival of the hospital. Mandates of PPS to reduce the length of stay along with corresponding reductions in patient days and occupancy rate of Medicare patients threatened the long-term financial viability of the institution.

In response the management initiated a number of changes. These changes were designed to either increase revenue through adding new programs and services, thereby changing the patient stay, or reduce cost through developing and implementing a cost containment program, including a modification of the final phase of the construction project. Intended revenue generating strategies included vertical integration through the establishment of an industrial medicine-occupational health program and a freestanding urgent care center and market share building through the creation of a women's health center, an adult health center, and the implementation of a state-of-the-art family-centered maternity program.

While each of these initiatives would eventually change the patient mix, more immediate actions were required for securing the hospital's financial future. To meet this challenge, management requested departments to describe their current cost containment efforts, quantify the outcomes of these efforts, and provide any additional suggestions for how the organization could further reduce costs. The results were compiled into a matrix-type chart and presented to the department heads at their monthly meeting. The objective was for each department to implement one new cost containment activity that had been suggested or had proven successful in another department. Actions included closer monitoring of overtime, revisions in policies regarding mandatory attendance at staff meetings and educational programs, revision of inventory levels and control systems, cross-training staff to increase versatility and improve scheduling flexibility, and encouraging staff to take vacations during periods of lowest census in order to reduce the need for supplemental staffing during census peaks.

In addition, management curtailed plans for the third phase of the construction project, thereby improving the hospital's capital position. By substituting renovation for new construction, several million dollars would be saved. The new plan changed the allocation of beds between services through a sequential displacement process of closing and reopening beds during the renovations, resulting in a net decrease of medical-surgical beds. From these changes emerged an overall retrenchment strategy downsizing the total number of beds in service and reducing full-time equivalents per occupied bed. While many challenges remain, Community Hospital was well on its way to meeting the requirements of a new and changing environment.

SOURCE: *Andrea Silvey, University of Alabama at Birmingham, Doctoral Program in Administration/Health Services, 1993.*

THE CHANGE PROCESS

Health care executives are involved in various types of changes and innovations ranging from the introduction of new pieces of equipment or programs to redefinition of the goals of the organization. Change is different from innovation. Change is a generic concept that deals with any modification in operations, structure, or ends of the organization. Innovation is more restricted and is defined as any idea, practice, or material artifact perceived to be new to a relevant unit of adoption—organization, work group, or individual.[1] Thus all innovation is considered change, but not all change is innovation.

Whether change or innovation, the organization or relevant unit within the organization is involved with a process. The process involves a number of distinct *stages.*[2]

• *Awareness* is the initial stage of the process in which individuals recognize that there is a discrepancy or gap between what the organization or work unit is currently doing and what it should or could be doing. This awareness may be sparked internally by the expectations of participants or externally by community or regulatory pressures affecting the performance of the organization.

• *Identification,* the second stage of the process, involves an attempt to address the discrepancies or performance gap identified in the prior stage. This may occur at various points within the organization, and the critical challenge is to assure that identified solutions are quickly moved to implementation.

• *Implementation* involves the very presence or operations of the change within the organization or the relevant work unit within the organization.

• *Institutionalization* refers to the integration of the change into ongoing activities of the organization. Many changes are implemented but fail to truly be internalized within the organization.

Figure 12.1 indicates a sequence of stages and the factors which influence each stage. Three points are critical. First, the stages involve a sequential process in which any change or innovation is at risk of not proceeding to the next stage of the process. Moreover, the process is interactive such that institutionalization

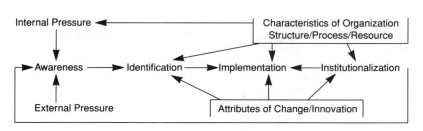

FIGURE 12.1. Attributes of change or innovation. Adapted from Smith, David and Kaluzny, Arnold, *The White Labyrinth: A Guide to the Health Care System,* p. 193, © Health Administration Press. Reprinted with permission.

is contingent on implementation; implementation is contingent on identification; and identification is contingent on awareness.

Second, the process is affected by a complex set of interacting factors. The prevailing structure and processes, such as degree of complexity and formalization as well as levels of communication, coordination, and availability of resources, all influence whether a change or innovation moves through the sequential stages of the process. These interactions may be paradoxical. For example, organizational complexity provides the diversity within the organization by which personnel are likely to be aware of any discrepancy between what the organization is doing versus what it could or should be doing along with the ability to identify solutions. However, this very same complexity may inhibit the actual implementation and institutionalization of the required change. The diversity of resources within the organization may create conflicting expectations and priorities, limiting the amount of change that actually occurs.[3] Moreover, change is not an undifferentiated phenomena. Certain types of innovation and change may be more consistent with a particular structure and set of processes and thus move through the various stages in a much easier manner.

Finally, change is a continual process. Given the dynamic environment within which the organization functions, changes are institutionalized and require continual assessment resulting in subsequent awareness of any discrepancy between what the organization

is currently doing versus what it should be doing, thus reinitiating the process.

TYPES OF CHANGE

Health services organizations experience technical change; product or service change; administrative, structural, or strategy change; and human resources change.[4] Some health service organizations are able to handle one type of change better than they are other types. For example, some organizations may identify, develop, and market new products or services quite easily while having great difficulty in adopting and implementing administrative changes. Senior health services managers need to understand the types of changes, their interactions, and the factors which influence or expedite the successful implementation and institutionalization of the various types of change.

Technical change is concerned with changing the basic methods that organizations use to deliver health services. This change may involve modifications in the practice patterns of physicians, changes in the flow of patients into or through the organization, change in job assignments and responsibilities of professionals within the organization, or change which results in the purchase of new equipment to provide existing services. For example, some rural hospitals have made a change in the technical manner in which services are provided by hiring cross-trained clinical technicians to do multiple functions within the hospital.

Product or service change is concerned with the introduction of new products or services by the organization. Teaching hospitals may be involved in research which results in the development of new methods for the diagnosis and treatment of disease. Community hospitals in competitive urban environments may learn of new services developed by other hospitals and begin providing those new services to attract patients to their facility.

Administrative, structural, or strategy change is concerned with the managerial or administrative activities of the organization. This area concerns changes in organizational structure, human resource policies, organizational strategy, use of integrating mechanisms within the institution, management and clinical information systems, and financial systems. For example, many health services organizations have restructured their institutions to provide product line or service line management. Other institutions have developed for-profit components and participated in joint ventures and outsourcing arrangements with vendors and other health care providers.

Human resources change refers to attempts to influence attitudes, behaviors, skills, and values of employees. Health services organizations, for example, may wish to improve the managerial capability of their department heads and midline managers or the level of their commitment to the organization's mission.

Below we examine each type of change in greater detail and suggest strategies to facilitate the change process. The strategies and types of change are not mutually exclusive, and effective management requires a blend of insight and judgement (see Debate Time 12.1).

Technical Change

The technical system is concerned with doing the primary work of the organization. James Thompson, for example, describes an organization in terms of "technical core" and a group of "boundary spanning units."[5] An organization attempts to reduce uncertainty for its technical core by sealing it from its environment so that its routine activities can be protected from change. Thus, the technical core standardizes work flows and work processes. It attempts to obtain slack resources by stockpiling or doing preventive maintenance so that its operations will not be disrupted. Individuals involved in the delivery of health services prefer routinization of such activities so that they are able to do repetitive tasks well. Thus, the challenge for health management is to introduce new methods which will improve the internal efficiency of their organization without unintentionally creating difficulties or disrupting the work patterns, norms, and values of professionals within the technical core.

DEBATE TIME 12.1: WHAT DO YOU THINK?

Change and innovation are not one dimensional or simple linear processes over time. Consider just a few of the changes occurring in various health service organizations

- unrelenting flow of technology such as the availability of extracorporeal membrane oxygenation (ECMO) and positron emission tomography (PET) scanners
- greater attention given to health promotion and early detection activities such as nutritional counseling and sigmoidoscopy screening
- new administrative arrangements including just-in-time management, outsourcing, joint ventures, and succession planning

- downsizing among existing personnel at the same time that new roles are being created

Is there a sequence to the types of changes which occur? Are some changes or innovations prerequisites for other types of changes? What factors affect each type of change? Is it likely that factors which facilitate problem recognition and thus lead to the identification of one type of change may limit implementation or institutionalization? Given the types of change and innovation, are some types more likely to occur easily in some organizations or in some units within organizations yet present major difficulties in other organizations or units?

Awareness of a *performance gap* and the need for technical change in a health services organization may arise internally. Management or health professionals in the organization may become aware of deficiencies in the technical core by a number of means. For example, quality management activities may challenge professionals by providing feedback that the level of care being provided is not at acceptable standards.[6] Or, patient satisfaction surveys may suggest that services are not being provided in a caring, sensitive manner acceptable to the population being serviced.

An organization may also become aware of the need for change because of regulatory pressures or competitive demands arising externally. For example, management may conclude that retrenchment and downsizing in operations must be done to allow the organization to remain viable. The need for cost reductions and efficiencies in technical operations may require that the organization reexamine its entire method of providing services in an attempt to streamline operations and provide care in a cost-effective manner.

Identifying solutions for technical performance problems, whether identified from internal or external sources, most frequently requires significant input from the professional staff. Health services organizations can make significant, successful change in patterns of work flow only with guidance and direction from those intimately involved in providing care.

Strategies

Management has a number of methods available for effecting technical change. One method used for facilitating technical change is *task analysis*. Task analysis focuses on the redesign of tasks within the organization to facilitate change and improve performance. Division of work into simple, specialized jobs was first suggested by the scientific management school to increase internal efficiency. This specialization allowed tasks to be differentiated, resulting in greater organizational control over individual behavior, selection of less skilled workers, and routinization of work flow to improve coordination.

However, routine jobs that require few skills and provide no challenge because of extreme specialization can lead to dissatisfaction, turnover and absenteeism, reduced motivation, and low quality performance.

Jobs may be redesigned by job enlargement (adding more activities) or job enrichment (adding more responsibility to the job).[7] The effect of job redesign to facilitate change has had mixed results, a positive relationship to change in some settings and little or no effect in other settings.[8] These and related issues of work design are discussed further in Chapter 7.

Successful technical change and innovation within an organization also may require that *specific roles* be designated to facilitate the change process. Organizations require the designation of an idea generator, a sponsor, and an orchestrator.[9] The idea generator recognizes a problem and develops a response to solve it. This individual may come from any level in the organization but, as an individual, lacks the resources or authority to develop and implement the changes. This situation creates the need for a sponsor to carry the idea through to implementation. Sponsors are usually middle managers who can take the idea and fund the increasingly disruptive and expensive development and testing efforts that it requires. Yet a third role is required to manage the political struggle that occurs with the organization against those who have authority and control of resources. The orchestrator, usually the chief executive officer (CEO), must protect idea people and provide the opportunity for change. This role is critical because new ideas often conflict with established programs within the organization. Health care organizations must recognize the various roles required for change. Ideas that arise within the technical core of the organization must receive support from the management structure for implementation to occur.

Total quality management (TQM), or *continuous quality improvement (CQI)* as it is sometimes called, is another approach to facilitate change. It requires a more systematic examination of the internal operations of the organization and focuses on identifying and implementing improvement in performance. It is a participative, systematic approach to planning and implementing a continuous organizational improvement process.[10–12]

This approach is focused on satisfying customers' expectations, identifying problems, building commitment, and promoting open decision making among workers. CQI uses a structured process often known as FOCUS to identify, analyze, and design process improvements and another known as PCDA to implement and institutionalize improvements.[13] Both FOCUS and PCDA are cyclical processes and provide a simple but effective short-hand for problem-solving and planning processes based on the scientific method. FOCUS specifies the steps to use in identifying and solving problems:

- Find process to improve.
- Organize the team.
- Collect information.
- Understand variation in the process.
- Select improvements.

PCDA reminds team members to:

- Plan and try out the change.
- Check the results.
- Do what it takes to implement the change.
- Act to secure the change and to identify new problems.

The analytical tools used in FOCUS-PCDA include Ishikawa (fishbone) diagrams, flow charts, check sheets, Pareto charts, and run and control charts. The process is also carefully designed to include decision and communication tools such as brainstorming, nominal group process and consensus formation to institute quality measures, and storyboards to communicate the results to others. An example of using TQM to change the way in which a hospital laboratory provides serum potassium results to the emergency room (ER) is shown in Figure 12.2.

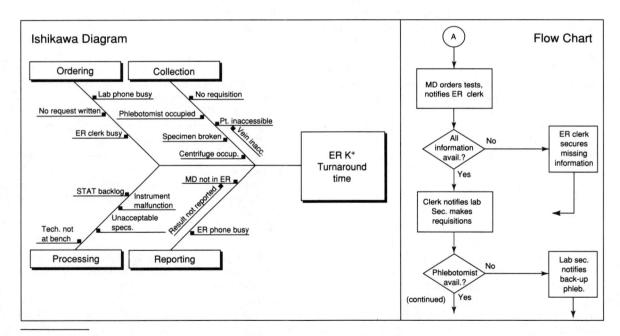

FIGURE 12.2. Analytical tools used in FOCUS-PCDA. Adapted from Simpson, Kaluzny, and McLaughlin, *Total Quality and the Management of Laboratories,* Clinical Laboratory Management Review, (November/December 1991), copyright © Clinical Laboratory Management Association, Inc. Reprinted with permission.

Check Sheet

Delays in production of Se K$^+$ results from 1/1/91 to 1/7/91

Code/Delay Type		Mon	Tue	Wed	Thur	Fri	Sat	Sun	Total
A	Request not written by physician	I	I				I		3
B	Lab phone busy > 2 min.	I		I		II		I	5
C	Phlebotomists unavailable	III	II	III	III	II	IIII	III	20
D	Requisition not ready	II	I	I	I	I	III	II	11
E	Patient inaccessible	I	I	II	I		II	I	8
F	Vein inaccessible	I		II		II			6
G	Centrifuge busy	II		I		I			4
H	Specimen broken	II		I				I	4
I	STAT backlog	III			I		II	I	7
J	Tech. not at bench	II		II		I	II	I	8
K	Unacceptable specimen	I	I		II		I	II	7
L	Lab. sec. unavailable to report	III		I		I	I		6
M	ER phone not answered			I		I	II		3
N	MD not in ER	II		I		II		I	6
O	MD not answer page	I	I	II		II		II	8
P	Results not reported by ER sec.	II	I	II	I	III	II	II	13

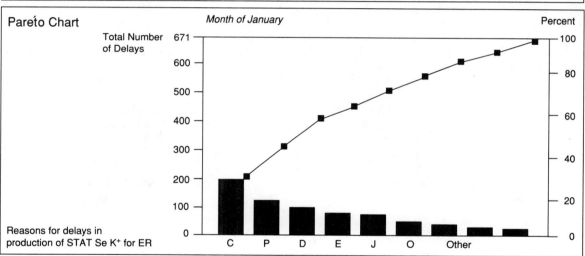

Pareto Chart

Month of January

Total Number of Delays — 671

Percent

Reasons for delays in production of STAT Se K$^+$ for ER

Bars (left to right): C, P, D, E, J, O, Other

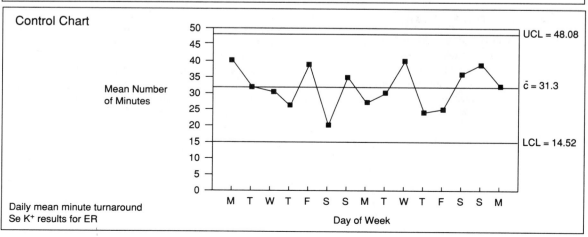

Control Chart

Mean Number of Minutes

UCL = 48.08

$\bar{c}$ = 31.3

LCL = 14.52

Daily mean minute turnaround Se K$^+$ results for ER

Day of Week — M T W T F S S M T W T F S S M

IN THE REAL WORLD
IDENTIFYING NEW SERVICES AT STORMONT-VAIL

Stormont-Vail Medical Center of Topeka, Kansas, has been using a strategic planning process for about ten years that is centered on major existing services within the hospital and the development of new programs and services. The major services have been identified as Heart Services, Women's and Children's Health, Behavioral Medicine, Geriatric Medicine, and Cancer Services. Annual planning retreats are used to determine new products and services for the organization, identify new ways of implementing change, and determine new directions and strategies.

The fiscal year for Stormont-Vail begins in October. The planning process is initiated with an administrative retreat in February which consists of the senior management of Stormont-Vail and administrators from the system's regional facilities. This retreat sets the direction for Stormont-Vail and identifies the organization's strategies and critical success factors (things that must be accomplished in order to achieve the mission).

The next step in the planning process involves members of middle management. There are approximately six planning groups which consist of a mix of managers from medical center departments and system activities. These groups each have a team leader and spend a half day brainstorming ideas for new services or modifications in current ones and reviewing the critical success factors. The Planning Department supplies team members with information (e.g., diagnosis related group (DRG), financial, market share) which might be helpful to the group in its deliberations.

The planning retreats are the beginning of the planning process for the organization. Other meetings are held by the groups after the retreats. The products produced by the process are:

- Planning groups develop goals for their area.
- Preliminary business plans are completed.
- Business plans are finalized with review by administration.
- Refined plans go to the board.

The business plan produced by the process identifies who will be administratively responsible and how the business will be conducted. Physicians are involved in new idea development by being included in small group planning teams which work on services in their specialty areas.

Product or Service Change

Health services organizations such as the Stormont-Vail Medical Center must constantly consider new products and services which it might provide, given advances in technology, consumer expectations, and the general competition for patients and physicians within its service area. Thus, the development and marketing of new products and services is a major activity for these organizations. The successful generation, evaluation, and implementation of new services involves numerous concepts and methods that might be employed whether the new undertaking is a radically unique product, a minor modification of an existing service, or an extension of a current product line.

The strategies for product and service development range from very informal and unstructured to formal and structured. Those strategies that are formal tend to be tied to formal planning systems for the organization while informal processes are on an ad hoc or entrepreneurial basis.

One strategy for product and service development is illustrated in Figure 12.3, which summarizes the

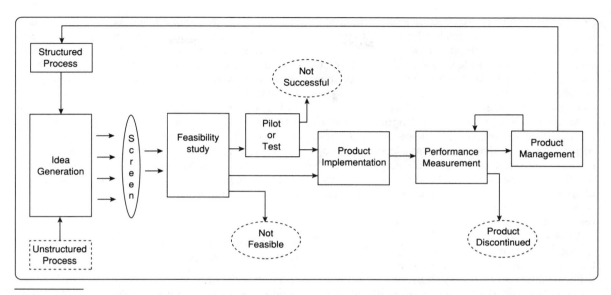

FIGURE 12.3. A model of product development. Adapted from Health Industry Forum, *Innovation Through New Product Offerings,* Birmingham: Health Industry Forum, Inc. 1987. Reprinted with permission.

elements of a new product development (NPD) process. The primary phases of the process include

- *idea generation*
- *idea screening*
- *feasibility study or business plan*
- *pilot or test program*
- *product implementation*
- *evaluation*
- *product management or product discontinued*

This process has a number of similarities to the innovation and change model described earlier in the chapter. In general, health services organizations are aware that they must constantly consider new products and services if they are to meet the needs of the community as well as remain financially viable in a competitive environment. Thus, the awareness and identification stages of the innovation model are portrayed in the idea generation and idea screening steps of NPD. The implementation stage occurs in NPD by develop-

ment of the feasibility study or business plan, the initiation of a pilot program, and product implementation. Finally, the institutionalization stage occurs with the NPD steps of evaluation and the final decision for product management or product discontinued.

Idea Generation

The initial step of product innovation is generating ideas to start the development process. Ideas are obtained from both structured and unstructured approaches. While the sources of ideas may be similar, the processes for identifying ideas may vary.

In some cases, a structured idea generation process is in place and is designed to provide a steady supply of product innovations. Formal idea generation processes include off-site retreats as part of a formal planning process involving all levels of management as well as clinician groups. For example, recalling the process at Stormont-Vail Medical Center, an annual planning retreat for a hospital may include brainstorming sessions with participants divided into planning groups that are assigned specific product lines for idea generation. Another structured approach is to assign responsibility for new product ideas to a product team or administrative people in the hospital as part of their ongoing management activities. Their responsibility is to improve or modify existing products.

An unstructured process depends upon ideas surfacing from various sources and being directed into a review process. Perhaps the key to success of this approach is creation of an atmosphere of innovation where people are encouraged and feel secure enough to bring up their ideas for consideration. This approach means that management will consider new product ideas as they arise.

Health services executives look to a variety of sources for new products as summarized in Table 12.1. Secondary sources of information include the published health management literature as well as the use of abstracting services for new product identification. Analysis of trends, not only in health care but among the general population, can generate ideas for products and services to be offered. Educational programs also serve as sources of ideas.

Existing models of services being delivered allow firsthand observation of the delivery of products or

services in the marketplace. Membership in multihospital or health services systems provide a source of ideas about products or services being used in other provider organizations. Scanning the industry to observe and evaluate experience of competitors may prove beneficial.

Existing personnel are another source as well as a processor of new ideas. Key individuals such as a marketing or planning personnel, are particularly important to idea generation in that they link to the organization's larger environment. Other stakeholders who may have an interest in seeing the organization do well are sources of ideas including consultants and vendors.

Specification of New Product or Service Features

Product features are the exact nature of how the product works (e.g., target market, pricing, operating characteristics). Origination of ideas for new services requires a management focus on the climate of innovation in the organization. An organization that creates the climate for "idea people" to be heard and for innovators to be recognized will allow more ideas to be developed.

If, for example, an organization defines idea generation as a stated management objective, recognition and rewards must be linked to the performance of this objective. If recognition is an intangible reward—such as recognition by management as an innovator or an entrepreneur—management creates an atmosphere of innovation and creativity but does not integrate or institutionalize the idea generation process into the operations of the organization.

Additionally, administrative support should be available to assist in development of innovative ideas. Individuals other than managers (e.g., clinicians, patients, employees) may have ideas for modification of current activities or development of new products and services, but these may require further management analysis such as development of market plans, pricing strategies, and related activities. Administrative support helps unstructured ideas to flow more freely.

A structured approach may also assist in the internal generation of ideas by encouraging new idea development. The use of brainstorming and nominal groups

TABLE 12.1. Sources of Product Ideas

Secondary Sources
  Published Literature
  Analysis of Trends
  Educational Programs and Seminars
Existing Models
  Affiliations
  Competitors
Management
  Senior Management
  Middle Management
  Product Line Management
Major Stakeholders
  Board Members
  Employees
  Physicians
  Patients
  Payors
Other Constituents
  Consultants
  Interested Individuals in the Market
  Entrepreneurs

in the strategic planning process helps foster innovative thinking and new idea development.

In contrast to origination, the basic features of adapted products are obtained from sources external to the organization such as secondary information or existing models. Data on the activity is supplied by management, stakeholders, or other groups. The adaptation process can be facilitated by a task force of involved parties who initially determine what aspects are or are not feasible.

Methods to improve information processing include assigning staff responsibility for scanning periodicals for new product ideas or subscribing to a clipping service. These methods insure more systematic exploration of published materials.

As noted, attendance at professional meetings and educational programs can provide new ideas. Facilitating the exchange of ideas may occur by requiring organizational personnel attending professional meetings to report new ideas at executive committee meetings. Alternatively, formal reports may be required to be drafted and circulated before individuals are compensated for travel expenses. Encouraging participation of medical and other professional employees in practitioner associations and national meetings improves the inflow of new ideas.

Borrowed products are less common because of the nature of health care delivery. Certain products are, in effect, borrowed when a hospital contracts for a franchised service to be replicated in the hospital. Borrowed products also involve installation of technology in a hospital without modification. Processes to facilitate borrowing include methods described as contributing to adaptation. The aim of these methods is to improve the flow of new ideas into the organization.

Regardless of source, the starting point for new product development is idea generation. Subsequent steps occur following the identification of new product or service concepts.

Idea Screening

Not every idea is a good one, yet it is important that each idea be reviewed. Creating an atmosphere of innovation will generate many ideas, some of which will not be appropriate, and some of which may become successful products or services. Health care organizations need screening criteria for determining which ideas deserve further management time and attention. In an era of heavy demands on management, early consideration of how many resources to expend on an idea is an important decision. A number of different criteria might be used to evaluate new products or services as shown in Table 12.2.

While initial screening may be viewed as the first hurdle to be overcome in the development process,

TABLE 12.2. Screening Criteria

Competition	Will it give us an edge over the competition? How is the competition likely to react?
Compliance with mission	Is this effort in line with the stated mission or purpose of the hospital? Will the service assist the organization in achieving its mission?
Ease of entry	How easily can we enter the market with this product? What are the barriers to entry?
Facilities	What plant and equipment resources are required?
Growth potential	Can the product or service experience growth in the future?
Location	Do we have the appropriate location to deliver this product or service?
Market assessment	Is there a market for the product? What is the size of the market? Will it improve market penetration?
Market share	Can we potentially hold or increase our market share with this product?
Medical staff acceptance	Is there a good physician base for the provision of the service? How will the physicians react to this idea?
Profitability	How do the financials look? Will it produce a profit? Are revenues generated by this service collectible?
Public relations	What will be the public relations opportunity created by this product? How will it affect our image with our publics?
Public acceptance	Does it meet a need in the community? Does the service advance the stature of the institution in the community?
Referral network	Will the product be a source of referrals for the hospital?
Resources required	What resources are necessary to undertake the idea? Do we have the staff to support this product? Are we, as an organization, capable of implementing the product? What must we invest to bring this product to market?
Utilization	Will it put more patients in the hospital or increase utilization of outpatient services?

it also informs personnel that every idea has a chance. The initial screens have to maintain a critical balance. Screening criteria should not restrict the flow of ideas which hold promise for the organization, but should be sufficiently rigorous to eliminate inappropriate ideas from further consideration.

The experience from other industries suggests that a considerable number of product and service ideas are never implemented. One large industrial firm, for example, found that for every 40 ideas that were generated, 6 made it through technical review, 2 were launched, and 1 was successful.[14] During a 10-year period General Foods similarly found that of 600 new product ideas—118 were developed, 40 were introduced, and 30 were considered a market success.[15]

Generalizing from the experiences of these other industries to health services organizations suggests that managers need to encourage the generation of many ideas so that the few potentially successful ideas can be implemented into product and service activities. Idea generation is not without risk. A critical managerial challenge is to appropriately allocate organizational resources and energy to achieve a balance between idea generation and successful implementation.

Involvement in the Review Process

Reviews take place throughout the product or service development process. At the idea screening stage, initially and throughout the process, various individuals and groups are involved in a review. Ideas are often presented at administrative or management meetings for a formal review at the management level. Task forces are often appointed to study issues and are selected to involve key players with specific insight or experience in the area under study. Some institutions use a formal screening committee, with specific criteria, which includes people from finance, management, and marketing. Physician input is often sought also.

Feasibility Study

After the screening process, feasibility studies are often conducted. The feasibility study must provide an in-depth assessment of whether to go ahead and introduce—as a test or as a full rollout—a product or service into the community. The feasibility study or business plan may show no rationale for further analysis or it may clearly define an opportunity. Feasibility studies begin with *market research*.

Market Research Organizations use both internal studies and contractual studies to examine the potential demand for new products. Specific methodologies include

- focus groups of former patients
- focus groups of people who have not used the organization's services to identify desires
- direct mail questionnaires
- market surveys
- physician input and physician contacts
- administrator market contacts
- Internal databases
- primary and secondary market information such as demographics and utilization data

Business Plan Development If a market exists for the proposed service, the business plan is then developed. Some elements of the business plan may have already been generated in an earlier phase of idea screening. However, more depth is needed in a final business plan. Data are reviewed for financial feasibility. In some cases, separate business plans are designed and developed for different scenarios or alternatives.

The typical feasibility study or business plan reports

- market research findings
- financial proformas
- marketing plans
- cost and pricing issues.
- tax issues
- other relevant information

Pilot or Test Program

Not every product or service is tested or piloted in the market. In some cases the use of a test depends on the investment required and the level of risk. Sometimes a trial phase aimed at market analysis or a small project is initiated. If a projected rate of return is marginal, the organization might minimize the risks and use a test. If it is a "sure winner," full scale implementation is generally undertaken. One-year and two-year pilots are often undertaken with evaluation at the end of the period.

The decision is then made whether or not to implement the service fully. Approval may be based simply on the business plan or on evaluation of the pilot or test. Approval for product introduction is generally at the board level but may be done by a designated management group. Depending on the magnitude of the service, the organization may involve the senior executive, the board, the medical staff, or a combination of these. The broader the impact, the higher level of involvement required.

Product Implementation

Once the decision is made, the business plan is implemented, and the product and service is introduced. Ongoing evaluation against the plan is required throughout the life cycle to assure institutionalization.

Administrative, Structural, or Strategy Change

The previous sections have identified change which is initiated and guided predominantly by the technical core of the organization involved in service delivery. Thus, revisions in the technical processes for service delivery and new product development activities frequently rely heavily upon professional staff for expertise. In contrast, administrative, structural, or strategy change is concerned with the fundamental design and structure of health services organizations. This change involves areas such as designation of departmental reporting relationships and authority; the clinical and managerial information systems of the organization; the management control systems used; and the goals, policies, and strategic direction for the organization.

Administrative, structural, or strategy change is initiated by senior management in collaboration with key professional and clinical personnel. This type of change is characterized as a top-down flow of influence. Top management decides that a change will be initiated and then designates the exact nature of the change

to be undertaken. Thus, administrative, structural, or strategy change is facilitated by the use of more bureaucratic mechanisms such as centralized decision making and formalization.

Senior management may become aware of the need for administrative change because of internal operating problems. For example, the CEO of a health maintenance organization (HMO) may feel that the decision-making process for the organization operates in a very slow, awkward manner. Further assessment reveals that this is placing the organization at a competitive disadvantage, given other HMOs in the area.

An examination of these issues may suggest several reasons for the inadequate decision-making process, as well as potential solutions. The management information system may not be providing managers with timely, useful information with which to make decisions. Thus, management may decide that a new information system is needed, identify the requirements for an improved system (with input from users throughout the organization), and then design the new system to better fit the organization.

The lack of a timely decision-making process also may result from the HMO having too many hierarchical levels or from involving too many groups in the decision-making process. Examination of the administrative ratio for the HMO and the decision-making process may require that the number of hierarchical levels be reduced.

Once a decision has been reached about the change that needs to be made, the process may in fact benefit from more bureaucratic features during implementation such as centralized control. Directives about time frames, operating features, and interfaces should be provided to expedite the activation of a new information system. The continuation of the administrative change (i.e., institutionalization) is aided by the existence of organizational support mechanisms such as training and orientation of employees to the new system and the use of policies and procedures manuals to reinforce desired behavior.

Strategies Management has a number of strategies for facilitating the administrative, structural, or strategy change process. One approach is called *stakeholder mapping*.[16] Stakeholder mapping attempts to provide a systematic assessment of the variance among personnel as stakeholders. The process involves three key steps

1. identifying relevant stakeholders (i.e., personnel who are affected or would be affected by the change
2. ranking each stakeholder based on attitudes toward the change, favorable or opposed
3. assessing each stakeholder's power within the organization to shape and affect its ultimate utilization

Based on this information, relevant personnel are identified and strategies are developed appropriate to each one. Individuals who are found to be in favor and clearly in a strong position within the organization should be mobilized to ensure support of this endeavor. It is critical that they be kept informed continuously of developments and planned activities in order to facilitate support of the activity.

Those individuals found to favor the approach but who are in a weak position within the power structure can be empowered, thereby giving them an opportunity to influence events. For example, to facilitate the implementation of CQI, physicians favoring the change, but marginal to decision making, could be appointed to various ad hoc or standing committees in the organization.

Individuals who oppose the idea but are weak may be coopted into a larger ongoing effort. More difficult, however, are those stakeholders who oppose and are in a strong position within the organization. Gilmore suggests "reframing" or redefining the issue so that they may see it in a different light.[16] For example, if someone in a large teaching hospital is opposed to a management information system, one might frame the change not as an administration control mechanism but as a mechanism to better assist the fundamental research mission of the organization.

If an organization wishes to change its decision-making process, *responsibility charting* is another approach to manage the change process. This technique identifies decision-making patterns among a set of actors—individuals, units, departments, or divisions within the organization.[18,19] Attention is given to identifying decision areas, actors, and the type of participation in the decision area. The approach provides an opportunity to compare responses of a specific participant about that person's own role in a decision with the response of one or more participants about the same participant role, compare responses across all actors on a specific decision, examine responses of each actor across a set of decisions, and compare actual decision patterns with desired activity.

An example of the use of responsibility charting is illustrated in Table 12.3. A broad range of decisions that are potentially made within Smith Medical Clinic is listed in the left-hand column of the chart. Major offices or groups involved in the decision process are shown on the top. In the legend are listed the roles that might be played in the decision-making process. These are

- D = Direct: set policy and allocate resources
- M = Manage: establish procedures
- S = Supervise: oversee operations
- I = Implement: responsible for performing actions
- R = Recommend: review and recommend a decision
- A = Approve: authority to authorize action

Within the squares are listed the role(s) that each group play(s) in each decision. As illustrated, some groups or individuals play multiple roles in a decision while other groups play no role. Examining the patterns of decisions allows the organization to determine if one or two groups have too much power and control within the organization. It also allows the organization to see if the pattern of decisions is rational and fits the culture of the organization

Responsibility charting is best used in combination with process type change strategies often associated with human resources change discussed in the next section. It is one thing to identify needed changes and quite another to be able to reorganize how decisions are made.

Human Resources Change

Human resources change is concerned with changing the attitudes, values, skills, and behaviors of employees within the organization. Health services organizations strive to create a work environment which

TABLE 12.3. Smith Clinic Decision-Making Responsibilities

	Physicians	President	Board of Directors	Department Chairmen	Executive Committee	Planning Committee	Personnel Committee	Recruiting Committee	Administration	Chief of Staff Med Executive	Hospital Board
Long-Range Strategy Development	A	I	A	DMIS			I		C		
Operational Planning Development				DMIS			R		C		
Analyze Opportunities	I										
Develop Business	I		A			R					
Analyze Financial Data		DMIS	IR		R						
Compile Performance Data				DMIS			D		IC		
Plan vs. Actual Reports Analysis							I		IC		
Billing	D			R							
Fees Policy		R	A		R						
Financial Policy and Programs		DR	RA		R				C		
Organizational Policy and Programs			RA	R'DMIS	R	R	R		I		
Compensation Policy			A		R						
Board Elections	A		R								
Officer Elections			IA								
Project Management	DMIS		A	DMIS					DMIS		
Continuity Policy	A	I	DR		D	D	D		C		A
Malpractice Insurance and Risk Management					R						
Work Loading Medical	IR			DMIS			I				A
Work Loading Non-Medical	S						S				
Manage Retirement Funds			DA								

Legend: D-Direct; M-Manage; S-Supervise; A-Approve; I-Implement; R-Recommend; C-Coordinate

Note: Any physician has the right to make any recommendations to the person who can do something about it.

MANAGERIAL GUIDELINES

1. Be clear about the type of change involved. Change is not an undifferentiated phenomenon. Each type of change has a specific set of attributes that need explicit attention from the health services manager. Moreover, these attributes interact with organizational characteristics to confound the change process. Thus, what may intuitively appear obvious, or at least similar to previous situations, may in reality be quite different and require caution because unanticipated consequences may develop.

2. Be conscious of the latent consequences of each type of change. Consider these latent consequences not as problems but as opportunities. While managers need to be specific about the particular type of change involved, they must also recognize that one type of change may lead to other types having their own anticipated and unanticipated consequences. For example, the introduction of medical educators within a community hospital results in an expansion and enhancement of managerial activity within the overall operations of the organization. This results in subsequent alterations in the basic power distribution within the organization.

3. Do not assume that the environment is a constant, not to be considered subject to intervention. Managers traditionally have taken a fairly parochial view of the change process. As a result, organizations are often considered the sole focus of change. Attempting to manage the interdependencies within the environment to enhance the operations of the organization may be a more viable strategy. Attention needs to be given to the context within which organizations operate. Enacting environments more compatible with existing organizational operations thus requires less change in the organization to enhance its overall performance. For example, efforts to increase or change the manner in which states reimburse health services organizations for indigent care is an effort on behalf of the providers to create a more friendly environment.

4. Consider intraorganizational change as a process involving a number of different

is conducive to the delivery of the highest quality service in an efficient manner. A work environment which is supportive, open, and responsive to organizational members provides such a setting. Management should monitor the climate within their organizations and initiate interventions to improve conditions which they perceive as harmful.

Recognition of the need to initiate a human resources change strategy can result from management's perception that the internal climate of the organization is not conducive to effective performance. Alternatively, management may believe that other changes being instituted by the organization such as downsizing, new service additions, or structural change may have a negative influence on employees and professional staff. Thus, a human resources change strategy may be viewed as critical for the success of other changes being initiated by the organization.

Strategies

A number of methods might be used by the organization to improve the attitudes, values, or behaviors of employees. Which method is chosen depends upon the problem that is perceived by management.

Survey feedback provides a mechanism for systematically gathering data on the ongoing social-psychological conditions of the organization and confronting work groups with the findings. Data usually deal with intergroup relations, communication, supervision, employee satisfaction, employee attitudes, and with more recent efforts, organizational culture.[20–23] This informa-

MANAGERIAL GUIDELINES

stages. Organizational change is a process involving a set of distinct stages. Managerial attention needs to be given to clearly identifying the stage at which a particular type of change is currently located and to designing interventions that will facilitate or limit the process, depending on the objectives of management vis-a-vis that particular change activity.

5. Recognize that the change process involves several levels of analysis. Organizational change and innovation occur at different levels within the organization. While we usually consider change and innovation as involving the entire organization, they in fact take place at various levels such as work groups, departments, or within individual roles. Attention should be given to clearly designating the level of the organization involved and to not confusing individual change with modifications in organizational variables.

6. Be aware that organizations are sometimes subject to large changes in the environment which managerial action can do little to affect. Managers need to be cognizant of their own limitations. Not all problems are tractable, and managers have only a limited amount of personal and organizational resources at their disposal. Attention should be given to those situations that are tractable rather than taking the position that resources are infinite and that all are applicable to facilitating or impeding the change process. Failure to make this distinction results at best in an inefficient use of limited resources and, more tragically, the burnout of managerial personnel.

7. Be conscious of time dimensions involved in change. Time, a difficult concept to understand, is particularly deceptive in an organizational setting. Shifting personnel and priorities contribute to the tendency to underestimate the amount of time involved in any change process. For example, what may be expected to take 6 months may take 12–18 months, or may never be completed. The pace of change must be managed—sometimes increased and sometimes decreased. The challenge for health services executives is the management of this process.

---

tion is usually gathered using questionnaire surveys of employees, but interview data can also be used. Results are fed back to individual work groups, starting at the top and moving down through the organization. Each group discusses survey results by analyzing potential problems, identifying possible causes, and agreeing upon solutions.

For effective results, three conditions must be met.[24] First, discussion of findings must occur in a factual, task-oriented atmosphere. Second, each group must have the freedom to consider implications of findings at its own level. Upper-level management should handle general problems, while problems affecting the work group should be handled at the source of the problem. Finally, reports of outcomes must be sent up the organizational hierarchy.

The assumption underlying these conditions is that management cannot directly influence the processes that exist within the organization.[25] Individuals and groups must be given the opportunity to see how their units compare with other units of the organization or how their current operations compare with desired expectations, thus understanding their own problems and initiating corrective action themselves.

Because health care requires coordination of many disciplines and complex tasks, conflict can arise within groups delivering or managing delivery of services. *Team development* strategies attempt to remove barriers to group effectiveness, develop self-sufficiency in managing group process, and facilitate the change process. These interventions differ from survey feedback techniques in that team development places greater emphasis upon the changing and refreezing stages of the change process and the importance of external consultation.[26]

External consultants are usually involved in all stages of this intervention strategy. Interventions begin with data gathering on leadership behavior, interpersonal processes, roles, trust, communication, decision making, task problems, and barriers to effective group functioning. After data are gathered, meetings are held during which problems are categorized and prioritized, selected problem areas are discussed, and action plans for change are developed.

The assumption underlying team development is that groups can solve their own problems if a catalyst is available to facilitate the process. Development activities require group participation, self-examination, problem confrontation, and goal setting.

A human resources tool considered part of the quality management initiative is *quality circles.*[27] Quality circles are small groups of employees from the same work area who work on a range of problems to increase their productivity and quality. The first-line supervisor, who is usually the team leader, receives special training in group dynamics and problem solving. Management supports quality circles by allowing team meetings on company time, training leaders, and responding to team proposals.

This technique relies upon a number of processes—such as the nominal group technique, multicriteria decision making, and critical incident technique—to identify and solve problems. Work groups also receive information on outcomes, such as productivity data and quality control information. Results of meetings are recorded, and reports are sent up the organizational hierarchy.

The use of quality circles is based on the assumption that those closest to problems should be responsible for the identification of issues and solutions. The approach also assumes that the use of group problem-solving techniques combined with data and reporting responsibilities will lead to changes that result in increased internal operating efficiencies.

Health services are experiencing rapid technological change in the provision of care. Changes require that personnel involved in service delivery stay abreast of innovations so that their organization can provide state-of-the-art care. It is assumed that participation in *continuing education* programs will provide health services personnel with the knowledge required to keep themselves and their organizations aware of new technology and service delivery programs. Change is assumed to be caused by the increased knowledge, awareness, and subsequent perception of a performance gap that results from continuing education activities.

Continuing education programs for physicians, however, have demonstrated no consistent association with quality of performance unless the program directly involved clinical leaders and face-to-face contact on data feedback based on individual physician performance.[28] A lack of association between continuing education programs and performance may occur for several reasons. First, participation in continuing education is mandatory in many states for most licensed health professionals. Professionals may attend continuing education programs without expecting substantive new knowledge to be gained from participation. Second, information acquired through these programs may not pertain to what the individual or organization is doing. Therefore, a stimulus for problem identification and corrective action does not exist.

If an organization faces an immediate threat or a need for rapid action, a *confrontation meeting* can provide direction in a much shorter time period than survey feedback. This technique brings together a large segment of the organization for problem identification and action planning.[30] Up to 60 people may be involved. The large group is then divided into small groups, each of which includes individuals from different organizational units. Supervisors are not placed in the same group with their own subordinates. Each group lists organizational problems that require attention. These problem lists are reported to the larger group of participants which combines the problems into categories with help from an external consultant. Next, new groups are formed along expert and functional lines in accordance with problem categories. The new groups select items to discuss and identify action steps to be initiated. Results are reported to the larger group.

Confrontation meetings provide rapid diagnosis, increase influence and commitment of lower-level personnel in problem identification and problem solving, reduce bureaucratic barriers in decision making, and improve decisions by having those with information solve problems. These meetings require a climate of openness for problems to be confronted by the organization.

Sensitivity training is designed to provide individuals with new experiences and data that disconfirm their perceptions of themselves and their environment. This training occurs in small unstructured groups that facilitate learning by nonevaluative feedback received by each individual from other group members. Feedback creates anxiety and tension, which causes the individual to unfreeze and eventually adopt alternative values, attitudes, and behaviors. These activities occur in the presence of a trainer who functions as a resource person and facilitator rather than as a formal leader.

This technique is intended to increase sensitivity, facilitate open communications, and encourage flexible role behaviors by individual organizational members. Sensitivity training conducted in groups that value personal risk taking and collaborative discussions is assumed to reduce defensiveness and resistance to self- and group-examination. Such examination leads to consideration of new attitudes and behaviors that may eventually be adopted.

Change and innovation also occurs through a better understanding of the personal, interpersonal, and group processes within the organization. *Process consultation* involves an outside consultant helping a client to perceive, understand, and act upon process events that are occurring.[31] Solutions can be developed to enhance the performance of the organization and can facilitate the overall change process. This technique focuses upon communications, role and function of group members, group problem solving and decision making, group norms, and the use of leadership and authority. The strategy, however, has limited effectiveness where individuals and/or groups with high levels of conflict involving disputes over major unresolved issues are involved.[32] For a further discussion of these issues, see Chapter 5.

KEY CONCEPTS

Administrative, Structural, or Strategy Change
Awareness
Business Plan
Confrontation Meeting
Continuing Education
Continuous Quality Improvement (CQI)
Evaluation
Feasibility Study
Human Resources Change
Idea Screening
Idea Generation
Identification
Implementation
Institutionalization
Market Research
Performance Gap
Pilot or Test Program
Process Consultation
Product Discontinued
Product Implementation
Product Management
Product or Service Change
Product or Service Review Process
Quality Circles
Responsibility Charting
Sensitivity Training
Specific Roles
Stages of Change or Innovation
Stakeholder Mapping
Survey Feedback
Task Analysis
Team Development
Technical Change
Total Quality Management (TQM)

DISCUSSION QUESTIONS

1. Four types of change have been identified in this chapter. Compare and contrast these types. Which of the four would you consider to be most critical for organizational success?

2. Select a change or innovation in health care delivery with which you are familiar and analyze it as either a technical; product or service; administrative, structural, or strategy; or human resources change. Describe the stages that the change would go through as it proceeds from concept to institutionalization.

3. What arguments can be made to support or refute the statement that "the worst feature of the American health care system is its resistance to change"?

4. As the chief operating officer for a large multispecialty group practice, you have been given the responsibility for selecting and managing the implementation of a new physician compensation program. What strategies might you consider to assure the successful awareness, identification, implementation, and institutionalization of a program?

REFERENCES

1. Rogers EM. *Diffusion of innovations.* New York, NY: Free Press; 1983.
2. Smith D, Kaluzny A. *The White Labyrinth.* Ann Arbor, Mich: Health Administration Press; 1986.
3. Scott WR. Innovation in medical care organizations: A synthetic review. *Medical Care Review,* Summer 1990;47(2):165–192.
4. Daft RL. *Organization Theory and Design.* 4th ed. St. Paul, Minn: West Publishing; 1992;249–282.
5. Thompson J. *Organizations in Action.* New York, NY: McGraw-Hill; 1967.
6. Kaluzny AD, McLaughlin CP, Kibbe DC. Continuous quality improvement in the clinical setting: Enhancing adoption. *Quality Management in Health Care.* 1992;1(1):37–44.
7. Gibson JL, Ivancevich JM, Donnelly JH. *Organizations: Behavior, Structure, Process.* 7th ed. Homewood, IL: Richard D. Irwin, Inc.; 1991.
8. Goodman PS, Kurke LB. Studies of change in organizations: A status report. In: Goodman PS and Associates, eds. *Change in Organizations: New Perspectives on Theory, Research, and Practice.* San Francisco, Ca: Jossey-Bass; 1982:1–46.
9. Galbraith JR. Designing the innovating organization. *Organizational Dynamics.* 1982;10:5–25.
10. Kaluzny AD, McLaughlin C, Simpson K. Applying total quality management concepts to public health organizations. *Public Health Reports.* 1992;107:257–264.
11. Berwick D. Continuous improvement as an ideal in healthcare. *New England Journal of Medicine.* 1988;32:53–56.
12. Berwick D, Godfrey A, Roessner J. *Curing Health Care: New Strategies for Quality Improvement.* San Francisco, Ca: Jossey-Bass; 1990.
13. Simpson KN, Kaluzny AD, McLaughlin CP. Total quality and the management of laboratories. *Clinical Laboratory Management Review.* 1991:448–462.
14. Fogg CD. New business planning—the resource allocation process. *Industrial Marketing Management.* 1976;5:3–11.
15. The rebuilding job at GF. *Business Week.* August 15, 1973;48–55.
16. Gilmore TN. *Managing a Leadership Change: How Organizations and Leaders Can Handle Leadership Change Successfully.* San Francisco, Ca: Jossey-Bass; 1988.
17. Ibid.
18. McCann J, Gilmore T. Diagnosing organizational decision making through responsibility charting. *Sloan Management Review.* 1983;24(2):3–15.
19. Gilmore TN. Building and maintaining effective working alliances. In: Sheldon R, Ginsburg L. *Managing Hospitals: Lessons from Johnson & Johnson—Wharton Fellows Program in Management for Nurses.* San Francisco, Ca: Jossey-Bass; 1991;201–231.
20. Van de Ven A, Ferry D. *Measuring and Assessing Organizations.* New York, NY: John Wiley; 1980.
21. Seashore S, Lawler III E, Mirvis P, Cammann C. *Assessing Organizational Change: A Guide to Methods, Measures, and Practices.* New York, NY: John Wiley; 1983.
22. Trice HM, Beyer JM. *The Cultures of Work Organizations.* Englewood Cliffs, NJ: Prentice-Hall; 1993.
23. Schneider E. *Organizational Climate and Culture.* San Francisco, Ca: Jossey-Bass; 1990.
24. Katz D, Kahn RL. *The Social Psychology of Organizations.* 2nd ed. New York, NY: John Wiley; 1978.
25. Bowers DG, Franklin JL. *Survey-Guided Development I: Data-Based Organizational Change.* La Jolla, Ca: University Associates; 1977.
26. Dailey R, Young F, Barr C. Empowering middle managers in hospitals with team-based problem solving. *Health Care Management Review.* 1991;16(2):55–63.
27. Lawler E, Mohrman S. Quality circles after the fad. *Harvard Business Review.* 1985;85(1):64–71.
28. Lomas J, Hayes RB. A taxonomy and critical review of tested strategies for the application of clinical practice recommendations: From "official" to "individual" clinical policy. In: Battista R, Lawrence R, eds. Implementing Preventive Services. *American Journal of Preventive Medicine.* 1988:77–94.
29. Eisenberg JM. Physician utilization: The state of research about physician practice patterns. *Medical Care.* 1985;3(5):461–483.
30. Beckhard R. The confrontation meeting. *Harvard Business Review.* 1967;45:149–155.
31. Schein EH. *Process Confrontation: Its Role in Organization Development.* Reading, Mass: Addison-Wesley; 1969.
32. Lewicki RJ, Litterer JA. *Negotiation.* Homewood, Ill.: Richard D. Irwin, Inc.; 1985.

CHAPTER

13

ORGANIZATIONAL PERFORMANCE: MANAGING FOR EFFICIENCY AND EFFECTIVENESS

Ann B. Flood, Ph.D.
Professor

Stephen M. Shortell, Ph.D.
Professor

W. Richard Scott, Ph.D.
Professor

LEARNING OBJECTIVES

After completing this chapter, the reader should be able to

1. understand the importance of assessing organizational performance
2. define performance measures for organizations
3. understand the important issues in defining, measuring, and using performance measures
4. evaluate professional work
5. compare management models based on quality assurance and quality improvement
6. manage for quality improvement in health care
7. understand management roles to create high performance organizations

CHAPTER PURPOSE

The demands for high performance in health care are increasing. This is reflected in the increasing demands from insurers—including public insurance programs like Medicare and self-insuring businesses—seeking discounted prices or other forms of cost containment in return for their business. At the same time, decreases in utilization such as dramatically shortened average lengths of stay, alternative sites for care such as same-day surgery and home care programs, and growth in provider availability have led to increased competition among providers. While these trends have stimulated health services

IN THE REAL WORLD

GOOD PRACTICE AND MALPRACTICE: SMITH vs ACE MANAGEMENT COMPANY

On May 19, 1992, at 9:30 P.M. at Jackson Memorial Hospital (JMH), Jay Smith was born severely mentally and physically handicapped. His 30-year-old mother, Mary Smith, had been admitted to the labor and delivery unit of the hospital at 11:00 P.M. on May 18, 1992; she was 17 days past her due date. At 10:30 A.M. on May 19, Mrs. Smith was examined by Dr. Wood, her personal obstetrician and chief of obstetrics at JMH, who ordered the administration by intravenous infusion of 10 milliunits per minute of Pitocin (oxytocin), a drug that stimulates uterine contractions. The normal dosage Dr. Wood usually gave was 1.0 milliunit—the dosage recommended by the drug manufacturer in the *Physicians' Desk Reference*. No one either preparing or administering the drug questioned the accuracy or appropriateness of the dosage for Mrs. Smith. Four hours before Jay was born, Dr. Wood attempted to further stimulate contractions by artificially rupturing Mrs. Smith's membrane, at which point meconium-stained amniotic fluid was identified, suggesting that the fetus may have suffered some distress.

The hospital's policy was to require electronic fetal monitoring only for high-risk pregnancies; however, the criteria for judging who was at "high-risk" were left largely to the physician. Following a recent uproar in the community about "excessive" use of fetal monitoring at area hospitals, a committee (including Dr. Wood as chair of the department) had reviewed the hospital's policy to be sure that it complied with accreditation standards. So, when Dr. Wood chose not to monitor Mrs. Smith's labor either before or after rupturing her membrane, no one in the labor room questioned the decision.

At delivery Jay was flaccid and could not breathe on his own. He was transferred to Delta Medical Center, a major medical center with extensive perinatal facilities, where he remained for one month. Jay's problems were severe and irreversible. Now seven years old, Jay has undergone extensive medical care throughout his young life and continues to exhibit signs of spasticity, cerebral palsy, mental retardation, blindness, deafness, and a variety of related conditions.

On October 14, 1993, the Smiths filed a $30 million suit against Dr. Wood, JMH, and ACE Management Company, Inc., the group from which JMH contracted for management services to run the hospital. In including the management company in the suit, the Smiths alleged that ACE was negligent in its management of the hospital—specifically, that the company failed to monitor and oversee the treatment and care provided by physicians and employees of the hospital, to enforce the standards of the Joint Commission on Accreditation of Healthcare Organizations, and to monitor, on an ongoing basis, the physicians of its medical staff.

How could this tragedy to Jay have happened? What roles should management have played in this situation to prevent it, to uncover the problem, and to take corrective actions to change the behavior of the providers and the system?

Given the complex nature of hospitals, staff errors with potentially tragic consequences such as those for Jay Smith are not surprising. Patient care in hospitals is characterized by highly subdivided tasks performed by numerous types of professionals and a culture that preserves the autonomy of physician decision making—factors that contribute to ambiguity and apathy about personal accountability and decision making in hospitals. Putting JMH in the hands of a management company responsible for all hospital operations gave a false sense of control but contributed little toward fostering a culture and a team approach which might have served to prevent the inappropriate orders or at least intervene before damage had occurred.

The fundamental nature of hospitals and the legal bases governing professional behavior make it impossible for management alone to implement a quality assurance (QA) program which can effectively prevent mistakes by identifying and disciplining providers—particularly physicians—not complying with good practice. Nevertheless, management has an important role in preventing such problems.

The classic definition of management's role in ensuring quality is to design an organization such that professionals are able to control their own performance. With this model, management focuses on the activities of the small groups operating within the hospital. This approach is important, but it is not enough by itself. Clearly this was inadequate to prevent the problems for Jay.

Several groups are promoting a new paradigm:

Quality must be viewed as a process, one that requires continuous improvement. That is, management throughout the organization must continuously endeavor to learn about all aspects of a process and use that knowledge to change the process, thereby improving service. What is required is a major shift in how organizations think of quality and how they define the roles of those participating in the processes.

A part of the redefinition needed involves recognizing the role of middle management. Middle managers traditionally have been neglected in favor of executives. For example, although much attention was given at JMH to reviewing the quality assurance standards, less attention was given to the day-to-day activities of the obstetrics and gynecology supervisor and to working relationships among nurses, administrators, and the physicians in department of obstetrics. A relationship characterized by information sharing and efforts at continuing improvement would have identified opportunities for improvement and initiated corrective action which could have prevented the medication error and identified Mrs. Smith as benefitting from monitoring.

Managers at JMH basically viewed quality problems as needing "control." Instead, greater emphasis was needed on day-to-day management involving: fostering and learning from individual initiatives, interdisciplinary skills, information sharing, and thoughtful participation within the larger organization. These types of middle management activities require the acquisition of new skills in the areas of group process, negotiation, and conflict resolution. Finally, middle management should understand that hospitals are behavioral systems that involve all the complexities of entangled interest groups and coalitions. One technique is for the administration to meet often with physicians, nurses, and other hospital staff to assess the dynamics of the hospital. However, a more formal level of assessment, involving multiple measurements over time and the comparisons of data from similar organizations, can assist hospital managers in the systematic diagnosis of problems and provide perspectives on an organization's performance.

In summary, the probability of the Smith case occurring could have been reduced if the hospital had

- emphasized practices designed to continuously improve quality rather than to satisfy accreditation standards

- recognized the important roles of middle management and other providers as well as physicians
- learned from systematic organizational assessment

SOURCE: Adapted from Kaluzny, AD *The role of management in quality assurance: The case of Smith vs. ACE Management Company.* Quality Review Bulletin. *April 1990:134–137. Copyright 1990 by the Joint Commission on Accreditation of Healthcare Organizations, Oakbrook Terrace, Ill. Reprinted from the April 1990* Quality Review Bulletin *with permission.*

managers to focus on the business of health services—that is, on market share, pricing policies, marginal costs, and productivity—a backlash in the form of reduced public confidence and threats to remove the tax-exempt status of hospitals have caused a renewed interest in serving the community—that is, in fulfilling a larger social function. The objective of this chapter is to review the major issues related to assessing organizational performance, compare and contrast the approaches of quality assurance and quality improvement, and describe the strategies to achieve an effective health care organization.

THE CHALLENGE OF PERFORMANCE

Clearly, a major challenge to the health care executive is to put together an organization that maximizes productivity, quality, and market share while not losing sight of the organization's mission to serve the health needs of the community. Because they operate in an environment of constrained resources, balancing these pressures has meant having to trade off some programs, services, and markets for others. For example, a hospital may agree to give up its maternity services in order to expand its medical-surgical services or may share high-technology resources with another hospital in order to concentrate more effort in expanding its ambulatory care programs. Alternatively, a hospital may agree to introduce a service critically needed in the community despite its being a net drain on resources. Such tradeoffs have meant that chief executive officers (CEOs) of today's health care organizations have to

manage their organizations in relation to other organizations and the community's needs in addition to considering the performance of individual subunits.

Another set of internal pressures comes from the concerns of committed health professionals—managers, nurses, physicians, and others—to improve professional practice by using their knowledge, skills, and technology to the best of their abilities and to the improved capabilities permitted by advances in medicine. This force is often neglected when considering the other, perhaps more visible, concerns.

Finally, in addition to these reasons for managers to attend to performance issues, outcomes research and clinical guidelines have gained a new prominence as the federal government also seeks to evaluate health care in an effort to minimize use of ineffective services, contain costs, and yet hold providers accountable for fairly distributed and well-performed services.

More than anyone else, the manager is responsible for the performance of the organization. In a real sense, all of the preceding chapters are building blocks for assisting the manager to improve organizational performance. As outlined in Chapters 1 and 2, the manager's role includes attending to the performance of the internal environment (i.e., the various departments and activities within the organization which serve each other) as well as attending to external customers. The successful manager needs to guide and oversee all of the subsystems of the organization, not just the maintenance or managerial subsystems, which have been traditionally emphasized in health administration. Thus the manager can improve performance not only through attending to productivity and maintenance of the human and capital infrastructure but also to boundary spanning activities, adapting the organization to its ever-changing environment and advances in medicine, and governing, or holding the organization accountable for its actions. The performance of health care organizations in the future may increasingly depend on the ability of health care managers to truly lead not just steer through obstacles—that is, to mold and innovate within their environment rather than passively react to external changes.[1]

All of these factors have helped spawn a variety of terms to describe performance in the delivery of health services: efficacy, effectiveness, appropriateness, productivity, and efficiency. Because these terms are often ill-defined, sometimes used interchangeably, and occasionally inappropriate for evaluating organizational performance, it is important to define them for present purposes. Their variety and occasionally contradictory results serve to illustrate why there cannot be a single criterion for organizational success. For example, a productive or efficient organization is not necessarily effective; and an organization which is efficient in some activities is not necessarily efficient at all.

Three terms widely used in assessing health services are generally used to describe the potential of a health service to produce the desired health benefit. *Efficacy* refers to the capability of a health service, under ideal conditions and applied to the right problem, to produce the desired effect. *Appropriateness* focuses on whether an efficacious treatment was applied to the right patient at the right time. *Effectiveness* in this context involves ascertaining the quality with which a service is carried out, assuming that the service was both efficacious and appropriate. Note that these terms, as defined, refer to the evaluation of a particular treatment or set of services or to a provider's ability to carry them out. They do not describe organizational performance.

Organizational performance is generally depicted using four interrelated concepts. The first two terms center on evaluating an organization in terms of the goods or services it produces for external consumption. Both terms characterize the inputs needed, either using dollars or units of resources expended, to produce these goods or services. Note that these inputs can depict labor or capital or both components. *Productivity* is defined as the ratio of outputs to inputs. An example of hospital labor productivity is the total number of admissions divided by the total number of nursing staff hours. *Efficiency* is defined as the cost per unit of output. An example is the average total labor costs per admission.

There are important and complex issues associated with assessing inputs. For example, should an efficiency measure include the costs of staff not directly involved in treating patients? Or, should productivity include physician hours when they are not paid by the hospital? Despite the difficulty of addressing these issues, the biggest challenge is the problem of measuring outputs. For example, consider the output: hospital stays. Since most of the variation in resources or dollars used during specific hospital stays depend on the reasons for hospitalizing the patients and whether they received surgery, two measures of efficiency—one based on 100 normal births and the other on 100 patients with coronary artery bypass surgeries—are clearly not directly comparable. The challenge is to create measures of efficiency or productivity which take into account such differences between patient stays which are due to patient-specific needs for care during an admission.

Given cost-containment pressures, all health care organizations face the challenge of becoming more productive and efficient. Existing studies suggest that the factors associated with increased productivity and efficiency include use of

- high standards and goals[2,3]
- information and feedback[4]
- interdepartmental coordination and resource sharing[5,6]
- compensation systems oriented toward rewarding productivity or efficiency[7,8]
- physician involvement in decision making and governance[9,10]
- efficient staffing and concentration of work activity[11–15]
- active governing boards that deal with environmental pressures[16]
- type of ownership[17–19]

Setting high standards for cost containment motivates organizational members, particularly when the compensation systems reinforce attainment of the productivity and efficiency standards. Productivity-based compensation incentives include sharing cost savings resulting from employee suggestions as well as year-end bonuses based on staying within budget or generating net profits beyond expectations.

The second set of terms to evaluate organizational performance is consistent with a broader, open-system perspective of what the organization is trying to accomplish. By *organizational effectiveness* is meant the degree to which organizational goals and objectives are successfully met. An organization goal to be achieved could be a subobjective (e.g., recruiting a coordinator for the organization's quality assurance-improvement program), an intermediate level objective (e.g., reducing nursing staff turnover on the units), or an ultimate objective (e.g., reduction in risk-adjusted mortality for acute myocardial infarction cases). *Cost effectiveness* is a composite measure that takes into account both cost as well as the degree of goal attainment.

Assessing effectiveness is complicated because of the problems associated with defining and measuring organizational goals. As Scott notes, assessing organizational effectiveness largely depends on the kinds of goals organizations adopt and their reasons for doing so.[20] Goals serve many purposes. They may

- motivate organization members to higher performance
- act as criteria for evaluating performance
- legitimize organizational activities
- indicate to external agencies what the organization is about

So how should success in reaching a goal be measured? Different goals may be developed to serve these different purposes; alternatively, the same stated goals may be used differently in different situations to serve any or all of the above functions—with varying degrees of success.

The following section examines the major approaches to assessing organizational performance, particularly in regard to effectiveness. It is organized to highlight three types of problems and issues in evaluating performance: definitional (what is measured), technical (how to measure), and managerial (why it is being measured). These sections include a review of the factors which affect performance, focusing particularly on

studies of health care organizations. The managerial issues focus on internal strategies aimed to assure quality and to improve it. The chapter concludes with a discussion of high-performing health care organizations and associated managerial guidelines.

ISSUES IN ASSESSING EFFECTIVE PERFORMANCE

Evaluation systems are the principal devices managers have for attempting to influence and improve the performance of their organizations. It is important for managers to become aware of the limitations of any particular system. As Haberstroh notes, "First, performance reporting is omnipresent and necessarily so. Second, almost every instance of performance reporting has something wrong with it."[21] These problems can be broadly classified into definitional, technical, and managerial issues of performance evaluation, although as Kanter remarks, "The most interesting questions in this area are not technical, they are conceptual: not *how* to measure effectiveness or productivity, but *what* to measure."[22] (Emphasis added.)

Definitional Issues in Assessment

Fundamental Perspectives about Organizations

The most important definitional issue in measuring organizational performance is related to one's view of the fundamental purpose and nature of organizations because these views affect the most critical assessment questions: *what* will be measured and *why* it is being evaluated? If organizations are conceived primarily as rationally designed instruments for the production of goods and services for external consumption, emphasis is placed on measures of productivity and efficiency. Alternatively, if organizations are viewed as collectivities capable of pursuing specific goals but primarily oriented toward their own survival—toward system maintenance—attention is diverted from output to support goals, such as members' satisfaction or morale or, more generally, the survival of the organization.[23,24] If organizations are envisioned to be open systems that are highly interdependent with their environments, the key strategies leading to an effective organization involve acquisition of scarce resources (e.g., through the fund-raising activities of volunteers and the choice of well-connected persons to serve on boards of trustees) and the capacity to adapt to a changing environment (e.g., through the creation of slack, or uncommitted resources).[25] This view, by recognizing both an external and internal reality for organizations, underscores the importance of knowing why an evaluation is being performed: for internal consumption (e.g., to take corrective action to solve a quality problem) or external (e.g., to demonstrate to an external group that accreditation standards were met).

Juxtaposing these different views of organizations not only exposes multiple ways to conceptualize effectiveness but highlights the potentially conflicting features of performance in an organizational system. Two issues leading to discrepancies help illustrate this point.

First, the measures may not be mutually compatible. For example, efficiency in the attainment of specific goals may not be consistent with maximizing participants' satisfaction. More specifically, a teaching hospital, organized to maximize opportunities to train and take advantage of the availability of residents, can lead to greater dissatisfaction of patients as they experience a depersonalized and discontinuous array of providers and of nurses as they relinquish some valued aspects of their roles to inexperienced residents.[26]

Second, different time frames for evaluating effectiveness can lead to discrepant evaluations. Particularly in a time of rapid environmental change, the organization that is well-suited to deal with today's demands may by that very fact be ill-equipped to handle tomorrow's challenges. Weick notes that organizational features that preserve adaptability "look ugly and wasteful" in the present context but can prove invaluable when conditions change.[27] Finally, the organization itself is seen as having a life cycle and all of its subunits are subject to changes that develop over time.[28] Cameron and Whetten propose that effectiveness varies according to the stage of organizational development.[29] Effectiveness in earlier stages depends primarily on creativity and mobilizing resources; later stages emphasize commitment and cohesion among members; still later, formal processes of control and efficiency come to the fore; and finally, structural elaboration, decentralization, and flexibility receive emphasis.

Domain of Activity

Once a general framework or model has been selected to guide the investigation, it is necessary to determine which particular functions or activities will be evaluated. Most complex organizations serve a variety of aims and objectives. Modern hospitals, for example, not only provide a variety of types of patient care, including broad categories of services such as outpatient, inpatient, and emergency care, but many also pursue educational goals (e.g., residency training), research goals, and preventive and community service goals. Departmental and work-group subdivisions often reflect—and protect—these differentiated purposes, with different subgroups and types of personnel performing quite divergent tasks and pursuing quite distinct objectives.

In some cases, these goals and the activities of the various groups are highly interdependent—in either negative or positive ways. Training objectives sometimes conflict with patient care as noted above, but they can also support and complement good care by making available advanced technology or encouraging providers to investigate unexpected results. In other cases, the goals and activities may be quite independent, the policies and practices of a labor and delivery center may be largely unaffected by those of the hospice program. In either situation—even if the same concept of effectiveness is being applied—the same organization may perform extremely well in one domain of activities but relatively poorly in another. Simply put, no organization can be equally effective with respect to all the objectives it pursues. Two implications are that there is no simple measure of overall effectiveness for a health care organization, but there is always room to continuously improve at least some aspect of performance.

Different Levels of Analysis

A third critical factor influencing conceptions of organizational performance is the level of analysis selected to guide the assessment. An important insight gained from open systems theory is that all complex systems tend to be nested units, systems within systems. Thus a hospital is composed of departments, and the departments are composed of work units, and the hospital as a whole is part of one or more larger systems, such as a multiunit hospital or regional health system. The boundaries that separate these levels are seldom clear and are often rather arbitrary. Further, many of these boundaries are not organized in neat concentric circles but frequently overlap and cross-cut one another. Individuals in modern societies are not completely contained within any single organization but instead are partially involved in several, and professional occupations and union organizations cross organizational boundaries in complex and unexpected ways.

Although there are obviously various possibilities, it is conventional to identify at least three system levels

- the organization itself, such as a health maintenance organization (HMO)
- a larger socially defined unit that contains the organization, such as a community, a health services region, or a system of hospitals
- subunits contained within the organization, such as individual departments or practitioners.

Nerenz and Zajac propose yet another unit of analysis to assess performance in a variety of vertically-integrated health systems.[30] They propose that the basic unit of data collection should not be a service or a patient but an episode of care that embraces services provided across multiple sites and involving numerous actors. They challenge traditional measures of performance as containing inappropriate assumptions for today's complex systems, such as the presumed association between utilization and revenue or the assumption that the system's effectiveness can be maximized by maximizing the effectiveness of each component organization. They propose new ways to collect information which can aid future attempts to understand the relationship between system performance and system characteristics.

The unit of analysis selected can have a profound effect on the assessment of performance. For example, a strategy to measure efficiency of emergency services at the community level may differ considerably from an assessment focused on one hospital's emergency room. Most analyses of organizational performance focus on one or more of these three levels. The critical

point, however, is that one should be as clear as possible about what level of analysis is selected.

It is also important to recognize that system performance at any given level may not be analyzable as a simple aggregation of system performance at lower levels. This is one of the principal features of any system, its performance is determined as much, if not more, by the arrangements of its parts—their relations and interactions—as by the performance of the individual components. A number of highly qualified physicians do not necessarily add up to a high-quality medical staff. Rather, how the staff members are deployed by level of privileges and types of service, how their work is monitored and information fed back to allow improvement, the arrangements for continuing education, and other similar factors may be more decisive for many aspects of medical effectiveness.

One must be careful not to confuse level of analysis with the issue of whose interests are reflected in the determination of assessment criteria. For example, it is possible to focus on the performance of the hospital as a complex system but to assess this performance from the standpoint of the interest of the larger community. Whose interests are served in assessing effectiveness is best treated as a separate topic, a fourth factor that affects one's view of organizational performance.

Stakeholders

Early performance measures, based on small entrepreneurial organizations, focused primarily on profit for the owners or their agents (managers). It was not long before analysts noted that the interests of owners and their agents were far from being perfectly aligned and that other groups—such as professional workers, the public, and external clients—had interests in the organization's performance.[31,32] Cyert and March described organizations in terms of shifting coalitions of interest groups—some internal, others external to the organization—that are constantly engaged in negotiating and renegotiating the conditions of their participation and thereby affecting the performance of organizations.[33]

In any organization, both internal and external interested parties—stakeholders—have different desires and needs to be met by the organization. They want the organization to score points on different things. They have varying expectations and criteria for effectiveness. For example, internal stakeholders in hospitals include employees, physicians, and boards of directors. Most employees want meaningful work, opportunity for growth, and a reasonable degree of job security. Physicians want up-to-date technology, and support services, and an environment in which they are free to practice medicine as they were trained. Physicians, while viewed primarily as internal stakeholders, can also be considered as external stakeholders, depending on the degree to which particular physicians identify with a given health care organization. Other external stakeholders include suppliers, regulatory groups, competitors, third-party payers, and community groups. Third-party payers expect care to be provided in the most cost-effective manner possible. Patients have varying expectations depending on the severity of their illness, their education, and their financial resources. Regulators will be concerned with the organization's ability to maintain standards and contain costs. Suppliers of capital focus on the institution's bottom line. Given this disparate set of demands and expectations, it is not possible for a given organization to be seen as equally effective by all of its stakeholders or constituent groups at a given point in time.

Recently researchers have examined performance issues which involve multiple interested parties and coalition formation in health care organizations. Fennell and Alexander note that a board of trustees is supposed to represent the external stakeholders' interests and monitor and contain any self-interested actions on the part of hospital management and internal stakeholders.[34] However, the stakeholders and customers in hospitals are often difficult to identify and sometimes to tell apart, resulting in continuous coalition formation among the interest groups.

This lack of clear-cut boundaries among the interests of various actors is further illustrated by proponents of quality improvement who argue that production of any service or product within the organization—such as filling a prescription or preparing a report for the government—involves a seemingly endless chain of suppliers, processors, and customers.[35] Rather than restrict the term "customers" to end users of an organization's product, this perspective emphasizes the complex web of parties with a stake in performance.

Of course, not all interests are equally powerful. In most organizations one can detect the presence of a dominant coalition whose interests carry more weight than others. But it is still important to note that in most organizations power is more widely dispersed today than in the past, and more diverse constituencies are perceived to be legitimate stakeholders in the enterprise.

To summarize, a number of factors have been identified that have clear relevance to the evaluation of organizational performance. Views of the nature of organizations and the impact of time frames, the domains of the activities being evaluated, the level of analysis, and the perspective of interested parties are sufficiently complex that one may expect to find little consensus in the selection of criteria employed to evaluate organizational effectiveness.[36–39]

Technical Issues in Assessment

Having described key definitional issues related to what should be measured, we now turn to problems of how to measure performance. The focus is on the generic problems and concerns that arise during the process of evaluating work performance.

Classes of Measures

Performance assessment requires that evidence be collected upon which evaluations can be based. More than 25 years ago, Donabedian noted that evaluators of the quality of health care answered the "how to" question by using one of three basic classes of measures: structural, process, and outcome measures.[40] Although he was referring to the evaluation of technical and psychosocial aspects of clinical care, these same categories are useful for evaluating nonclinical performance as well. Table 13.1 provides examples of each class of indicators applied to financial management, clinical care, and human resources management.

Structural Measures Structural indicators are based on assessments of organizational features or participants' characteristics that are presumed to have an impact on organizational performance. They measure

TABLE 13.1.   Examples of Performance Measures by Category

	Domain of Activity		
	Clinical Care	Financial Management	Human Resources Management
Structure	*Effectiveness* • Percent of active physicians who are board certified • JCAHO accreditation • Number of residencies and filled positions • Presence of council for quality improvement planning	*Effectiveness* • Qualifications of administrators in finance department • Use of preadmission criteria • Presence of an integrated financial and clinical information system	*Effectiveness* • Ability to attract desired registered nurses and other health professionals • Size (or growth) of active physician staff • Salary and benefits compared to competitors • Quality of inhouse staff education
Process	*Effectiveness* • Rate of medication error • Rate of nosocomial infection • Rate of postsurgical wound infection • Rate of normal tissue removed	*Effectiveness* • Days in accounts receivable • Use of generic drugs and drug formulary • Market share • Size (or growth) of shared service arrangements	*Effectiveness* • Grievances • Promotions • Organizational climate
	Productivity • Ratio of total patient days to total full-time equivalent (FTE) nurses • Ratio of total admissions to total FTE staff • Ratio of physician visits to total FTE physicians	*Productivity* • Ratio of collection to FTE financial staff • Ratio of total admissions to FTE in finance department • Ratio of new capital to fund-raising staff	*Productivity* • Ratio of line staff to managers
	Efficiency • Average cost per patient • Average cost per admission	*Efficiency* • Cost per collection • Debt/equity ratio	*Efficiency* • Cost of recruiting
Outcome	*Effectiveness* • Case-severity-adjusted mortality • Patient satisfaction • Patient functional health status	*Effectiveness* • Return on assets • Operating margins • Size (or growth) of federal, state, or local grants for teaching and research • Bond rating	*Effectiveness* • Turnover rate • Absenteeism • Staff satisfaction

an organization's capacity to permit or promote effective work. For example, in the opening scenario of Jackson Memorial Hospital, *structural measures* would portray the quality and number of staff in the labor and delivery room and the forms of coordination to carry out doctor's orders. Other indicators include the number and types of specialized equipment, such as fetal monitoring; the presence of an active peer review program; and the proportion of the medical staff that is board certified. Until recently, accreditation and certification reviews relied almost exclusively on either structural or process measures of performance; note too that accreditation itself can be used as a structural indicator of performance.

Process Measures *Process measures* are based on evidence relating to the performer's activities in carrying out work. Examples include quality assurance activities such as reviews of physician decision making and orders provided to all patients dying in-hospital or reviewing nurse and physician conformance with standards for cleanliness on units with outbreaks of nosocomial infections. Process measures can be directed at an organization or system of care as well—a review of the system for conducting and reporting the results of urgently requested laboratory tests. Process measures can also be used to assess the nonclinical aspects of performance. Examples in the financial area include liquidity ratios, such as the ratio of current assets to current liability, and activity ratios, such as the ratio of total operating revenue to total assets.[41]

Outcome Measures *Outcome measures* are based on evidence gathered from the objects upon which the work is performed. Assessments are made to determine whether changes have occurred in their characteristics that can be attributed to the work performed upon them. Thus, for clinical care, changes in the patient's health status (to measure technical aspects of care) or satisfaction (to assess the interpersonal care) are assessed; and for training institutions, changes in the student's knowledge, skills, or attitudes may be examined. In the financial area, outcome might be measured by the operating margin (ratio of operating income to operating revenue) or the return on assets.[42]

These three classes of measures are not independent measures of performance, but linked in an underlying model. Structural measures of quality are valid to the extent that they motivate and encourage providers to choose efficacious, appropriate, or cost-effective actions. Process measures in turn are valid if they lead to improved products or better outcomes. This model overstates the simplicity of these relationships, which are loosely coupled at best and certainly should not be mistaken as substitutes for each other. It is important to recognize that each of these types of indicators is imperfect—subject to bias and misinterpretation. Process measures focus on energy and effort expended but neglect effects achieved. Moreover, measures based on process alone can only compare performance values with some specified standard; they cannot themselves assess the appropriateness of the standards employed. If process measures are once removed from effects, then structural indicators are twice removed, since they do not assess work performed or effort expended but only the organization's capacity for work. Presumed competencies may in practice turn out to be ineffectual, and existing capacities may on specific occasions be unemployed or underemployed. Outcome measures have the advantage of focusing attention on changes produced and results achieved. Their drawback is that they do not in themselves provide evidence that can

connect observed outcomes to the effects of performance. Particularly in arenas such as medical care, it is common for poor outcomes to occur in spite of superior performance, and vice versa. Causal factors that are beyond the control of the caregiver are at work. And at a more general organizational level, a high proportion of good outcomes—patient recoveries, student achievements, profitability—may be more a function of selection procedures—admitting only the easiest patients or brightest students—than what the organization does.

It is also important to distinguish objective measures of quality from people's perceptions. For example, a given home health agency may have the highest possible accreditation rating and best patient functional health status outcomes (objective measures) but be perceived by the community as having relatively low quality, perhaps owing to problems of convenience and access to services or an occasional war story of poor care. In the same vein, it is important to recognize that the public's perception of quality may differ from those of physicians and caregivers. For example, the public may give greater weight to access, convenience, comfort, and interpersonal relationships while the professional caregiver places greater emphasis on technical skill. In part, this is due to the public's relative inability to evaluate technical expertise. As a result, they use other criteria as proxy measures or assume technical quality as a given and then make choices based on the non-technical criteria discussed above.

Preferences for Classes of Performance Measures

Associations are likely to exist between these classes of indicators and broadly defined categories of constituencies in organizations.[43] Executives and managers typically prefer to employ structural measures of effectiveness since these are the types of indicators over which they have most control. Similarly, caregivers are likely to emphasize process measures because these activities are more under their control. By contrast, clients and representatives of the various external publics may prefer to focus attention on outcomes; never mind capacity or effort, what results were actually achieved? Patients, for example, are much more likely to be concerned about remission of symptoms and restoration of function than about the technical correctness of the procedures employed or the formal qualifications of personnel. Despite this preference, patients seldom can obtain good information about the average patient's experience with outcomes and must rely on the physician's judgment or structural indicators like accreditation. Indeed, for these reasons, executives need to be attentive to such visible indicators of quality—whether or not they reflect true differences in patient care—since these indicators may be used by prospective customers to choose where they go for care.[44] More broadly, licensing, accreditation, tort law, and regulations associated with quality control abound in health care. Even when they use standards based on widely held beliefs rather than on evidence of their import for quality, they have an ability to influence organizational performance regardless of the validity of the claim.

Factors Associated with Effective Performance

Despite the difficulties involved, studies have identified a number of factors generally associated with higher quality of care

- quality of professional staff[45-47]
- high standards[48-50]
- experience with other cases of the same type[51-55]
- more formally organized professional staffs with well-defined coordination and conflict management processes[56-61]
- participative organization cultures emphasizing team approaches[62-66]
- timely and accurate performance feedback[67-73]
- active management of environmental forces[74,75]

Evidence related to peer review through quality assurance and continuous quality improvement is discussed in the following section.

In regard to the quality of professional staff, key factors are recruitment, retention, and having people work within their professional abilities.[76,77] This involves concentrating the work of professionals in such a fashion that greater experience produces better patient-care outcomes over time. As noted several studies have found higher volume of patients treated by both institutions and individual physicians to be associated with more positive patient-care outcomes.[78-81]

Setting high standards is compatible with professional values. A key factor involves strict admission requirements and exerting strong control in enforcing standards.[82-84] More tightly organized professional staffs assist in this process by providing regular forums for problem management and conflict resolution.[85,86] Coordination also plays an important role in overall effectiveness.

A participative organizational culture emphasizing team approaches is particularly important when the environment is changing rapidly.[87] An ongoing team approach allows ideas to be communicated and discussed quickly by the professionals that will be most affected by the changes involved. A participative culture helps to develop good work habits on the part of all involved and reinforces appropriate peer group pressure. Further, teams generally do a better job of solving complex problems than individuals.[88] For example, work focused on hospital intensive care units found that efficiency of utilization and perceptions of higher quality of care were related to good conflict management—including communication, problem solving, and leadership—combined with a patient orientation.[89]

Timely and accurate feedback raises the visibility of behavior in the organization such that accountability requirements are met and deviation from performance standards is assessed.[90-92] A good clinical-financial management information system enables corrective action to be taken more quickly.[93] Finally, more active management of the external environment enables the organization to educate external groups (e.g., licensing and accreditation bodies, regulatory groups, third-party payers) about quality objectives and practices and the associated challenges involved. For example, university teaching hospitals, which have established their own hospital-specific governing boards separate from the university governing boards, have been better able to negotiate with relevant external groups and more clearly communicate their mission and objectives.[94]

As the incentives to form more integrated delivery systems grow, there is great need to assess the performance of such systems from both an efficiency and effectiveness perspective. The existing evidence is largely mixed while the issue of quality of care provided by such systems is largely unexplored.[95-99]

In sum, managers must recognize the limitations of each class of performance indicator as well as understand the interests of the various constituency groups—including their own—that have a stake in the functioning of their organization. Only such awareness will enable them to correct for these biases and balance the often conflicting interests of the several parties involved.

Managerial Issues in Assessing Performance

The need for managing quality is central to any organization. Health care organizations, coming under increasing pressure to be cost-effective, have been turning away from old models of assuring quality to a new model of quality improvement which has been effective in helping industries world-wide to improve their products or services. The old model in health

---

IN THE REAL WORLD
DECISION SUPPORT SYSTEMS FOR OUTCOMES MANAGEMENT

The decision support systems of the future must be able to analyze the performance of complex, integrated systems with multiple provider types, facilities, and access points. And they will be person—not patient—focused to enable the tracking of health status over time.

Decision support systems will employ analytical tools such as rules-based processing (also known as expert systems) and artificial intelligence programs to perform retrospective and concurrent analyses. Artificial intelligence applications using neural networking programs under development in several health care organizations show promise in their ability to identify optimal patterns of care, accurately predict outcomes for individuals or populations of patients, and optimize the use of resources.

Future applications are likely to include real-time clinical decision support. The ability to display the best available options and the risk-benefit analyses for interventions on a particular patient are the logical evolution for decision support systems.

Measurement of performance does not by itself influence outcomes. To achieve the goal of continuous improvement in the structures and processes of health care, effective feedback of outcome measures to providers is vital. This can be done prospectively through the use of practice guidelines and assessments, concurrently through the use of expert systems, and retrospectively by analyses of patterns of care outcome.

If outcome measures are to drive the process of continuous improvement, outcomes-based feedback strategies must be acceptable to clinicians. Educationally oriented programs based on the principle of "measure, don't mandate" are achieving increased acceptance and resulting in significant improvement in health care outcomes. The alignment of physicians with health care delivery systems through outcomes-based educational programs will likely be a strategic success factor for outcomes management.

Outcomes-based feedback offers opportunities to understand what really works in clinical practice and can be used to validate and update practice guidelines. Providers will be better able to assess and choose therapies, counsel patients on expected outcomes, follow progression of health conditions, and estimate resources to be expended on treatment. In turn, payers will become better purchasers of care, and patients will become better informed consumers of healthcare.

SOURCE: *Geehr EC. The search for what works. Healthcare Forum Journal. July/August 1992:33. Reprinted with permission.*

care relegated quality to the quality assurance (QA) department; the new model emphasizes quality improvement (QI) teams which cut horizontally across functions and reach vertically across hierarchical lines to involve the entire management and staff. The old model solved problems and held individuals culpable for mistakes; the new one prevents problems by continuously improving the true source of defects—the process. The old model was based on peer review and focused on upholding minimally acceptable standards of care; the new borrows from principles applicable to any industry and encourages striving for excellence. The form and function of the old model was required by external accreditors and third-party payers for quality of care; the new permeates all processes and requires a strong internal culture to support it. The differences are profound enough to require a major paradigm shift—not necessarily to displace all of the activities of QA but to restructure most of the way quality is managed. In this section both models are presented and their strengths and weaknesses contrasted. To set the stage, general issues in evaluating professionals and other staff and unintended responses to evaluation are presented.

Evaluating Professional Performance: The Professional Model

In the classic professional model, the foremost means to ensure that professionals produce high quality work is to give them the skills, training, and values needed to produce life-long devotion to excellence. However, to weed out any "bad apples" and to inspire them to continue learning, professional workers can be held accountable by making their work visible to others whose opinion counts. In professional work, peer review is needed because only peers can truly judge the quality of one's work.[95] These notions, for physicians in particular and nurses to a more limited extent, are backed up by a potential for malpractice litigation against substandard care and by financial fines or professional reprimands for poor performance.[100]

Health care organizations have always operated by using both professional and bureaucratic forms of control. Some have argued that there are two independent lines of authority, one for physicians and the other for

everyone else. In their exposition of work in hospitals, Georgopoulos and Mann implied that these two lines of authority acted more like a lobotomized brain rather than an integrated right and left brain in coordinating activities.[101] But others, like Scott, describe three alternative models which can be used to embed professionals effectively into an organization: autonomous, in which professionals retain independent authority to control and evaluate themselves as a group; heteronomous, in which professionals are subject to more line-authority control; and conjoint, in which professionals and administrators coexist in a mutually interdependent setting in which each group is roughly equal in power and in the importance of their functions.[102] The hospital that Georgopoulos and Mann were describing fit the autonomous model. But the modern health care organization is moving toward the third model, in which mutual understanding and cooperation play key roles for organizational effectiveness.

In health care organizations, because of the high percentage of professionals involved and their diversity, health care executives need to understand and accommodate the varying professional requirements of each group. Physicians, in particular, have high need for achievement and autonomy in clinical decision making. Other groups have less highly developed claims to autonomy but desire organizational settings in which they can practice their full range of professional skills. Job autonomy, for example, is associated with less conflict, increased job satisfaction, and greater client satisfaction.[103]

Almost all professionals have high standards of excellence, and therefore organizations and managers that emphasize high performance expectations and provide the necessary support for obtaining excellence are likely to be more effective.[104] Achieving such standards is a function of both specification of rules and procedures as well as informal communication and use of ad hoc task forces which involve relevant groups.[105,106] Rules and procedures help to define and handle many problems, but because of the complexity and uncertainty of much professional work, informal and ad hoc mechanisms must also be used to deal with nonroutine problems. Examples include emergency cases; patients with multiple diagnoses; elderly patients with chronic care needs that cut across many specialties and even organizations; and patients with illnesses involving complicated moral, legal, economic, or ethical issues.

Involving professionals in the development of standards, norms, rules, policies, and practices is essential. Studies indicate that such involvement is associated with greater professional satisfaction and can play an important role in staff retention.[107,108] Increasingly, professionals want to be involved not only in deciding what will have an immediate impact on their work but also in some of the larger organizational issues that may affect their future practice. Examples include the organization's relationship with third-party payers, regulators, and competitors. Thus there exists growing physician involvement in management and governance issues and new forms of joint venture relationships (also see Chapters 9 and 11).[109–111]

In sum, existing studies suggest that evaluating and coordinating professional work is facilitated by high standards and clear expectations, specified rules and procedures combined with job autonomy, flexibility in coordinating work, and a high degree of professional involvement in decision making. These practices place a premium on the manager's conflict management (see Chapter 5), communication and coordination (see Chapter 8), and organization design skills (see Chapters 6, 7, 9, and 10).

Evaluating Nonprofessional Work: The Bureaucratic Model

Comparing observed performance values with established standards is also seldom a simple mechanical process but one requiring experience and judgment. It is to accommodate these skills that the appraisal function is typically assigned to a supervisor—a person selected on the basis of seniority or merit and located close to the work site. Experience and proximity allow these individuals to detect nuances in performers' activities and to take into account special circumstances that affect performance values and their associated outcomes. Many of the complaints and problems associated with supervisor-worker relations may be attributed to disagreements over performance appraisal and may signify both the complexities and the sensitivities associated with this process.

In the modern health care organization, these tasks

of evaluating performance—particularly in the context of maximizing organizational performance—are made more difficult by the complexity of occupations and people involved in providing care. More and more, in recognition of the different skills and perspectives necessary to perform such tasks, interdisciplinary teams rather than individuals become the basic accountability unit within the organization, necessitating new means for evaluating work and improving the process.

The Impact of Evaluation on All Types of Performers

All attempts to evaluate a performance may be expected to have effects on that performance. The setting of standards, the selection of indicators, the sampling of performance, and the comparison of performances with standards all affect the performance itself.[112] The primary purpose of any evaluation system is to exert influence on the performances of participants—if not the performance immediately under review, then subsequent ones. But equally important and less obvious are the unintended effects of performance evaluation. People basically prefer to receive a good evaluation; therefore, workers will seek to improve their evaluation irrespective of whether that change actually improves the quality of their performance. Ideally, of course, the evaluations made are accurate and appropriate; but if not, *reactivity* to the performance criteria can result in an appearance of improvement in performance rather than motivating the worker to seek true changes in quality. Or, as W. Richard Scott once paraphrased an old song, "When you're not near the goal that you love, you love the goal that you're near."

These biasing or diverting effects occur because it is often difficult or overly costly to devise evaluation systems and indicators that accurately reflect the complexity of desired outcomes to which the performance is addressed. Thus although examinations are developed to test learning, their repeated use is likely to influence what is taught or, more importantly, what is learned. And if diagnostic thoroughness is signified by the number of laboratory tests ordered, then the number of tests ordered may far exceed the number required by the patient's medical condition. In particular, hard measures—measures that are specific, capable of being quantified, and easy to observe—tend to drive out soft measures.

Nonetheless, there is some evidence that physicians will respond to evaluations by peers for its own sake. For example, physicians have responded to internally imposed peer review.[113] Dyck and his colleagues found that rates of healthy tissue removal associated with appendectomy dropped significantly when criteria about "acceptable" rates were made explicit, absent any need to reprimand physicians.[114] However, physicians knew that peers were going to monitor their rates in the future with undetermined consequences. Physicians have also responded by dropping the rate of prescribing drugs when a computerized system with the capability to monitor prescriptions was introduced, even though the system was intended for another purpose.[115]

Finally, the work by the Maine Medical Foundation (MMF) and the Minnesota Clinical Comparison and Assessment Project provides many examples of how a study group of physicians, when given feedback on utilization with evidence that some physicians were unusually high, can result in a reduction of the outlier rates over time.[116-118] However, there is some recent evidence that suggests that physician profiles showing the relative use rates of services, when divorced of any apparent consequences, appear to have no effect on behavior.[119]

Two Models for Changing Performance

Quality Assurance *Quality assurance (QA)* refers to "the formal and systematic exercise of identifying problems in medical care delivery, designing activities to overcome these problems, and carrying out follow-up steps to ensure that no new problems have been introduced and that corrective actions have been effective."[120] In reviewing 25 years of QA activities, Williamson notes agreement on five principles for assuring quality.[121]

- Successful QA requires individual and organizational commitment to develop the values and incentives of excellence.

- Responsibility for excellence must be decentralized so that the professionals and staff responsible for the care have the power to review and implement necessary changes.

- At the same time, QA requires an approach which is comprehensive of all the groups in the hospital which can affect quality, including education, administration, and support services.

- At the same time, QA is best targeted toward prioritized, specific needs rather than being based on a shotgun approach to identifying problems.

- QA itself should be continuously monitored for its effectiveness and adaptiveness to current organizational needs to insure that its contributions outweigh its costs.

The evidence that QA has been successful in changing physician's behavior is scant.[122-124] As Luke, Krueger, and Modrow remark, "It is clear that quality assurance has until now been both expensive and, in general, marginally effective."[125] The general conclusion is that the primary problem has been a failure to focus on the means to secure changes in organizations or physicians rather than on the techniques to assess quality.[126-129] In reviewing the evidence on changing physician's behavior and assuring quality, Eisenberg discusses the importance of an environment conducive to high quality, including strong professional leadership and diffusion of up-to-date innovations in medicine as well as face-to-face interactions with colleagues—not necessarily found in most QA activities.[130] These arguments have been supported by work based on QA in a primary care setting.[131,132]

Many are calling for greater integration and coordination of QA activities as well. For example, a recent study by the U.S. General Accounting Office found several reasons for concern about the systems for monitoring quality in Medicare. There is little evidence of the effectiveness of the review methods being used; there is poor coordination across groups reviewing quality with little or no sharing of information; the data used are of questionable accuracy and generalizability; and there are inadequate strategies for developing the methods and knowledge needed to correct the situation and inadequate resources being allocated to redress these concerns.[133]

While most have called for increased coordination and integration of these activities as well as standardization of the procedures, others have warned of information overload which overwhelms the system and stymies action and largely symbolic evaluations—going through the motions of QA—which can attend too centralized and extensive of reviews.[134-138]

Quality Improvement Quality improvement is the promise put forward to address the problems—real and imagined—in quality assurance in American health care delivery. *Quality improvement (QI)* is a management philosophy to improve the level of performance of key processes in the organization. It was developed originally by several industrial quality experts and applied successfully in a variety of industries world-wide.[139-141] The principles espoused by these experts differ little but have helped spawn several terms used interchangeably with QI: total quality management (TQM), industrial quality control, and continuous quality improvement (CQI). Key philosophical concepts include:

DEBATE TIME 13.1: WHAT DO YOU THINK?

An article in the *Journal of the American Medical Association (JAMA)* described a study of serious medical "missteps" based on anonymous responses from 114 interns and residents regarding their own most significant errors in the previous year. The main categories of serious missteps and examples of each are indicated below.

It is possible that the problems may *not* have been due to individual error but rather to underlying processes and systems involved in patient diagnosis and treatment. For each category of missteps, develop an argument that the error was due to problems in the underlying process rather than from the individual physician's mistake.

Example	Outcome*
ERRORS IN DIAGNOSIS 38 Cases (33%)	
Failed to diagnose bowel obstruction in patient with fluid buildup in abdomen	Death
Failed to examine and diagnose fracture in crack cocaine user	Delayed treatment
EVALUATION AND TREATMENT 24 Cases (21%)	
Treated malignant hypertension on the ward instead of in an intensive care unit	Stroke
Incompletely cleaned a diabetic foot ulcer	Amputation
PRESCRIBING AND DOSING 33 Cases (29%)	
Did not read syringe and gave 50 times the correct dose of a thyroid drug	None apparent
Inadvertently stopped asthma medication at time of hospitalization	Respiratory failure
PROCEDURAL COMPLICATIONS 13 Cases (11%)	
Removed pulmonary artery catheter with the balloon inflated	Small amount of bleeding
Placed intravenous line in main vein without a follow-up X-ray	Fatal lung collapse
FAULTY COMMUNICATIONS 6 Cases (5%)	
Failed to put do-not-resuscitate order in chart and failed to inform spouse	Resuscitation performed against patient's wishes
Failed to obtain consent before placing intravenous line in main vein	Fatal complication after procedure

* Cause and effect cannot be determined.

SOURCE: Adapted from Wu AW, Folkman S, McPhee SJ, Lo B. Do house officers learn from their mistakes? JAMA; 265,(16):2090. Copyright 1991, American Medical Association.

- Productive work involves processes. Most work implies a chain of processes whereby each worker receives inputs from suppliers (internal or external to the organization), adds value, and then passes it on to the customers who are defined to include everyone internal or external who receives the product or service of the worker.
- The customer is central to every process. Processes are improved to meet the customer's needs reliably and efficiently.
- There are two ways to improve quality: eliminate defects in the process and add features that meet customers' needs or preferences better.
- The main source of quality defects is problems in the process. Workers basically want to and succeed in carrying out the process correctly. The problems derive from the process being wrong.
- Quality defects are costly in terms of internal losses by lowered productivity and efficiency, increased requirements for inspection and monitoring, and dissatisfied customers. Preventing defects in the process by careful planning saves resources.
- Focus on the most important processes to improve. Use statistical thinking and tools to identify desired performance levels, measure current performance, interpret it, and take action when necessary.
- Involve every worker in QI. Use new structures like teams and quality councils to advise and plan QI strategies.
- Set high standards for performance; go for being the best.

Benchmarking is the process of establishing operating targets based on the leading performance standards for the industry or what the Japanese call *dantotsu,* the "best of the best." But it should not simply be a metric—determining a standard against which to measure performance; benchmarking is a philosophy to guide the process of proactive, structured practices needed to achieve excellence. Camp describes this process in four steps.[142]

1. Know your operation. That is assess your organizational strengths and weaknesses.
2. Know the industry leaders or your direct competitors.
3. Incorporate the best. Don't hesitate to copy or modify, but be sure you start with the best.
4. Gain superiority.

An example of this philosophy applied to a clinical situation in a hospital is illustrated in the case of Jackson Memorial Hospital.

The philosophical approach of QI in some senses is similar to that of groups like the MMF.[143] Both start with the premise that wide variation in practice indicates that something is amiss—not all rates can be right, even if one doesn't know which rate is right. But the two part company in their philosophical approaches to which rate is right—in the sense of being desirable. The MMF approach targets the outliers (usually high utilization) with the view that outlying providers should alter their performance to look more like the typical performance of their peers. All others are okay as is. The QI approach, in contrast, argues that the outliers on the side of good quality should become the benchmark against which everyone else should strive—to try to be the best, not typical.

The evidence that QI will help improve performance in health care comes mostly from other industries since its application is so new to the health industry. Many groups have turned to QI, and accreditation bodies like the Joint Commission of Healthcare Organizations has revised its accreditation rules to foster this approach.[144] Berwick, Godfrey, and Roessner report on demonstrations carrying out QI in 21 health care organizations including hospitals, group practices, and HMOs.[145] While some organizations did not complete their reports and few tackled clinical quality of care issues, most felt that they had made significant progress. The authors conclude:

> The evidence that quality management can help in manufacturing and business processes is overwhelming, and it is a very safe bet that the analogous processes in health care (billing, information transfer, equipment maintenance, and the like) stand to gain as much. . . . The same goes for *service* processes, like making appointments, providing telephone access, and moving patients efficiently from place to place. . . . It requires a little more imagination to see how quality management can help

IN THE REAL WORLD

BENCHMARKING IN SETTING GOALS TO DISCUSS PATIENT PREFERENCES FOR LIFE-SAVING PROCEDURES

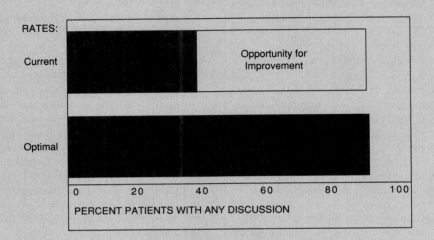

At Jackson Memorial Hospital, all adult patients with serious chronic illnesses and a life expectancy of less than one year or their family members were surveyed to determine how many had had discussions with any provider regarding their preferences about when or whether to use life-sustaining procedures. They found that even among this seriously ill group, only 40 percent had had any such discussions. About 30 percent—some who had had such discussions and some who had not—actually had do-not-resuscitate (DNR) orders placed in their charts during the hospitalization. Arguing that ascertaining preferences for these seriously ill patients was especially important, the QI team set as a benchmark goal for the future that 90 percent of these patients or their surrogates should have had such discussions no later than the first few days of hospitalization.

SOURCE: *Adapted from SUPPORT: Study to Understand Prognosis, Preferences for Outcomes, Risks, and Treatment project. Journal of Clinical Epidemiology. 1990;43(suppl).*

technical medical care . . . yet these areas still await complete exploration.[146]

In the process of implementing QI, a balance between the basic components—implementing the technique, establishing the culture, and planning appropriate strategy—needs to be maintained to be effective.[147] Sometimes proponents try to implement only one component, such as data gathering and problem solving by the interested parties. But evidence from other industries suggests that the package, to be successful, requires implementing all features. Based on the experiences with QI at the Henry Ford Health

System, Sahney identified several major barriers to successful implementation and urged preventive or corrective attention be paid by managers.[148]

• Middle management is unsure of its role and lets teams tackle insignificant processes or complex problems with insufficient support.
• The pace of improvement is often glacially slow as people brainstorm and flounder on how to proceed. Feedback and rewards for time invested are insufficient.
• Changing the culture is difficult and members can lose faith in the process.
• Evangelistic devotion to QI can block free discussion and inventive solutions. Likewise, cynical use of QI can divert resources and energy with no real benefit to the organization as a whole.
• Time availability to carry out QI must be sufficient at all levels, including senior and middle management.
• Results of QI, if not shared broadly internally to the organization, are unknown beyond the few people involved.

A basic premise of QI is that every process has variation in how well it produces a service or product. In order to reduce the variation, the first step involves a careful and information-driven analysis of what can cause a failure of the process, with what frequency such problems occur, and the extent to which problems vary over time. Understanding the process and developing and implementing corrective action by a group process requires being able to communicate the information effectively. Simple and direct statistical tools, such as histograms, bar charts, and scattergrams, help ensure that anyone throughout the organization can understand and use them. In addition, some tools have been developed specifically to help QI teams, such as flow charts, Pareto diagrams, and control charts.[149–152] They serve multiple purposes in the process of improving quality: gathering information about processes and probable causes of problems, displaying information and testing theories, and monitoring and controlling a process after a remedy has been applied.[153,154] One such tool, the cause-and-effect diagram, is used to condense a large array of information about processes in an organized way. The ultimate effect (e.g., an adverse event like medication errors) is at the end of the arrow. Each major antecedent cause is represented by a branch attached to the arrow. Figure 13.1 is a cause-and-effect diagram portraying the overall process of producing health services.

Finally, both advocates and critics of QI note the special challenges presented by involving professionals—particularly physicians—in QI systems to evaluate clinical processes. Combining general lessons about how to implement innovations in organizations with the special requirements of professionals, Kaluzny, McLaughlin, and Kibbe advise taking several precautions when designing QI strategy in health care organizations.[155]

• Use physicians' time wisely. Use them as consultants or on subteams that focus on clinical issues needing their expertise. Recognize that their involvement will be episodic and related to specific interests and topics.
• Peak physicians' interests. Capitalize on physicians who are most interested in QI, nurture their involvement, and focus on issues that make them curious.

DEBATE TIME 13.2: WHAT DO YOU THINK?

Figure 13.1 provides a framework for thinking about quality improvement in health services organizations. Some people believe that the greatest improvement opportunities lie with increasing clinicians' competence and skills. Others believe greater improvement results from changes in the organization and management of patient care units. Still others believe that the quality of care is largely a function of the availability of sophisticated technology or the degree of teaching activity going on. What do you think? Where would you place the most emphasis? What factors, conditions, or variables influence your decision?

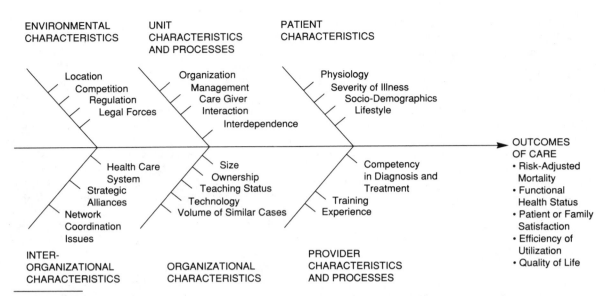

FIGURE 13.1. Cause-and-effect diagram for continuous improvement in health services organizations. Copyright 1992 by the Joint Commission on Accreditation of Healthcare Organizations, Oakbrook Terrace, Ill. Reprinted from *Quality Review Bulletin,* May 1992, p. 151, with permission.

• Empower physicians' participation. Involve them early on in the process.

• Respect professional values. Avoid statistics and reviews that threaten physicians' competency. Be flexible. Balance the needs for autonomy with the requirements of QI initiatives.

• Diagnose and capitalize on which of the four stages of adoption specific units and groups have reached: recognizing a problem in need of a solution, identifying QI as a valued solution, implementing QI strategies related to the problem, or institutionalizing QI thinking and techniques into everyday clinical practice.

THE MANAGER'S ROLE IN CREATING HIGH PERFORMANCE HEALTH CARE ORGANIZATIONS

The problems in defining and measuring performance, which occur in all organizations, are particularly challenging for health care organizations. This is because, as noted in Chapter 1, the product of health care organizations is frequently difficult to define and measure. In addition, many of the activities that influence the performance of health care organizations are not directly controllable by managers but rather are under the direction of physicians and other health care professionals. Add to this the environmental forces of inflation, regulation, competition, new technology, and changing consumer preferences, and it's no wonder that some have referred to the health care executive's job as attempting to steer a wayward bus down a hill in which physicians control the brakes and other groups (trustees, third-party payers, etc.) have their foot on the accelerator. Thus it is tempting to wave the white flag and conclude that there is relatively little that managers can do to define, measure, or influence performance. Nothing could be further from the truth.

It is precisely because the task of defining, measuring, and influencing performance is so difficult that management can play a key role. As discussed in Chapter 4, defining the organization's core values and reasons for being and translating these into operational reality lies at the heart of *transformational leadership.* Transformational leaders think about performance in terms of controllable and noncontrollable factors and constantly work to convert uncontrollable factors into factors that can be controlled. Figure 13.2 provides a continuum of such factors.

As shown, events such as natural disasters, international relations, and national economic policy are relatively uncontrollable by health care executives. In contrast, issues concerning the organization's wage and salary administration, marketing plans, and patient care policies and practices are, for the most part, directly controllable by executives. In between are factors involving intermediate degrees of control. These include factors largely internal such as the organization's mission and culture, labor mix, and organization design as well as external factors such as system consolidation, growth, and third-party payment trends on the one hand and external regulation, competition, and new technological developments on the other. A major point of Figure 13.2 is that more effective managers not only focus on variables on the right side of the page that are most directly controllable but also attempt to extend their influence over factors moving to the left, involving health industry trends and external regu-

latory, competitive, technological, and legal forces. They do this by refusing to accept these forces as givens and viewing them instead as opportunities for expanding their organization's mission and potential effectiveness. For example, many health care companies have developed, on their own or in joint ventures with insurance companies, the ability to provide health insurance services and other third-party financing which can channel more patients into their delivery system. Many hospitals are changing their size by reducing their inpatient bed capacity and converting formerly unused capacity to long-term care beds or outpatient programs. Other organizations have gained control over new technological developments through linkages with medical schools and research centers and through investment in biomedical and biological product companies. In similar fashion, these organizations are proactive in shaping consumer preferences and tastes through market research and new product development strategies rather than merely reacting to changes in consumer preferences.

These attempts to broaden the influence base involve macropolitical strategies of networking, coalition building, and joint venturing (see Chapters 9–11 for related discussions). They involve actively managing

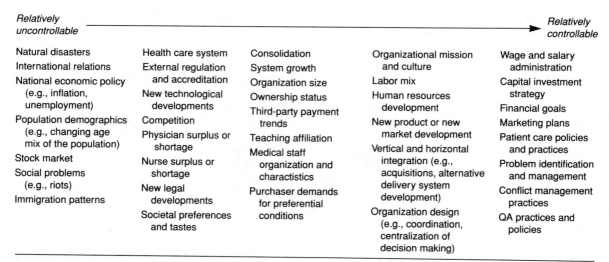

Relatively uncontrollable				Relatively controllable
Natural disasters	Health care system	Consolidation	Organizational mission and culture	Wage and salary administration
International relations	External regulation and accreditation	System growth	Labor mix	Capital investment strategy
National economic policy (e.g., inflation, unemployment)	New technological developments	Organization size	Human resources development	Financial goals
Population demographics (e.g., changing age mix of the population)	Competition	Ownership status	New product or new market development	Marketing plans
Stock market	Physician surplus or shortage	Third-party payment trends	Vertical and horizontal integration (e.g., acquisitions, alternative delivery system development)	Patient care policies and practices
Social problems (e.g., riots)	Nurse surplus or shortage	Teaching affiliation		Problem identification and management
Immigration patterns	New legal developments	Medical staff organization and charactistics	Organization design (e.g., coordination, centralization of decision making)	Conflict management practices
	Societal preferences and tastes	Purchaser demands for preferential conditions		QA practices and policies

FIGURE 13.2. Factors affecting health care organizational performance arranged on a continuum of the degree to which managers can exert control.

the environment and not merely managing one's own organization. Priorities must be set and tradeoffs must be made. Nonetheless, all stakeholders would agree that the organization needs to obtain necessary resources (people, money, legitimacy) for its continued existence; to coordinate, manage, and integrate these resources in providing desired services and products; and to achieve a reasonable degree of goal attainment in those areas that are deemed most important. Thus the discussion and guidelines that follow are organized around the issues of acquiring necessary resources, making wise performance tradeoffs, and managing a high performance health care organization for the twenty-first century.

Resource Acquisition

The way in which health care organizations obtain resources has changed radically in the past few years. Philanthropy has declined to the point where it is no longer a major source of support, and much greater emphasis is given to the debt and, for investor-owned organizations, equity markets. At the same time, mergers, consolidations, affiliations, and opportunities to join multihospital systems have enabled many hospitals to obtain resources otherwise not available.[156] As a result, it has become increasingly important for health care organizations to have positive operating margins and strong balance sheets regardless of whether they are investor owned or not-for-profit. Overall, *resource acquisition* needs to be more carefully targeted than in the past to conform with the organization's overall strategic plan (see Chapter 14). New areas for strategic growth include same-day surgery, satellite clinics, home health care, diagnostic imaging, ambulatory alcoholism and psychiatric care, health promotion, sports medicine, and related ventures.[157]

The forces listed above have meant a different role in the resource acquisition process for the organization's board of directors. Previously, effective health care organizations selected board members primarily for their ability to provide and maintain rapport with community groups as a linkage to philanthropic sources; today's boards require greater experience and expertise in marketing, finance, risk taking, and entrepreneurship.[158] Taking hospitals as an example,

bridges to the community and other links to the external environment are still important, but the linkage requires board members to possess expertise and experience to help hospitals make the transition from acute care inpatient institutions to more diversified health care organizations emphasizing outpatient and primary care. The emphasis shifts from board members being the stewards of the hospital's assets to becoming active builders of a more diversified resource base. This is a particular challenge for rural, inner-city, public, and some university teaching hospitals.[159,160] These groups face a variety of resource acquisition issues: low occupancy and financial instability (e.g., many rural hospitals), a high percentage of Medicaid and medically indigent patients (e.g., many inner-city and public hospitals), and diminished revenues from state governments coupled with increased competition from surrounding community hospitals (e.g., many teaching hospitals affiliated with state medical schools).

The issue of resource acquisition is particularly important in competitive environments. A study focused on hospitals found that organizations in competitive environments whose boards are entrepreneurial tend to be more successful in obtaining needed resources (money, patients, and staff) than those with boards not so oriented.[161] This study also suggests that in any environment, whether competitive or noncompetitive, effectiveness in obtaining resources is increased when there is greater congruence of interests between the CEO and the board chairperson.

Failure of a given organization to attract sufficient resources on its own may result in corporate reorganization, consolidation, merger, affiliation membership, or multihospital system membership. With the exception of internal corporate reorganization, all of these represent to varying degrees a networking strategy designed to attract capital, strengthen political clout, create possible economies of scale, compete for managed care contracts and perhaps most importantly, achieve integration of clinical services. Failure to successfully negotiate such relationships is likely to result in suboptimal performance and possible closure.

A second important resource acquisition issue involves the ability to recruit and retain physicians, nurses, and related professional staff, which in turn can help attract patients. The existing shortage of primary care physicians represents a major new challenge not only to acquire such staff but potentially to restructure and retrain current staff to meet these needs. To meet this challenge, recruitment efforts need to be carefully targeted. Restructuring efforts may involve nurses playing an even greater role in delivering primary care or some specialists retraining to provide general care. Such restructuring of the professional staff, to be successful, needs to be extra sensitive to issues of control and motivation in professional work (see Chapters 3–5).

Managing Tradeoffs

Health care organizations are confronting an increasingly competitive environment in which the public will hold managers accountable not only for the cost of care but for the quality of care provided within their institutions. A natural reaction to this type of demand is to tighten existing controls, define lines of authority, clarify role definitions, and implement a range of performance evaluation systems. These actions may symbolically fulfill the expectations of those within and outside the organization that somebody is finally taking control. In reality, however, this approach may camouflage serious problems.

What is really needed is a shift in paradigms away from the mechanical model of control based on surveillance, inspection, and discipline to a new model of commitment and a cycle of continuous improvement as previously discussed. Each department in the organization determines who its customers are and what they want. The department then develops systems to meet the needs of its constituent groups and to monitor performance, assuring continuous improvement in the quality of services provided.

Many observers believe that there are inherent tradeoffs between efficiency and effectiveness—between containing costs and providing high-quality care. It is felt that attempts to become more efficient and productive will be made at the expense of quality. For example, patients may be discharged too soon, they may receive fewer services, the quality of the services they receive may be reduced, and hospitals may not keep up with the latest technology advances to provide state-of-the-art care. All of these behaviors may indeed erode the quality of care provided as perceived by one group or another.

But a contrasting view may also be taken. Specifically, it is possible that attempts to become more productive and efficient may be associated with improvements in quality. For example, productivity improvements that reduce length of stay may facilitate patient discharge to more appropriate outpatient settings or home environments, which may facilitate the healing process and reduce patients' susceptibility to hospital-acquired infections and illnesses. Fewer tests and procedures reduces the risk of possible side effects and mistakes. It also requires that caregivers be better diagnosticians and provide more focused treatment. Given the lack of evidence supporting strong relationships between process and outcomes of care, it is uncertain how changes in the process of care may affect outcomes, although it is recognized that there are thresholds beyond which outcomes may not improve and may, indeed, even deteriorate. Reductions in the quality of inputs involving patient-care amenities may reduce patient satisfaction but are not likely to affect mortality or functional health status measures. Finally, the fact that not all hospitals will be able to have state-of-the-art technology may actually improve quality by channeling patients to selected high-tech hospitals where more qualified professionals exist to use the technology appropriately and where sufficient volume of cases exist to promote better patient outcomes.[162–164]

Which of the scenarios described above is most likely to occur depends on a number of key variables. It would appear that the greatest potential for diminished quality exists in health care organizations that are financially stressed, serve a relatively high percentage of uninsured patients, operate in highly competitive markets, have difficulty recruiting highly qualified staff, and serve a patient population in which there is inadequate home and social support networks.

Existing studies, for the most part, suggest that tradeoffs between efficiency and effectiveness need not occur. Some studies find that efficiency is associated with higher quality of care.[165–172] A common thread underlying these results is effective management. In brief, these organizations have developed many of the management and organization practices discussed in this chapter. For example, several Rochester area hospitals identified patients who could be tube-fed rather than IV-fed. This resulted in a significant cost reduction while improving patient treatment.[173] A study of the nursing home industry in New York State revealed that labor-intensive aspects of care involving the quality of nursing and rehabilitation services did not increase costs, perhaps because of careful screening of nurses (which reduces turnover), better staff training, and better coordination.[174] However, capital-intensive aspects of patient care quality were associated with higher costs, which is consistent with results from some hospital studies as well.[175,176]

Existing knowledge regarding the tradeoff issue must be viewed with caution. First, it is important to note that almost all of the studies have been done prior to the widespread introduction of Medicare's Prospective Payment System and related incentive reimbursement arrangements. Thus health organizations were not feeling the pressure to contain cost to the degree they are today. Second, all the studies have been cross-sectional at a single point in time, and thus have not been able to assess the issue of whether a strategy to cut costs at time T1 actually results in a change in quality at time T2. Third, all studies have struggled with the problem of developing valid measures of quality which adequately take into account the case-mix severity of patients. While great strides have been made, considerable more work needs to be done. Finally, it is important to remember that high cost does not necessarily mean inefficient management but may simply reflect management's desire to provide more amenities to patients and staff, resulting in higher patient and staff satisfaction. More recently, however, the margins for such behavior are being reduced.

It is clear that the tradeoff issue will not go away. It places health care managers squarely in the center of the tension between those who view health care primarily as an economic good and those who view it primarily as a social good. We end the chapter by considering future management and organizational practices that appear to be associated with truly high-performing health care organizations. These are organizations that recognize the inherent tensions involved and see them as opportunities for greater achievement. They are high performing in the sense of enjoying outstanding reputations in their communities for high-

quality cost-effective patient care; financial integrity; and innovative approaches to service delivery.

Leadership Strategies for High-Performance Health Care Organizations

High-performing health care organizations are both aware and able to act on the basis of their awareness. Truly high-performing health care organizations have both the ability and willingness to be outstanding.[177] Contrary to findings from other industries, the basic form of strategic adaptation to a changing environment appears to play an important part in successful performance for hospitals in systems.[178,179]

> It appears that in rapidly changing industries such as health care, proactive strategies such as the prospector and analyzer, which emphasize experimentation, innovation, risk-taking, diversification, and continual differentiation of new products and services, are likely to be more effective.[180]

Some organizations have the desire but not all of the ability required. They require additional talent and staff development to move out of the ranks of the mediocre. Other organizations have the ability but lack the willingness. They lack strategic vision of what they can become. They are underachievers. Still others lack both the willingness and ability. Without a radical transformation, their chances of survival are minimal.

A synthesis of existing research and observations suggest that high-performing health care organizations

- stretch themselves by setting high standards
- maximize learning
- take risks
- exhibit transformational leadership
- incline toward action
- create a chemistry among top management teams
- manage uncertainty and ambiguity
- remain loosely coordinated
- possess a strong culture
- signify meaningful values and beliefs to themselves and others

Some of these characteristics are better documented than others. Nonetheless, they provide suggestive in-

IN THE REAL WORLD
LOCATION AND GOOD MANAGEMENT MAKE THE DIFFERENCE

A 1991–1992 study conducted by ICF/Lewin for the Prospective Payment Assessment Commission (ProPAC) of Medicare winners and losers highlights the importance of both location and effective management to hospital performance. The winners were defined as hospitals whose Medicare operating margins remained in the top 25 percent for three consecutive years. In 1989, for example, the average margin for the top quartile was 7.1 percent, while the average margin for the bottom quartile was −15 percent. Among the key findings were the following:

• Winning hospitals were located in stable economic areas with less competitive markets and greater availability of nurses and physicians. Losers also had to hire more nurses from outside agencies which is more costly and inefficient.

• Hospitals having a larger proportion of patients who remain in the hospital beyond the standard Medicare stay were more likely to be losers.

• Hospitals with strong management that had a long-standing commitment to cost containment and to forging good relationships with their medical staffs also were more likely to be winners.

• Facilities with post acute services such as a skilled nursing unit also did better largely because they could manage resources better and shift a portion of their overhead costs to those units.

• Winning hospitals also maintained a high occupancy rate but, in addition, monitored their intensive care units to minimize utilization. They also had strong discharge planning and utilization review.

SOURCE: Adapted from Modern Healthcare. April 27, 1992:2, with permission from MODERN HEALTHCARE. Copyright Crain Communications, Inc., 740 N. Rush Street, Chicago, IL 60611

sights into what differentiates truly high-performing organizations from others. Of these factors, the first four appear to be particularly important.

Stretching

High-performing health care organizations set very high standards. They are constantly raising the high jump bar. An example is provided by one health care system in which it is corporate policy to give people responsibilities which they can't possibly fulfill. This is intentionally done to stretch people to their fullest capability and is an integral part of the organization's human resources planning. To prevent burnout and undue frustration, the organization has a strong management development program tied to its strategic plan.

Stretching is a core value of the organization's culture, and people's efforts are reinforced and supported. In addition to setting high standards, stretching is facilitated by the development of overarching goals which can be bought into by individual divisions and departments. For example, one HMO's goal of emphasizing consumer convenience was translated into the appointment-reception department's objective to reduce appointment and visit waiting times to a minimum. Toward this end, they worked for months to develop a computerized appointment and scheduling system which significantly reduced both appointment and visit waiting times. The system enabled one staff member on each shift to work the reception area answering patient's questions, providing information, and playing with children. As one patient commented, "I've never seen such personal attention in a waiting room."

MANAGERIAL GUIDELINES

Maintaining and Improving Quality of Care

1. Develop a participative, team-oriented organizational culture that encourages input from professionals and other workers from all levels of the organization.
2. Establish high standards that appeal to professional standards. Link professional values and goals to those of the organization.
3. Develop information systems that provide relevant, timely, and accurate data for purposes of taking corrective action and reaching ever-higher standards. Use statistical thinking and tools to identify desired performance levels, measure current performance, interpret it, and take action when necessary.
4. Look for opportunities to improve quality by detecting and preventing potential problems in the process. Focus on the most important processes to improve.
5. Design work to make the best use of professionals' experience and expertise.
6. Develop reward systems that reinforce participation and high performance. Don't blame individuals for defects in the process.
7. Develop organizational structures that promote communication, coordination, and conflict management.

8. Actively manage the external environment to recruit the best available talent.

Evaluating Professional Work

1. Professionals working in health care organizations are largely self-motivated. Thus setting high standards consistent with professional norms of excellence promotes effectiveness.
2. Any organization requires rules and procedures. In health care organizations the rules and procedures must be based as much on professional needs, values, and aspirations as on the needs, values, and aspirations of the organization.
3. The professional's need for autonomy must be kept paramount in all organization design decisions.
4. The special needs of professional work demand that flexible mechanisms be used to coordinate such activity.
5. Professionals want to participate in decisions that will affect the professional nature of their work.
6. Increasingly, professionals want to participate in larger issues that will affect the nature of their work in years to come.

In their commitment to high standards and overarching goals, high-performing health care organizations emphasize management development. Their executives are trained to resist always being the hero or orchestrator of solutions and, instead, to use every problem solving situation as an opportunity to develop one's subordinates.[181] Performance appraisal and reward systems are established to reinforce such behavior. As subordinates' skill levels increase along with their confidence and commitment to the organization, the organization is rewarded by having available a richer array of management skills than any single leader can alone possess.

Maximizing Learning

The winning health care organizations in the twenty-first century will be those that learn quickly, observe accurately, and have the ability to put their learning to use.[182] They are both proactive (i.e., plan ahead) and enactive (i.e., learn by doing) in their approaches. They engage in wide searches, conduct experiments to facili-

MANAGERIAL GUIDELINES

Acquiring Resources

1. Boards of directors need to adopt more corporate forms of organization with emphasis given to strategic planning, entrepreneurial, and risk-taking activities.
2. Linkages must be formed with new types of stakeholders, including employers, business coalitions, and special interest consumer groups.
3. Executives need to make more use of macropolitical strategies involving the negotiation of network relationships which will form larger resource pools.
4. The effective health care organization needs to become more proactive in managing its environment in order to compete more effectively.
5. The organization needs to become adept at developing specialized market niches and initiating products and services for targeted market segments where sufficient resources exist to gain a distinctive long-run competitive advantage.
6. In order to be effective in the long run, organizations need to learn how to continuously differentiate their product or service relative to competitors.

Improving Productivity and Efficiency

1. Develop accurate, timely, and useful management information systems. Remember that all data is not useful information.
2. Concentrate productivity improvement programs in large departments where big payoffs will result.
3. Consider streamlining and consolidating departments and functions.
4. Develop scheduling systems consistent with professional values. Focus on areas where quality can be maintained or even enhanced through better scheduling of staff and support resources.
5. Cross-train staff to gain greater flexibility.
6. Develop productivity-based incentives based on work activities under the control of organizational members.
7. Set high standards by establishing "best practices" in one's own organization as well as using comparisons from competitors and industry leaders.
8. Involve organizational members, particularly professionals, in the development, implementation, and monitoring of productivity and efficiency initiatives.
9. Focus energy on working smarter, not necessarily harder.

tate learning, have market-driven information systems, and create redundancies that emphasize effectiveness over efficiency.

High-performing health care organizations search their environments for opportunities and hidden threats. This involves what Argyris calls "double loop" learning, which goes beyond existing organizational practices and policies to question the underlying causes of present behavior and to imagine future behaviors in response to changing environmental circumstances.[183] An example is provided by a west coast hospital which recognized the need for an upgraded physician referral service. Instead of simply looking at examples in their immediate area, they set as their goal to learn about the best system in the country. Their search led to the discovery of a system in an eastern hospital which enabled patients who phoned in to communicate with a specific physician and lock in the appointment at the time of the call.

Because learning is a core value for high-performing health care organizations, they are continually conducting experiments. They undertake new initiatives based not only on the likelihood of success but on the amount of learning that can be derived. An HMO in the early 1980s experimented with providing coverage to retirees. It was not particularly successful at the time, but what was learned from the experience enabled the HMO to be among the first to successfully participate in a federally funded HMO waiver experiment to provide care to Medicare beneficiaries. Another example is represented by a hospital that failed in its initial attempts to create a home health care program, but learned so much from the experience that two years later, it became the market leader of home health services in its area because it was in a position to create a joint venture with another organization.

Market-Driven Information Systems Obtaining useful information and feedback is critical to the manager's ability to take corrective action. Most health care organizations have invested heavily in improved management information systems. These systems enable the organization to assess the true cost and integrate financial and accounting data with clinical data on a diagnosis-by-diagnosis basis. This has allowed organizations to assess the productivity, efficiency, and profitability of specific service lines and, therefore, compete more effectively.

As health care becomes more price-competitive, organizations need ways of linking information about consumer wants and needs (including third-party payers and businesses) with the fiscal and human resources of the organization designed to meet those demands and needs. Market-driven information systems must be based most fundamentally on the organization's overall strategic plan (Chapter 14). It must also create the necessary links between the marketing plan (which specifies the products or services for a particular market; determines "packaging", price, and distribution channels; and sets the advertising and promotion policies), the operation plan (which specifies who does what, when, with what special resources to deliver the services), and the financial plan (which specifies the financial resources and capital needed overall and by the marketing and operation plans).[184] The information needs to be pushed down in the organization to the physicians, nurses, and other health professionals who are closest to patients and therefore can most readily act on the information.

Strategy of Redundancy—Choosing Effectiveness over Efficiency Existing analysis suggests that some amount of redundancy (i.e., inefficiency) appears to be associated with higher performance.[185,186] This is because redundancy facilitates learning, particularly when undertaking programs that are new and different from what the organization has done before. For example, in undertaking ambulatory care joint ventures with physicians, successful hospitals were found to use both hospital and clinic personnel policies, purchasing policies, budgeting practices, and information systems. While not efficient, it enabled each hospital to learn more quickly about what systems worked best. In the long run, it was a more effective strategy than those that decided on a one-best-way approach that offered little opportunity for learning by doing.

Risk Taking

- Nothing ventured, nothing gained.
- Analysis should not lead to paralysis.
- Sometimes, it is better to ready, fire, aim.
- It is better to be roughly right than precisely wrong!

High-performing health care organizations believe in the above ideologies. *Risk taking* is one of the major ways these organizations learn. They are concerned only if they fail to learn from their mistakes.

Unlike studies in other industries, high performers in health services do not necessarily "stick to their knitting"—that is, do things they know and do well.[187] Instead, they recognize that the health care industry has undergone so much change that for organizations to operate as they have in the past begs mediocrity and failure. They recognize the need to develop new programs and services outside of their traditional areas of expertise and experience. They recognize the need to become something other than they have been. If they do not have the necessary expertise or experience, it can be purchased or developed, either internally or through networking with other organizations.

While recognizing the need to take risks, these organizations distinguish between prudent and foolish risk taking. They attempt to reduce uncertainty and maximize the probability of a positive outcome through careful analysis of their environment, their competition, their strengths and weaknesses, and the development of both collaborative and competitive strategies that will enable them to best serve their communities over the long run. They also involve a wide network of individuals (trustees, physicians, department directors) in the strategic planning and management process. This facilitates consideration of multiple perspectives, incorporation of additional knowledge and information, and most importantly, support for projects that involve a high degree of risk. It also helps to instill a risk-taking culture, perhaps best captured by the words of Walter Wriston, ex-president of CitiCorps Bank in New York, who frequently told his employees, "When I make a mistake, the first thing I try to do is go back out and make an even bigger one. If you're not making mistakes, you're not learning."

Transformational Leadership

The effects of leadership are most pronounced in difficult times. In benign environments, most organizations do relatively well and there is relatively little performance differentiation among them. But in times of great change and uncertainty, truly outstanding organizations are revealed, and a primary reason as noted in Chapter 4 is often the presence of transformational leadership.[188] This involves spending a great deal of time on developing, communicating, and role modeling the new strategic vision required to be successful. It involves showing how the organizational changes needed will help to promote the personal and professional growth of those involved. It involves assisting people in making career transitions. It involves paying attention to meanings and symbols. It involves helping people let go of the past while showing new ways for success in the future.

While most examples of transformational leadership involve people at the top of the organization, outstanding organizations try to instill such qualities in key individuals throughout the organization. A culture develops in which members show a high degree of responsibility for each other and give and take meaning from each other.

It is important to recognize that improving the performance of individual health care organizations is not the same as improving an individual's performance or the overall ability of health care systems and communities to deliver cost-effective services. Nonetheless, as the delivery of health care becomes more consolidated both horizontally and vertically, improvements in individual organizational performance are likely to have ripple effects. Conversely, failure to improve performance has pervasive negative effects throughout the system. Thus a major challenge for health care managers in the future lies not only in improving individual organizational performance but in improving the performance of networks, coalitions, affiliations, and systems. In the process, it will be important to remember that there is something wrong with every available measure of performance. Thus effective managers will use many indicators to assess individual, group, organizational, and network performance.

KEY CONCEPTS

Appropriateness
Benchmarking
Cost Effectiveness
Effectiveness
Efficacy
Efficiency
Organizational Effectiveness
Outcome Measures of Quality
Process Measures of Quality
Productivity
Quality Assurance
Quality Improvement
Reactivity
Resource Acquisition
Risk Taking
Stretching
Structural Measures of Quality
Transformational Leadership

Discussion Questions

1. Take the perspective of an HMO executive. Describe three major ways that you could manage the HMO plan to improve the access, quality, and cost containment for your patients. Critique your solutions regarding the extent to which your solutions may cause other problems to surface (what kind?) and the extent to which you as a CEO could (or should) have the power to accomplish these changes.

2. Using a health care organization that you know well, provide three examples each of possible structural, process, and outcome measures of effectiveness. Would you expect these measures to be highly associated? Why or why not?

3. Consider a community hospital, a major teaching hospital, and an HMO. For each, list the major constituency groups (both internal and external). Indicate what kinds of effectiveness criteria each group would be most likely to promote.

4. Hospital A and Hospital B both have as their major goal for this year the implementation of a QI program. Hospital A hired a consultant firm and sent its top managers to a program to learn how to change the corporate culture and to set up quality teams to investigate problems. They formed teams to plan strategies of meaningful QI in two specific areas: billing and use of the emergency room. Hospital B, lacking funds, tried to have study groups and use self-teaching but involved everyone from the CEO to the janitor. Which hospital do you think will succeed in implementing QI? Why?

5. Clinic Q was a large multispecialty group practice with a major emphasis on specialist care. Because they were worried about not having enough referrals for specialist care, their major goal for the year was to set up two new branches of primary care providers. To attract primary care providers, they discovered that they had to offer salaries higher than the average salary of other physicians at the clinic. Start up costs were also high. Using concepts like strategic planning, effectiveness, productivity, and efficiency, discuss how to evaluate whether this expansion was a "success" for the organization.

REFERENCES

1. Weick KE. Enactment processes in organizations. In Staw BM, Salancik GR, eds. *New Directions in Organizations and Organizational Behavior.* Chicago, Ill: St. Claire Press; 1977.
2. Schulz RI, Greenley JR, Peterson RW. Differences in the direct cost of public and private acute in-patient psychiatric services. *Inquiry.* Winter 1984;21:380–393.
3. Shortell SM. High performing health care organizations: Guidelines for the pursuit of excellence. *Hospital and Health Services Administration.* July-August 1985;30:7–35.
4. Neuhauser D. *The Relationship Between Administrative Activities and Hospital Performance.* Chicago, Ill: Center for Health Administration Studies, University of Chicago; Research Series 28; 1971.
5. Schulz, et al., op. cit.
6. Shortell SM, Becker SW, Neuhauser D. The effects of management practices on hospital efficiency and quality of care. In: Shortell SM, Brown M, eds. *Organizational Research and Hospitals.* Chicago, Ill: Blue Cross Association; 1976.
7. Sloan F, Becker E. Internal organization of hospitals and hospital costs. *Inquiry.* 1981;18:224–240.
8. Luft HS. *Health Maintenance Organizations: Dimensions of Performance.* New York, NY: John Wiley & Sons; 1981.
9. Schulz, et al., op. cit.
10. Shortell SM. Physician involvement in hospital decision-making. In: Gray B, ed. *The New Health Care for Profit: Doctors and Hospitals in a Competitive Environment.* Washington, DC: National Academy Press, Institute of Medicine; 1983:73–102.
11. Schulz, et al., op. cit.
12. Pauly M. Medical staff characteristics and hospital costs. *Journal of Human Resources.* 1978;13 (Suppl).78–111.
13. Garg ML, Mulligan JL, Gliebe WA, et al. Physicians' specialty, quality and cost of in-patient care. *Social Science and Medicine.* 1979;13C:187–190.
14. Sherman HD. Hospital efficiency measurement and evaluation: Empirical test of a new technique. *Medical Care.* October 1984;22:922–938.
15. Alexander JA, Rundall TG. Public hospitals under contract management: An assessment of operating performance. *Medical Care.* March 1985;23:209–219.
16. Choi T, Allison RF, Munson F. *Governance and Management of University Hospitals: External Forces and Internal Processes.* Ann Arbor, Mich: Health Administration Press; 1986.
17. Institute of Medicine. *For Profit Enterprise in Health Care.* Washington, DC: National Academy Press; 1986.
18. Levitz GS, Brooke PP. Independent versus system-affiliated hospitals: A comparative analysis of financial performance, cost, and productivity. *Health Services Research.* August 1985;20:315–339.
19. Coyne JS. Hospital performance in multi-hospital systems: A comparative study of system and independent hospitals. *Health Services Research.* Winter 1982;17:303–329.
20. Scott WR. Effectiveness of organizational effectiveness studies. In Goodman PS, Pennings JM, eds. *New Perspectives on Organizational Effectiveness.* San Francisco, Ca: Jossey-Bass; 1977.
21. Haberstroh CJ. Organization design and systems analysis. In: March JG, ed. *Handbook of Organizations.* Chicago, Ill: Rand McNally; 1965:1182.
22. Kanter RM. Organizational performance: Recent developments in measurement. *Annual Review of Sociology.* 1981;7:321.
23. Gouldner AW. Organizational analysis. In: Merton RK, Broom L, Cottrell Jr LS, eds. *Sociology Today.* New York, NY: Basic Books; 1959.
24. Etzioni A. Two approaches to organizational analysis: A critique and a suggestion. *Administrative Science Quarterly.* 1960;5:257–278.
25. Yuchtman E, Seashore S. A system resource approach to organizational effectiveness. *American Sociological Review.* 1967;32:891–903.
26. Fleming GV. Hospital structure and consumer satisfaction. *Health Services Research.* 1981;16:43–64.
27. Weick KE. Re-punctuating the problem. In: Goodman PS, Pennings JM, eds. *New Perspectives on Organizational Effectiveness.* San Francisco, Ca: Jossey-Bass; 1977.
28. Kimberly JR, Miles RH, eds. *The Organizational Life Cycle.* San Francisco, Ca: Jossey-Bass; 1980.
29. Cameron K, Whetten DA. Perceptions of organizational effectiveness across organizational life cycles. *Administrative Science Quarterly.* 1981;26:525–544.
30. Nerenz DR, Zajac BM. *Indicators of Performance for Vertically Integrated Health Systems: Final Report of 1990 Ray Woodham Visiting Fellowship.* Detroit, Mich: Center for Health System Studies, Henry Ford Health System; 1991.
31. Berle AA, Means GC. *The Modern Corporation and Private Property.* New York, NY: Macmillan; 1932.
32. Burnham J. *The Managerial Revolution.* New York, NY: John Day; 1941.
33. Cyert RM, March JG. *A Behavioral Theory of the Firm.* Englewood Cliffs, NJ: Prentice-Hall; 1966.
34. Fennell ML, Alexander JA. Governing boards and profound organizational change in hospitals. *Medical Care Review.* 1989;46:157–187.
35. Berwick DM, Godfrey AB, Roessner J. *Curing Health*

Care: New Strategies for Quality Improvement. San Francisco, Ca: Jossey-Bass; 1991.

36. Price JL. *Organizational Effectiveness.* Homewood, Ill: Richard D. Irwin, Inc.; 1968.

37. Steers RM. Problems in the measurement of organizational effectiveness. *Administrative Science Quarterly.* 1975;20:546.

38. Campbell JP. On the nature of organizational effectiveness. In: Goodman PS, Pennings JM, eds. *New Perspectives on Organizational Effectiveness.* San Francisco, Ca: Jossey-Bass; 1977.

39. Flood AB. The impact of organizational and managerial factors on the outcomes and effectiveness of health services. Urbana-Champaign, Ill: University of Illnois at Urbana-Champaign, Institute of Government and Public Affairs; Working Paper Series, 1991.

40. Donabedian A. Evaluating the quality of medical care. *Milbank Memorial Fund Quarterly.* 1966;44(2): 166–206.

41. Cleverly WO. Financial ratios: Summary indicators for management decision making. *Hospital and Health Services Administration.* 1981;26:26–47.

42. Ibid.

43. Scott, 1977, op. cit.

44. Scott WR. *Organizations: Rational, Natural, and Open Systems.* 3rd ed. Englewood Cliffs, NJ: Prentice-Hall, 1992.

45. Georgopoulos BS, Mann FC. *The Community General Hospital.* New York, NY: Macmillan; 1962.

46. Rhee SO, Luke R, Lyons TF, Payne BC. Domain of practice and the quality of physician performance. *Medical Care.* January 1981;19:14–23.

47. Payne BC, Lyons TF, Neuhaus E. Relationships of physician characteristics to performance quality and improvement. *Health Services Research.* August 1984;19:307–332.

48. Rhee SO. Relative importance of physician's personal and situational characteristics for the quality of patient care. *Journal of Health and Social Behavior.* March 1977; 18:10–15.

49. Flood A, Scott WR. Professional power and professional effectiveness: The power of the surgical staff and the quality of surgical care in hospitals. *Journal of Health and Social Behavior.* 1978;19:240–254.

50. Rhee SO, Luke RD, Culverwell MB. Influence of client/colleague dependence on physician performance in patient care. *Medical Care.* August 1980;18:829–841.

51. Pauly, op. cit.

52. Flood, Scott, op. cit.

53. Flood AB, Scott WR, Ewy W. Does practice make perfect? Part I: The relationship between hospital volume and outcomes for select diagnostic categories. *Medical Care.* February 1984;22:98–114.

54. Luft HS. The relation between surgical volume and mortality: An exploration of causal factors and alternative models. *Medical Care.* September 1980;18:940–959.

55. Shortell SM, LoGerfo JP. Hospital medical staff organization and quality of care: Results for myocardial infarction and appendectomy. *Medical Care.* October 1981;19:1041–1055.

56. Georgopoulos, Mann, op. cit.

57. Flood, Scott, 1978, op. cit.

58. Flood, Scott, Ewy, op. cit.

59. Shortell, LoGerfo, op. cit.

60. Argote L. Input uncertainty and organizational coordination in hospital emergency limits. *Administrative Science Quarterly.* 1982;27:420–434.

61. Roemer MI, Friedman JW. *Doctors in Hospitals: Medical Staff Organization and Hospital Performance.* Baltimore, Md: Johns Hopkins University Press; 1971.

62. Neuhauser, op. cit.

63. Shortell, LoGerfo, op. cit.

64. Holland TP, Konick A, Buffum W, et al. Institutional structure and resident outcomes. *Journal of Health and Social Behavior.* 1981;22:433–444.

65. Denison DR. Bringing corporate culture to the bottom line. *Organizational Dynamics.* 1985:5–22.

66. Mark B. Task and structural correlates of organizational effectiveness in private psychiatric hospitals. *Health Services Research.* June 1985;20:199–224.

67. Neuhauser, op. cit.

68. Mark, op. cit.

69. Morlock L, Nathanson C, Horn S, Schumacher D. Organizational factors associated with the quality of care in seventeen general acute hospitals. Presented at the Annual Meeting of the Association of University Programs and Health Administration; 1979; Toronto, Canada.

70. Morrow PC. Explorations in macrocommunication behavior: The effects of organizational feedback on organizational effectiveness. *Journal of Management Studies.* 1982;19:438–446.

71. Keeler EB, Kahn KL, Draper DM, et al. Changes in sickness at admission following the introduction of the Prospective Payment System. *Journal of American Medical Association.* 1990;264:1962–1968.

72. Kosecoff SB, Brook RH. Comparing outcomes of care before and after implementation of the DRG-based prospective payment system. *Journal of American Medical Association.* 1990;264:1984–1988.

73. Rubenstein LV, Chang BL, Keeler EB, Kahn KL. Measuring the quality of nursing surveillance activities for five diseases before and after implementation of the DRG-based Prospective Payment System. In: *Payment Outcomes Research: Examining the Effectiveness of Nursing Practice,*

Proceedings of the State of the Science Conference. Bethesda, Md: National Institutes of Health publication 93-3411; October 1992.

74. Choi, et al., op. cit.
75. Mosely SK, Grimes RM. The organization of effective hospitals. *Healthcare Management Review.* Summer 1976;1:13–23.
76. Payne, et al., op. cit.
77. Rhee, op. cit.
78. Pauly, op. cit.
79. Flood, Scott, Ewy, op. cit.
80. Luft, 1980, op. cit.
81. Shortell, LoGerfo, op. cit.
82. Rhee, op. cit.
83. Flood Scott, 1978, op. cit.
84. Flood, AB, Scott WR. *Hospital Structure and Performance.* Baltimore, Md: Johns Hopkins Press; 1987.
85. Shortell, LoGerfo, op. cit.
86. Argote, op. cit.
87. Denison, op. cit.
88. Ibid.
89. Shortell SM, Zimmerman JE, Gillies RR et al. Continuously improving patient care: Practical lessons and an assessment tool from the National ICU Study. *Quality Review Bulletin.* May 1990;5:150–155.
90. Sherman, op. cit.
91. Morlock, et al., op. cit.
92. Morrow, op. cit.
93. Rubenstein, et al., op. cit.
94. Choi, et al., op. cit.
95. Biggs EL, Kralewski J, Brown G. A comparison of contract-managed and traditionally-managed non-profit hospitals. *Medical Care.* 1980;18:585–596.
96. Ermann D, Gabel J. Multihospital systems: Issues and empirical findings. *Health Affairs.* 1984;3:50–64.
97. Zuckerman HS. Multi-institutional systems: Their promise and performance. In: Zuckerman H, Weeks LE, eds. *Multi-Institutional Hospital Systems.* Chicago, Ill: Hospital Research and Educational Trust; 1979.
98. Friedman B, Shortell SM. The financial performance of selected investor-owned and not-for-profit system hospitals before and after Medicare prospective payment. *Health Services Research.* 1988;23:237–267.
99. Shortell SM, Morrison EM, Friedman B. *Strategic choices for America's hospitals: Managing change in turbulent times.* San Francisco, Ca: Jossey-Bass; 1990.
100. Hall MA. Institutional control of physician behavior: Legal barriers to health care cost containment. *University of Pennsylvania Law Review.* 1988;137:431–536.
101. Donabedian, op. cit.
102. Scott WR. Managing professional work: Three models of control for health organizations. *Health Services Research.* 1982;17:213–240.
103. Weisman CS, Nathanson CA. Professional satisfaction and client outcomes: A comparative organizational analysis. *Medical Care.* October 1985;23:1179–1192.
104. Hetherington R, Soroko S, Bidle I. *Quality Assurance and Organizational Effectiveness in Hospitals.* Hyattsville Md: National Center for Health Services Research, Division of Intramural Research; Report 17(2); 1982.
105. Georgopouluos, Mann, op. cit.
106. Argote, op. cit.
107. Price JL, Mueller CW. A causal model of turnover for nurses. *Academy of Management Journal.* 1981;24:543–565.
108. Barr JK, Steinberg M. Professional participation in organizational decision making: Physicians in HMOs. *Journal of Community Health.* Spring 1983;8(3):160–173.
109. Shortell, 1983, op. cit.
110. Shortell SM, Morrisey MA, Conrad D. Economic regulation and hospital behavior: The effects on medical staff organization and hospital-physician relationships. *Health Services Research.* December 1985;20:597–627.
111. Alexander JA, Morrisey MA, Shortell SM. The effects of competition regulation and corporatization on hospital-physician relationships. *Journal of Health and Social Behavior.* September 1986;27:220–235.
112. Dornbusch SM, Scott WR, with Busching BC, Laing JD. *Evaluation and the Exercise of Authority.* San Francisco, Ca: Jossey-Bass; 1975.
113. Wennberg JE, Blowers L, Parker P, Gittelsohn AM. Changes in tonsillectomy rates associated with feedback and review. *Pediatrics.* 1977;59:821–826.
114. Dyck FJ, Murphy FA, Murphy JK, Road DA, Boyd MS, et al. The effect of surveillance on the number of hysterectomies in the province of Saskatchewan. *New England Journal of Medicine.* 1977;296:1326–1328.
115. Cohen SN, Flood AB, Himmelberger DU, Mangini RJ, Moore TN. *Development, Implementation, and Evaluation of the Monitoring and Evaluation of Drug Interactions by a Pharmacy Oriented Report System (MEDIPHOR) HS00739.* Springfield, Va: National Technical Information Service; 1980; Final Report to the National Center for Health Services Research.
116. Keeler RB, Chapin AM, Soule DN. Informed inquiry into practice variations: The Maine Medical Assessment Foundation. *Quality Assurance in Health Care.* 1990;2:69–75.
117. Keeler RB, Soule DN, Wennberg JE, Hanley DF. Dealing with geographic variations in the use of hospitals: The experience of the Maine Medical Assessment Foundation Orthopedic Study Group. *Journal of Bone and Joint Surgery.* 1990;72(A):1286–1293.
118. Borbas C, Stump MA, Dedecker K, et al. The Minnesota Clinical Comparison and Assessment

Project. *Quality Review Bulletin.* February 1990;16:87–92.

119. Wones RG. Failure of low-cost audits with feedback to reduce laboratory test utilization. *Medical Care.* 1987;25:78–82.

120. Brook RH, Lohr KN. Efficacy, effectiveness, variations and quality: Boundary-crossing research. *Medical Care.* 1985;23:710–722.

121. Williamson JM. Future policy directions for quality assurance: Lessons from the health accounting experience. *Inquiry.* 1988;25:67–77.

122. Komaroff AL. Quality assurance in 1984. *Medical Care.* 1985;23:723–738.

123. Jessee WF. Quality assurance systems: Why aren't there any? *Quality Review Bulletin.* 1984;10:408–411.

124. Mittman BS, Siv AL. Changing provider behavior: Applying research on outcomes and effectiveness in health care. In: Shortell SM, Reinhardt UE, eds. *Improving Health Policy and Management.* Baxter Health Policy Review, Ann Arbor, Mich: Health Administration Press; 1992.

125. Luke RD, Krueger JC, Modrow RE. *Organization and Change in Health Care Quality Assurance.* Rockville, Md: Aspen System Corporation; 1983.

126. Jessee, op. cit.

127. Fifer WR. Integrating quality assurance mechanisms. In: Luke RD, Krueger JC, Modrow RE, eds. *Organization and Change in Health Care Quality Assurance.* Rockville, Md: Aspen System Corporation; 1983.

128. Shanahan M. The quality assurance standard of the JCAH: A rational approach to patient care evaluation. In: Luke RD, Krueger JC, Modrow RE, eds. *Organization and Change in Health Care Quality Assurance.* Rockville, Md: Aspen Systems Corporation, 1983.

129. Wyszewianski L. The emphasis is on measurement in quality assurance: Reasons and implications. *Inquiry.* 1988;25:424–436.

130. Eisenberg JM. *Doctors' decisions and the cost of medical care: The reasons for doctors' practice and ways to change them.* Ann Arbor, Mich: Health Administration Press Perspective; 1986.

131. McCoy CE, Kind EA, Fowles J, Schned ES. Measuring quality in an HMO: The primary care practice profile. In: *Managing Quality Health Care in a Dynamic Era.* Washington, DC: The Group Health Association of America, Inc.; 1987:112–117.

132. Kind EA, Fowles J, McCoy CE. Effectiveness of the primary profile in changing physician practice styles. Presented at the American Medical Review Research Center Annual Meetings; September 1987; Washington, DC.

133. *Medicare: Improving Quality of Care Assessment and Assurance: Report to the Chairman, Subcommittee on Health, Committee on Ways and Means, House of Representatives.* Washington, DC; US General Accounting Office; 1988:GAO/PEMD-88-10.

134. Fifer, op. cit.

135. Shanahan, op. cit.

136. Rosen HM, Feigin W. Medical peer review and information management: The deadend phenomenon. *Health Care Management Review.* 1982;7:59–66.

137. Vuori H. Optimal and logical quality: Two neglected aspects of quality of health services. *Medical Care.* 1980;18:975–985.

138. Heatherington RW. Quality assurance and organizational effectiveness in hospitals. *Health Services Research.* 1982;17:185–201.

139. Deming WE. *Out of the Crisis.* Cambridge, Mass: Massachusetts Institute of Technology; 1986.

140. Crosby PB. *Quality is Free.* New York: New American Library; 1979.

141. Juran JM, ed. *Juran's Quality Control Handbook.* 4th ed. New York, NY: McGraw-Hill; 1988.

142. Camp RC. *Benchmarking: The Search for Industry Best Practices that Lead to Superior Practices.* Milwaukee, Wis: American Society for Quality Control, Quality Press; 1989.

143. Keeler, et al., op. cit.

144. Roberts JS. Peer review and continuous quality improvement. In: *Bridging the Gap Between Theory and Practice.* Chicago, Ill: Hospital Research and Educational Trust; 1992.

145. Berwick, et al., op. cit.

146. Ibid., 25.

147. Berwick DM. Blazing the trail of quality: the HFHS quality management process. *Frontiers of Health Services Management.* Summer 1991;7(4):47–50.

148. Sahney VK. Implementation, observed barriers, and management of continuous quality improvement (CQI). In: *Bridging the Gap between Theory and Practice: Exploring Continuous Quality Improvement.* Chicago, Ill: Hospital Research and Educational Trust; 1992.

149. Ishikawa K. *What is Total Quality Control?* Englewood Cliffs, NJ: Prentice-Hall; 1985.

150. Stewart WA. *Statistical Method from the Viewpoint of Quality Control.* New York, NY: Dover Publications; 1986.

151. Wheeler DJ, Chambers DS. *Understanding Statistical Process Control.* Knoxville, Tenn: Statistical Process Controls, Inc.; 1987.

152. Batalden PB, Buchanan ED. Industry models of quality improvement. In: Goldfield N, Nash DB. *Providing Quality Care: The Challenge to Clinicians.* Philadelphia, Pa: American College of Surgeons; 1989.

153. Plsek PE, Onnias A, Early JF. *Quality Improvement Tools.* Wilton, Conn: Juran Institute, Inc.; 1989.

154. Plsek PE. Resource B: A primer on quality

improvement tools. In: Berwick DM, Godfrey AB, Roessner J, eds. *Curing Health Care: New Strategies for Quality Improvement.* San Francisco, Ca: Jossey-Bass; 1991.

155. Kaluzny AD, McLaughlin CP, & Kibbe DC. Continuous quality improvement in the clinical setting: Enhancing adoption. *Quality Management in Health Care.* 1992;1:37–44.

156. Ermann, Gabel, op. cit.

157. Shortell SM, Morrison EM, Hughes SL, et al. Diversification of health care services: The effects of ownership, environment and strategy. In: Rossiter L., Schecter R, eds. *Advances in Health Economics and Health Services Research.* San Francisco, Ca: JAI Press; 1986.

158. Pfeffer J. Size, composition, and function of hospital boards of directors: A study of organization-environment linkage. *Administrative Science Quarterly.* 1973;18:349–364.

159. Elling R, Halebsky S. Organizational differentiation and support. *Administrative Science Quarterly.* 1961;6:185–209.

160. Choi, et al., op. cit.

161. Barrett D, Windham SR. Hospital boards and adaptability to competitive environments. *Health Care Management Review.* Fall 1984:11–20.

162. Flood, Scott, Ewy, op. cit.

163. Luft, op. cit.

164. Shortell, LoGerfo, op. cit.

165. Neuhauser, op. cit.

166. Shortell, Becker, Neuhauser, op. cit.

167. Longest BB. An empirical analysis of the quality/cost relationship. *Hospital and Health Services Administration.* 1978;23:20–35.

168. Schulz R, Greenley JR, Peterson RW. Management cost and quality in hospitals. *Medical Care.* September 1983;21:911–928.

169. Morse EV, Gordon G, Moch M. Hospital costs and quality of care: An organizational perspective. *Milbank Memorial Fund Quarterly.* 1974;52:315.

170. Scott WR, Flood AB. Costs and quality of hospital care: A review of the literature. *Medical Care Review.* Winter 1984;213–261.

171. Clinical services improved. *Human-Size Hospital Economics.* Beverly Hills, Ca: American Medical International; July/August 1982:4.

172. Ullmann SG. The impact of quality on cost in the provision of long-term care. *Inquiry* 1985;22(3):293–302

173. Clinical services improved, op. cit.

174. Ullmann, op. cit.

175. Scott, Flood, op. cit.

176. Flood AB, Ewy W, Scott WR, et al. The relationship between intensity and duration of medical services and outcomes for hospitalized patients. *Medical Care.* 1979;17:1088–1102.

177. Shortell, 1985, op. cit.

178. Miles R, Snow CC. *Organizational Strategy, Structure, and Process.* New York, NY: McGraw-Hill; 1978.

179. Hambrick DC. Environment, strategy, and power within top management teams. *Administrative Science Quarterly.* 1981;26:253–276.

180. Shortell, Morrison, Friedman, op. cit., 282.

181. Bradford DL, Cohen AR. *Managing for Excellence.* New York, NY: John Wiley & Sons; 1984.

182. Songe P. *The Fifth Discipline: The Art and Practice of the Learning Organization.* New York, NY: Free Press; 1990.

183. Argyris C. *Reasoning, Learning, and Action.* San Francisco, Ca: Jossey-Bass; 1982.

184. *Managing Hospital Marketing at AMI.* Beverly Hills, Ca: American Medical International; June 1984.

185. Landau M. On the concept of a self-correcting organization. *Public Administration Review.* 1973;33:533–542.

186. Shortell SM, Wickizer TM, Wheeler Jr JRC. *Hospital-Physician Joint Ventures: Results and Lessons from a National Demonstration in Primary Care.* Ann Arbor, Mich: Health Administration Press; 1984.

187. Peters TK, Waterman Jr RA. *In Search of Excellence.* New York, NY: Harper & Row; 1982.

188. Burns JM. *Leadership.* New York, NY: Harper & Row; 1978.

THE NATURE OF ORGANIZATIONS: FRAMEWORK FOR THE TEXT

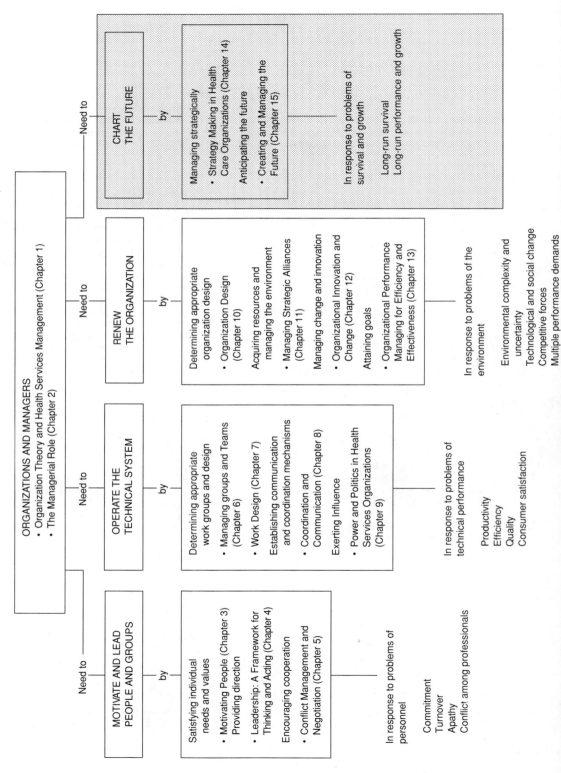

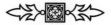

PART FIVE

CHARTING THE FUTURE

Organizations are components of a larger environment and are influenced by an unfolding series of events over time. Success of an organization depends upon its ability to chart the future given the events of time. The two chapters in this section highlight a number of future trends that will influence health care and various approaches to manage the organization given these trends.

Chapter 14, Strategy Making in Health Care Organizations, focuses on the idea of strategic management and how the principles of strategic management can increase the effectiveness of the organization in its changing environment. Specifically, the chapter addresses the following questions:

- What is strategic management, and how does it relate to competitive advantage, corporate structure, and market structure?
- What are the major structural features of markets and market structure, and how does this affect the development of a management strategy?
- What strategic models are available, and how might they be used within the health care setting?

The last chapter, Creating and Managing the Future, identifies the major trends likely to affect the delivery of health care over the next decade. Attention is given to understanding the changing role of health care providers and, specifically, the challenges facing management. Questions include:

- What larger societal forces are shaping the health care system?
- How are the changing roles of physicians, nurses, and other health professionals likely to influence the delivery of health care?
- What are the major future challenges to health care managers?

Upon completing these final two chapters, readers should be able to identify the major trends likely to affect the operations of health services organizations and the strategic approaches required to meet these challenges over the next decade.

CHAPTER

STRATEGY MAKING IN HEALTH CARE ORGANIZATIONS

Roice D. Luke, Ph.D.
Professor

James W. Begun, Ph.D.
Professor

CHAPTER TOPICS

Elements of Strategy
Strategic Management
Strategy
Strategy and Market Structure
Sources of Competitive Advantage and
    Market Structure

LEARNING OBJECTIVES

After completing this chapter, the reader should be able to

1. define the concepts of strategic management, strategy, competitive advantage, corporate strategy, and market structure
2. understand the major schools of thought in strategic management and how the relevance of each might be dependent upon the degree of turbulence in the environment
3. understand the major sources of competitive advantage, some major examples of these sources, and why they are important in the design of strategy
4. understand how multiorganizational structures can facilitate implementation of health care strategies
5. identify the major structural features of markets and be able to apply them in the analysis of health care strategies
6. identify the major sources of threat in the Porter framework and be able to use them in conducting strategic analyses
7. understand the relationship between strategy and market structure and be able to apply this understanding to the analysis of health care markets

CHAPTER PURPOSE

While at first glance the health care and grocery store industries may appear very different from one another, they do share some important market characteristics that, if properly understood, could impart valuable insights to the health care strategic analyst. They both engage in retail enterprise and provide an essential product or service to meet basic needs of the public. But perhaps more importantly, they face similar patterns of strategic threats and opportunities. Both industries have experienced significant attempts by competitors to consolidate nationally, with grocery store firms having considerably more success in this regard. At the same time, many consolidated firms within the two industries have discovered that the ponderous advantages they assumed would accompany large-scale enterprise are often offset by the more focused and carefully directed strategic moves of smaller, locally-oriented businesses. The case presented at the beginning of this chapter illustrates clearly how one small local firm (Ukrops) has competed most effectively against larger regionally (Food Lion) and nationally (Safeway) distributed rivals.

While it is not always the case that local firms win over industry goliaths, the many examples of this occurring make the investigation into the reasons why

IN THE REAL WORLD

FROM GROCERIES TO GURNIES—LEARNING FROM THE GROCERY STORE BUSINESS

Just about 50 years ago, in 1937, Joe and Ldevia Ukrop opened their first 16-foot by 32-foot grocery store. These were difficult times in the general economy, but the owners of this new store nevertheless gave high priority to customer service. They readily gave credit to shoppers and had an active delivery service. Having been successful with their special blend of quality products and personal service, the Ukrop family enlarged their small store in 1942 to 3,000 square feet, thereby becoming Richmond's first independent, full self-service grocery store. During the ensuing

20 years, the Ukrop family expanded their store still further, added new management staff, and became one of the highest volume supermarkets in the Richmond metropolitan area.

Then came a major change in the Ukrops strategy. In 1963, realizing that they had a winning formula for success, the Ukrops opened a second store. Then within the next ten years, they added three more, one of which included their first move north of the James River, an important barrier that historically had divided the core of Richmond from important suburbs to the south.

The Ukrops company now has 22 stores in the Richmond metropolitan area and has established a leadership position in the market. As a local chain, it has been able to compete with its larger regional and national competitors by sticking to the basic formula that sustained its original steady growth. Today Ukrops is broadly recognized for its high level of customer service and product quality. In recent surveys of shopper attitudes, Ukrops consistently ranked at the very top on all quality and service-oriented measures (e.g., friendliness of personnel, attractiveness of interiors, quality of meats and produce, cleanliness, convenience, selection, speed of check out service, value, orderliness of arrangements). Ukrops is also distinguished by its own particular brand of family values—it remains closed on Sundays, does not sell alcohol products or lottery tickets, offers financial incentives in support of local charities, and promotes church attendance.

But the family orientation of this local store has not caused it to be conservative in its strategic maneuvering. Ukrops has consistently led competitors in the introduction of new product and service innovations such as scanning, Valued Customer Cards (discount cards), and a wide variety of on-site prepared food and other new product lines. With its combination of customer orientation, aggressive innovation, and persistent but slow growth, Ukrops has moved from a market share 10 years ago of 25 percent to a share in 1992 of 32 percent. Clearly, Ukrops is attempting to be a dominant firm in a single market.

The achievements of Ukrops have not come easily, nor is a similar pattern of growth guaranteed in the future. With the recent downturn in the economy, low cost positions have been aggressively pursued by Ukrops' competitors, causing Ukrops to experiment with both high quality and service and low price positions. Heading the list of Ukrops' competitors is a Virginia company known as Farm Fresh, which also trades under the name of The Grocery Store. Beginning in 1958, Farm Fresh has expanded to 35 stores throughout the state of Virginia and now has a 16 percent share of the Richmond market. Farm Fresh, a publicly owned chain, has pushed for a

middle ground between high quality and service and low prices. It has also attempted to offer a wide range of products at reasonable prices. And it has stressed the advantages of geographic contiguity by opening stores only in Virginia.

In third place in market share is Food Lion, a rapid growth regional grocery store chain. Since its origins in 1957, Food Lion has experienced an almost meteoric expansion to the point that it now has over 300 stores located mostly in southern markets ranging from Pennsylvania to Texas. The company is projected to have as many as 500 stores by the end of 1995. The key to Food Lions' success has been its ability to establish low price position in most of its markets. Through a strategy of rapid growth, it has been able to capture all-important economies of scale. Food Lion claims that when it moves into an area, it will lower the prices in that area by as much as 15 percent (via price competition thereby stimulated). To do this, Food Lion has aggressively introduced management, production, and delivery strategies including computerized management of energy, labor controls, avoidance of promotional gimmicks, and use of its own fleet of trucks that are designed for fuel efficiency. It also has maintained the practice of expanding only on its geographic margins, emphasizing the need to reduce the costs of transportation and coordination. Importantly, Food Lion has recently been flailing about in search of a proper response to an unfavorable story aired by ABC's *Prime Time* about the quality of its meats and other products.

In fourth place is a major nationally-distributed company, Safeway, Inc., that has steadily lost position in the Richmond market over the past several decades. With just over 1,100 stores in the United States and Canada, Safeway has the potential to be a powerful competitor in any city in which it might be located. But in Richmond, despite its 31 stores (about the same number as the leader, Ukrops), it has fallen from a 30 percent share in 1982 (then the leading position in the market) to a 13 percent share in recent surveys. Safeway has no particularly distinctive position in the market except, perhaps, that it has a highly recognizable national identity.

In addition to a few other grocery store competitors in the area that hold relatively small market shares, Ukrops' leading position in the market is being threatened by big discount stores, especially by the recently entered discount shopping clubs that offer bulk purchases of food products at very low prices.

As Ukrops looks to the future, it will need to assess how, as a relatively small, local firm, it can maintain or even expand its current position of dominance. It will also need to consider whether its strong quality and service position and pattern of aggressively introducing market innovations will hold up under the stress of price competition, the continuing threats of major regional and national companies, and a cloudy economy.

---

a most useful strategic exercise. This is especially important in health care since the industry is now only beginning to consolidate. Powerful forces are driving many health care firms to consider joining with others in order to gain the strategic advantages of larger scale organization. But which of the many available configurations will prove the most advantageous will depend on a firm's own capabilities as well as local market conditions.

In this chapter we examine directly the concept of strategy as applied to health care organizations and the fit between a health care organization's strategy and its competitive environment. We accomplish this in four steps. First, we introduce the concept of strategic management, drawing on Mintzberg's interpretation of the major schools of thought that were prominent at the beginning of this decade. Second, having established a general frame for understanding strategy formulation and its subset, strategic analysis, we develop the concept of strategy itself. We offer our own definition of the concept and investigate some major sources of competitive advantage. Third, we consider the marketplace, the primary arena in which strategy is executed, by exploring the dimensions of market structure as well as some of the important interrelationships that exist between strategy and market structure. We apply the concepts of strategy and market structure to health care by examining them within an increasingly important competitive context, the local health care market. In this section it will become clear that health care organizations face very distinctive strategic challenges, depending upon the competitive structures they encounter in their own local markets.

ELEMENTS OF STRATEGY

Brutus   . . . What do you think
           Of marching to Philippi presently?
Cassius I do not think it good.
Brutus Your reason?
Cassius . . . 'Tis better that the enemy seek us:
           So shall he waste his means, weary his soldiers,
           Doing himself offence; whilst we, lying still,
           Are full of rest, defense, and nimbleness.
Brutus Good reasons must, of force, give place to better.

           Our legions are brim-full, our cause is ripe:
           The enemy increaseth every day;
           We, at the height, are ready to decline.
           There is a tide in the affairs of men
           Which, taken at the flood, leads on to fortune;
           Omitted, all the voyage of their life
           Is bound in shallows and in miseries.
           On such a full sea are we now afloat;
           And we must take the current when it serves
           Or lose our ventures.
Cassius Then, with your will, go on;

        William Shakespeare, *Julius Caesar*, Act IV

In this famous scene from Shakespeare's *Julius Caesar,* Brutus and Cassius debate how they should go up against the troops of Octavius Caesar and Mark Anthony that are marching upon Philippi. Cassius argued that they should maintain their well-established defensive positions, but he ultimately and mistakenly succumbed to Brutus' arguments that they "take the current when it serves" and attack.

Embedded in this fatal exchange between two conspirators in the death of Caesar are several essential elements of *strategy*. The exchange reveals not only the options of battle, the specific actions to be taken (attack now or hold off on the attack) but the reasons why those actions might prove victorious ("'Tis better that the enemy seek us: So shall he waste his means, weary his soldiers"). Just as Brutus and Cassius did before choosing from among the major options available to them, health care strategists must explore both the available options and their underlying sources of advantage and then choose courses of action they hope will bring success. Here Brutus' eloquent arguments won the day. They took the offensive, but unfortunately for their side, they lost.

Even though the eloquence or effectiveness of strategic reasoning is no guarantor of success, such reasoning nevertheless is fundamental to the making of strategy. Strategic decisions are highly important (as proved true for Brutus and Cassius) and must not be taken lightly. Any important decision calls for careful analysis and provision of the rationale for action.

The responsibility for articulating the conceptual structures and for choosing from among the alternative courses of action clearly rests with the leaders of organizations. They are the ones who not only are in the best position to see the "big picture," but they bear the primary responsibility for assuring the long-term survival of their organizations. The cognitive structures that support the formation of strategies thus flow from the insights gained by an organization's leaders as they search for answers as to how they might ensure their organization's survival in hostile environments. The soundness of those insights, though, depend greatly upon the degree to which they understand the bases upon which relative marketplace advantages can best be achieved.

Strategic management embodies many managerial elements that range from the formulation to the implementation of strategy. This chapter focuses on the formulation side, particularly on the analysis of strategy, the core concern of strategic management. Many of the elements that best fit under the heading of implementation have been covered in considerable detail in other chapters within this book. For example, Chapter 10 discusses essential concepts of organization structure; Chapter 4, the shaping of a supporting culture; and Chapter 11, the design of multiorganizational forms.

STRATEGIC MANAGEMENT

All organizations that operate within competitive environments must engage in the management of strategy. Organizations use the techniques and ideas of strategic management to mediate their struggles with rivals over the patronage of valued consumers. This can also include collaborative activities and strategic alliances (see Chapter 11). Strategic management is thus intensively external in its orientation. But at the same time, if it is to be successful, it must carefully meld competitor and market analyses with the shaping of internal structures, cultures, management systems, and essential organizational competencies.

Strategic management is also inherently militant—it deals with the tactics of winning territory and defeating enemies. As a result it is common for the roots of strategy to be traced to the maneuvers of war making, even as far back as the antiquities.[1] Quinn, for example, reached back to 338 B.C. for insights, to the stratagems of Philip and his son Alexander who attempted to free Macedonia from the influence of the Greeks and then to dominate the northern part of Greece.[2] One need not go back quite so far, however, to discover the origins of strategic thinking in the management field. While the rudiments of business strategy appeared very early in management literature, the fundamentals took root from the mid-1950s through the mid-1960s. Important early works included three books written respectively by Drucker, Chandler, and Ansoff.[3-5] Despite a tenuous military pedigree and rapidly growing business literature, strategic management is a very young field, still in considerable flux and evolution.

While not coined by them, the concept of strategic management received considerable prominence when Schendel and Hofer proclaimed it the new paradigm of business strategy: "Today, the policy field is in need of a new paradigm that can end the continual and pointless redefinition of concepts used in both practice and teaching. . . . The new paradigm we propose . . . is that of "Strategic Management," and it rests squarely on the concept of strategy."[6] Strategic management, they explained, involves those entrepreneurial processes that ultimately lead to organizational growth and renewal. Six such processes were identified in their groundbreaking work[7]

- goal formation
- environmental analysis
- strategy formulation
- strategy evaluation
- strategy implementation
- strategic control.

In the ensuing years, the number of identified processes have been expanded and contracted many times. As an example, Figure 14.1 displays one fairly detailed elaboration of strategic management processes, as published in a recent book on health care strategy.[8] But in their essence, all such formulations seek to link the external analyses of competitors and markets to the needed internal adjustments organizations must make to assure the success of decisions derived from those analyses.

By asserting that strategic management "rests squarely on the concept of strategy," Schendel and Hofer attempted to differentiate strategic from other forms of management. Strategic management is distinguished by its focus on the most critical and, quite possibly, the most challenging of decisions—organizational strategies. It has been argued, on the other hand, that the singular emphasis on strategy may be too restrictive. Leontiades, for instance, acknowledged that, while strategy may be the most consequential decision to be made, it is only one of three types of decisions that ultimately fit within the realm of strategic management[9]

- mission—what to become
- strategy—what strategy to follow
- plans—what steps to take

Thus, while we take direct aim on strategy in this chapter, it is important to recognize that this constitutes only a part, albeit a critical part, of the overall focus of the strategic management process.

Schools of Thought

The schools of thought about strategy making tend to be either prescriptive, emphasizing how strategies should be formulated, or descriptive, characterizing how strategies actually get made. Table 14.1 summarizes ten schools of thought identified by Mintzberg and fits them within these two groupings.[10] The first of three prescriptive schools, the *design school,* views strategy as the product of the conceptual and analytical efforts of chief executives. Strategy in this school flows most effectively from the full implementation of SWOT analyses—assessments of an organization's Strengths, Weaknesses, Opportunities, and Threats. Strategy is conceived as embodying explicit and simple principles that organizations use to guide them in their organizational structuring and resource allocation processes.[11–14] This school especially typifies the approach taken by many management consultants working in the field.

The *planning school,* by contrast, focuses more on the technical processes of strategy analysis. While this perspective recognizes the ultimate role played by chief executive officers (CEOs) in making decisions, it gives considerable weight to the role of planning staffs in developing the plans and supporting rationale for whatever strategies are adopted. Consequently, the executive role is more one of approving than of designing. In this school strategic planning is both formal and complex. It is a process in which detail and thoroughness become the hallmarks of successful performance. The expected end result of the rather rational, machine-like strategic planning process is a detailed blueprint for action, backed by extensive analyses of data (often financial).[15]

The *positioning school* is in one sense "the new kid on the block" and in another, the oldest school of them all. It derives its newness from Porter's enormously influential book, *Competitive Strategy,* published in 1980.[16] In this work, Porter drew upon the frameworks of industrial organization economics, which is perhaps best known for the following simple paradigm:

$$\text{Market} \rightarrow \text{Firm} \rightarrow \text{Performance}$$
$$\text{Structure} \quad \text{Conduct}$$

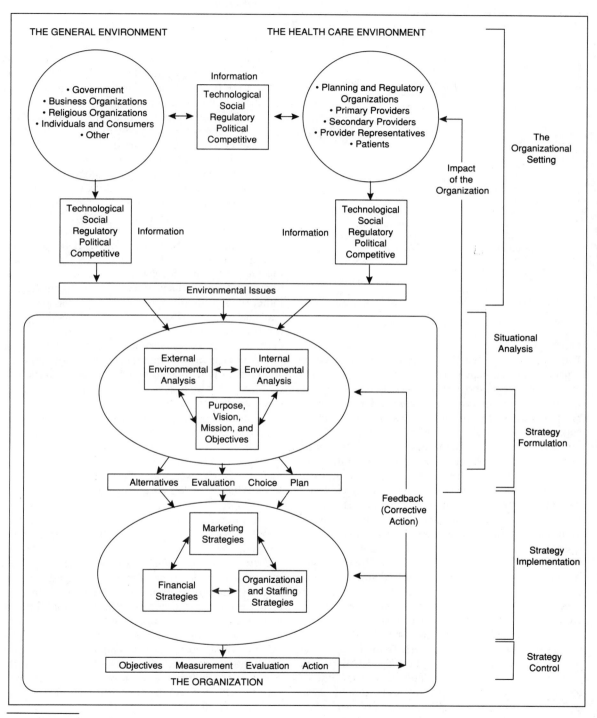

FIGURE 14.1. The strategic management process in health care organizations. SOURCE: Adapted from Duncan JW, Ginter PM, Swayne LE. *Strategic Management of Health Care Organizations.* Boston, MA: PWS-Kent Publishing Company, 1992:43.

TABLE 14.1 Mintzberg's Ten Schools
of Thought in
Strategy Formulation

School	Strategy Formulation as a
Prescriptive Schools	
Design	conceptual process
Planning	formal process
Positioning	analytical process
Descriptive Schools	
Entrepreneurial	visionary process
Cognitive	mental process
Learning	emergent process
Political	power process
Cultural	ideological process
Environmental	passive process
Configurational	episodic process

SOURCE: Adapted from Mintzberg H. "Strategy Formulation
Schools of Thought." in *Perspectives on Strategic Management*
(Fredrickson JW, ed.). New York: Harper Business, 1990:108.

The logic here is that firm conduct, which is where organizational strategy is found, is driven by the structures of markets; and performance is driven by the combined effects of *market structure* and firm conduct. The positioning school thus has links to the much older and very well established field of industrial organization economics. Through the years, the industrial organization field has placed heavy emphasis on the relationships that exist between market or industry structures and performance. Porter directly explored the relationships between unique market structures and individual firm strategies. He adapted important industrial organization concepts to the more micro, specific firm and market levels. In so doing, he provided important new insights into how strategy might be conceived and formulated within competitive contexts. Market structure concepts and relationships between strategy and the structures of health care markets are developed in later sections of this chapter.

As can be seen from Figure 14.2, the design and planning schools formed the early foundations of the field. They grew rapidly throughout the 1970s, only to see a precipitous decline in interest with the rise of the positioning school. After 1980 and the publication of Porter's book, the positioning school, according

to Mintzberg's assessment, has dominated the field. Mintzberg further predicts that the positioning school "shows the potential for making an even greater [contribution] in the next decade."[17] This chapter emphasizes and applies Porter's work to the health care field.

These three schools suggest that successful strategies can be conceived, planned, and analyzed in advance of their being implemented.[18-20] The counterargument is that organizational strategy is more the outcome of *learning* than of carefully reasoned strategic decision making.[21] Figure 14.3 presents Mintzberg's characterization of the process by which strategies evolve. So-called realized strategies, he reasoned, are the combined product of intended, deliberate, and emergent (unintended) strategies.[22,23] He suggested that the emergent strategies may be the most important as they are the products of learning and reality testing rather than of unduly optimistic conceptual, planning, and analytical processes. The design, planning, and positioning schools, he argued, create unfounded expectations that strategy can be designed in the abstract. This could rigidify commitments to intended strategies and create blind spots to new information in the face of unpredictable, highly complex, and everchanging external environments.

While we emphasize the positioning school, which Mintzberg characterized as the rising star of the current schools of thought, it is important to assess where the major perspectives fit within the arsenal of a strategic manager. First, we acknowledge that each of the schools has merit. We also recognize that the selection of an approach to develop and manage strategy will depend upon a number of factors, possibly the most important of which is the level of turbulence in the environment.

Environmental turbulence plays a very important role in determining how strategy is managed in health care organizations. Certainly, the health care environment can be characterized as having been highly turbulent, given the many changes that have been occurring in the field during the past 25 years. Also, it should be safe to assume that the uncertainties in the industry will continue well into the foreseeable future. In the next section we explore the implications of environmental turbulence on the approach one might take to strategic management.

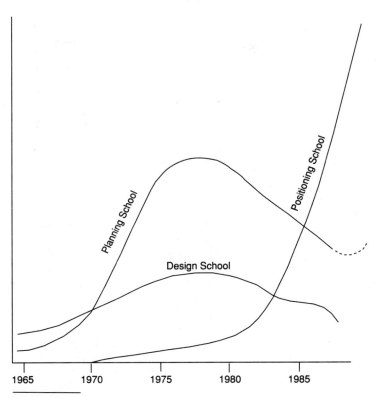

FIGURE 14.2. Evolution over time in prescriptive schools of thought in strategy formulation. SOURCE: From "Strategy Formulation Schools of Thought" by Henry Mintzberg from PERSPECTIVES ON STRATEGIC MANAGEMENT by James W. Frederickson. Copyright © 1990 by HarperBusiness. Reprinted by permission of HarperCollins Publishers Inc.

Strategy and Environmental Turbulence

It is common to conceive of two types of external environments—those that are relatively predictable and those that are fraught with turbulence.[24,25] In the more predictable environments, approaches selected for making strategy will likely be linear. They will tend to focus more on the maintenance and fine tuning of existing, successful strategies than on the remaking of strategies. In addition, they will emphasize the control of strategy in order to assure the proper functioning of the organizational subsystems that are involved in the implementation of established strategies.[26] In predictable environments, science will likely take precedence over art in strategy making. Thus, the more mechanistic approaches to strategy formulation will be the most applicable in such situations. Such was the case during the 1960s, when the health care industry experienced increased funding and growing prosperity.

By contrast, in turbulent environments—which typify the health care industry since the late 1970s—competing organizations need to rethink and possibly redirect their courses of action and corresponding allocations of scarce resources. They are challenged

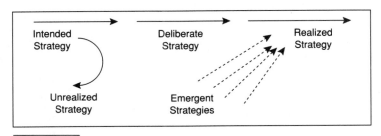

FIGURE 14.3. Mintzberg's pattern of learning in the formulation of strategy. SOURCE: Adapted from Mintzberg H. "Patterns in Strategy Formulation." *Management Science* 1978;24(9):934.

to find winning strategies in environments in which all competitors will be searching aggressively for strategic approaches to assuring their own survival. The simultaneity of search by all competitors will tend to exaggerate the level of unpredictability and threat in the environment over what otherwise might exist were conditions more tranquil. The methods of strategic planning thus may be the least useful in such situations. There simply will be few readily accessible formulae that will not have already been considered or attempted by a given organization or its competitors. Strategic planning, as a formal process for decision making, may also be too sluggish for timely responses to rapidly changing environmental conditions.

In turbulent times, the spoils of victory will likely flow to those who will have engaged either in careful analysis or, simply, are the beneficiaries of luck. It is said that Napoleon liked generals who were lucky. But because few gamblers win in the long run, thorough analyses—combined with nimbleness, innovativeness, speed, and directiveness—will be required if an organization hopes to outmaneuver tenacious competitors. To do this, the leaders of organizations will need well-honed capacities to analyze the markets in which they operate and assess the relative advantages and possible actions of major rivals. This is the domain of the positioning school.

It is important also to consider how strategy is made in turbulent environments. In such environments, creative processes take precedence, drawing heavily on the gifts of the entrepreneurial mind. Thus to the extent that strategic ideas emanate, perhaps even mystically, from entrepreneurial enterprise, attention will be di-

rected to an organization's leaders and their innate skills. Successful leaders will be those who are best able to generate innovative ideas that enlighten the road to success.

Unfortunately, the more visionary approach to strategy making is not easily acquired. Either it is in the genes or it simply must come with experience and learning. Our emphasis in this chapter is on the latter—on the need to be capable of applying analytical skills that enhance one's understanding of the workings of markets. The trick is for leaders to be capable of seeing beyond the complexities, that is, to be able to grasp the subtle interrelationships that exist between strategy and environmental conditions, to be able to assess the distinctive competencies of rivals, and to be aware of emerging trends in the marketplace. Such skills are essential for good strategists, especially for those who must lead large, complex organizations in highly competitive environments—which, after all, is the challenge facing most health care leaders.

What do we learn from this? We learn that one very important ingredient of strategic leadership in turbulent times is a willingness to change and modify organizational strategy when careful analysis suggests that such may be necessary. We also learn that the information required for decision making may not be extractable from the standard planning mechanisms but will be the derivative of thoughtful analyses conducted by top executives. The tools necessary to conduct these analyses fall directly within the domain of the positioning school. It should also be noted that the design school of thought essentially stretches across all schools as it emphasizes the steps to be taken in the management of strategy, steps which apply to all schools of thought.

In sum, assuming that significant environmental turbulence exists in the health care industry and should continue for the foreseeable future, it follows that the making of strategy in health care will involve more art than science. It should also involve somewhat less formality and be based more on ideas, conceptualizations, visions, and other nonlinear patterns of strategic thinking than on the products of formal analytic processes. The formal processes, as encompassed in strategic planning methodologies however, will have their place even under such conditions. In particular, they will be useful for confirming strategic decisions and assisting in the control of strategies once implemented. But they will have only limited utility in generating new ideas or repositioning organizations that face highly unstable environmental conditions. For this, the leaders of organizations must be well equipped to engage personally in strategic analyses of their own markets and competitors.

STRATEGY

Strategy means different things to different people.[27] Porter's definition perhaps captures the prevailing viewpoint best. His definition—". . . positioning a business to maximize the value of the capabilities that distinguish it from its competitors"—draws attention to what is increasingly becoming the central focus of strategy, to achieve *competitive advantage.*[28-31] Two important points can be taken from Porter's definition. First, competitive advantage is a relative concept, that is, advantage has meaning only by comparison to the advantages of rivals. Ulysses S. Grant is quoted as having said in 1860 that "strategy [is] the deployment of one's resources in a manner which is most likely to defeat the enemy."[32] Strategy and, correspondingly, competitive advantage has little meaning if it is not juxtaposed against the strategies and advantages of competitors. Second, competitive advantage has important, identifiable sources which need to be understood. Porter defines competitive advantage specifically in terms of positioning: "At the heart of positioning is *competitive advantage.*"[33] By positioning, he means creating goods and services whose characteristics are more highly valued than are those of competitors. As is discussed

below, we suggest that Porter focuses too narrowly on positioning per se, though he is correct in emphasizing the need to identify major sources of competitive advantage as the key to formulating and defining strategy.

Others have conceptualized competitive advantage in terms of its outcomes, most commonly as being equivalent to achieving a desirable financial performance or higher than expected profits.[34] Again, all such approaches beg the question of what competitive advantage actually is. We define competitive advantage in terms of market power, which varies directly with a competitor's ability to resist threats from buyers and sellers and to take market actions without fear of reprisal. It is to gain and sustain more market power than is enjoyed by competitors that ultimately is the objective of a market-oriented strategy. As is discussed later, cooperation and collaboration strategies may be part of such pursuit. Positioning, Porter's concept of strategy, is directly focused on building market power. Firms that are successful in differentiating their products, diminish the effect of competitors and thereby increase their own power in the market place. This and other sources of competitive advantage discussed below, if successfully pursued, help build an organization's power in the market and thereby contribute to the achievement of competitive advantage.

Having argued that the essence of strategy is achieving competitive advantage, we offer our own definition of strategy: Strategy is an integrating set of ideas and concepts that guide an organization in its attempts to achieve competitive advantage over rivals. Consistent with Porter, we suggest that the object of strategy is to achieve competitive advantage over rivals. Importantly, the definition recognizes that strategy is conceptual and not a plan, policy, or specific intended investment. It is an expression of those highly proprietary concepts and ideas that an organization hopes will help it achieve advantage. In the following two sections, we discuss strategy as an integrating set of concepts and ideas and then explore some major sources of competitive advantage.

Strategy as an Integrating Set of Concepts and Ideas

In addition to its most obvious purpose of achieving competitive advantage, strategy, properly formulated, should provide the central rallying point around which an organization's members can unite to assure that the organization survives and thrives over the long term. To achieve its potential as a unifying force, any strategy should have at its core a foundation of logic that expresses how the organization hopes to achieve advantage in its markets. In a way, this is what Brutus provided in his debate with Cassius over military strategy. The core of his argument was that their troops were ripe and at their peak. To delay the attack would have invited a decline from their current state of readiness and placed them in a relatively weak position vis-a-vis the enemy. Their readiness and the timing of attack constituted the core of Brutus' strategic reasoning. Once accepted, this core framed the specifics, the strategic choices, and presumedly marshaled the resources of the troops so that they were able to mount an imminent attack.

The foundation of logic is what Ansoff referred to as the "common thread," that set of concepts that integrates the activities of a business.[35] This common thread, he explained, provides the rationale for many strategic considerations including determining in which products and markets a firm should invest, the patterns by which it will grow (i.e., into new product or market areas or stick to existing areas), how it distinguishes itself from its competitors, and how multiple business activities might be combined so as to maximize synergies among them.

The foundation of logic is also what Schendel and Hofer called the *key idea,* or the idea that provides the fundamental rationale for how a firm will develop and ultimately survive.

> Any successful business begins with a "key idea". . . The "key idea," that product of the entrepreneurial mind, is the central concept . . . Without it, there is no business . . . and it is a good strategy that insures the formulation, renewal, and survival of the total enterprise that in turn leads to an integration of the functional areas of the business and not the other way around . . .[36]

In some organizations, it may be sufficient for the key idea to remain in the head of the entrepreneur or leader of an organization. But if other members of the organization are to draw together in the pursuit of the strategy, the leader must share with them, in clear and convincing terms, the essential ideas and concepts that underlie the unique approach the organization will take to achieve competitive advantage.

On the other hand, given the highly entrepreneurial nature of strategies, it may be necessary for the leaders of organizations to keep confidential the core of their ideas and to reveal them in varying degrees depending upon who the audience might be. Hax has pointed out that even top management and boards of directors may not be privy to the inner-most concepts and ideas being considered by the leaders of organizations.[37] The expression of strategy serves many purposes, not the least of which is to provide guideposts for the achievement of competitive advantage. But which guideposts are emphasized, again, will depend upon the audience. Expressions of strategy by hospital CEOs to boards of directors, for example, may stress financial over tactical issues. Or a CEO concerned with possible reactions of physicians may promote motivational objectives more than share critical market assessments of rivals. Certainly, strategy as expressed in an annual report might provide a general sense of where an organization is going. But it also will likely emphasize positive performance expectations and obscure the more proprietary considerations inherent in strategy.

Once embraced by an organization's members, a key idea can take on an almost evangelical aura, replete with all the symbolism of inspired thought. In their book on leadership, Kouzes and Posner, discussed the almost visionary role of strategic ideas.

> Every organization . . . begins with a dream. The dream or vision is the force that invents the future.
>
> Leaders spend considerable effort gazing across the horizon of time, imagining what it will be like when they have arrived at their final destinations. Some call it vision; others describe it as a purpose, mission, goal, even personal agenda. Regardless of what we call it, there is a desire to make something happen, to change the way things are, to create something that no one else has ever created before.[38]

As they point out, there are many terms—purpose, dream, mission, agenda—that embody the vision or key idea of an organization. But in its essence, the key idea provides both the frame for decision making and a basis for inspiring coordinated action.

Sources of Competitive Advantage

Having defined strategy as those ideas and concepts that guide an organization in its attempts to achieve competitive advantage over rivals, we now explore some of the more common sources of competitive advantage. In his discussion of strategy, Quinn reviewed what he called "the most basic principles of strategy" or the "key concepts and thrusts" of strategy. Drawing on classic writings from about 300 B.C., Quinn illustrated some of these basic principles.[39]

- establishment of dominance
- joining a coalition
- avoiding overwhelming superiority
- emphasis on distinct advantages
- deceptive maneuvers
- surprise attack
- assessment of relative strengths
- mobility
- command of key positions
- concentration of forces
- overwhelming power

He then translated these military-like phrases into a selected list of principles for business strategy

- clear, decisive objectives
- maintaining the initiative
- concentration
- conceding selected positions
- flexibility
- coordinated and committed leadership
- surprise
- security
- communications

In effect, Quinn attempted to identify sources of competitive advantage, as could be derived from military literature. Unfortunately, his list mixed administrative tactics (clear, decisive objectives; communications) with what might be fundamental strategic principles (flexibility, surprise, concentration).

The strategy literature is replete with fundamental principles that comprise the essential sources of competitive advantage. We suggest, however, that these can be clustered into three groups, each differentiated by the primary underlying logic required for attaining advantage. For ease of remembering the three, we label each with a word beginning with a *P*. The three Ps of strategy or the three primary sources of competitive advantage are

- power: competitive advantage gained through the accumulation and effective combination of mass
- pace: competitive advantage gained through managing the timing and intensity of actions
- position: competitive advantage gained by achieving distinctive value in the minds of consumers

All organizations draw upon each of these sources of advantage, however effectively or consciously they may be employed. One or two may be emphasized over the others. For example, an organization may pursue large organizational scale (power) so that it can project a low cost image in the minds of consumers (position). But all sources of advantage are embodied in any organization's competitive strategy. In the following, we consider each in greater detail, but in reverse order from how they are listed above.

Position

Strategies that derive their advantage from the achievement of distinctive value in the marketplace are labeled *position strategies*. According to Porter, distinctive value can be achieved by pursuing one or more of the following three positions, Porter's "generic" strategies[40]

- low cost
- high differentiation
- distinctive niche

It has long been recognized that the achievement of a *low cost position* relative to rivals makes it possible for organizations to price their goods and services such that the market shares of rivals can be eroded and potential entrants into markets deterred. Less than optimal cost positions can also be maintained, but only if an organization is able to protect its position by producing goods and services that consumers perceive to have distinctive value or by limiting its markets to specific niches where competition might be somewhat less intense. Organizations are able to achieve low cost positions in many ways, including capturing the advantages of economies of scale and learning or introducing tight managerial controls and lean operating systems. In the 1970s and 1980s, the desire to achieve low cost positions led many hospitals to join multihospital systems (a power strategy). It is unclear, however, whether that tactic proved successful in helping participating hospitals actually achieve low cost positions or whether it merely made it possible for them to ensure survival or higher profits.[41,42] This point is developed further in the discussion of power as a source of competitive advantage.

Positions of *high differentiation* are achieved by modifying the characteristics (quality, service support, technological sophistication, etc.) of goods and services for the purpose of projecting distinctive value to consumers. Differentiation opportunities can be found throughout most organizations. This is especially true in health care and many other service industries where consumption and production are often performed simultaneously.[43] The simultaneity of production and consumption means that consumers come into contact with organizations at many points and levels. Differentiation is therefore far more than a matter of product design; it is a matter of designing the very character of the organization itself. Kaiser Health Plan, the large health maintenance organization (HMO) company headquartered in Oakland, California, has learned this important lesson. Having enjoyed a low cost position in the health insurance market for decades, Kaiser recently adopted a strategy designed to improve its overall quality image. To do this, in 1991 they initiated a major program of total quality improvement, which they labeled "A Quest for Quality" (see the discussion of Kaiser in Chapter 1). Leaders in the Kaiser system were very aware of the simultaneity of production and consumption and the need, therefore, to focus quality concerns at many levels within their delivery organizations. A recognition of the relationship between consumption and production may, in general, account for the ground swell of interest within health care in total quality improvement concepts and approaches.

Ultimately, whether or not the pursuit of quality or any other approach to position strategy will produce competitive advantage should depend on the determinants of market structure. This is a very timely point, given the tremendous interest that is currently being paid to quality in almost all industries, including health care. The thoughtful strategy analyst will recognize, of course, that industries and markets vary significantly from one another and thus that the relative value of pursuing position versus pace versus power strategies vary as well. The reader can address this issue in Debate Time 14.1.

Niching positions are achieved by selecting distinctive segments in the market and orienting one's appeal uniquely to them. That appeal can draw upon one or both of the other two approaches to achieving distinctive positions—low cost and high differentiation. Specialty, public, teaching, and many other types of hospitals offer good examples of where niching has produced relatively safe strategic positions. Such strategies have often proven highly successful in health care where a great diversity of products, services, and client preferences have long existed. Despite the complexity and high levels of specialization required of those who would occupy such niches, they have become increasingly vulnerable to attack in the increasingly competitive environment of the past decade. Major teaching centers, for example, have learned that many of their specialty niches are now subject to successful assault by other, often smaller and far less technologically advanced hospitals that choose selectively to enter their markets.

Niching has traditionally been a favored strategy of small competitors that face larger, often dominating rivals.[44] Increasingly, this has also been true for small or simply unaffiliated hospitals that reside in markets where large local hospital systems have evolved. Lacking the size necessary to go head-to-head with large local competitors, they find safe havens focusing on specialized products and services (e.g., rehabilitation care) or narrow consumer groups (e.g., rural or suburban populations).

Pace

Porter's "generic strategies," of course, emphasize only one of several key sources of competitive advan-

DEBATE TIME 14.1: WHAT DO YOU THINK?

In the last several years, a considerable interest has been devoted to upgrading quality in organizations at all levels. Variously labeled as total quality management and continuous quality improvement, this new managerial approach to improving the internal workings, quality, and productivity of organizations is also considered by many to be a major tool for strengthening strategic positions in markets. Put simply, the view holds that, by imbuing an organization's members with a powerful commitment to continuous quality improvement, efficiency will advance, the quality of goods and services sold to the public will improve, morale among employees will be enhanced, and the consuming public will become more satisfied, thereby increasing overall demand and the prospects for the organization's survival.

Alternatively, there are those who would argue that in most markets the issue is not how best to appeal to a wary consuming public but how best to defeat a determined competitor bent on improving its position at its competitors' expense. This latter approach argues that organizations should assume a competitive stance and be ever ready to engage in nihilistic battles against competitors in order to achieve positions of dominance in their markets.

Behind such orientations are a number of issues. One has to do with determining the strategies that might be most effectively applied under various market structural conditions. Another has to do with values. On the one hand, there is the perspective that health care is not like other industries, that it is imbued with a delicate admixture of *public and private interests,* and therefore that overt competitive battling does harm to the consuming public as well as to those who might engage in such actions. An alternative perspective holds that the only way for a firm to be really strong in the long term is to steel itself in the heat of competitive battle, that competition is the best way in the long run to improve quality, and that giving excessive attention to quality improvement and cultural enhancements wastes vital organizational energies that might better be spent on winning the competitive war.

Which orientation to strategy fits best within the health care field in the 1990s? Which will prevail in the long run?

---

tage. Another critical source is grounded in the timing and intensity of strategic action. It was a question of timing that Cassius and Brutus debated. Clearly that old cliche that "timing is everything" has great application in the arena of strategy.

Miles and Snow's now well-recognized typology provides one of the best conceptualizations of strategy as a matter of timing and intensity of action.[45] They suggested that organizations can be classified by how aggressively they respond to environmental uncertainty or competitor threat. They grouped the particular response patterns into four orientations, each differentiated by the degree to which an organization is willing to incur risk or assume aggressive postures in their pursuit of market opportunities.

- *Prospectors* are organizations that frequently search for new market opportunities and regularly engage in experimentation and innovation. They are, as a result, not often the most efficient competitors.
- *Analyzers* are organizations that maintain stable operations in some areas, usually their core product or business, but also search for new opportunities and engage in market innovations. Characteristically they watch competitors and rapidly adopt those strategic ideas that appear to have the greatest potential.
- *Defenders* are organizations that engage in little search for additional opportunities for growth and seldom make adjustments in existing technologies, structures, or strategies. They devote primary attention to improving the efficiencies of existing operations.
- *Reactors* are organizations that perceive opportunities and turbulence but are not able to

adapt effectively. They lack consistent approaches to strategy and structure and make changes primarily in response to environmental pressures.

These patterns characterize not only approaches to strategy but also orientations that are often deeply embedded within an organization's culture and strategic history. In health care, recent evidence suggests that hospitals that are more prospector-like in their strategic orientations are better performers in regard to profitability and market share, particularly when compared to those with a defender orientation.[46] Evidence also exists that many hospitals do change their strategies when faced with strong environmental pressures.[47] However, Shortell et al. assert that these changes are more likely to result in improved performance when they are made within the organization's "strategic *comfort zones*"—that is, they are not too dissimilar in terms of accustomed patterns of action. As represented in Figure 14.4, organizations may choose to modify their strategic orientations, but only by adopting new orientations that are marginally different from the old ones in terms of aggressiveness or willingness to accept risk. Should defender organizations, therefore, wish to become more aggressive in the market-

place, they would be expected to shift to the analyzer rather than all the way to the prospector orientation. The reverse would be true for prospector organizations. Analyzers, since they are found in the middle of the continuum, would be expected to move to any of the other orientations. Reactors, since they characteristically flip flop from one position to another, could also be expected to move to any of the other orientations, with perhaps a slightly greater likelihood of shifting to the more rational, analyzer position. While there was no short-run support for the comfort zone concept in the study of hospitals, it has been supported in a study of major tobacco firms.[48,49] The concept is important because it reminds managers of the need to balance external environmental pressures for change against the organization's existing culture and internal capabilities to implement the change.

Other useful strategic concepts that fall under the heading of pace include management of surprise, signaling of strategic actions, managing momentum, as well as a variety of strategies associated with deterring entry and initiating countermoves in response to the strategic actions taken or threatened by competitors, potential entrants, and recent entrants.[50–54] Surprise has often been the key to successful military as well

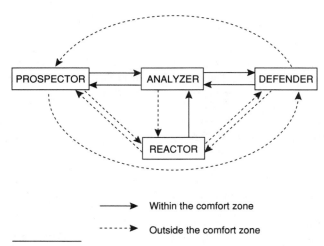

→ Within the comfort zone

---→ Outside the comfort zone

FIGURE 14.4. Strategic comfort zones for shifting pace strategy orientations. SOURCE: Adapted from Shortell SM, Morrison EM, Friedman B. *Strategic Choices for America's Hospitals.* San Francisco: Jossey-Bass Publishers, 1990:37.

as business strategies. Unexpected attacks catch rivals unprepared, thus producing critical advantages for the initiators of surprise that would not otherwise be possible were their moves telegraphed ahead of time. It is vital in the management of surprise that organizations have a clear understanding of the landscape of competition. In particular, they need to be aware of competitor capabilities, difficulties or possibilities of entry, and the broader trends in the market. Vulnerability to surprise is especially acute for competitors engaged in niching, market segmentation, and other position strategies. While the advantages inherent in position strategies are clear, competitors focusing narrowly on their own business areas often become vulnerable to surprise attacks from without. Specialty hospitals, for instance, risk becoming so myopic about and centered on their specific areas of activity that they do not recognize moves on the part of general hospitals to offer substitute products or compete directly with them.

There is also, of course, a place for announcing strategic actions well in advance. A competitor just beginning to invest heavily in a particular strategic move could choose to make an early announcement of its plans in order to scare away potential rivals. A hospital could announce plans to build a satellite hospital in a suburb, for example, thus signaling to rivals that they should look elsewhere to find opportunities for market expansion. A competitor, however, could also use such announcements to detract attention away from other moves that are being initiated in secret or simply to cause competitors to react unnecessarily to feigned strategic action.

Power

Perhaps the most important source of competitive advantage, and the one that receives the greatest attention in the strategy literature, is the amount of raw power an organization is able to amass in the competitive arena. Relative mass was the source of advantage that the Philistines assumed was on their side when they sent Goliath to challenge the armies of Israel:

> And there went out a champion out of the camp of the Philistines, named Goliath . . . whose height was six cubits and a span. And he had an helmet of brass upon his head, and he was armed with a coat of mail; and the weight of the coat was five thousand shekels of brass. And he had greaves of brass upon his legs, and a

target of brass between his shoulders. And the staff of his spear was like a weaver's beam; and his spear's head weighed six hundred shekels of iron; and one bearing a shield went before him.
> —1 Samuel 16:4–7

The story of David and Goliath illustrates all three of the major sources of competitive advantage: strength on the part of Goliath (power strategy) and quickness and accuracy on the part of David (pace and position strategies, respectively). It also shows how effectively timed moves, even well-positioned ones, might be used to overcome the advantages of sheer strength. By moving early and positioning a smooth stone in the center of Goliath's head, David was able to defeat a competitor who otherwise must have appeared rather invincible. But it is easy to imagine how, if the stone had not hit its mark, the outcome might have been very different. Goliath mistakenly assumed that his source of advantage, his might, was sufficient for him to win no matter what other sources of advantage could be brought against him.

Might has been at the very core of many military and business strategies. General Motors used it to great advantage for years, of course, before the Japanese countered by adopting a superior positioning strategy of building fuel efficient, high quality, and very reliable automobiles. The battle between IBM and Macintosh similarly has been based largely on might versus pace (innovativeness) versus positioning (product quality and niching). The pursuit of competitive advantage by power is perhaps best represented in the health care field by the steady increases since the 1970s in the numbers of hospitals that have become members of multihospital systems, purchased contracts for management services, joined hospital consortia, or expanded into a great variety of health care and health insurance businesses.

Power strategies derive their advantages from one or both of the following sources: economies that come from *size,* whether formed from scale or scope expansions and economies that come from the *synergies* that accrue when business units are combined into larger organizational entities. Table 14.2 lists some of the more common strategies that involve the amassing of resources to gain advantage and highlights the types of synergies that are the focus of each. To differing degrees and in divergent ways each of the strategies listed in Table 14.2 draws upon the advantages of size

TABLE 14.2. Major Power Strategy Options

Strategy	Definition	Example
Horizontal expansion	Expansion in the scale of existing business activities	The merger of two or more hospitals
Horizontal integration	The pursuit of synergies among different types of businesses (other than among those that are vertically related); could include business combinations that are either	
	related (have in common similar technologies, markets, or product functions)	The combination of hospital and nursing home businesses and centralizing many management functions for both organizations
	or	
	unrelated (have in common few or no similarities in technological, market, or product functions)	The combination of hospital and furniture store businesses and sharing marketing and information system capacities
Vertical integration	The pursuit of synergies among different types of businesses that share input-output relationships with each other along the production chain	The combination of hospital and insurance companies to produce HMO products
Portfolio	The pursuit of financial synergies among different types of businesses, regardless of whether related or not	The combination of hospital and furniture store businesses either to diversify investments or to facilitate excess cash flows to be drawn from one to support growth in the other

and synergy. The logics that support *vertical* and *horizontal integration,* for example, are identical, with the exception that the former takes advantage of synergistic potential among different stages of the production process while the latter emphasizes synergies across the same stage of the process. *Horizontal expansion* is also similar to these, except that synergies are achieved by combining units that share the same production logics. It is here where the highly important economies of scale and learning are the most prominent. In *portfolio* strategies, any types of businesses, however related or unrelated they may be, are combined primarily to take advantage of financial interdependencies. Such strategies include the spreading of risk across businesses and the restructuring of financial flows from established businesses to those that have great potential for growth but may be lacking the funding needed to support that growth. Health care examples of each of these important approaches to building power are also provided in Table 14.2.

Which of the four power strategies—horizontal integration, vertical integration, horizontal expansion, and portfolio—is being pursued at any given point in time cannot easily be determined merely by examining the particular businesses in which an organization has

invested. The joining of nursing home and hospital businesses, for example, could involve horizontal integration, vertical integration, or portfolio strategies, depending on how advantages are being pursued among the combined businesses. While it is common in the health care field to characterize such strategies as vertical, few in practice involve much coordination in production flows (the hallmark of vertical integration) or even the pursuit of synergies across the business units (the essence of horizontal integration). One reason for this is that the costs of pursuing coordination or synergies are often substantial (e.g., costs of coordinated decision making, communications, and overcoming interorganizational resistances), and as a result, such multibusiness combinations often amount to little other than mere investment (portfolio) strategies.[55] Likewise, the advantages of horizontal expansion may not always be realized, even in instances where the rationale for coordination may be very great. To date, few of the local hospital systems that have been forming in and around metropolitan areas across the country have been successful in capturing the numerous advantages that so clearly are the potential of these combinations.[56–58] The transformation of synergies into meaningful strategic advantage thus represents a major managerial challenge, especially in the health care field where there are so many highly institutionalized autonomies and organizational complexities that serve as significant barriers to interorganizational coordination (see Chapter 11).

Absolute Versus Relative Power. It is important to note that power as derived from size can be expressed in either absolute or relative terms. The building of *absolute power* focuses directly on economies of scale, learning, and scope. Further, large organizations simply are capable of directing more economic strength to any given competitive skirmish than are small organizations. It is possible, however, for smaller organizations to capture some of the advantages attributable to absolute power by pursuing high market shares within specific markets, which is the essence of *relative power*. For instance, a small firm that has captured a substantial share of a local market can often compete effectively with rivals, regardless of the level of absolute power to which those rivals may have access (i.e., from their parent companies).

There are many examples within the health care field of firms that possess high relative but low absolute power and that compete very effectively against firms that have low relative but high absolute power. In the early 1980s, many nonprofit hospitals joined hospital consortia in the hopes of duplicating the advantages available to hospitals that were members of large, multihospital systems. But what both types of hospitals did not fully appreciate at the time was that these advantages could be countered quite easily by the building of dominating positions in local markets. The advantages of relative power were, perhaps, best recognized by nonprofit hospitals, which more frequently have formed into local multihospital clusters in local markets than have hospitals in other ownership categories.[59] By consolidating and thereby capturing significant market shares locally, they have been able to muster significant market power, thus enabling them to compete aggressively against competitors backed by absolutely large parent companies.

The contrast between the advantages of relative and absolute power is illustrated by the hospital market on the Virginia side of the Washington, D.C., metropolitan area. INOVA, a four-hospital, nonprofit system that was formed at the initiative of Fairfax Hospital, competes directly and forcibly with HCA Reston Hospital Center,

which is owned by the multibillion dollar (in annual revenues) Hospital Corporation of America (HCA). Reston with its 135 beds has only one percent of the local market compared to an 11 percent share for INOVA, which has a combined total of over 1,100 beds in the D.C. market. Because of its relatively greater local share, the INOVA system dominates the market—at least, on the Virginia side of the D.C. area—and the Reston Hospital plays a more niched role. The use of relative power, of course, is not restricted to nonprofit systems. Many of the large systems of all ownership types are now combining the advantages of both relative and absolute power in many markets.

Hybrid Organizations and Power Strategies. Organizational structure can often play a major role in facilitating the amassing of strategically important resources. This is especially true in the health care field where there reside numerous determined sources of resistance to interorganizational consolidation. Many hospitals, physicians, and other health care organizations and providers who have traditionally enjoyed high levels of autonomy are reluctant to give up prized independencies in exchange for gains in strategic power. A new organizational form—the *hybrid organization*—has become the method of choice in health care and many other fields for combining multiple organizations without having to resort to formal ownership changes in those organizations.[60] Using a wide variety of contractual and other interorganizational linking mechanisms, many health care organizations and providers have formed into loosely coupled or hybrid organizational forms.

The primary rationale for the hybrid organization is that it preserves long-held autonomies. Possibly the most significant strategic advantage is that contractual arrangements can be both arranged and undone with relative ease, by contrast to what might be involved were it necessary for ownership changes to be made. This is especially valuable in an environment of rapid change, where there is great potential for strategic errors to be made. Rapid entry or exit can be facilitated by the relative ease with which complex organizations can be created by contract. A number of commercial insurance companies, for example, have used contractual mechanisms to create highly competitive managed-care products with which they have been able to enter rapidly selected local markets. Kaiser

Health Plan, by contrast, has been very slow to enter new markets since their model requires more formal structures than would be possible with the looser, contractual arrangements. In just the last few years, the terms networks and managed collaboration have come into vogue as characterizations of the new hybrid organizational forms being created in the health care field.

The advantages of the hybrid forms, however, may be offset by a number of critical strategic disadvantages.[61] Since hybrid organizations involve loose forms of coupling between cooperating organizations, they will typically lack two organizational features critical to effective strategic performance: a decisive and powerful strategic head and strong interorganizational linkages and integrative mechanisms.[62] Because the combined organizations generally retain intact their own decision-making structures, the collective will generally not be sufficiently empowered to make difficult and controversial strategic decisions. As a result, hybrids are prone to react slowly to environmental change or competitive threat. Also, lacking strong and well-developed interorganizational linkages, hybrids may not be able to achieve valued synergies or to realize sufficiently the promise inherent in the increased organizational scale. Possibly, the best illustration of how loose linkages among otherwise independent organizations lead to slow and ineffective responses are found in the performance records of the United Nations or the Organization of Petroleum Exporting Countries (OPEC).

Hierarchy in Strategy. Since many power strategies involve combinations of businesses or business units rather than merely expansions of existing businesses, they fall within the domain of corporate strategy. It is important to note the differences between corporate, business unit, and other levels of strategy.

In many ways, strategies are prisms. What one sees in them will vary dramatically by the angle from which they are perceived. Perceptions of strategy will differ significantly by the level within an organization at which strategy is considered. There are at least four levels at which strategies can be viewed in most organizations: enterprise, corporate, business, and functional.[63] The first, enterprise strategy, deals with the social-legitimacy concerns of an organization—that is, with the approaches organizations take to deal with threats that emanate from their broader, nonmarket

environments. When expressed as a response to environmental threat, this form of strategy has been labeled "domain defense."[64] Faced by significant threats from government and other sources within their external environments, tobacco firms have during the last half century been forced to invest considerable resources in efforts to preserve the legitimacy of their products—a defense or enterprise strategy. Similarly, though perhaps to a lesser degree, for-profit hospitals have had to defend against charges that they are more concerned with profits than patients and nonprofit hospitals have had to justify why they still should be granted nonprofit tax status, given the significant excess revenues they are able to generate. In the future many health care providers may face significant enterprise strategy concerns if, in the successful pursuit of competitive (corporate or business) strategies, they fail to take proper consideration of how their hard-earned market power might or might not translate into measurable public good. We return to this vital point in the concluding section of this chapter.

Corporate and business-level strategies both deal with the efforts of organizations to achieve competitive advantage within markets. In his early work, Ansoff suggested that corporate strategy deals with the question, What business(es) should we be in and business strategy with, How should a firm compete in a given business?[65] Corporate strategy is now recognized as dealing with far more than deciding in what businesses to invest. It extends beyond the strategies of single markets, industries, or businesses, where individual business strategies are formed. Corporate strategy becomes important once the interplay between an organization's business activities is so complex that real advantages can be gained from the effective coordination of those activities. In effect, corporate strategy might best be defined as involving those concepts and ideas that guide an organization in its efforts to achieve competitive advantage through multibusiness combinations. Business-unit strategy, by contrast, focuses on the achievement of competitive advantage for a single business activity. Finally, functional-area strategies address the ways in which subunits within an organization individually and collectively assist in achieving the objectives of the three other levels of strategy (enterprise, corporate, and business unit).

Of the four, enterprise strategy has historically been the most important for health care organizations. Efforts to lobby governmental entities for the purpose of maintaining control over either or both technical and economic domains of health care delivery are tactics driven by enterprise-level strategies. Corporate strategy, by contrast, has lately become a critical concern since health care organizations have in recent decades engaged on a broad scale in multibusiness activities. The pursuit of corporate strategy has become a major challenge for health care executives, especially because it concerns bringing together a complex array of organizations and professional groups that have historically been highly protective of established autonomies. Certainly, with the continuing and steady movement toward consolidation, health care executives more than ever must have a clear understanding of the essentials of multibusiness activity, especially the distinctive challenges involved in deriving advantages from the integration of those activities. This in turn leads to greater attention being paid to business- and functional-level strategies.

STRATEGY AND MARKET STRUCTURE

The structure, conduct, and performance paradigm suggests that the performance of firms depends upon the organization of "economically significant features" of markets—market structure—and "the acts, practices, and politics pursued by firms in markets as they strive for profits"—firm conduct.[66–70] Second, it recognizes the direct effect of market structure on conduct and, in particular, the effects of specific market structural factors on the strategic behaviors of individual firms.[71] This is very important for the strategic management field, as it brings the wealth of insights accumulated in the industrial organization literature directly into the strategy arena.

We point out that the analysis of market structure applies most directly to the analysis of business rather than corporate strategy. Market structure analyses focus directly on the interplay of all major actors within a single market context. This also is relevant to corporate strategy since a major portion of corporate strategy analysis involves assessing the strategic positions of individual business units.

The following sections highlight the dimensions of market structure and apply *Porter's framework* to the analysis of strategy in health care markets.

Dimensions of Market Structure

The market features of greatest interest include[72]

- the degree of seller concentration, described by the number and size distribution of sellers in the market
- the degree of buyer concentration, defined in parallel fashion
- the degree of product differentiation among the various sellers in the market or, the extent to which their outputs (though similar) are viewed as imperfect substitutes by buyers
- the condition of entry to the market, referring to the relative ease or difficulty with which new sellers may enter the market, as determined generally by the advantages that established sellers have over potential entrants.

Each of these features reflects degrees to which market actors possess and are able to exercise market power. Individual sellers in the highly concentrated markets are assumed to have far greater market power than those that operate within more fragmented markets. As a result, any economic action competitors in the more concentrated markets may take (e.g., raising prices) will likely have major impacts on rivals, causing the latter to react and engage in countermaneuvers. By contrast, since sellers in less concentrated markets are numerous and relatively small in size, their strategic actions are not expected to produce strong reactions among rivals. Accordingly, sellers in these markets can be expected to concentrate their strategies directly on consumers, giving only limited attention to the actions or possible reactions of competitors. This distinction between the actions and reactions of sellers according to the degree to which their markets are concentrated has important implications for strategy. In large measure, the sources of threat determine on which of the major sources of competitive advantage an organization should concentrate.

It is important to emphasize that some *dimensions of market structure* appear to have direct parallels in the sources of competitive advantage discussed earlier. This is not coincidental. Recall that the objective of strategy is to achieve competitive advantage or to gain market power. If, for example, an organization is successful in the pursuit of product differentiation, it will also have been successful in increasing its market power. By definition, product differentiation increases distinctiveness, reduces real competitors, and thereby increases the market power of effectively differentiated firms. Likewise, a market that is characterized structurally as having high levels of product differentiation will be made up of competitors that have few direct competitors and, again, would be one in which the competitors collectively possess relatively high levels of market power.

Markets vary dramatically from one another by various structural dimensions, even within the same industry. Thus it would be useful to have in hand a classification of markets based upon the major structural dimensions in order to improve the ability to analyze the strategic implications of structure variations. In one such classification, Bain focused exclusively on three of the above four dimensions that specifically captured characteristics of the sellers themselves (i.e., he dropped the buyer concentration dimension).[73] In developing his classification scheme, Bain divided the first and perhaps most important dimension—the degree of seller concentration—into the following three subcategories

1. atomistic: many small sellers (low level of interaction to one another)
2. oligopolistic: few large sellers (high level of interaction to one another)
3. monopolistic: single seller

The second dimension emphasized by Bain was the presence of product differentiation. He used two categories to represent this dimension

A. with homogeneous products: products nearly identical
B. with product differentiation: products differentiated by design, quality branding, etc.

The third dimension, ease of market entry, Bain divided into three levels

a. easy entry: no barrier to entry
b. moderately difficult entry: appreciably high, but not high enough to permit sellers to act like monopolists
c. blockaded entry: barriers high enough to permit monopoly pricing without attracting additional entry

Using the degree of seller concentration as the primary organizing characteristic, he was able to identify nine general market types. These are summarized in Table 14.3. It is recognized, of course, that within and between each of these, the actual structural characteristics of markets will vary widely.

While examples of all nine market types can be found in the health care field, those involving undifferentiated products are the least likely to be observed. This is because virtually all health care markets involve considerable degrees of product differentiation. Competitors in hospital markets, for example, differ by their complexity, specialization, ownership (e.g., church-operated, for-profit, nonprofit), teaching status, quality reputation, physician affiliations, and, location (e.g., rural, suburban, urban, spatial isolation vs. clustering).

TABLE 14.3. Bain's Market Typology, Based upon Three Major Dimensions of Market Structure: Seller Concentration, Product Differentiation, and Conditions of Entry

Market Structure Dimensions	Type
1. Atomistic	
A. Without product differentiation	1-A
B. With product differentiation	1-B
2. Oligopolistic	
A. Without product differentiation	
a. With easy entry	2-A-a
b. With moderately difficult entry	2-A-b
c. With blockaded entry	2-A-c
B. With product differentiation	
a. With easy entry	2-B-a
b. With moderately difficult entry	2-B-b
c. With blockaded entry	2-B-c
3. Monopolized	3

SOURCE: Adapted from Bain, JS, Qualls PD. *Industrial Organization: A Treatise*, Part A. Greenwich, CN: JAI Press, 1987:23–24.

Location is perhaps the most important characteristic for differentiating hospitals.[74] Nursing home, physician, and other markets draw upon similar bases for achieving product differentiation.

In addition to the above commonly stressed features of market structure, there are others that also are likely to play major roles in shaping strategic behaviors in markets. Of special importance to the health care field is the rate of growth in the market, which is often expressed using the well-known stages of market or product life cycle.[75] Usually four stages are identified, including introduction, growth, maturity, and decline. The important point is that the effects of the above market structural features will be moderated by the stage or rate of growth in the market. This point will be illustrated in the discussion to follow.

Porter Framework

Of the many "sources of competitive pressure" that exist within any given market, Porter identified five that he argued must be understood by strategic analysts.[76] The five, exhibited in Figure 14.5, include threats from competitors, potential entrants, buyers, substitutes, and suppliers. While all five are important in analyses of health care markets, their effects vary widely across the great variety of markets that exist within the industry.

The Competitors

Porter identified a number of factors that will directly impact the intensity of rivalry within a market, including all that are identified above in the Bain classification scheme. We selectively discuss these in regard to health care markets.

Market Concentration. The degree of concentration within a market refers to the proportion of market power held by the leading firms. As already discussed, the more concentrated a market, the more power individual competitors will be able to wield in attacks against their rivals. A number of concentration ratios are commonly used to measure the degree of concentration in a market.[77] Two of the most popular are the *four-firm ratio* and the so-called Herfindahl-Hirschman Index (HHI). The former is simply the sum of market shares controlled by the top four firms in a market, and the latter is measured as follows

$$\text{HHI} = \sum_{i}^{N} S_i^2$$

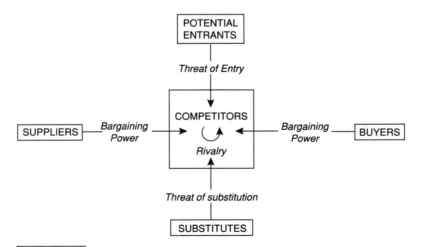

FIGURE 14.5. Porter's framework of five forces that affect the level of rivalry in a market. Reprinted with the permission of the Free Press, a Division of Macmillan, Inc. from COMPETITIVE STRATEGY: Techniques for Analyzing Industries and Competitors by Michael E. Porter. Copyright © 1980 by the Free Press.

where, S_i^2 equals the share for the ith competitor squared.

By squaring each competitor's shares (percentages of the market), the shares of the larger firms are more heavily weighted. This has the advantage of emphasizing the strength of the most powerful firms in a market, thus giving a good indicator of a disproportionate distribution of power.

Regardless of which measure is used, it is critical that they be applied at the proper geographic level—national, regional, or local. For some industries, especially service and retail markets, concentration is best measured at the local level. This is primarily because transportation costs in such markets limit market exchanges among buyers and sellers within proximate geographic space. This is also true in health care markets, with the possible exception of tertiary care markets which often reach well beyond local boundaries. Applying the four-firm ratio to the analysis of hospital markets, we illustrate the effect of market level on measured concentration. If computed at the national level, the top four hospital firms would be shown to control somewhere in the range of six to eight percent of the total national market. Measurement at this level clearly would lead to the mistaken conclusion that the hospital market is very fragmented. Were it calculated at the local level, on the other hand, a very different picture would emerge.

Table 14.4 summarizes the mean four-firm ratios within four population-size groups for each of the metropolitan statistical areas (MSAs) in the U.S. In this illustration, a firm would be a combination of hospitals if they were under the same ownership or a single hospital if it had no local partners. As can be seen in the table, average ratios for the top four firms in the two smaller population-size categories ($<$ 250,000 and 250,000–499,999) exceed 90 percent. And the average for the largest markets ($>$ 999,999), in which there is a mean of 45 hospital firms per market, is just under 50 percent. Table 14.4 also presents the mean number of firms per market, which provides a direct indicator of why the concentration scores are so high. In the smaller population group, in which nearly half (49 percent) of the MSAs are found, the average market has just under three hospital firms. And in the three smallest population size categories, which constitutes about 86 percent of the MSAs, the average ranges from 2.8 to 9.2 firms per market.

What does all of this mean? It means that, if hospital concentration is measured at the local level, the level at which patterns of exchange between buyers and sellers generally occur, hospital markets will be seen to be highly concentrated. This shows that, in most markets, individual hospital firms exercise considerable power. When considered in the context of their other sources of market power—for example, product differentiation—hospitals can thus be seen to be increasingly capable of resisting the *threats* not only *of rivals* but of other economic actors, especially including the increasingly powerful health insurance companies.

A serious complication inherent in the application of concentration at the local level is that concentration varies inversely with the total number of competitors in an area, which itself varies directly with an area's population. Thus comparisons across areas that have different population levels usually will amount to little more than an analysis of population variation rather than of concentration per se. The key is thus to examine relative concentration, that is, to compare concentration levels across similarly-sized local markets, as is done in a subsequent section.

Gradation in Market Shares. This second structural feature is very important for the analysis of oligopolistically-structured markets. Distributions in market shares, with competitors arrayed from highest to lowest, could take on a number of very distinctive shapes, some of which could have important strategic implications. Two of the more noteworthy patterns are presented in Figure 14.6.[78] Continuing with the hospital example, the first pattern would be characterized by

TABLE 14.4. Average Four-Firm Ratios by Market (MSA) Size Categories

MSA Size	Number of MSAs	Average Four-Firm Ratio	Average Number of Firms
1. <250,000	156	99%	2.77
2. 250,000-499,999	69	90%	5.43
3. 500,000-999,999	50	74%	9.20
4. >999,999	45	48%	27.02

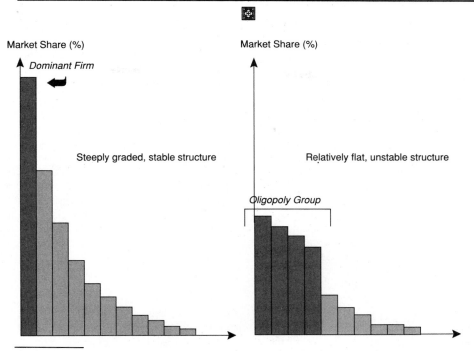

FIGURE 14.6. Market structure patterns differentiated by gradients in market shares. Shares are calculated as the percent of beds in the market. SOURCE: Adapted from Shepherd WG. *The Economics of Industrial Organization.* New York: Prentice Hall, 1979:199.

a large, dominating hospital or hospital firm (which could include either a single hospital or a combination of two or more hospitals that are members of the same company and located in the same market) and a steeply descending distribution of market shares among the remaining hospitals or hospital firms. The second pattern typically would be headed by what has been called an oligopoly group or, in the hospital case, by a small group of dominating hospital firms whose shares differ little from one another.

Ironically, the first of the two patterns may be the more stable of the two since it has a clearly established pecking order among competitors. Such a clear ordering of market power will tend to reduce the prospects that any one rival will significantly threaten any other. The second, flatter pattern should be somewhat less stable than the first. The relative equality in power existing within the oligopoly group can be expected to invite group members to vie with one another for

positions of dominance—that is, to determine which of the peers will ultimately be crowned "king of the hill." Positions of dominance could be achieved in a number of ways, the most dramatic of which would be for one rival to merge with one or two others, thereby rapidly adding to its market share. Were this to occur, the structure would evolve toward the first pattern, producing reductions in competitive tensions and overt rivalry. Notably, the smaller members with much lower market shares in both patterns, given their relative inability to exercise power, can be expected to strategically seek safe positions or niches where they hope to be free from the threats of the other, larger competitors. And dominant firms in the steeply graded pattern will likely assume the role of enforcers, pressing for discipline among competitors, especially in the volatile area of price competition.

In those markets in which few hospital combinations have occurred to date, the *gradation of shares* will be flat, reflecting primarily simple differences in hospital bed capacities. But in those areas where mergers have occurred or multiple acquisitions by a single hospital company have been accomplished, the pattern will likely appear as the dominant firm model. Examples of both patterns will be presented in the last section of this chapter.

Slow Industry Growth. Slowed industry growth is often a characteristic of a sluggish economy, a maturing market, or both. Whatever the cause, the effect is often the same—intensified competition for market share. One common result is that competitors will emphasize position strategies, especially low cost positions, in direct attempts to maintain or even widen shares. But in a market in which there is great potential for *consolidation* to take place—which is true for many health care markets—emphasis will often be on power strategies. These include efforts to build shares through mergers, acquisitions, pursuit of vertical integration, portfolio diversification, and the creation of complex hybrid organizations. Clearly, power strategies have been a major and very effective strategic response taken by many U.S. hospitals in reaction to a slowed economy and a maturing acute care industry. The payoff for overcoming fragmentation can be very significant if there exists sufficient economic basis for pursuing consolidation (e.g., there is a potential for achieving economies of scale, raising *entry barriers,* or creating a stronger base to pursue vertical linkages with managed care firms). But where these conditions do not exist, the pursuit of consolidation could prove to be a significant strategic trap.

Presence of Switching Costs. Another factor influencing rivalry is the presence of *switching costs* (the costs inherent in switching from one seller to another). If there are few switching costs, the potential for buyers to shift among sellers will increase the intensity of rivalry and overall instability in the market. The costs of switching, on the other hand, can be significant and, as a consequence, serve to stabilize buyer-seller relationships and dampen competitive pressures. Switching costs are very significant at many points within the health care industry and, therefore, may play a major role in diminishing rivalry among health care competitors. For example, because referral relationships among physicians, between physicians and hospitals, or among hospitals are difficult to create, involve

important elements of trust, are critical components in increasingly integrated delivery systems, and often require complex information system arrangements to manage them, once established they will often evolve into semi-permanent arrangements. Similarly, arrangements between health care providers and insurance companies, especially in a world of expanding managed care systems, can entail significant switching costs. Therefore, they too can engender rather permanent interorganizational relationships. Possibly for this reason alone, current efforts on the part of insurance carriers to create networks of hospitals and physicians will, after an initial period of jockeying for position and price negotiations, resolve into almost unalterable structures, thereby significantly reducing competitive pressures within those markets.[79]

Diverse Competitors. Porter argued that "competitors diverse in strategies, origins, personalities, relationships to their parent companies . . . have a hard time reading each other's intentions accurately and agreeing on a set of 'rules of the game' for the industry."[80] As a result, they may more frequently make wrong strategic choices than would be the case in an environment involving less diversity. Continuing the hospital example, it could be argued that congruencies in goals between any two hospitals (e.g., of the same ownership type—both nonchurch, nonprofit hospitals) could do much to facilitate cooperation among them.[81] Conversely, consistent with Porter, a lack of goal congruency could stimulate rivalry. On the other hand, if linked to differentiation strategies, diversity could serve to reduce competitive tensions. Consider, for example, the great variation in ownership types and products that exists within the health insurance industry (e.g., the Blues, commercial insurers, large HMO companies, and hospital-based HMOs). Similar differences in ownership and function exist in the hospital and other sectors of the health care industry. To the extent that these translate into product differentiation, rivalry among the firms could be less than what might otherwise be expected in this highly diverse industry.

High Exit Barriers. Markets with high *exit barriers* retain some competitors that otherwise might be driven out by competition. When such remain, excess capacity in the market is not eliminated and competitive pressures are increased. There is good reason to believe that exit barriers in some health care sectors may indeed be very high. Despite the closure of some hospitals over the past 10 to 15 years, excess capacities appear resistant to economic downturns in many U.S. metropolitan areas. There are a number of economic, social, emotional, and other reasons why a hospital might not exit from a market. Despite poor or negative returns or even poor quality, many hospitals play such crucial roles in serving particular populations (e.g., inner-city poor, suburban, religious or special ethnic groups) that resistance to their closure could be very substantial. The barriers to exit, on the other hand, might not be quite so high for the nursing home sector. Thus the exiting of weaker competitors could serve to dampen competitive pressures in that sector.

The Buyers

The most significant threats facing most health care organizations may well issue from the buyer side. For over a decade, health insurance companies have been intensely engaged in their own strategic maneuvers in response to powerful challenges from their own buyers, the primary effect of which has been to increase competitive pressures upstream on providers and, ultimately, on health care suppliers. The threat coming from health insurance companies will vary, however, depending on the degree to which providers are dependent upon the financing they provide. Dentists still are little dependent upon insurance companies. Their patients perform essential buyer functions, and the powerful insurance companies play a secondary third-party role. The degree to which providers are dependent upon individual buyers, however, is only one of several factors Porter suggested that determine the strength of *buyer threats*. We summarize some of these here.

Seller Dependency. If a substantial percentage of a seller's goods or services are purchased by a single buyer, that buyer will obviously be in a position to exercise substantial leverage over the seller. This indeed is a calculation many insurance companies have been making in their attempts to build preferred provider organizations (PPOs) and provider networks, especially with hospitals. To date, most hospitals have been able to diversify provider contracts, but the trend is clearly toward more and more exclusive contracting.

As a result, hospitals will need not only to manage more purposefully their relationships with insurance companies but also to pursue strategies that will neutralize the effect of the power amassed by their buyers. Certainly, horizontal expansion in the local market (i.e., the formation of local hospital systems) is one strategy that would provide hospitals with a kind of countervailing power to balance the growing potency of insurance companies.

Buyer Threat of Backward Integration. In the health care field, few health insurance companies as yet pose a very credible threat of full backward integration. But threats of at least partial or quasi integration—as represented by the increasing role being played by managed care arrangements and network formations—are real. Again, health care provider organizations will need to pursue a variety of strategies, including horizontal expansion in local markets, to ward off this growing threat. One important countermove, of course, would be to threaten forward integration, as illustrated by providers—mostly hospitals—creating their own HMOs.

Market Information Controlled by Buyers. To the degree that buyers have good access to strategically important information about the businesses of their sellers, they will be able to exercise leverage in their negotiations with those sellers. This is a very important consideration in the relationship between health insurance companies and health care providers and, in similar ways, between hospitals and physicians. With the continuing expansion and growing sophistication of managed care systems, insurance companies are increasingly able to obtain unusual amounts of information about the demand structures, prices, and production capabilities of their buyers. When viewed in light of the growing dependencies many providers have on individual insurance companies, this factor takes on an even greater strategic significance.

The Entrants

Entrant threats involve elements of surprise, true and false signaling of strategic moves, predatory pricing, and other hostile behaviors on the part of incumbent competitors. But, as noted by Porter, the most common sources of barriers to entry include economies of scale, product differentiation, capital requirements, switching costs, access to distribution channels, and other cost advantages independent of scale. In addition to these, barriers can be created artificially (e.g., by government regulation such as, certificate of need in health care). These are all important in health care markets, but to varying degrees. Certainly, the barriers to entry are very substantial in local hospital markets. By contrast, the barriers limiting entry into the markets for services of physicians, dentists, and other health professionals are relatively low (as are the exit barriers). On the other hand, the need to establish referral relationships, to gain privileges, or to obtain licensure and other barriers all inhibit entry of professional workers into health professional markets and participation in vital informal referral structures.

The Substitutes

Substitute products or services are those that serve the same function as existing services or products within an industry. One prominent health care example of situations where substitutes create significant competitive pressures is found in the competition that takes place among health professional groups.[82] New, emerging health professional groups have occasionally vied with established professions for turf. But recently, with the powerful combination of demands for cost containment, rising power of buyer groups, growing technological sophistication (especially with the advance of computers and other information processing technologies), and, generally heightened competitive pressures in the health care field, significant opportunities for substitution have emerged. Hospitals appear the most vulnerable to rising *threats from substitute products and services*. The movement toward the unbundling of hospital services, including the spin off of such vital services as ambulatory surgery and high-tech diagnostic procedures, is an example of substitution-creating activity. Interestingly, hospitals, given their considerable financial and human resource capabilities, have been able to exercise considerable control over this process. In many cases, they themselves have been able to finance and run many of the substitute activities as new businesses. But the era of substitution in health care is still ahead of us. With the continuing

and, even heightening, need to reduce costs and to eliminate waste and redundancies, opportunities to offer substitute products and services will certainly increase, thereby increasing still further the overall level of competitive threat within the health care industry.

The Suppliers

Seller threats are the inverse of those that emanate from buyers. They primarily take the form either of threats of forward integration or the exercise of economic power in the exchange between sellers and buyers. For most health care providers, threats of integration from buyers are relatively remote. Few suppliers offer credible threats of forward integration, though they do have significant capacity to negotiate effectively over prices and other product characteristics. One prominent example of suppliers that have achieved significant economic power over providers is found in the case of the pharmaceutical industry versus the pharmacy profession. The pharmaceutical industry not only exerts considerable control over prices at the retail level but has, through its control over research and development, diminished the pharmacy profession's technical functions, limiting it essentially to the performance of more mundane distributive activities.

The relationship between pharmacists and the pharmaceutical industry, however, may provide a hint of future threats that could come from the supply side. With the explosion of technology coming on the heels of critical developments in computing, lasers, genetic engineering, and the like, many suppliers could find themselves in a position of altering the relative power positions not only of selected health professionals but of other key actors that are identified in the Porter model. For one, the increasing potential of supplier-controlled innovations could threaten the positions of academic health care institutions, the traditional citadels of technological innovation and experimentation. Rapid technological innovation, particularly coming from sources outside provider sectors, could also increase the threats of substitute products. This would especially be true if the innovations make it possible for the otherwise indeterminate technologies controlled by the professions to be transformed into more technical and systematized products. On the other hand, some provider groups could benefit from the transfers of control over evolving health care technologies. Hospital pharmacists, for example, are among those most likely to benefit from the evolution of computerized drug utilization and control systems. This could over time, however, significantly alter the roles of physicians, nurses, and pharmacists in the area of drug therapy within hospitals.

SOURCES OF COMPETITIVE ADVANTAGE AND MARKET STRUCTURE

The general relationships expected between strategy and structure are summarized in Table 14.5. Since sellers in the *atomistically-structured markets* pose little threat to one another, it is suggested in the table that their strategies will more likely focus on position rather than pace or power strategies. One exception to this, however, needs to be mentioned. Some atomistically-structured markets have within them the economic fundamentals essential for successful consolidation. This might be the case, for instance, in markets that historically have not experienced sufficient competitive pressure to provoke the pursuit of power strategies. Were such markets then to experience increased turbulence, competitors within them might be driven to find ways to consolidate those markets. Ambulatory care offers a good example of a market in which this might be a possibility. Heightened competitive threats from hospitals, insurance companies, and other sources have caused some ambulatory firms to pursue growth strategies, and there has been a steady move

TABLE 14.5. The Importance of the Three Sources of Competitive Advantage in each of the Three Market Types Differentiated by Degree of Seller Concentration

	Power	Pace	Position
Atomistic	L	M	H
Oligopolistic	H	M	L
Monopoly	L	L	L

toward the group practice mode of medical delivery. While to date, these and other trends have reduced the overall fragmentation in the market, there remains much potential for the ambulatory care market to consolidate still further. Whether and how this will happen will depend on a variety of factors, not the least of which will be the reaction of the medical community to the growing power of hospitals in the local health care markets.

The primary challenge facing competitors in *oligopolistically-structured markets* is to improve their positions of dominance relative to threatening rivals. As indicated in Table 14.5, therefore, they can be expected to pursue any number of power strategies with somewhat greater vigor than might be the case in the other two structural forms. But as with the atomistically-structured markets, the degree to which this may be true will vary by a number of other factors. As has already been discussed, such markets vary importantly by the steepness of the gradient in market shares. In the flatter gradient structures in which there might exist a fairly balanced oligopoly group, the expectations expressed in Table 14.5 would apply. The leading competitors, perhaps all of them, could be expected to seek ways in which to gain dominance through the pursuit of power strategies. On the other hand, in situations in which the gradient is far steeper and one firm occupies an unassailably dominant position, several different patterns of strategic response can be expected. First, the dominant firm, content with its relative market power, may adopt rather passive, shares-maintaining strategies, perhaps focused more on position strategies than power or pace. The smaller, fringe firms, on the other hand, themselves possibly accepting the existing divisions of power, could be expected to act in a manner more consistent with an atomistically-structured market. Not feeling threatened by the relatively passive dominant firm, they could give somewhat more priority to position strategies, especially those involving product differentiation or niching.

Such differences in gradients are common in U.S. hospital markets. Figure 14.7 contrasts two very different patterns within two similarly-sized metropolitan areas: Salt Lake City, Utah, and Rochester, New York. The Salt Lake pattern, a steeply-graded oligopolistic structure, represents the consolidation

MANAGERIAL GUIDELINES

1. Develop a clear understanding of the concepts of and interrelationships among strategy, competitive advantage, and market structure. Strategy is not the mere selection of business opportunities that might have the best financials. Rather, it is a collection of concepts, ideas, and interrelationships that should assist leaders of organizations to better visualize and give meaning to their complex and often very threatening external environments. The vagaries and indirections of market competition can only be understood if interpreted within the context of a valid and workable framework. Such a framework is provided by the positioning school of thought within the strategic formulation field. In the framework, such concepts as strategy, competitive advantage, and market structure can be woven into a powerful set of strategic tools. In particular, Porter's structural framework provides a simple checkoff of major market forces and the interplay among them that should prove useful for those involved in strategic analysis.

2. Develop a clear understanding of the important relationship between organizational structure, implementation capabilities, and strategy. While discussed only briefly in this chapter, a strategic analyst will ultimately be confronted with the challenge of creating an organizational structure and implementation capabilities that will facilitate and sustain the objectives of intended strategies. This is especially important for complex organizations in which strategy often leads to the combination of multiple business units to achieve identified strategic ends. And it may be even more important for a health care field that is becoming ever more integrated and elaborate. With the many interorganizational relationships that will need to be managed in the modern health care firm, new structures and approaches to implementation may well become the linch pin of a successful strategy. It will likely be of little value, for example, to visualize the strategic power of a regionalized health system if there is no way to bring physicians, partnering hospitals, and other health care providers into a unified whole. Structure and implementation skills thus could be the keys to unlocking the full potential of well-conceived strategic ideas in the health care field.

3. Grasp the close linkage between strategic objectives and the public interest in health care. Strategy may well be the equivalent of an ill-shapen suit when fitted onto health care organizations. While health care organizations

strategies of two medium-sized hospital companies: Intermountain Health Care (IHC), a 23-hospital nonprofit firm headquartered in Salt Lake City, and Holy Cross Health System Corporation, a nationally-distributed 16-hospital Catholic system headquartered in South Bend, Indiana. By combining four hospitals in the Salt Lake City metropolitan area, IHC has achieved a dominating position totaling approximately 1,200 beds and a nearly 43 percent market share. Holy Cross maintains a strong second position with its three urban hospitals, which combine almost 500 beds and have a 20 percent share. Of IHCs total of 23 hospitals, 19 are located within the state of Utah and two each are in the states of Idaho and Wyoming. In addition to their four hospitals in the Salt Lake City metropolitan area, IHC owns five more hospitals that are located within 60 miles of the flagship hospital in Salt Lake City, three of which are in the very nearby Provo market (IHC has an approximately 80 percent market share in that city) and two are in proximate rural areas. Thus, IHC not only enjoys a dominant position in and around Salt Lake City but an even more dominating position throughout the state. By contrast, the Rochester, New York hospital market is very flat and much more fragmented. No hospital clusters have been created in the Rochester metropolitan area. Therefore, the 14 Roches-

MANAGERIAL GUIDELINES

pursue their individual strategies, they will often be confronted by the question, But does this serve the community interest? For example, while power strategies may prove very effective in assuring survival in highly competitive and oligopolistically-structured hospital markets, they may not necessarily add to an objective of maximizing competition. A low cost strategy may not prove to be in the best interest of patients whose lives hang in the balance of critical resource allocation decisions. Or an aggressive expansion in health care business lines could simply add to the duplication of an already too costly health care system.

Strategy need not, however, be in conflict with the public good. The pursuit of a power strategy in a local market, for instance, could lead to the integration of otherwise fragmented and highly duplicative health care delivery units, as reflected in the American Hospital Association's and the Catholic Hospital Association's proposals to create integrated health delivery units as the key features of a reformed health care system.[83,84] Health care providers operate in a unique environment in which there will inevitably exist a tenuous balance between public and private interests. Health care strategists,

therefore, must not carry out their roles with a blind eye to how their decisions will impact the cost, quality, and access of care available to local populations. And for this, collaborative rather than competitive strategies will often offer better prospects for serving local community needs.

4. As a final precautionary note, we would point out that once commitments are made to particular strategic courses of action, one risks becoming deeply immersed in strategic implementation and control at the expense of engaging in ongoing strategic analyses and reconsiderations of those courses. Strategic analysis should indeed be dynamic. Thinking while doing and doing while thinking should be the hallmark of effective strategy making.

It should now be clear that neither the prescription of Cassius—" 'Tis better that the enemy seek us: So shall he waste his means, weary his soldiers"—nor that of Brutus—"we must take the current when it serves"—will necessarily apply to any one situation. The diversity of circumstances is very great and the possible responses, countless in their number and variations. It is the challenge of the successful strategic analyst to bring coherence and meaning out of the chaos of inexorably changing and often turbulent external environments.

ter firms are made up of 14 hospitals, which compares with the six firms that comprise the 11 hospitals in the Salt Lake area.

The considerable implications such differences might have for the pursuit of strategy should be clear. We point out that in addition to the two clusters holding first and second place positions in the Salt Lake City market, there is a university hospital, four for-profit hospitals (one each belonging to HCA and Humana and two owned by Health Trust), and several federal government hospitals (not shown in the distributions). Such diversity in ownership, as it inhibits further inter-organizational collaboration or combinations, likely

contributes to the rigidity of the overall structure of the Salt Lake City market. All of these factors, when considered together, suggest that the Salt Lake City market is fairly well-established and unlikely to be modified were any hospital company to aggressively pursue a power strategy. Therefore, the prediction that firms in such markets can be expected to concentrate on the margin by stressing position strategies should hold. In the Rochester market, on the other hand, there remains great potential for a power strategy to alter the structure of the market. Not only is there a very flat and relatively fragmented structure, but all but one (a Catholic hospital) of the 14 hospitals in that market

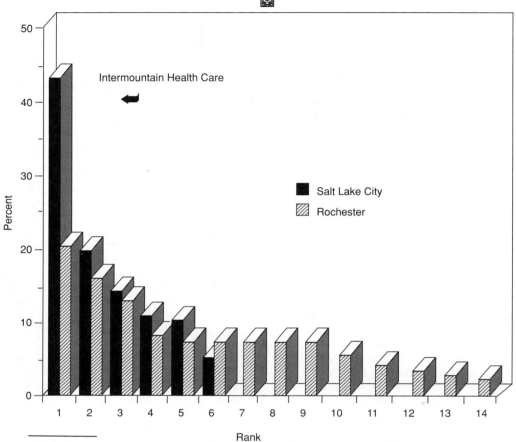

FIGURE 14.7. Hospital firm market shares for Salt Lake City, Utah, and Rochester, New York. Firms constitute either single hospitals or the combination of those hospitals that are owned, managed, or sponsored by the same multihospital company (e.g., the Intermountain Health Care firm combines a total of five hospitals). Shares are calculated for each as the percent of beds in the market.

are nonprofit. There exists a relatively high degree of goal congruency among the competitors, and the potential for some combinations to occur in this market is therefore very great.

Since by definition monopolists have no active rivals, they can be expected to place somewhat less emphasis on any particular sources of competitive advantage, as indicated in Table 14.6. Having achieved the ultimate in power strategies, complete dominance, strategic maneuvering may play a relatively minor role in determining their ultimate survival. On the other hand, despite having positions that may appear to be

free of competitors, many monopolists actually face rather serious competitive threats from one or more of four of the sources of threat identified by Porter. (By definition, they face no threats from direct rivals.) Monopolists can be threatened by the countervailing moves of powerful buyers or suppliers or by the challenges of substitutes or potential entrants. The Hill Rom Corporation headquartered in Evanston, Indiana, offers a good example of a firm that enjoys a near monopoly position but is still very aggressive strategically. Hill Rom dominates the general medical-surgical bed and patient room support system businesses. Their market shares in these areas are in the 95 percent range. They do have one major competitor, Stryker, which is headquartered in Kalamazoo, Michigan. In contrast to Hill Rom, Stryker has concentrated its efforts in a variety of niches in and around the acute care bed business. In some markets such as orthopedic beds, Stryker has even captured over 60 percent market share. Hill Rom is very aware that their own overwhelming market share is vulnerable to attack. Technological change in the industry, for example, could alter the formulas currently determining how beds, furniture, and wall patient-support systems are combined in patient rooms. Future advances in computer and other medically-related technologies could easily make it possible for competitors to enter the market thereby eroding Hill Rom's powerful market position.

The upshot is that Hill Rom, despite enjoying near-monopoly positions in its markets, has developed a highly sophisticated capacity to conduct strategic analyses. They regularly monitor trends in new technologies and medical applications, assess consumer attitudes and preferences, and measure the advantages of existing and prospective rivals. They also provide a good example of a firm that, despite an overwhelming power position, recognizes the need to pursue an aggressive pace strategy. In sum, we would characterize Hill Rom, a near monopolist, as an analyzer, perhaps even a prospector at times, that attempts to preserve its strong absolute and relative power positions by pursuing aggressively a highly consumer- and quality-oriented position strategy. It illustrates as well the critical interplay and interdependence between power, pace, and position approaches to strategy.

KEY CONCEPTS

Absolute vs. Relative Power
Analyzers
Atomistically-Structured Markets
Buyer Threats
Comfort Zones
Competitive Advantage
Consolidation
Defenders
Dimensions of Market Structure
Diverse Competitors
Entrant Threats
Entry Barriers
Environmental Turbulence
Exit Barriers
Four-Firm Ratio
Gradation of Shares
High Differentiation
Horizontal Expansion
Horizontal Integration
Hybrid Organization
Key Idea
Learning

Low Cost
Major Schools of Thought in Strategic Management:
  Design, Planning, Position
Market Structure
Monopolists
Niching
Oligopolistically-Structured Markets
Pace Strategies
Porter's Framework
Portfolio
Position Strategies
Power Strategies
Prospectors
Public and Private Interests
Reactors
Rival Threats
Seller Threats
Size vs. Synergy
Strategic Management
Strategy
Switching Costs
Threats from Substitution
Vertical Integration

DISCUSSION QUESTIONS

1. The Ukrops grocery store company (see the introductory case) has asked you to consult regarding what it should do to maintain and, hopefully, expand its share in the Richmond, Virginia market. Review its current strategy using the concepts developed in this chapter, analyze similarly the strategies of its competitors, and recommend what strategic actions it should take to achieve its objectives. Be sure to explain all of the major points in your analysis, especially your recommendations for the future.

2. Select two metropolitan areas in your region and, using the most recent issue of the *AHA Guide to the Health Care Field,* identify the hospitals that reside there; the systems that own them, if any; and their market shares (using the ratio of their total beds to the total in the market). Be sure to determine what suburban areas and counties are also included within those metropolitan areas so that all competing hospitals are identified. Using this information, develop an analysis of the structure of the hospital markets in those areas and a prediction of what strategies might most likely be followed by each hospital located in those areas. Defend your analyses.

3. Redo Table 14.5 by replacing the existing structural forms with the following

   Atomistic: no possibility for consolidation
   Atomistic: possibility for consolidation
   Oligopolistic: steep gradient in shares
   Oligopolistic: flat gradient in shares
   Monopolistic

   Using the same three sources of competitive advantage as are listed there, indicate for each of the resulting 15 cells, the relative importance of the sources of competitive advantage. Again, defend your analysis.

4. Select a major health care system or hospital in your area and a major merger or acquisition target (hospital or other type of health care organization) in or around the area. Using the insights gained in the preceding chapters, identify three major categories of actors within each organization that might have a strong interest in and could have a powerful effect on the success of the proposed interorganizational combination. Once identified, assess their likely responses to the proposal and suggest managerial actions that should be taken by the leaders of the system initiating the change to assure the cooperation of each of the identified categories of actors.

REFERENCES

1. Bracker J. The historical development of the strategic management concept. *Academy of Management Review.* 1980;5(2):219–224.
2. Quinn JB. Strategies for change. In: Quinn JB, Mintzberg H, James RM, eds. *The Strategy Process: Concepts, Contexts and Cases,* Englewood Cliffs, NJ: Prentice-Hall; 1988:2–9.
3. Ansoff HI. *Corporate Strategy: An Analytic Approach to Business Policy for Growth and Expansion.* New York, NY: McGraw-Hill; 1965.
4. Chandler Jr AD. *Strategy and Structure: Chapters in the History of The Industrial Enterprise.* Cambridge, Mass: MIT Press; 1962.
5. Drucker PF. *The Practice of Management.* New York, NY: Harper & Brothers; 1954.
6. Schendel D, Hofer C. *Strategic Management: A New View of Business and Policy and Planning.* Boston: Little, Brown, and Co.; 1979:2.
7. Ibid, 14.
8. Duncan WJ, Ginter PM, Swayne LE. *Strategic Management of Health Care Organizations.* Boston, Mass: PWS-Kent Publishing Co.; 1992.
9. Leontiades M. The confusing words of business policy. *Academy of Management Review.* January 1982;7(1):48.
10. Mintzberg HI. Strategy formation schools of thought. In: Fredrickson JW, ed. *Perspectives on Strategic Management.* New York, NY: Harper Business; 1990:105–236.
11. Andrews KR. *The Concept of Corporate Strategy.* 3rd ed. Homewood, Ill: Richard D. Irwin, Inc.; 1987.
12. Ansoff HI. *Corporate Strategy: An Analytic Approach to Business Policy for Growth and Expansion.* New York, NY: McGraw-Hill; 1965.
13. Christensen CR, Andrews KR, Bower JL, Hamermesh RG, Porter ME. *Business Policy: Text and Cases.* 6th ed. Homewood, Ill: Richard D. Irwin, Inc.; 1987.
14. Selznick P. *Leadership in Administration: A Sociological Interpretation.* New York, NY: Harper & Row; 1957.
15. Steiner GA. *Strategic Planning: What Every Manager Should Know.* New York, NY: Free Press; 1979.
16. Porter ME. *Competitive Strategy: Techniques for Analyzing Industries and Competitors.* New York, NY: Free Press; 1980.
17. Mintzberg 1990, op. cit., 137.
18. Ansoff I. Critique of Henry Mintzberg's "The design school: Reconsidering the basic premises of strategic management." *Strategic Management Journal.* 1991;12(6):449–461.
19. Goold M. Design, learning, and planning: A further observation on the design school debate. *Strategic Management Journal.* 1992;13(2):169–170.
20. Mintzberg H. Learning 1, planning 0: Reply to Igor Ansoff. *Strategic Management Journal.* 1991; 12(6):463–466.
21. Quinn JB. *Strategies for Change: Logical Incrementalism.* Homewood, Ill: Richard D. Irwin, Inc.; 1980.
22. Mintzberg H. Patterns in strategy formation. *Management Science.* 1978;24(9):934–948.
23. Mintzberg H, Waters JA. Of strategies, deliberate and emergent. *Strategic Management Journal.* 1985;6:257–272.
24. Drucker PF. *Managing in Turbulent Times.* New York, NY: Harper & Row; 1980.
25. Ansoff HI. *The New Corporate Strategy.* New York, NY: John Wiley & Sons; 1988.
26. Lorange P, Morton MFS, Ghoshal S. *Strategic Control.* St. Paul, Minn: West Publishing Co.; 1986.
27. Bracker, op. cit.
28. Porter, 1980, op. cit., 47.
29. Fiegenbaum A, Karnani A. Output flexibility—A comparative advantage for small firms. *Strategic Management Journal.* 1991;12(2):101–114.
30. Porter ME. *Competitive Advantage: Creating and Sustaining Superior Performance.* New York, NY: Free Press; 1985.
31. Powell TC. Organizational alignment as competitive advantage. *Strategic Management Journal.* 1992;13(2):119–134.
32. Mintzberg H. Opening up the definition of strategy. In: *The Strategy Process: Concepts, Contexts, and Cases.* Quinn JB, Mintzberg H, James RM, eds. Englewood Cliffs, NJ: Prentice-Hall; 1988:17.
33. Porter ME. *The Competitive Advantage of Nations.* New York, NY: Free Press; 1990:37.
34. Fiegenbaum, Karnani, op. cit.
35. Ansoff, 1965, op. cit.
36. Schendel, Hofer, op. cit.
37. Hax AC. Redefining the concept of strategy and the strategy formation process. *Planning Review.* 1990;18(3):34–40.
38. Kouzes JM, Posner BZ. *The Leadership Challenge: How to Get Extraordinary Things Done in Organizations.* San Francisco, Ca: Jossey-Bass; 1990:9.
39. Quinn, 1988, op. cit.
40. Porter, 1980, op. cit., Ch 2.
41. Gray BH, ed. *For-Profit Enterprise in Health Care.* Washington, DC: National Academy Press; 1986.
42. Ginsberg E. For-profit medicine: A reassessment. *New England Journal of Medicine.* September 1988;319:757–761.
43. Carman JM, Langeard E. Growth strategies for service firms. U.C. Berkeley, Berkeley, Ca: Institute of Business

and Economic Research, University of California at Berkeley; November 1978. Working paper.

44. Bowring J. *Competition in a Dual Economy.* Princeton, NJ: Princeton Press; 1986.

45. Miles RE, Snow CC. *Organizational Strategy, Structure, and Process.* New York, NY: McGraw-Hill; 1978.

46. Shortell SM, Morrison EM, Friedman B. *Strategic Choices for America's Hospitals: Managing Change in Turbulent Times.* San Francisco, Ca: Jossey-Bass; 1990.

47. Zajac EJ, Shortell SM. Changing generic strategies: Likelihood, direction and performance implications. *Strategic Management Journal.* 1989;10:413–430.

48. Shortell, Morrison, Friedman, op. cit.

49. Miles R. *Coffin Nails and Corporate Strategies.* Englewood Cliffs, NJ: Prentice-Hall; 1982.

50. Amburgey TL, Miner AS. Strategic momentum: The effects of repetitive, positional, and contextual momentum on merger activity. *Strategic Management Journal.* June 1992;13:335–348.

51. Harrigan K. *Strategic Flexibility: A Management Guide for Changing Times.* Lexington, Mass: Lexington Books; 1985.

52. Macmillan IC. Seizing competitive initiative. In: Lamb R, ed. *Competitive Strategic Management.* Englewood Cliffs, NJ: Prentice-Hall; 1984:272–296.

53. Porter, 1985, op. cit.

54. Rothschild WE. Surprise and the competitive advantage. *The Journal of Business Strategy.* 1984;4(3):10–18.

55. Porter, 1985, op. cit.

56. Anderson HJ. Hospitals seek new ways to integrate health care. *Hospitals.* April 5, 1992:26–36.

57. Berwick DM. Seeking systemness. *Healthcare Forum Journal.* March-April 1992;35:22–28.

58. Greene J. Do mergers work? New study questions hospital industry's claim of benefits to consumers. *Modern Healthcare.* March 19, 1990;20:24,25,30,33.

59. Luke RD. Local hospital systems: Forerunners of regional systems? *Frontiers of Health Services Management.* 1992;9(2):3–51.

60. Powell WW. Neither market nor hierarchy: Network forms of organization. In: Straw BM, Cummings LL, eds. *Research in Organizational Behavior, XII.* Greenwich, Conn: JAI Press, Inc.; 1990;295–336.

61. Jarillo JC. On Strategic Networks. *Strategic Management Journal.* 1988;9:31–41.

62. Luke RD, Begun JW, Pointer DD. Quasi firms: Strategic interorganizational forms in the health care industry. *Academy of Management Review.* 1989;14:9–19.

63. Schendel, Hofer, op. cit.

64. Miles, op. cit.

65. Ansoff, 1965, op. cit.

66. Mason ES. Price and production policies of large scale enterprise. *American Economic Review.* March 1939:61–74.

67. Bain JS. *Barriers to New Competition.* Cambridge, Mass: Harvard University Press; 1956.

68. Bain JS. *Essays on Price Theory and Industrial Organization.* Boston, Mass: Little, Brown; 1972.

69. Bain JS, Qualls PD. *Industrial Organization: A Treatise.* Greenwich, Conn: JAI Press, Inc.; 1987.

70. Caves R. *American Industry: Structures, Conduct, and Performance.* 5th ed. Englewood Cliffs, NJ: Prentice-Hall; 1982.

71. Bain, Qualls, op. cit., 7.

72. Ibid, 5.

73. Ibid, 23,24.

74. Luke RD. Spatial competition and cooperation in local hospital markets. *Medical Care Review.* 1991;48(2): 207–237.

75. Porter, 1980, op. cit.

76. Ibid, Ch 1.

77. Scherer FM, Ross D. *Industrial Market Structure and Economic Performance.* 3rd ed. Boston, Mass: Houghton Mifflin; 1990.

78. Shepherd WG. *The Economics of Industrial Organization.* New York, NY: Prentice-Hall; 1979 199.

79. Hurley RE, Luke RD. Patterns of hospital affiliation with national provider networks: Precursors to a purchased-designed delivery system? Williamson Institute Working Paper; 1992.

80. Porter, 1980, op. cit., 19.

81. Luke, 1991, op. cit.

82. Begun JW, Lippincott RC. *Strategic Challenges in the Health Professions.* San Francisco, Ca: Jossey-Bass. In press.

83. *Overview: AHA's National Reform Strategy.* Chicago, Ill: American Hospital Association; 1992.

84. *Setting Relationships Right: A Working Proposal for Systemic Healthcare Reform.* St. Louis, Mo: Catholic Health Association; February 2, 1992.

CHAPTER

15

CREATING AND MANAGING THE FUTURE

Arnold D. Kaluzny
Professor

Stephen M. Shortell
Professor

CHAPTER TOPICS

The Organization and the Environment
Individuals and Groups Within the
   Organization
The Managerial Role

LEARNING OBJECTIVES

After completing this chapter, the reader should be able to

1. identify the major trends likely to affect the delivery of health care
2. understand the changing role of physicians, nurses, and other allied health care providers within health services
3. understand the changing role of management and the competencies required to function in the managerial role

CHAPTER PURPOSE

Like so many health care organizations, NMC is trying to create, or at least manage, its future. Whether it succeeds or fails will depend, in part, on larger secular trends. Some of their options may be influenced by the *future scenarios* summarized in Debate Time 15.1.[1]

It is likely that elements of each scenario will combine to influence the future provision of health services and the future of NMC. A number of forces will play a key role in the emerging health care sys-

IN THE REAL WORLD

NEUMANN MEDICAL CENTER

The Neumann Medical Center (NMC) is a 200-licensed-bed hospital located in a close-knit section of northeast Philadelphia, called Fishtown. NMC prides itself on providing affordable health care alternatives and serving as the largest employer in Fishtown. Initially founded in 1860 by the Franciscans as St. Mary Hospital, in 1988 the Franciscan Health System announced that St. Mary was closing and filing for bankruptcy. Area residents, employees, and other concerned individuals led a successful protest against the closing; and in January 1989 the hospital was acquired by a real estate development firm, renamed, and managed as a for-profit hospital. After the first year, near bankruptcy once again, NMC was acquired on April 19, 1991, by the Northeastern Hospital Foundation.

The Foundation owns NMC and Northeastern Hospital, a 231-bed community hospital located in the neighboring section of the city called Port Richmond. The Foundation assumed control of NMC in order to keep it from bankruptcy. Although both hospitals compete, NMC serves an adjacent community that is largely Medicare- and Medicaid-eligible. NMC inpatients are approximately 54 percent white, 26 percent black, and 18 percent Hispanic. NMC's role in serving the health care needs of the Philadelphia Latino community is particularly significant. Dur-

ing the past 10 years, the Hispanic population of the city of Philadelphia has grown 39 percent, while both the white and black populations have actually decreased. If NMC were to close, Northeastern Hospital would face the possibility of seriously eroding its health maintenance organization (HMO) and charge-based payer mix.

Almost a year after the Foundation subsidiary began management, NMC was still struggling to remain a viable health care institution. It faced a weak financial position and a host of management problems, including poor employee morale, need for an active physician recruitment program, and lack of medical program development and market penetration outside of NMC's immediate neighborhood. The outlook remains bleak. Hospitals to the north and south of NMC are also in financial crisis, and all are competing for patients in a city saturated with hospitals all easily accessible by Philadelphia's strong transportation system. Not only does NMC's patient volume need to increase, but costs also need to be controlled. The strict reimbursement rates imposed on hospitals by Medicare, Medicaid, and other insurers make cost containment critical. At the same time, nursing salaries are rising, and attracting quality physicians for the medical staff has become even more competitive.

NMC is truly a community hospital, drawing the majority of its patients from the surrounding neighborhoods. Approximately 73 percent of the inpatients served by NMC come from just 10 communities. Not surprisingly, the largest market served is the Fishtown community. Fishtown is a white, working, middle-class neighborhood whose residents, mostly of Polish-Irish Catholic descent, have lived and worked in Fishtown their entire lives. Because of all the chaos surrounding NMC's ownership and viability, and increasing health needs of the community, employees have become frustrated and skeptical about their future and the future of the hospital.

SOURCE: Woods K, and McLaughlin C. Kenan-Flager School of Business, University of North Carolina at Chapel Hill, 1992.

tem. This chapter begins by considering changes likely to occur in the organization and its environment, discusses the future of individuals and groups within organizations, and ends with consideration of the managerial role. The intent is to be provocative yet realistic, building on issues developed in preceding chapters. A central theme is that health services organizations and their leaders can actively influence their environment and thereby create and actively manage their future.

THE ORGANIZATION AND THE ENVIRONMENT

Health services organizations, functioning as corporate actors, are the major repository of power within health services. Health care expenditures represent a significant percentage of the gross national product, and as federal and state governments continue to be major purchasers of care, the influence of health services corporate actors will increase. The collective decisions of individual hospitals, multihospital systems, alternative delivery systems, nursing home chains, regulatory groups, suppliers, and other corporate actors within the health services field will significantly affect the basic structure and characteristics of services provided.

Moreover, these organizations will be operating in and affected by an increasingly complex and unpredictable environment, an environment characterized by the difficulty of predicting both the occurrence and content of change. For example, decisions about health care may in fact be made on factors quite independent of the substantive issues involved with health care. Specifically, as health services consume greater portions of the gross national product, their effects on other sectors of the economy are pervasive. Thus, other criteria, such as local employment or employment in a variety of other support ancillary areas, become important criteria affecting decisions within heath services.

Along with increasing complexity and unpredictability of the environment will come a demand for greater organizational responsiveness and accountability from different groups. The organization will face the problem of reconciling incompatible objectives. For example, the federal government often defines accountability in terms of cost control, while local consumer groups may see accountability in terms of added facilities and services and greater consumer participation in decision making. In short, the future involves major issues centering on the organization's ability to adapt to divergent demands. This effort will require innovation, the ability to manage external dependencies, and at the same time the ability to restructure relationships. A number of major trends and their implications are presented below.

Changing Social Norms and Expectations

The underlining *norms and expectations of society* are important guides to behavior within health services, and changing norms and expectations will serve to shape the fundamental questions and issues that will guide the public policy debate regarding the future character of health services. Questions of access and accountability will play a central role and be shaped by fundamental norms and expectations. As a society,

DEBATE TIME 15.1: WHAT DO YOU THINK?

- **Continued Growth and High Technology**
  National health care reform never did occur, but expensive advancing technology in therapeutics, including function enhancing bionics, helps the health care share of the gross national product grow to 17 percent by 2001. Health care providers shift to predicting and then managing illness far earlier and more successfully. Poverty and lack of access to health care persists.

- **Hard Times and Government Leadership**
  Recurrent hard times and a political revolt against health care leads to a frugal Canadian-like national insurance system. Most states follow Oregon in consciously setting priorities. Heroic measures for terminal patients decline, and a more frugal approach to innovation is adopted. Health care percentage of the gross national product is reduced to 11 percent by 2001. Thirty percent of Americans "buy up" to affluent, higher tech care, and two different systems of health care emerge.

- **Buyers Market** Many thought the 80s was the decade of health care entries into the marketplace—that competition would lead to better, less expensive service. What failed during the 80s worked well during the next two decades. Markets, including health care, now do a much better job of giving consumers a range of high quality service, delivered in convenient ways, at relatively low cost over the long term while maintaining a high degree of innovation. These amazing changes are coupled with better social policies to block the inequities and lack of access that accompany the stronger market approach.

- **A New Civilization** Dramatic changes in the paradigm of science, technology, society, and government hasten health care change. Health care broadens its focus from the individual to the community and the environment. National health care reform favors managed care, particularly social HMOs, which are effective at predicting and often preventing various personal and community health problems. High tech and alternative therapies are common. Health care consumes 12 percent of the gross national product by 2001.

- **Healing and Health Care** This option shares the fundamental characteristics of the new civilization—dramatic changes in the paradigms of science, technology, society, and government, but with a different emphasis. The role of the spirit and its integration to health care lead to a greater focus on healing. Health care providers, particularly those running hospitals, take an early and active role in moving health care toward real personal, community, and environmental health rather than allowing it to continue to simply cure individuals. Poverty, other social problems, and environmental causes of ill health are dealt with more systematically. Health care structures have changed dramatically, merging with a variety of other community organizations. Healing the planet, particularly the environment, for our children is a dominant issue.

Which of the above scenarios do you believe is most likely to occur? What are the most important implications for health services managers?

---

we have valued equality of access and opportunity as well as placing a great deal of emphasis on individualism. While it is unlikely that the future will see a resolution between the values of universal access to health care and individual freedom, it is equally unlikely that new initiatives will not be presented. As described by the Pew Commission:

What seems likely is that we will equivocate the values of freedom and individualism on the one hand, and equality and public intervention on the other hand, by advancing a range of incremental pluralistic responses—rather than one solution for all (these issues) we are more likely to see many experiments involving efforts to limit and manage care and extend access.[2]

There is growing recognition that accountability must include both clinical and financial criteria. Simply holding down costs without paying attention to the quality of services provided or the impact on patient health status is unacceptable. The new accountability will emphasize value—the relationship between quality and cost or between benefit and cost that meets purchaser and consumer needs and demands. Whether or not the locus of accountability is centralized in the federal government, decentralized in the state or local level, or shared among the various levels is not clear. Most likely the country will evolve toward a system of shared accountability at multiple levels requiring the active participation of many parties.

Demographic Composition and Epidemiology

Managing the future requires a thorough understanding of the evolving demographics and epidemiological characteristics of the population. Perhaps most far reaching is the changing character of the population, and specifically, the increase in percentage of elderly people in the population. The proportion of the total population composed of those over age 64 is expected to increase from 12.2 percent in 1987, to 13 percent in the year 2000, and to 21.8 percent by the year 2030. Just as the overall population is aging, the elderly are aging. While 9.6 percent of the elderly population was over age 85 in 1987, this percentage will grow steadily to 15.5 percent in the year 2010.

Equally important for managing the future is the racial and *ethnic composition* of the population. Two groups of particular importance that will affect our ability to manage the future are Afro-Americans and Hispanic-Americans. Both groups currently remain outside the mainstream of health services and will greatly challenge the ability of the health system in the future. It is expected that Afro-Americans will grow as a percentage of the population from 11.8 percent in 1980 to 13.2 percent in the year 2005. Although in 1980, the Hispanic-American population was roughly half of the total Afro-American population, by the year 2005, the two groups will be equal in size and together represent 26 percent of the U.S. population. Both groups will represent the youngest part of the population requiring services which are fundamentally different from those required by the elderly portion of the population.

The demands of the population will be further reflected in the epidemiological trends of the population. Diseases of aging, lifestyle, and behavior will present major challenges to the delivery system. Although mortality from cardiovascular disease has declined 39 percent since 1964, it still remains the most common cause of death and will remain a major disease of aging well into the twenty-first century. While cardiovascular diseases have been declining, there has been a steady increase in the age-adjusted incidence in national death rate for all forms of cancer. It was estimated that about 30 percent of Americans now living will develop cancer.[3] Alzheimer's disease will also present major challenges to the system as the population increases in age. The U.S. Office of Technology Assessment reported a prevalence of 1.4 million in 1980, and a projected 2.4 million people will have Alzheimer's in the year 2000 and 3.3 million in the year 2020. Total costs are estimated to exceed $30 billion.[4,5]

Diseases of lifestyle and behavior will present the most difficult challenges to the health services system. Perhaps most traumatic will be the continued toll taken by Acquired Immune Deficiency Syndrome (AIDS). More than 200,000 Americans have already been diagnosed with AIDS with an estimated 1.5 million thought to be Sero positive for the human immune deficiency virus (HIV). The cost in human suffering is immeasurable, and the medical expenses associated with AIDS treatment are estimated to be more than $75,000 per person. Current total health care expenditures for AIDS exceed $2.3 billion yearly and will place an increasing burden on health service providers.[29]

Technology Development, Assessment, and Outcomes

Technology development in both treatment, prevention, and early detection activities will continue to have a major impact on health services in the future. Such developments will raise questions involving who will have access to new technological developments; to what degree the decision to use new technology will be centralized, what effect new technology will have on provider-patient relationships, and what new ethical considerations must be considered.

New developments will change our paradigm of disease. The paradigm of diagnosis and treatment will be replaced by one of prediction and early stage management of the illness. Such projects as the Human Genome Project in which geneticists around the world will be conducting a massive cooperative research effort to completely map or at least partially sequence the entire human genome. This process will define the form and function of most of our genes; and thus, instead of diagnosing diseases late in the disease process, we will be predicting disease risk based on our genetic inheritance and attempting to manage that risk before symptoms emerge. While the challenges are great, proponents of this project, and particularly those who speculate about its implications for health services, suggest that "within 15 years it will be morally and fiscally untenable to continue to think of disease as an inexorable act of God."[6]

New developments in prevention, early detection, and health promotion activities will have similarly important implications. Although, not as dramatic or as heroic as the basic technological development described above, significant progress is occurring in the control of hypertension, coronary disease, cancer, and certain disabling forms of mental illness. For example, the development of biomarkers and chemoprevention agents, such as the breast cancer prevention agent, tamoxifen, for women at increased risk of developing breast cancer, are important developments having profound implications on the health services system.

Developments of both basic as well as preventive and health promotion technologies will be accompanied by greater concern for assessment of cost and efficacy. Increasingly, attention will be given to outcomes with emphasis on both outcomes assessment and *outcomes management.*[7] Outcomes assessment focuses on the relevant effectiveness of different interventions. Outcomes management is concerned with how this information is used within an operating setting to assure the elimination of unnecessary procedures and to improve quality of care provided. This focus will be institutionalized and reinforced among a variety of federal and private agencies. For example, within the federal government the Agency for Health Care Policy Research (AHCPR) is expected to "conduct and support research with respect to the outcomes, effectiveness, and appropriateness of health care services and procedures in order to identify the manner in which disease, disorders, and other health conditions can effectively be prevented, diagnosed, treated and managed clinically."[8] These developments will be reinforced by the Joint Commission for the Accreditation of Health Care Organizations' *Agenda for Change* and its emphasis on clinical outcome indicators. As described by Dennis O'Leary, "The payoff is performance—are you getting done the things that you should be getting done, and are you getting them done well?"[9]

Organizational Arrangements

While evolving social norms and expectations, demography, epidemiology, and technologies will affect organizational arrangements, the very nature of the organizations themselves and their interactions will affect the management challenges of the future. New organizational forms will be developed, and existing forms will change, forging new relationships with other organizations in the environment. In the world of health services, increasing attention will be paid to the configuration of service delivery organizations transcending existing organizational entities. While both *vertical and horizontal integration* represent interorganizational efforts, to be more responsive to changing environmental conditions, the unrelenting demand of cost containment, improving quality, and assuring technology transfer and accountability will force managers to increasingly consider other forms of organizational arrangements. Several options are available, including the development of *organized delivery systems, community care networks,* or more loosely coupled alliances. An organized delivery system is a collection of organizations which provides, or arranges to provide, a coordinated array of services to a defined population and is willing to be held financially and clinically accountable for the health status of the population served. This system shares a common ownership, and efforts are made to achieve levels of clinical and functional integration to maximize the value or service delivered to the patients. Organized delivery systems are not necessarily community care networks. The latter would include broad-based health and social services, such as those typically associated with public health departments and social service agencies. Their locus of control would be at the community level.[10]

Alliances—loosely coupled arrangements among existing organizations including networks designed to achieve some long-term strategic purpose not possible by any single organization—will have important implications for management.[11] While these alliances are not unique to health services, they are clearly different organizational forms from those historically characterizing health services and thus, in profound ways, will change how existing health care organizations operate. Emphasis is given to the interaction process in which there is a constant exchange of products, information, money, and social symbols with the emphasis being on interaction and interdependency on each other in various ways. Clearly these are fragile relationships with the critical challenge being the way management deals with issues of commitment, control, performance, communication, participation, and stability over time.

Along with these new emerging forms will be significant realignment of existing organizations. While health services organizations, particularly hospitals, have prided themselves as being citadels—self-contained units that function under all adversity—the push for efficiency will force attention to new configurations with suppliers and vendors and further experimentation with subcontracting functions to other organizations in the community. For example, "Just In Time" management (JIT), which has received a great deal of attention from industrial-type organizations, may have applicability to health services.[12] The basic premise is that the organization can benefit from synchronizing inventory with workflow needs. The efficiency in operations is attributable to decreases in inventory levels, smoother workflows, and lower storage costs.[13] Similarly, subcontracting—or, as it is sometimes known, outsourcing—provides an opportunity to have other organizations perform functions, thereby increasing efficiency. For example, subcontracting of emergency medical services and dietary services is well established. However, other activities such as managing employee benefits and inservice training, which have traditionally been considered parts of management, may be likely candidates for outsourcing in the future.

Financing

The changing demographics and epidemiology and new organizational forms will put added stress on the financing of health services and the manner in which providers are reimbursed. Major segments of the population are without health insurance coverage, and health care expenditures continue to consume a growing portion of the gross national product. For example, the number of people without health insurance in the United States increased at four times the rate of the population growth from 1977 to 1987.[14] In 1989 alone, between 34 and 40 million people were without health insurance coverage for all or part of the year, and an additional 65 million were underinsured.[15] During this period, national health expenditures continued to consume a growing portion of the U.S. gross national product and is expected to reach 17 percent by the year 2000.

Several initiatives are underway that will have important implications for the financing and reimbursement of health services. The increasing visibility that the United States is the only industrialized country with the exception of South Africa that does not guarantee financial access to health care for all of its citizens has resulted in a growing interest, at both national and state levels, in expanding financial access to assure a basic set of benefits for all Americans. Major considerations in developing such a program are what benefits should be considered basic, what the benefits will cost, how they should be financed, and what incentives should be developed for the delivery system to provide cost-effective care in meeting the increased demand.[16]

As the percentage of gross national product devoted to health spending grows, increasing attention will be given to financial and clinical accountability. For example, the development of the Resource-Based Relative Value Scale (RBRVS) for paying physicians, which in turn will be tied to expenditure targets, will receive increasing scrutiny as a means for cost accountability. In addition, there is the likelihood of the incorporation of capital payments into the Medicare (DRG) formula and renewed discussion of limiting prices charged for prescription drugs.

The development of regional systems or networks will give further importance to the development of risk-adjusted capitated payments. Capitation—a set fee paid to the regionally-integrated network or system—establishes a budget for delivering care to the enrolled community. The implications for health care organizations are substantial. Revenue is generated up front with the negotiation of the capitated premium dollar or established target budget. Everything else then becomes a cost center, such that incentives are created to manage patients' care in as cost-effective a way as possible. This will force clinicians and health services managers to work together more closely to figure out at what point in the continuum of patient care the greatest value is added. Increasingly, this will be in outpatient settings, in the work place, and in homes. As noted later, it will involve fundamental transitions in managerial roles.

Social Experimentation

Evaluation and experimentation will extend beyond technology assessment to encompass a wide variety of new approaches, programs, and organizations for delivering more cost-effective health care. The demands for greater accountability under an environment of constrained resources will push the health care system further in the direction of Campbell's "experimenting society," in which new demonstration programs are rigorously evaluated.[17] Emphasis will be placed not only on results but also on the process by which the results were obtained. A contemporary version of this with specific application to health services is known as Clinical Firm Trials Research.[18] Initiated in the 1980s at the Cleveland Metro Health Center and, more recently, ongoing in several hospitals throughout the country, firm research provides an opportunity to evaluate various changes in programmatic initiatives in the delivery of health care with the rigors of a randomized clinical trial.

An important effect of this research is that health services managers will increasingly become part of more formal program evaluation efforts. Examples include programmatic initiatives such as alcohol counseling activities within a general medicine clinic to more global evaluations such as the evaluation of managed care programs; defining the specific kinds of patient populations, delivery settings, and health conditions for which managed care programs are effective; and

determining the impact of the RBRVS.[19,20] In these kinds of evaluations, there are four areas in which managers will be called upon to play a major role: initiation of the evaluation process, facilitation of the evaluation process, mediation of the relationship between the evaluators and program staff, and implementation of the evaluation results.[21]

In the initiation stage, managers will be responsible for determining the purposes of the evaluation. Is the organization willing to commit the resources required for valid evaluation? What are the likely payoffs? Are ulterior or covert purposes involved? These are some of the questions that managers will have to articulate and assess. In addition, managers will be faced with the issue of selecting an inside or outside group to conduct the evaluation. At the same time, the manager must determine whether and when the organization is ready for the evaluation. Premature evaluation serves no one's ends. The manager will also play an important role in facilitating the implementation of the evaluation. This is particularly true in regard to formulating program objectives, which should be clearly understood by all involved.

The manager can also play an important role in mediating relationships between program staff members and evaluators. These relationships are frequently characterized by conflict. Program staff understandably view their activities as beneficial and as contributing to the organization's goals. Evaluators, on the other hand, are charged with maintaining the integrity of the evaluation design and taking an independent view as to whether or not and to what degree the program's objectives have been achieved. Further, the evaluation may consume resources that program staff members feel may be better spent on direct services. Managers can help minimize these conflicts by ensuring that sufficient time is allocated for discussion and development of mutual understanding and by engaging in direct problem-solving and conflict-resolution strategies as needed.

Finally, managers play a key role in making use of the evaluation results. Managers who work closely with evaluators can help to ensure that the key questions are being answered in a manner that makes sense to the eventual users. This includes suggesting to the evaluators that the report be written in a language and format understandable to the intended audience.

Past, Present, and Future

Table 15.1 presents each of the major trends involving the organization and the environment. As can be seen, both the organization and environment are faced with increasing risk and uncertainty. Organizations are increasingly being challenged, requiring greater adaptability and creativity. The future obviously will involve activities that have not been done before and will require efforts that have not yet been tried.

INDIVIDUALS AND GROUPS WITHIN THE ORGANIZATION

As an organization functions within a larger environment, individuals and groups function within a larger organizational setting. This interaction is critical to the overall performance of health care institutions in the future role of managers within these organizations. Several developments likely to affect the interaction of individuals and groups within organizations having profound implications on the managerial role are discussed below.

Changing Role of the Physician

Changing demographics and epidemiology, new technologies and their emphasis on assessment and outcomes, and fundamental changes in the configura-

tion of health services resulting in increased scrutiny of health care costs are all factors that are redefining the role of the physician and are likely to affect the basic role that physicians will play in the emerging health care system. The implications are expected to be reflected in greater attention to prevention, the incorporation of consumer preferences into medical decision making, and greater involvement in managerial activities, either as a knowledgeable clinician or a physician executive.

The shifting patterns of morbidity and mortality as well as changes in the demographic composition of the population are increasingly forcing medical practice to focus on the treatment of diseases associated with specific lifestyles or behaviors and chronic degenerative diseases of aging. Cardiovascular and pulmonary diseases, trauma, substance abuse, AIDS and other sexually-transmitted diseases, cancer, chronic cognitive impairment, and diabetes are among the major health problems facing the population. Today and into the future, prevention will be the primary focus, and the physician will increasingly be at the vanguard of this movement.

Changes in the organization and delivery of health services and the results of health services research efforts are reflected in outcomes research. Outcomes research will produce more knowledge about the consequences of alternative treatments for specific conditions and provide recognition of the importance of

TABLE 15.1. Environmental Trends

	Past (1950s–1970s)	Present (1990s)	Future (1995 and beyond)
Social Norms and expectations	Provider dominated	Changing consumer expectations	Provider-consumer-employer partnerships
Demographics and epidemiology	Aging of population not an issue Infectious diseases	Aging as an emergent issue Chronic diseases	Aging a major focus of activity Diseases of lifestyle and aging Afro-American and Hispanic-American influences
Technical development, assessment and outcomes	Rapid development and implementation	Emerging efforts at assessment	Use of randomized trials and meta analysis
Financing and reimbursement	Not an issue; retrospective reimbursement	Emergent concern and shift to prospective reimbursement	Global budgets and development of a fully capitated system
Organizational arrangement	Cottage industry; large number of individual providers	Systems and emerging organizational forms	Regionally-integrated systems, networks, and alliances
Social experimentation	Emerging efforts	Pressure on accountability	Collaborative efforts among policy makers, researchers, and managers

consumer participation in the choice of treatment options available. The empirical documentation that all treatment is not equal and the explicit recognition that there are tradeoffs will give increasing focus to what Wennberg and his colleagues refer to as "shared decisions."[22]

Finally, the emerging trends within the larger environment will force physicians to become increasingly knowledgeable about the organizational and managerial environment within which they function. Some physicians may become active participants in the decision-making process and will join the growing ranks of physician executives. The development of organized delivery systems and community care networks—let alone alliances—and perspective reimbursement for all services will force a merger of clinical and financial data and place a premium on the role of the physician executive. "Clinical decisions are increasingly viewed as managerial decisions," and the physician executive will be critical to the integration of these traditionally disparate decision processes.[23] The challenge for the health services executive is to develop a working partnership with the physician community—one that fully recognizes the role of physicians in the managerial process.

Changing Role of the Nurse

The dominant coalition in health services management of the past 30 years has consisted of the governing board, management, and the medical staff. Within the next 5 to 10 years, it is likely that nursing will join this coalition. Two key features of the nurse's role have significantly influenced this trend. First, as a professional group and clearly recognizing its heterogeneity, nurses are pervasive throughout the health care delivery system. While more than two-thirds of nurses work in hospital settings, employment outside the hospital continues to grow, with much of this growth occurring in HMOs and group practice settings. Secondly, the nurse is the primary resource coordinator and, given the greater emphasis on information management, the linking of financial and clinical information will become a critical component in the managerial decision process. Both features clearly place nursing at the center of both conceptual and methodological issues critical to assuring organizational productivity.

Many of the trends affecting physicians will affect the changing role of nurses in the future. The emphasis on cost-effective care, changes in the demographics and epidemiology of the population, and the various organizational arrangements within the larger system will continually challenge the role of nursing within the health care system. To meet the challenge, nursing will demand a larger voice in management and governance. The challenge for management is to join in partnership with nursing and implement appropriate roles for nurses, clearly recognizing their professional heritage as well as their importance to emerging health care issues. Several approaches need to be considered. A key role in hospitals today is that of first line management. First-line unit-level managers, traditionally known as head nurses, are key players in ensuring organizational productivity. These individuals have traditionally been chosen because of their clinical expertise and out of respect for their ability to make patient-level decisions, but they frequently lacked education or skills in management. In structuring organizational systems to enhance their contribution to management, it is important to clearly identify role expectations and then provide didactic and experiential support for their success. In the ideal setting, unit-level managers have received the education needed to successfully manage a nursing unit in an academic setting; there is an increasing trend, at least in teaching hospitals, to require education at the master's level for these individuals.

Utilizing nurses as case managers is a way to utilize nurses in a new role. In this system of care delivery, a non-line management nurse manages a patient's care throughout an entire episode of illness. Traditionally, a nurse's contact with a given patient has been limited to the amount of time spent on a given patient unit. In *case management,* the nurse is not subject to geographic restrictions and directs a patient's nursing care on any nursing unit and in the home and community environment. Consistent interventions by a case manager greatly facilitate continuity of care, thereby enhancing patient satisfaction and organizational productivity.

A third new role for nurses in delivery of patient care is as participants in the development of *critical paths.* When developing a critical path, practitioners from all disciplines collaborate to define specific goals and activities that are to be accomplished on each day of a patient's hospital stay. For example, progressive ambulation targets are set by physicians, nurses, and physicial therapists. These targets are then utilized to evaluate a patient's care progress. If they are not met, variance analysis is done and early interventions are implemented to decrease the likelihood of increased lengths of stay. Nurses are usually the facilitators of critical path development and serve effectively as coordinators of this process.

There are many countervailing forces to these changes. In some cases, new roles may not be workable or even wise to implement. In other cases, these approaches will be welcome. Nonetheless, the challenge from the nursing profession is well underway, and the ultimate challenge is forging a new partnership between the governing board, management, physicians, and the nursing community.

Expanding Role of Allied Health Professionals

Comprising more than 60 percent of the entire health care workforce and expanding over 200 distinct disciplinary groups, allied health is the largest and most complex health professions constituency in the United States.[4] Defined broadly, allied health includes all of the health-related disciplines, with the exception of nursing and the so called MODVOPP disciplines: medicine, osteopathy, dentistry, veterinary medicine, optometry, pharmacy, and podiatry. This group includes more than three million health professionals providing services in a range of settings including hospitals, clinics, physicians' offices, hospices, extended care facilities, HMOs, community programs, and schools.

As with nursing and medicine, the realities of financing, reimbursement, demography, epidemiology, technology, and organizational arrangements will have profound implications on this group of health care providers with subsequent implications for health services management. Perhaps its distinguishing feature is its heterogeneity and size, and thus the emerging forces within the larger system will greatly affect the role of this particular group of providers. Personnel shortages, understaffing in hospitals and other health care settings, inadequate funding for educational programs, inability to recruit and retrain personnel in

underserved areas are all factors that will challenge the ability of allied health to respond.

Dynamic Nature of Individual and Group Configurations

Effective management recognizes the dynamic nature of disciplinary and interdisciplinary work groups and individuals interacting within the organization. Clearly, the emerging and dynamic roles of nurses, physicians, and the range of allied health professionals within the context of the larger trends affecting health services delivery will place a premium on the ability to understand and manage these individual and group configurations.

The implications are substantial. First, the recognition that health services organizations are composed not only of work groups, but a range of interest groups and coalitions that are constantly shifting in order to compete for resources, provides an opportunity for managers to develop leverage between and among these interest groups and coalitions to enhance the overall operations of the organization. The recognition of these dynamics provides an opportunity to structure situations so that individuals and groups can more effectively monitor and control their own activities.

Secondly, the increasing role of interdisciplinary groups and work units in the provision of health services raises the issue of work group effectiveness. While the business of providing health services is usually done within the context of some group setting, the ability of these groups to function effectively is limited by the individual's own disciplinary perspective and lack of appreciation for the dynamics involved as well as other disciplinary perspectives. The overall effectiveness of the group is constantly threatened by the tendency of one disciplinary perspective to dominate and by a fundamental lack of group dynamics.

Finally, given the importance of interdisciplinary activity and the increasing emphasis given to total quality management which attempts to focus on the horizontal flow of activities within the organizations, individuals will increasingly occupy boundary spanning roles involving various work groups, interest groups, or coalitions. Boundary spanning involves considerable conflict, and increased attention will be given to the development of skills required for negotiation and conflict management.

Health Services Policy and Management Research

Health services research has come of age and clearly has made major contributions to the policy issues facing the health services system.[25] Moreover, it is likely that the synthesis and dissemination of health services research will play an important role in the process of formulating policy. Future considerations, however, need to be given to the interdisciplinary nature of health services research and the utilization of research by managers.

While clearly the substantive issues facing health services at this point focus on cost containment, increasing attention needs to be paid to the configuration and organizational aspects affecting managerial decision making. The interdisciplinary nature of health services delivery and the critical issues of understanding the process of health services delivery will increasingly place a premium on analytical questions that go beyond simply those of cost and reimbursement. The management of groups, the motivation of personnel, and the integration and coordination of services at various delivery levels require the attention of a wide variety of social science disciplines within the health services research community.

A second challenge is the utilization of health services research in the decision-making process. More than anything else, the health services manager of the future must be an innovator, at times a visionary, and also be able to apply health services management research and bring a research perspective to all management decisions. A partnership is needed between managers and researchers, whereby the health services research community will be acutely aware and sensitive to the substantive issues facing managers, and managers in turn will be a beneficiary of greater insight and strategies derived from the research process. In a sense, this partnership represents an alliance in which both managers and researchers work collaboratively to provide an opportunity to assess performance of ongoing activities, develop predictors of performance, and specify the conditions under which various approaches to health services delivery are most effective. Perhaps most importantly, the development of the partnership provides an opportunity to truly develop meaningful and relevant guidelines for effective management.

Information Management

While emerging trends at the larger environmental level such as outcomes management and the development of guidelines are occurring, it has been recognized that existing data systems within organizations are inadequate to meet the information needs and strategies inherent in many of these important developments. Information systems within health services organizations often have a programatic or categorical character and thus are greatly hindered in their attempt to integrate clinical outcomes, process of care, and financial information. Existing systems either

- do not collect and store the right information
- are not automated or computerized
- are not integrated, or
- lack sufficiently sophisticated computer hardware, software, and data entry support to permit retrieval and analysis of information.[26]

Nevertheless, the fact that health services organizations and providers will be held increasingly responsible for a clear definition of service area and will then be held accountable for the health status of people in these areas will require the development of such systems. While discipline and resources are required, the implications for management are substantial. Such integrated systems will facilitate accountability, provide tools for increased productivity, have direct clinical applications, and provide an opportunity to actively manage clinical care.[27]

Past, Present, and Future

Table 15.2 summarizes the trends dealing with individuals and groups within the organizations. As with the environment and larger organizations, individuals and groups within organizations are confronting in-

TABLE 15.2. Individual and Group Trends

	Past (1950s–1970s)	Present (1990s)	Future (1995 and beyond)
Physicians	Solo practice	Group practice	Corporate practice and active involvement in managerial activity
Nurses	Clinical practice	Emerging as a political force	Active participation in managerial structure and policy
Allied health	Not an issue	Emerging issue	Key participants in teams that manage care across episodes of illness and pathways of wellness
Management research and assessment	Not an issue	Increased recognition	Integral part of managerial and organizational effectiveness
Dynamic nature of groups	Individual and disciplinary groups dominate	Emergence of interdisciplinary groups	Dominance of interdisciplinary groups
Information management	Not an issue	Emerging efforts	Clinical and financial networking

creasing complexity and uncertainty. The future will require the active participation of physicians, nurses, and allied health professionals with the major challenge being to motivate and preserve human resources available to the organization. These resources will be increasingly involved in interdisciplinary groups and will be informed by a developing research base that will permit new designs and managerial strategies.

THE MANAGERIAL ROLE

Developments at the environment-organizational level, and the individual-group level of the organization provide a clue to future demands on managers. These demands involve three assumptions and three fundamental implications. The first assumption is that health care will continue to have features of both an economic and social good. Since it is financially impossible to provide unlimited care, there must be a mechanism for allocating resources, and it is likely that this will continue to include some marketplace features. At the same time, health care is an intensely personal, human service which most Americans believe ought to be available to people in need, who are without the ability to pay for the service. A major responsibility and challenge of health services executives and managers of the 1990s will be to manage the inherent tension between health care as both an economic and a social good.

The second assumption is that the world will not become simpler but, if anything, more complex, ambiguous, and uncertain. If past is prologue, managers of health services organizations will encounter continued, if not increasing, stress; this stress will be reflected in the turnover rates among chief executive officers (CEOs). In 1983 hospital CEO turnover rate, for example, was 12.8 percent; it rose steadily at an annual rate of 7.5 percent to peak at 18.4 percent in 1988. Since then the rate has declined so that in 1990 it was again at 12.8 percent.[8] It is fully expected that this rate will continue into the foreseeable future.

The third assumption is that health services executives and managers working together and with other health care providers can create the future for themselves and their organization. It is precisely because health care delivery will become even more complex, ambiguous, and uncertain that it is possible for managers to shape their destiny. The external environment not only influences managerial and organizational decision making, but the decisions made by managers on behalf of their organizations will help to shape and influence the environment.

From the three assumptions come three fundamental implications, each involving a major transition in the managerial role.

- The first involves a transition from managing an organization to managing a market or network of services. Health services executives of the future will increasingly be called upon to manage across boundaries. This will require increased skills in coalition building, negotiation, and the ability to put together strategic alliances and partnerships to serve defined populations. It will require executives who see any given organization as part of a broader whole.

- For middle managers it involves a transition from managing a department to managing a continuum of care. In brief, the job of the pharmacy department head, laboratory department head, radiology department head, or any other hospital department head is no longer that of a department head but rather a manager of pharmaceutical, laboratory, or radiology services across the continuum of care—most of which will be provided outside hospital settings. This will require these individuals to discard the hospital mindset and develop a broader community-based approach to delivering services. It will place a premium on interpersonal skills and the ability to develop collaborative relationships.

- The third transition involves moving from a mentality of coordinating services to a new mindset of actively managing quality across the continuum of care. This involves adopting a broader view of one's responsibilities. For example, the main focus is no longer on whether intensive care services are coordinated with those of step down units but rather on coordinating care along the entire episode of illness or pathway of wellness leading from the patient's home, to the physician's office, to the relatively short stay in the intensive care unit, and back out again to the after-care units and into the home. It does little good to coordinate only part of this continuum of care if it has no resulting lasting value or impact on the overall episode of illness or ultimately the patient's health status. Actively managing quality will require health services managers at all levels to move beyond suboptimization and consider the overall interdependent processes involved in patient care—again, most of which will occur outside the hospital.

Role Performance and Emerging Challenges*

The managerial role within health services is perhaps one of the most complex administrative assignments. Role performance will become even more challenging as managers attempt to deal with integrated networks, resource constraints, and increasing emphasis on health and preventive services that are customer-focused, information-driven and outcome-based. To meet these emerging trends, the managerial role requires

- new competencies
- a recognition that the rapidly changing environment and the scope and depth of competencies needed by health services administrators cannot be provided only at career entry level and requires a life-long commitment
- a recognition that managerial competencies must be shared with clinical colleagues to form a partnership to meet the changing demands of the future.

Adequate role performance requires new skills and competencies in leadership, coalition building, policy and political acuity, quality improvement and assurance, sensitivity to cost-quality relationships, research utilization, innovation, and problem solving. Specifically, managers must reaffirm the commitment to leadership which is the fundamental characteristic of management and requires the development of skills to facilitate change and assure flexibility, the ability to act in ambiguous and unstable environments, and the true recognition of the constancy of change in health services organizations.

Secondly, managers require new skills and competencies in coalition-building and a perspective which facilitates networking. Given the emergence of multi-specialty group practice and multidisciplinary health care delivery organizations in complex structures will

---

* Based on material prepared for Pew Panel on Health Care Management. Pew Commission, Health Care Management Advisor Panel Report, 1992.

be the dominant practice pattern, and thus for optimal performance, administrators need skill and vision to integrate the clinical professions and institutions into organizations which provide predictable, cost-effective care through comprehensive service delivery systems. The managerial role here will require group leadership skills, coalition building, negotiation, and conflict management, as well as an overarching systems perspective.

A third competency is in the area of policy and political acuity. While currently managers know how to make improvements, they often lack access to the levers to change the system. Often they are not rewarded for doing the right thing and are punished for thinking globally. Managers of the future will require political skills including interagency analysis, coalition building, and understanding the realities of partisan politics.

Similarly, the entire area of quality improvement and assurance will be fundamental to role performance in the future. Purchasers—whether individual consumers, third party payers, or governmental units—increasingly demand accountability of health services providers for an appropriate return on investment and increasingly expressed in terms of improved health status and outcome. To function within this set of expectations, managers will require skills in the area of quantitative, statistical, and epidemiological reasoning, outcome interpretation, and application.

Future role performance also requires that managers have a sensitivity to the cost-quality relationship. Individual consumers, third-party payers, and governmental units increasingly demand the provision of health services within the constraints of budgetary limits in all their diversity. Increasingly managers will be called upon to demonstrate their abilities in budget-based resource management, resources creation and allocation, and management within limits and constraints.

New dimensions of role performance are also required in research utilization and innovation. Future role performance will require practitioners to have skills in the area of health services research, management assessment, and application. Many health services managers fail to recognize problems which are, in fact, researchable and fail to apply knowledge from existing research to enhance organizational performance.

There is a serious and growing need for managers to become informed consumers of health services management research to improve organizational performance and services outcomes. Finally, future role performance requires that managers apply knowledge to assure benefit. In an area where the demand for greater productivity and improved outcomes with finite resource limitations predominate, the health services administrator must create workable solutions to operational and system problems.

Another challenge facing the future of role performance of the administrator is the recognition that, given the rapidly changing environment, the scope and depth of competencies needed by health service administrators cannot be provided only at career entry level. The acquisition of new competencies will be needed throughout their entire careers. Health services managers will increasingly come from a variety of educational backgrounds, and thus enhanced lifelong learning is required to equip the manager to address the issues in a rapidly changing environment.

Finally, role performance in the future will increasingly require the support and participation of clinical professions. Clinicians have increasing impact on the management of the health service system. Thus, if the managerial role is to meet its expectations, it must join in a partnership with the clinicians exposing them to the basic core of the organization and policy knowledge to support role performance in the future. At a minimum, clinical colleagues require a basic understanding of the health services system and the impacts of clinical practice and decision making an organization, delivery, and cost.

Preparing Future Managers*

Much like orange juice not being just for breakfast anymore, health services managers are playing an increasing role in all segments of the health services delivery system. Initially developed to improve the management of large acute care hospitals, the demand for professional administrators has expanded greatly

---

*   Based on material prepared for Pew Panel on Health Care Management. Pew Commission, Health Care Management Advisor Panel Report, 1992.

to include all the private and public organizations that are involved in financing, regulating, assessing, supplying, assisting, and generating policies for health services. While limited training is provided at the undergraduate and doctoral levels, major effort in health administration education is at the master's degree. Although commonly referred as the MHA, the degrees conferred include health administration specialization within the MBA, MPH, MPA, MS, MA, MSHA, and others. The degrees reflect a variety of settings in which the programs are based, including schools of medicine, public health, management, public affairs, and graduate schools. It is these educational arrangements which carry the burden of meeting the changing challenges and expectations for health services management. Several strategies need to be considered to better meet the expectations of the future.[8]

- Core Curriculum Reform: Develop a paradigm for core health administration curriculum which embraces the new competencies including leadership, coalition building, policy and political acuity, quality improvement, cost-quality relationships, research utilization, and problem solving. Model curricula which convey the essential values, competencies, and skills must be developed and educational institutions challenged to undertake the required reforms. The development of educational materials and methods must emphasize adaptability and the development of skills to manage the characteristics of the health care system of the future. Given the demographic changes in the community and the workforce composition of health service organizations, it is imperative that students and academic faculty reflect this diversity.
- Quality Partnerships between University and Practice Personnel: Expand the university-practice interface to assure the relevance of health services administration curricula to broader health care fields and return the research and educational products which yield improved administrator and organizational performance. The practitioner-academic interface requires a major expansion of the range or provider organizations involved and a redefinition of the

mutual benefits accruing to each party. Special emphasis needs to be given to identifying and establishing a broad range of relationships with operating health services organizations, particularly those exhibiting the characteristics of the system of the future, and using these as teaching and research models and focal points for training administrators. Idealized relationships with the future include

- experiential learning opportunities such as mentoring, internships, residencies, postgraduate fellowships, and administrator training programs
- middle management congresses by academic programs for provider organizations participating in experiential learning programs
- executive-in-residence or visiting-health-care-executive programs bringing operational managers to the classroom
- leadership forums for multidisciplinary management teams from health care organizations, providing them with training in areas of self-identified skill and competency deficiencies
- collaborative research efforts between faculty and health care systems which focus on operational problems
- Stage Career Competency: Management education for health services administrators must be tied to critical career transitions and linked to specific competencies. Given the dynamics of the health care system, managers will be in constant need to update and expand their ability to function within the system. The challenge is to create new partnerships and structures between the field of practice, professional associations, and academic programs that will develop training and opportunities to assure the highest quality educational product.
- Management for Clinical Professions: Health administration programs need to serve as key managerial-policy education resources by supporting and teaching health care organization and management to the clinical professions. This obviously is a collaborative endeavor, taking a variety of forms including joint appointments,

TABLE 15.3.   Managerial Trends

	Past (1950s–1970s)	Present (1990s)	Future (1995 and beyond)
Role performance and changing values	Coordinating role subordinate to professional providers	Ascendance of managerial ability; financial and strategic expertise	Continued prominence of managers and recognition of role in managing human resources vs. simply financial resources
Preparing future managers	Relatively isolated from mainstream management and organizational theory	Emerging integration yet differentiated from industrial management	Fully integrated into management training and life-long learning

collaborative teaching, research, and service activities, but also serving as a resource to prepare clinical faculty to teach their students health services management and policy issues. As our industrial colleagues have learned so long ago, the world is too complex to go it alone.

Past, Present, and Future

Table 15.3 presents the summary of trends dealing with the managerial role. As can be seen, the role has made a number of major transitions, and more will be required to meet the challenges of the 1990s and beyond. The field is rich with challenges and opportunities, and as never before, the manager is truly a significant player in determining the future provision of health services.

Returning to the challenges being faced by NMC options for health services, NMC managers are likely to face elements of all five alternative futures as they deal with the organization and the environment, individuals, groups within the organization, and their own roles. The challenge will be to identify tractable elements within each option and their inevitable combinations and to direct limited resources and energy to those elements that make a difference in the provision of health services. Issues of quality and efficiency will remain paramount, confounded by fundamental moral and ethical choices heretofore considered only in the abstract. Our ability and contribution to determining the future provision of health services will depend on a critical mix of abilities, insight, and courage. Failure to meet the challenge will sideline managers to simply observing rather than influencing the future.

KEY CONCEPTS

Case Management
Community Care Networks
Critical Paths
Ethnic Composition
Future Scenarios
Horizontal Integration
"Just in Time" Management
Organized Delivery Systems
Outcomes Management
Social Experimentation
Social Norms and Expectations
Technology Assessment
Vertical Integration

Discussion Questions

1. Recalling the five alternative futures presented at the beginning of the chapter, speculate on the implications of each scenario as it affects efforts at cost containment, changing the organization's culture, and the role of management.

2. Design an idealized educational program for incumbent managers to enhance their overall effectiveness. Be specific about the types of problems you anticipate and how the training program will resolve or mitigate these problems.

3. Compare and contrast how an organized delivery system would be most likely to respond to the challenges outlined in this chapter. Compare the most likely responses of the organized delivery system with those of an individual hospital. Specifically address issues related to cost containment, changing social norms and demographic composition, technology development and social experimentation, changing roles of physicians and nurses, organizational culture, and the incorporation of women and minorities into management positions.

4. Return to the opening scenario regarding NMC. One option would be for NMC to close—to go out of business as an acute care facility. Develop a coherent argument for this option. What would be the advantages and disadvantages to the various stakeholders involved—Northeastern, the community, NMC employees, and others?

REFERENCES

1. Bezold, C. Five Futures. *Healthcare Forum Journal.* 29 May/June 1992;29:29–42.
2. *Healthy America: Practitioners for 2005.* Durham, NC: Pew Commission; 1991.
3. *Cancer Facts and Figures.* Atlanta, Ga: American Cancer Society; 1989.
4. *Losing a Million Minds: Confronting the Tragedy of Alzheimer's Disease and other Dementias.* (OTA-BA0323). Washington, DC: US Congress; 1987.
5. Ernst RL, Hay JW. The economic cost of Alzheimer's disease. 1987;77:1169–1175.
6. Goldsmith JC. The reshaping of healthcare. *Healthcare Forum Journal.* May/June 1992:14–27.
7. Nash DB, Markson L. Managing outcomes: The perspective of the players. *Frontiers of Health Services Management.* 1991;8(2):3–31.
8. Omnibus Budget Reconciliation Act of 1989.
9. O'Leary D. Accreditation in the quality improvement mold—A vision for tomorrow. *Quality Review Bulletin.* March 1991:74.
10. *National Health Care Reform: Refining and Advancing the Vision.* Chicago, Ill: American Hospital Association; May 1992.
11. Zuckerman H, Kaluzny A. Strategic alliances in health are: The challenges of cooperation. *Frontiers of Health Service Management.* 1991;7(3):2–23.
12. Freudenheim M. Removing the warehouse from cost-conscious hospitals. *New York Times.* March 5, 1991:5.
13. Hall EH. Just-in-time management: A critical assessment. *The Academy of Management.* Vol III 1989;3(4):315–318.
14. Short P, Cornelius L, Goldstone D. Health insurance of minorities in the United States. *Journal of Health Care for the Poor.* 1990;1:9–24.
15. Short P, Manheit A, Beauregard R. "A profile of uninsured Americans." Rockville, Md: National Center for Health Services Research, National Medical Expenditure Survey; September 1989.
16. Shortell S, Reinhardt U, eds. *Improving Health Policy and Management: Nine Critical Research Issues for the 1990s. Health Administration Press.* Ann Arbor, Mich: 1992.
17. Campbell DT. Reforms as experiments. *American Psychologist* 1969;24:409–429.
18. Research on the delivery of medical care using hospital firms. *Medical Care* July 1991 (suppl);29(7).
19. Goldberg H, et al. Alcohol counseling in a general medical clinic: A randomized controlled trial of strategies to improve referral and show rates. *Medical Care.* July 1991 (suppl);29(7):49–56.
20. Shortell, Reinhardt, eds, op. cit.
21. Ibid.
22. Kasper J, Mulley Jr. A, Wennberg J. Developing shared decision making programs to improve the quality of health care. *Quality Review Bulletin.* June 1992;18(6):183–190.
23. Schneller E. The leadership and executive potential of physicians in an era of managed care systems. *Hospital and Health Services Administration.* 1991;36(1):43–55.
24. Pew Commission, op. cit.
25. Ginzberg E, ed. *Health Services Research: Key to Health Policy.* Cambridge, Mass: Harvard University Press; 1991.
26. Lonberg R, Fenster F. Value assessment and enhancement: The link between outcome management and CQI. *Quality Sources for Group Practice.* 1992;1(4):1–6.
27. Shortell, Reinhardt, eds, op. cit.
28. American College of Healthcare Executives. "Hospital Chief Executive Officer Turnover, 1981–1990." *Foundation of the American College of Health Care Executives,* Chicago, Ill, 1991.
29. Pew Commission, op. cit.

AUTHOR INDEX

SUBJECT INDEX

A

B

C

T